WILL MACLEAN
JANE LYTTLETON

CLINICAL HANDBOOK of INTERNAL MEDICINE

The Treatment of Disease with Traditional Chinese Medicine

Volume 1

Foreword by Alan Bensoussan
Author of *The Vital Meridian* and *Towards a Safer Choice*
Chinese Medicine Unit, Faculty of Health,
University of Western Sydney

UNIVERSITY OF WESTERN SYDNEY

Clinical Handbook of Internal Medicine
copyright © 1998 University of Western Sydney

This work is copyright protected. All rights reserved. Apart from any permitted use under the Copyright Act of 1968, no part of this publication may be reproduced, stored in a retrieval system, or transmitted in any form or by any means without the prior written permission of the publisher. Requests and inquiries concerning reproduction and rights should be addressed to the Chinese Medicine Unit of the University of Western Sydney.

First published 1998   Fourth printing 2007
Second printing 2000   Fifth printing 2008
Third printing 2003

National Library of Australia Cataloging-in-Publication data:
Maclean, Will and Lyttleton, Jane
    Clinical Handbook of Internal Medicine
    Bibliography
    Includes Index
    ISBN 978-1-875760-93-0
    ISBN 1-875760-93-8

    1. Internal diseases 2. Medicine, Chinese

Published by
    Chinese Medicine Unit
    College of Social and Health Sciences
    University of Western Sydney
    Locked Bag 1797
    Penrith South DC
    NSW, Australia 1797

Distributed by Redwing Books, Taos NM USA ~ www.redwingbooks.com

Distributed in Australia by
    Pangolin Press
    PO Box 199
    Katoomba 2780

Cover Design: Yolande Gray Design
Photography: Louise Lister
Illustrations: Karen Vance

THE AUTHORS

Will Maclean BSc (Syd), D.TCM (NSW, China)
Will Maclean is a practitioner and teacher of Chinese medicine. He studied Chinese Medicine both in Sydney and China. In Australia, he was apprenticed under the late great Chris Madden, well known for his unique perspective on life and Chinese medicine. Chris Madden was especially influential in laying the foundations of Chinese medical thought and practice, and in showing how much pleasure can be derived from critical and rigorous practice. In China, Will did an internship at the Red Cross Hospital in Hangzhou under the renowned Dr. Li Dong-sen. Since graduating in 1987, Will has been teaching and practising TCM in Sydney. He developed the idea for this book in the early 1990s while attempting to teach a course in internal medicine and finding that the available English literature based on western clinical experience was virtually nonexistent. He teaches seminars in Australia, New Zealand, the US, UK and South Africa.

Jane Lyttleton BSc (Hons) NZ, MPhil (Lond), D.TCM (NSW, China)
In the mid 1970s Jane Lyttleton left a career in science and medical research to pursue the study of a traditional medicine that she felt could fill some of the gaps left by the approach to health of our complex and technological modern medicine. She has spent time working and studying in the acupuncture and herbal medicine departments in hospitals in Nanjing, Hangzhou and Guangzhou and has taught TCM students in Australia, New Zealand and England. Since the early 1980s she has run busy TCM clinics in various parts of Sydney where she has had first hand opportunity to observe the effects of both working class and corporate city lifestyles on health. She has worked closely with Western trained doctors, including surgeons and specialists, always trying to find the best mix of therapies for her patients.

Contents

Acknowledgements xv
Foreword xvi
Translation and Terminology xix
Introduction xx

Part 1. Lung Disorders

1. ACUTE EXTERIOR DISORDERS (*gan mao* 感冒) 2
1.1 Wind Cold 6
1.2 Wind Heat 10
1.3 Summer Heat and Dampness 12
1.4 Wind Dryness 16
1.5 Exterior Wind Cold with Interior Heat 18
1.6 Exterior Disorders with deficiency 20
    1.6.1 *Qi* deficiency (and external Wind) 20
    1.6.2 *Yang* deficiency (and external Wind Cold) 23
    1.6.3 Blood deficiency (and external Wind) 25
    1.6.4 *Yin* Deficiency (and external Wind) 27
Summary of guiding formulae for acute exterior disorders ... 29
Appendix – Warm Diseases (*wen bing* 温病) 30
1. *Wei* level 30
2. *Qi* level 30
    2.1 Heat in the Lungs 30
    2.2 Heat accumulating in the Stomach and Intestines
    (*yang ming*) 32
        2.2a Heat in the *yang ming* channels 32
        2.2b Heat and Phlegm in the chest and *yang ming* ... 33
        2.2c Strong Heat in *yang ming* with constipation 34
        2.2d Damp Heat in *yang ming* 35
    2.3 Heat lingering in the chest and diaphragm 37
3. *Ying* level 38
    3.1 Heat entering the Pericardium 38
    3.2 Heat obstructing the Pericardium 39
4. Blood level 41
    4.1 Heat causing the Blood to move recklessly 41
    4.2 Hot Blood and Blood stasis 42

Appendix – Febrile diseases caused by Cold (*shang han* 伤寒) 46
1. *Tai yang* syndromes 48
    1.1 *Tai yang* channel syndrome 48
    1.2 *Tai yang* organ syndrome 49
    1.3 Wind Cold with retention of Phlegm Dampness 50
    1.4 Wind Cold with pre-existing internal Heat 51
2. *Shao yang* syndrome 54
3. *Yang ming* syndrome 55
4. *Tai yin* syndrome 56
5. *Shao yin* syndromes 58
    5.1 Heart and Kidney *yin* deficiency 58
    5.2 Heart and Kidney *yang* deficiency 59
6. *Jue yin* syndromes 62
    6.1 Classical presentation 62
    6.2 *Jue yin* channel syndrome 63

2. COUGH (*ke sou* 咳嗽) 68
2.1 Wind Cold 74
2.2 Wind Heat 77
2.3 Wind and Dryness 80
2.4 Lung Heat 84
2.5 Phlegm Damp 87
2.6 Phlegm Heat 90
27 Liver Fire Invading the Lungs 93
2.8 Lung *yin* Deficiency 96
2.9 Lung *qi* Deficiency 100
2.10 Kidney (and Spleen) *yang* deficiency 103
2.11 Blood stagnation 105
Summary of guiding formulae for cough 107
Appendix – Lung Abscess (*fei yong* 肺痈) 108
1. Early Stage 109
2. Middle Stage (suppuration, rupture stage) 111
3. Convalescent Stage 114

3. WHEEZING (*xiao chuan* 哮喘) 118
3.1 Wind Cold 122
3.2 Wind Cold with Phlegm Fluids 124
3.3 Wind Cold with Internal Heat 126
3.4 Wind Heat 128
3.5 Phlegm Damp 131

3.6 Phlegm Heat 135
3.7 *Qi* Stagnation damaging the Lungs 138
3.8 Lung *qi* and *yin* deficiency 142
3.9 Lung and Spleen *qi* deficiency 144
3.10 Lung and Kidney *yin* deficiency 147
3.11 Kidney *yang* deficiency 150
Summary of guiding formulae for wheezing 154
Appendix – Asthma 155
Appendix – Paediatric Asthma 157

4. EPISTAXIS (*bi nü* 鼻衄) 164
4.1 Wind Heat, Lung Heat 168
4.2 Toxic Heat 170
4.3 Stomach Heat 172
4.4 Liver Fire 174
4.5 Liver and Kidney *yin* deficiency 177
4.6 Spleen *qi* deficiency 180
Summary of guiding formulae for epistaxis 182

5. HAEMOPTYSIS (*ke xue* 咳血) 184
5.1 Wind Heat 187
5.2 Dryness affecting the Lungs 189
5.3 Wind Cold 191
5.4 Lung Heat 193
5.5 Phlegm Heat 195
5.6 Liver Fire 197
5.7 Lung and Kidney *yin* deficiency with Heat 201
5.8 Spleen *qi* deficiency 204
Summary of guiding formulae for haemoptysis 206

6. LOSS OF VOICE (HOARSE VOICE) (*shi yin* 失音) 208
6.1 Wind Cold 212
6.2 Wind Heat 214
6.3 Lung Dryness 218
6.4 Phlegm Heat 221
6.5 Liver *qi* stagnation 223
6.6 Lung and Kidney *yin* Deficiency 226
6.7 Lung and Spleen *qi* Deficiency 228
6.8 *Qi*, Blood and Phlegm Stagnation 230
Summary of guiding formulae for loss of voice and hoarse voice 232

7. SINUSITIS AND NASAL CONGESTION (*bi yuan* 鼻渊) 234
7.1 Wind Cold 238
7.2 Wind Heat 240
7.3 Liver *qi* Stagnation With Stagnant Heat 242
7.4 Liver and Gall Bladder Fire 244
7.5 Phlegm Heat 246
7.6 Lung *qi* deficiency 249
7.7 Spleen *qi* deficiency 252
7.8 Kidney deficiency 255
7.9 Blood stagnation 258
Summary of guiding formulae for sinusitis and nasal congestion 260

8. RHINITIS (*bi qiu* 鼻鼽) 262
8.1 Wind Cold 265
8.2 Lung *qi* deficiency 268
8.3 Lung and Spleen *qi* deficiency (with Phlegm) 272
8.4 Kidney deficiency 275
Summary of guiding formulae for rhinitis 279

9. SORE THROAT (*hou bi* 喉痹) 282
9.1 Wind Heat 285
9.2 Lung and Stomach Heat 289
9.3 Lung and Kidney *yin* deficiency 292
9.4 Spleen *qi* deficiency 296
Summary of guiding formulae for sore throat 300
Appendix – Throat abscess (*hou yong* 喉痈) 301

10. TUBERCULOSIS (*fei lao* 肺痨) 306
10.1 Lung *yin* Deficiency with Heat 310
10.2 Lung and Kidney *yin* deficiency 312
10.3 Lung *qi* and *yin* Deficiency 314
10.4 *Yin* and *yang* both deficient 316
10.5 Symptomatic treatment 318
   10.5.1 Nightsweats, spontaneous sweating 318
   10.5.2 Bone steaming, tidal fever 319
   10.5 3 Haemoptysis 319
   10.5.4 Cough 320
   10.5.5 Chest pain 320

Part 2. Kidney Disorders

11. LOWER BACK PAIN (*yao tong* 腰痛) 324
11.1 Cold Damp 330
11.2 Damp Heat 333
11.3 Wind (Damp, Cold or Heat) 335
11.4 Blood stagnation 339
11.5 Liver *qi* stagnation 341
11.6 Spleen Damp 343
11.7 Kidney deficiency 346
Summary of guiding formulae for lower back pain guiding formulae . 349

12. PAINFUL URINATION SYNDROME (*lin zheng* 淋证) 352
12.1 Heat Painful Urination Syndrome 358
    12.1.1 Damp Heat 358
    12.1.2 Heart Fire 363
    12.1.3 Liver Fire 365
12.2 Stone Painful Urination Syndrome 367
    12.2.1 asymptomatic stones 367
    12.2.2 stones with Damp Heat 370
    12.2.3 stones with Blood stagnation 372
    12.2.4 stones with Kidney Deficiency 373
12.3 *Qi* Painful Urination Syndrome 376
    12.3.1 Liver *qi* stagnation 376
12.4. Blood Painful Urination Syndrome 379
    12.4.1 Heat, Damp Heat 379
    12.4.2 Blood stagnation 382
    12.4.3 Kidney *yin* deficiency 384
12.5 Cloudy Painful Urination Syndrome 386
    12.5.1 Damp Heat 386
    12.5.2 Kidney *qi* deficiency 388
12.6 Exhaustion painful urination syndrome 390
    12.6.1 Kidney deficiency 390
    12.6.2 Spleen *qi* deficiency 394
    12.6.3 Heart and Kidney *qi* and *yin* deficiency 396
Summary of guiding formulae for painful urination guiding formulae 398

13. CLOUDY URINATION (*niao zhuo* 尿浊) 400
13.1 Damp Heat 402
13.2 Spleen *qi* deficiency with sinking *qi* 404
13.3 Kidney *yin* deficiency 406

13.4 Kidney *yang* deficiency 408
Summary of guiding formulae for cloudy urination guiding formulae 411

14. DIFFICULT URINATION AND URINARY RETENTION
(*long bi* 癃闭) 414
14.1 Damp Heat 418
14.2 Obstruction of Lung *qi* 422
14.3 Liver *qi* stagnation 425
14.4 Blood stagnation 428
14.5 Spleen *yang* deficiency 430
14.6 Kidney *yang* deficiency 433
14.7 Kidney *yin* deficiency 436
Summary of guiding formulae for difficult urination and
urinary retention 438

15. FREQUENT URINATION AND INCONTINENCE
(*yi niao* 遗尿) 440
15.1 Damp Heat 444
15.2 Liver *qi* stagnation 446
15.3 Kidney (*qi*) *yang* deficiency 449
15.4 Kidney *yin* deficiency 452
15.5 Spleen (and Lung) *qi* deficiency 454
Summary of guiding formulae for frequent urination and
incontinence of urine 456

16. HAEMATURIA (*niao xue* 尿血) 458
16.1 Damp Heat 462
16.2 Heart Fire 466
16.3 Liver Fire 468
16.4 Blood stagnation 470
16.5 Kidney *yin* deficiency with Heat (Fire) 473
16.6 Spleen and Kidney *yang* (*qi*) Deficiency 475
Summary of guiding formulae for haematuria 478

17. IMPOTENCE (*yang wei* 阳痿) 480
17.1 Liver *qi* stagnation 483
17.2 Damp Heat 485
17.3 Kidney *yang* Deficiency 488
17.4 Kidney *yin* deficiency 490
17.5 Heart Blood and Spleen *qi* deficiency 493

17.6 Heart and Gall Bladder *qi* deficiency 495
Appendix – Nocturnal Seminal Emission (*yi jing* 遗精) 497
Summary of guiding formulae for impotence and nocturnal
seminal emission 504

18. TINNITUS AND DEAFNESS (*er ming* 耳鸣, *er long* 耳聋) 506
18.1 Wind Heat 510
18.2 Liver *qi* stagnation 513
18.3 Liver Fire 515
18.4 Phlegm Heat (Fire) 518
18.5 Blood Stagnation 521
18.6 Kidney deficiency 523
18.7 Spleen *qi* deficiency (with Phlegm Damp) 526
18.8 *Qi* and Blood deficiency 529
Summary of guiding formulae for tinnitus and deafness 531

Part 3. Liver Disorders

19. DIZZINESS, VERTIGO (*xuan yun* 眩晕) 534
19.1 Liver *qi* stagnation 540
19.2 Liver *yang* rising, Liver Fire 542
19.3 Liver and Kidney *yin* deficiency with *yang* rising 545
19.4 Phlegm Damp 548
19.5 Blood stagnation 552
19.6 *Qi* and Blood deficiency 554
19.7 Kidney deficiency 557
Summary of guiding formulae for dizziness 561

20. HYPOCHONDRIAC PAIN (*xie tong* 胁痛) 564
20.1 Liver *qi* stagnation 566
20.2 Damp Heat in the Liver and Gall Bladder 571
20.3 Liver *yin* (Blood) deficiency 573
20.4 Blood stagnation 576
Summary of guiding formulae for hypochondriac pain 580
Appendix – Gallstones (*dan shi bing* 胆石病) 581

21. JAUNDICE (*huang dan* 黄疸) 590
21.1 Damp Heat (Heat greater than Dampness) 594
21.2 Damp Heat (Darnpness greater than Heat) 597
21.3 Damp Heat with exterior symptoms
    (early stage external Damp Heat) 599

21.4 Liver and Gall Bladder stagnant Heat
(Bile duct obstruction with Heat) 601
21.5 Toxic Heat 604
21.6 Cold Damp 607
21.7 Spleen *qi* and Blood deficiency 609
21.8 Blood stagnation 611
Summary of guiding formulae for jaundice 614

22. SHAN QI (*shan qi* 疝气) 616
22.1 Cold *shan qi* 618
22.2 Watery *shan qi* 620
22.3 Liver *qi* stagnation *shan qi* 623
22.4 *Qi* deficiency *shan qi* 625
22.5 Foxy *shan qi* 627
24.6 Phlegm and Blood stagnation *shan qi* 629
Summary of guiding formulae for *shan qi* 631

23. TREMORS (*chan zheng* 颤证) 634
23.1 Liver and Kidney *yin* deficiency 636
23.2 *Qi* and Blood deficiency 639
23.3 Phlegm Heat generating Wind 642
Summary of guiding formulae for tremor 644

24. WIND STROKE (*zhong feng* 中风) 646
Channel syndromes 652
24.1 Emptiness of the channels with Wind invasion 652
24.2 Liver and Kidney *yin* deficiency with rising
Liver *yang* and Wind 655
24.3 Phlegm Heat with Wind Phlegm 658
Organ syndromes 660
24.4 Closed syndrome 660
24.4.1 *Yang* closed syndrome 660
24.4.2 *Yin* closed syndrome 662
24.5 Flaccid collapse syndrome 665
Sequelae of Wind stroke 667
24.6 Hemiplegia 667
24.6.1 *Qi* deficiency with Blood stagnation 667
24.6.1 Liver *yang* rising with Blood stagnation 669
24.7 Dysphasia 672
24.7.1 Wind Phlegm 672
24.7.2 Liver and Kidney *yin* and *yang* deficiency 673

24.8 Facial paralysis 675
Summary of guiding formulae for Wind stroke 677

25. EPILEPSY (*dian xian* 癫痫) 680
25.1 *Yang* seizures 685
25.2 *Yin* seizures 688
25.3 Spleen deficiency with Phlegm 690
25.4 Liver Fire with Phlegm Heat 693
25.5 Liver and Kidney *yin* deficiency 696
25.6 Blood stagnation 698
Summary of guiding formulae for epilepsy 701

26. SPASMS, CONVULSIONS (*jing bing* 痉病) 704
26.1 Febrile convulsions 707
    26.1.1 Acute phase 707
    26.1.2 Post acute phase (*yin* and Blood deficiency) 713
    26.1.3 Post acute phase (Chronic childhood convulsions
    due to Spleen *yang* deficiency) 716
26.2 Wind Toxin tetany (Muscular tetany) 718
26.3 External Cold Damp (Damp Heat) 720
26.4 Phlegm obstruction 722
26.5 Blood stagnation 724
26.6 *Qi* and Blood deficiency 726
Summary of guiding formulae for convulsions and spasms 728

27. ASCITES (DRUM LIKE ABDOMINAL DISTENSION)
(*gu zhang* 臌胀) 730
27.1 *Qi* and Damp stagnation 733
27.2 Cold Damp 735
27.3 Damp Heat 737
27.4 Blood stagnation 740
27.5 Spleen and Kidney *yang* deficiency 742
27.6 Liver and Kidney *yin* deficiency 744
Summary of guiding formulae for ascites 746

Part 4. Heart Disorders

28. CHEST PAIN (*xiong bi* 胸痹) 748
28.1 Heat scorching and knotting the chest 761
28.2 Phlegm obstruction 764

28.3 Liver *qi* stagnation 770
28.4 Cold congealing Heart Blood circulation 774
28.5 Heart *yang* deficiency 777
28.6 Blood stagnation 781
28.7 Heart (Lung and Spleen) *qi* deficiency 785
28.8 Heart (and Kidney) *yin* deficiency 787
Summary of guiding formulae for chest pain 793

29. PALPITATIONS (*jing ji* 惊悸, *zheng chong* 怔忡) 796
29.1 Heart *qi* deficiency 801
29.2 Heart *yang* deficiency 803
29.3 Heart *yin* deficiency 806
29.4 Heart Blood and Spleen *qi* deficiency 810
29.5 Heart and Gall Bladder *qi* deficiency 813
29.6 Phlegm Heat 815
29.7 Spleen and Kidney *yang* deficiency 818
29.8 Blood Stagnation 821
Summary of guiding formulae for palpitations 824

30. INSOMNIA (*bu mei* 不寐) 826
30.1 Liver *qi* stagnation, stagnant Heat, Fire 834
30.2 Heart Fire 838
30.3 Stomach disharmony 841
30.4 Phlegm Heat 843
30.5 Blood stagnation 846
30.6 Heart Blood and Spleen *qi* deficiency 849
30.7 Heart and Kidney *yin* deficiency 852
30.8 Heart and Gall Bladder *qi* deficiency 856
30.9 Liver *yin* (Blood) deficiency 858
Summary of guiding formulae for insomnia 860

31. SOMNOLENCE (*duo mei* 多寐) 862
31.1 Dampness wrapping the Spleen 864
31.2 Phlegm obstruction 866
31.3 Blood stagnation 868
31.4 Spleen *qi* (and Blood) deficiency 870
31.5 Spleen and Kidney *yang* deficiency 873
Summary of guiding formulae for somnolence 875

32. FORGETFULNESS (*jian wang* 健忘) 878
32.1 Heart Blood and Spleen *qi* deficiency 881
32.2 Heart and Kidney *yin* deficiency 884
32.3 Kidney *jing* deficiency 887
32.4 Blood and Phlegm stagnation 889
Summary of guiding formulae for forgetfulness 892

33. ANXIETY (*you lü* 忧虑) 894
33.1 Heart *qi* deficiency 899
33.2 Heart and Kidney *yin* deficiency 901
33.3 Heart Blood and Spleen *qi* Deficiency 904
33.4 Heart *qi* and *yin* deficiency 907
33.5 Heart and Gall Bladder *qi* deficiency 909
33.6 Phlegm Heat 911
Summary of guiding formulae for anxiety 913

Appendix A Original unmodified formulae 914
Appendix B Processing methods for herbs; modifications to prescription; herbs that require special treatment 934
Appendix C Delivery methods for herbal medicine 937
Appendic D Herbs contraindicated during pregnancy 941
Appendix E Incompatible and antagonistic herbs 943
Appendix F Toxic herbs 944
Appendix G Medical substances derived from endangered species 948
Appendix H Medical substances derived from animals 950
Index 953
Source texts and references 993

ACKNOWLEDGEMENTS

A book of this size is impossible without the help, input and patience of many people. My sincere thanks to all those who were integral to, or involved in some way with, this project. Particular thanks and gratitude are due to my co-author Jane Lyttleton. Without her dedication this work would have been impossible. Thanks also to Dr Tony Goh, Alan Bensoussan, Helen Gordon, David Legge, Dr Li Dong-Sen, Chris Madden, Kathryn Taylor, Christine Flynn, Janine Coleman, Peter Townsend, Karen Vance, David Moor, Yolande Gray, Alex Evangelinidis and especially Bill Maclean. My deepest appreciation and gratitude to Aretha Franklin and John Coltrane.

Thanks are also due to all those patients who allow us to practise on them and continue to encourage us to learn some humility and compassion. This book would never have happened without their support, and also the probing curiosity and sometimes awkward questions asked by our students.

All care has been taken to ensure the accuracy of the information in this book and any errors remaining are wholly my own.

Note to the second printing
Since this book was first printed, both Peter Townsend and Chris Madden have sadly passed away. Both these men were very influential on me and the development of my understanding of Chinese medicine, as well as being good friends. This book is dedicated to their memory.

W.M

I would like also to make grateful acknowledgement to all the above mentioned people for their invaluable advice, support and contributions. Next I would like to acknowledge the principal author of these volumes, Will Maclean. Not only was it his initial inspiration that began and then drove a work of this magnitude, but also his great talent for unlocking the treasures contained in those extensive and daunting collections of modern and ancient TCM texts. It is his skill in translating written Chinese combined with the experience gained from application of the original material that has produced this work of indisputable authority. We bring to this collection 40 years of study and practice we have between us–perhaps significant given the newness of TCM in the West but in truth providing a thin veneer of Western context to the wealth of Chinese material Will has laboured many long hours to translate.

A work of this nature consumes many hours of many days and could not have been sustained without the continuing and sometimes divine patience of my husband, David, and my daughter Lara's boundless enthusiasm for the present moment.

J.L

FOREWORD

There is a legend in China of a peasant deity *Shen-Nong*, to whom the origins of Chinese pharmaceutical literature (in the form of the *Ben Cao Jing*) are ascribed. *Shen-Nong* (circa 300 B.C.) was claimed to have tasted hundreds of plants, including many that were poisonous, so that medicines could be discovered and classified. As a result, 120 drugs were graded as non-toxic and nourishing or supportive to life but without strong therapeutic properties; 120 drugs in the middle category were deemed partly tonics and partly therapeutic; whilst the lower class of 125 drugs have marked medicinal effectiveness and cannot be taken over long periods of time. This legend in many ways encapsulates the ongoing search of the right cure for the right disease. This all too familiar activity is reflected in our contemporary searches for cures for cancer, HIV and other chronic illnesses.

However, in the migration of Chinese medicine to the West, little recognition has been given to this fundamental human behaviour. Patients when ill and in discomfort will do virtually anything in search of a successful remedy and recovery of health. Whilst in the beginning they may choose conventional approaches with which they are familiar, a lack of positive response will soon trigger a wider quest. However, in recent studies, which aim to make sense of the growing usage of complementary medicine, including Chinese medicine, medical sociologists have explored a range of patient characteristics. They identify by and large that patients who use complementary medicine belong to a 'new age' trend, and exhibit particular associated values. But inevitably these conclusions miss the purpose of medicine. They ignore the practical results offered by Chinese medicine or any successful therapy.

The practice of Chinese medicine is fundamentally very pragmatic. Treatment formulae have been modified over the centuries to suit changing clinical presentations and, in its day-to-day application, formulae are routinely modified in immediate response to the patient's changing condition. But clearly, modern Western medicine also provides solutions that are often very simple, accurate and immediate. So why has there been an increase in usage of Chinese medicine? How does Chinese medicine arrive at providing new and different solutions?

Chinese medical theory turns the conventional medical diagnosis upside down. The particular language, theory and diagnostic processes of Chinese medicine create fresh options for understanding the causative factors and the way lifestyle may have impacted on the disease process. The main outcome is a totally different perspective of the patient's condition. An unexpected window of opportunity for treatment emerges. For example, insomnia is described in Chinese medical terms as either of an *excess* or *deficient* nature. Either way, the conventional medical management of insomnia relies on the prescription of sedative drugs, which have a dulling effect on the nervous system. Yet *deficient* presentations of insomnia are common and require appropriate tonics to initiate a cure. Hence, what may be viewed as nourishing, (*yin* supporting) Chinese herbal drugs are prescribed in lieu of calming, sedating pharmaceutical medications. The Chinese diagnostic process has resulted in quite a converse approach to treatment. Readers will find many further examples in this handbook.

Recent medical interest in Chinese medicine is international and has resulted in providing substantial clinical evidence of its efficacy in the treatment of eczema, chronic hepatitis C, and irritable bowel syndrome. In each of these cases reported in the medical literature, formulae were designed based on the theory and diagnostic language of Chinese medicine, and not on the basis of known active pharmacological compounds in herbs.

The practice of Chinese medicine is well established and fully integrated into the health care systems of a number of nations, most notably the People's Republic of China, South Korea, North Korea, and Japan. In China and Korea, Chinese herbal medicine and acupuncture play a significant role in the treatment and prevention of a wide range of common and chronic diseases. Chinese statistics in the mid 1980s revealed that 80 per cent of the one billion population used various forms of herbal preparations in the treatment of a wide range of diseases as well as for preventative purposes. Chinese or oriental herbal medicine accounted for 33.1 per cent of the pharmaceutical market share in China in 1995, and 28 per cent of national expenditure on drugs in the Republic of Korea in 1996.

Western nations are also reporting high levels of usage of Chinese medicine. With the support of the World Health Organisation, governments in the Western Pacific region are moving towards increasing the regulation, formal recognition and integration of indigenous herbal medicine of which Chinese medicine is a major component. In all corners of the globe, acupuncture and Chinese herbal medicine are gaining wide acceptance amongst the public and medical and government personnel.

With the growth of usage of Chinese medicine comes an increasing demand for better, well organised texts for students and practitioners. Will Maclean and Jane Lyttleton have produced a strong reference text that makes sense of many of the internal medicine concepts in Chinese medicine and they relate these to modern medical concepts. The three volumes that make up the set represent an important clinical reference for all students and practitioners providing an enriched resource that is easily accessible and coherent. The three volumes cover a comprehensive range of clinical presentations and diagnostic patterns. Will Maclean and Jane Lyttleton both have strong clinical practice backgrounds, which they have used to enrich and contextualise information drawn from the Chinese source texts.

Chinese medicine represents a constant challenge to students and practitioners. Dialogue between health care professionals is often difficult because of contrasting medical concepts and language to express those concepts. These volumes represent a significant step toward improving our understanding, communication and use of Chinese medicine.

Maybe it is worth taking a lesson from the pages of a 16th century Chinese text (*I Xue Qi Ch'eng*), a chapter most aptly entitled 'Medical learning must combine the best from all writings'.

> 'Illnesses may appear in countless variations ... the (basic) symptoms may be identical, but the treatment must, in fact, be different. Those who study (medicine) have to take the best from many books, combine it with what they see with their own eyes, and apply it in medical practice. This way (their learning and their therapies) will be right.'

1998 Alan Bensoussan
Sydney

TRANSLATION AND TERMINOLOGY

Translation from original Chinese sources is a task fraught with difficulty. There are numerous technical terms for which there are no satisfactory English equivalents, and attempts at translation often fall short of all the subtleties and implications of the term in Chinese. A certain ambiguity is inherent in the language of TCM, even in the Chinese literature there is debate about the precise meaning of certain terms, particularly in ancient texts. This ambiguity is relevant to another translation issue, attempts to capture the 'poetic spirit' of the original material. We believe that an attempt to retain the fluidity of the original language is as important to accessing the material as accurate translation of terms. At the time of writing, a satisfactory standardised translation terminology that embodies both principles, accuracy and spirit, has not yet been developed.

Having thus considered these issues, we have decided to retain and italicise terms in common useage–*qi, shen, yin, yang, jing, jiao, san jiao, tai yang, shao yang* and so on. Our experience is that these terms are more readily and accurately understood as they are. In some cases we have kept the Chinese term rather than the widely accepted translation, because again, the translation fails to convey the full meaning. An example of this is *shan qi* (疝气), usually given as Hernial disorders (Bensky and Barolet 1990). *Shan qi* in fact, refers to a number of conditions not related to hernia, as well as certain types of hernia.

Translated technical terms with precise meaning specific to Chinese medicine, like Blood, Liver, Wind and Damp, are capitalised.

In instances where an English rendering captures the meaning accurately, and has been widely adopted elsewhere in the English TCM literature, we have retained that rendering. Examples of this include painful obstruction syndrome for *bi zheng* (痹症), atrophy syndrome for *wei zheng* (痿证), and indeterminate gnawing hunger for *cao za* (嘈杂).

In general, we have attempted to render the language and spirit of Traditional Chinese medicine into plain English, hopefully making the text easy to read and the material easy to access. All comments and suggestions for improvement will be gratefully received.

INTRODUCTION

Traditional Chinese medicine (TCM) is growing in popularity and importance throughout the world, and is now being taught at university level in several countries outside China. The English language literature that has supported this development has, until the last decade, been scant and has tended to be Sinocentric, which is natural enough for a medical system that has grown out of and is rooted in the perceptions and culture of the Chinese. However, as TCM has expanded into the Western world, it has had to confront cultural and lifestyle differences that give rise to a different clinical reality, a non Chinese presentation of disharmony. These differences can cause pattern variations that don't appear in the Chinese model, and which require a different type of response. The process that we are now faced with, of taking the essence of the TCM analytical model and making it our own, has occured in other countries over the centuries. Japan, Korea and Vietnam have developed their own unique styles of acupuncture and herbal medicine, firmly rooted in the ancient Chinese classics, but adapted to suit the cultural and sociological features of their own people.

Similarly, in the West, with our different perceptions of the world and our relationships, diets, environmental and genetic influences, TCM cannot be successfully applied in exactly the same way as it is in China. The lengthy process of accumulation of clinical experience (in the rich light of China's millenia of experience) has only just begun, and our learning curve is steep. This is quite an exciting time to be practicing TCM in the Western world, as new ideas and understanding enrich the classical model, and we discover just how far we can go with what is a very powerful and effective medical system.

Aim of this book

For the reasons noted above, the way Chinese medicine is practised in the clinics of the Western world is somewhat different to the way it is in China. As practitioners, we are all too aware of the gaps in the English language TCM literature, and the Chinese cultural bias that flavours much of the material available. For this reason, we felt that a clinical handbook that at least began to take our cultural and social differences into account was required. Our clinical experience is shaped by the climatic and social environment in which we practise. The collaborators of this handbook live and work in Sydney, Australia, with a temperate climate, mild winters and hot humid summers, and a predominantly Anglo-Saxon culture (although this is changing rapidly). Australia is an affluent country with a tendency to overconsumption of fats and high protein diets, and an excess of sedentary behaviour relative to physical exercise. The types of illnesses patients present with in our clinics, and the way these illnesses present, are sometimes quite different to those we observe in China. Presumably practitioners in other parts of the world with different cultural backgrounds and environments will have different experiences and expertise in different types of pathology.

We believe that TCM could take its next developmental step in the West, and the gathering and recording of our accumulated experience is an important part of that process. Because TCM is relatively new to the West, and from a cultural point of view we are still quite inexperienced, we can only get better and more mature in our profession. Our learning curve is steep, so we consider this book to be very much a *work in progress*, and one which will grow as we gather experience as a profession. In future editions of this work, we would like to include other pieces of clinical information, such as detailed prognosis, other therapies, patterns that may be more prevalent in some parts of the world and case histories, and to this end contributions from readers are encouraged.

Using this book

The purpose of this handbook is to provide easy access to the clinical information needed to treat a patient. This book is not a substitute for a solid background in the theory of TCM, indeed a good understanding of TCM theory is essential for efficient use of this handbook. The main body of the text is the description of 'patterns' of disharmony. In this context, a pattern is defined as a group of signs and symptoms that point to a particular imbalance in the function and/or structure of the body. The patterns described here are not in reality discrete entities (or 'diseases'). Rather, they attempt to describe and give clinical meaning to the many ways the body's *yin, yang, qi* and Blood can be out of balance.

Furthermore and importantly, the clinical treatment approaches described in this book represent the accumulated experience of generations of physicians who recorded their knowledge in so many classical texts. Those texts have in turn been modernised and modified by contemporary physicians and the treatments adapted for use in the West. The majority of treatments outlined in this book are not the fruits of contemporary research in the form of randomised controlled trials, animal studies or laboratory experiments, but rather the oral and written legacy of Chinese medical masters and the experienced gained from centuries of application and practice.

Internal medicine has historically been the province of the herbalist, so the treatment emphasis in this book is on herbal medicine. This is not to suggest that acupuncture is not effective in internal medicine, it is, and in many cases remarkably so. However, for certain types of disorder, most notably chronic deficiencies of Blood, Fluids and *yin*, acupuncture, which must replenish the deficiency through improved organ function, generally takes second place to herbs, which can directly supplement the deficiency at the same time as improving organ function. The way that TCM is developing in the West is towards the integration of treatment with both herbs and acupuncture, a situation not common in China or Japan, where patients usually receive one or the other and get them from different practitioners. In the West, practitioners are being trained in both skills, and developing the knowledge to combine them clinically to greatest advantage. Precise and effective herbal medicine, however, relies on the emphasis of diagnostic tools not commonly used for acupuncture, and diagnostic or therapeutic error is more likely to produce side effects or adverse effects with herbs than with needles. Acupuncture treatment tends to be more forgiving. Manipulation of the *qi* with an acupuncture needle usually produces a positive response, regardless of the point selected, simply because moving *qi* is therapeutic. A review of the diagnostic tools relevant to herbal medicine (and acupuncture) can be found in Box 1.

Diagnostic procedure

The starting point of the effective clinical application of TCM is a reasonable diagnosis. Diagnosis and the selection of appropriate treatment can be a complex process. The interaction of *qi* and Blood, *yin* and *yang* is a dynamic process, constantly in a state of flux, and so different patterns frequently co-exist, overlap and transform into one another, producing a confusing constellation of signs and symptoms. The subtle shadings of a pattern may suggest several different pathologies. For this reason, diagnosis has been developed and formalised over the centuries into a series of logical steps that guide the analysis. In addition, practitioners have a variety of diagnostic tools at their disposal, each of which has a specific usefulness depending on the aetiology and presentation of the disorder. Because of the complexity of accurate diagnosis and prescription, several formal steps have been laid down to guide the process.

Step 1. The first step (after gathering all the information available using the four methods of diagnosis *si zhen* 四诊) is to decide on the 'disease'. This is known as disease differentiation (*bian bing* 辨病). In TCM the 'disease' is the main symptom with which the patient presents. The chapter headings in this and Volumes 2 and 3 (to be published in 2001), represent the starting point for the analysis of all TCM internal disorders. For example, patients with gallstones will likely present in clinic with pain under the ribs and therefore starting point for analysis will be 'hypochondriac pain'. Patients with cystitis will usually present with 'painful urination', but sometimes with 'urinary retention' or 'urinary frequency', without pain. Some patients will have insomnia, palpitations and anxiety, and one of these three 'diseases', usually the main presenting or most prominent one, must be chosen as the starting point for analysis. The correct choice determines the diagnostic route the practitioner will then follow. The 'diseases' insomnia, palpitations and anxiety have varying patterns (and subsequently treatments) associated with them.

Step 2. Once the disease has been selected, the next step is to differentiate the pattern (or patterns) that are giving rise to it (*bian zheng* 辨证). Once a general overview of the pattern is obtained using the Eight Principles, a more specialised tool (see Box 1) will be selected, depending on the nature and location of the illness. The selection of a specific pattern diagnosis leads directly to the next step.

Step 3. Once pattern diagnosis is complete, the next stage is selection of a treatment principle. This step is crucial in focusing the therapeutic goal of the prescription and aiding in the selection of formula modifications.

Step 4. The final step is the selection of guiding herbal formula, acupuncture prescription or both, with appropriate modifications to suit the individual case.

Structure of the handbook

The body of the text is arranged in the traditional groups of TCM defined 'diseases' associated with one of the internal organ (*zang fu* 脏腑) systems, the channels, or physiological substances. Beginning with disorders associated with the 'metal' phase of the Five Phase generative cycle, this volume deals with disorders of the Lungs (metal), Kidney, Liver and Heart. The second volume of this series will contain disorders of the Spleen, Stomach and Intestines, channels, and *qi*, Blood and Body Fluids. When understood from a strictly TCM point of view, these groups are natural and intuitive[1] so disorders associated with the Kidney system include (for example) disorders of urination, lower back pain and tinnitus; Heart disorders include (for example) chest pain, palpitations and those associated with disturbance of the *shen* and so on.

Traditionally, internal medicine texts have focused on the *zang* rather than the *fu* organs and pathologies of the *fu* will usually be included in the appropriate *zang* chapter. Thus Urinary Bladder disorders are found in the Kidney section, Gall Bladder disorders in the Liver section and *san jiao* disorders in the *qi*, Blood and Body Fluids section. The Stomach *fu* is included in the Spleen section by convention.

At the beginning of each chapter a brief account is given of the

---

1. The traditional groups do have a degree of arbitrariness, however. For example, in some sources epilepsy (*dian xian* 癫痫) appears in the Heart section, in others the Liver section; because of the Wind association, and to contrast it with convulsions and tremors, we have decided to include it in the latter.

Fig 1. Example of application of diagnostic method

A patient presents with:
right sided hypochondriac pain worse for pressure, accompanied by fever, irritability, nausea, bitter taste in the mouth, constipation, malaise and mild jaundice. The tongue has a thick, greasy yellow coat and the pulse is wiry and rapid.

Step 1
Decide on the guiding TCM disease, usually the presenting complaint, or where there are multiple symptoms, the one that is most acute or distressing to the patient. In this case we could begin with either hypochondriac pain or jaundice. The pain is distressing, so we select hypochondriac pain.
Possible patterns: Liver *qi* stagnation, Blood stagnation, *yin* deficiency, Damp Heat

Step 2 Eight principles overview
Is the pattern internal or external?
 –there are no clear exterior signs, no chills or floating pulse, therefore Internal
Is the pattern Hot or Cold?
 –fever, rapid pulse, yellow tongue coat, bitter taste point to Heat
Is the pattern deficient or excess?
 –pain worse for pressure, wiry pulse, thick tongue coat, therefore Excess
The overview points to an Internal Excess Heat pattern

Selection of diagnostic tool – *zang fu bian zheng* – because the internal organs are affected - hypochondriac pain is the cardinal sign of Liver dysfunction
What is the nature of the Excess Heat? – Damp Heat
Which organ system is affected? – the Liver

The diagnosis – Damp Heat in the Liver (and Gall Bladder)

Step 3 Selection of treatment principle
1. Clear Damp Heat from the Liver (& Gall Bladder)
2. Stop pain, relieve jaundice, relieve nausea, open the bowels etc. depending on the accompanying signs and symptoms

Step 4 Treatment
Selection of guiding formula and modifications
Representative formula for Liver Damp Heat hypochondriac pain
LONG DAN XIE GAN TANG 龙胆泻肝汤, plus herbs to stop pain, relieve jaundice etc.
Appropriate acupuncture prescription, with reducing method,
 i.e. Liv.14 (*qi men* -), SJ.6 (*zhi gou* -), GB.34 (*yang ling quan* -), GB.24 (*ri yue* -), Liv.3 (*tai chong* -), GB.43 (*xie xi* -), Bl.18 (*gan shu* -), Bl.19 (*dan shu* -)
 • with severe fever add Du.14 (*da zhui* -) and Ll.11 (*qu chi* -)
 • with nausea add PC.6 (*nei guan* -)
 • with jaundice add Du.9 (*zhi yang* -)

BOX 1. DIAGNOSTIC TOOLS OF TCM

THE EIGHT PRINCIPLES (ba gang)
The eight principles are the broadest analytical brushstrokes summarising the overall nature of a pattern or patterns. They describe the yin or yang nature of a pattern, its location, hot or cold nature and the relative strength or weakness of zheng qi or pathogenic qi. This analysis is the most general of all diagnostic procedures and is applicable to all patients. Typical summaries are external, excess and Cold (in the case of a Wind Cold surface pattern) or internal, deficient and Hot (in the case of yin deficiency). Following this general assessment, further refinements using more specialised tools are used to focus the precision of the diagnosis.

1. FOR DISEASES DUE TO EXTERNAL PATHOGENS
1.1 The Six Channel system (liu jing bian zheng)
The Six Channel system is used for analysing the effect of external Wind Cold and its progression into deeper levels of the body. This system is summarised in Appendix 2 of Chapter 1 (Acute External Disorders, p.46).
1.2 The Four Level system (wei qi ying xue bian zheng)
The Four Levels analyse the progress of febrile diseases, primarily due to Wind Heat. This system is summarised in App. 1 of Chapter 1 (Acute External Disorders, p.30).
1.3 The *san jiao* system (san jiao bian zheng)
This method of analysing the progress of febrile diseases follows their progress from the upper *jiao*, through the middle and lower *jiao*. Upper *jiao* patterns are similar to those of the *wei* level (1.2), middle *jiao* patterns involve Damp Heat and are similar to *yang ming* level patterns (1.1), and lower *jiao* patterns involve Liver and Kidney *yin* deficiency.

2. FOR DISEASES AFFECTING THE CHANNELS
2.1 The Channel and collateral system (jing luo bian zheng)
This system is used to identify channels or collaterals disrupted by obstruction or deficiency. This system is mostly applied in painful obstruction syndrome (*bi zheng*) and atrophy syndrome (*wei zheng*). These syndromes will be discussed in detail in Volume 3.

3. FOR DISEASES AFFECTING THE INTERIOR OF THE BODY AND ORGAN SYSTEMS
3.1 The Qi, Blood and Body Fluid system (qi, xue, jin ye bian zheng)
The *qi*, Blood and Body Fluid system identifies problems in the circulation, metabolism or distribution of fluids and *qi* that bathe all parts of the body. It involves generalised disorders that have not involved the internal organ network. For example, Heat in the Blood, Phlegm Damp, Body Fluid deficiency, rebellious *qi* and so on, are systemic conditions that do not involve specific *zang fu*. This system can overlap with the *jing luo* system or the *zang fu* system, for example rebellious *qi* can be specific to the *chong* or Stomach channel, Phlegm can stagnate in the channels, *qi* deficiency may be focused in the Spleen, and stagnant Blood may be located primarily in the Liver.
3.2 The Internal Organ System (zang fu bian zheng)
The Internal Organ system identifies disorders at the deep functional level of the *zang fu*. This analytical method overlaps with other systems. For example, *qi*, Blood and Fluid disorders can be localised in a specific organ system (for example Phlegm Heat affecting the Heart). Similarly, disorders originating as Wind Cold (thus analysed by the Six Channel system) become identical to internal organ disorders once in the interior (that is, *tai yin* syndrome involves *qi* or *yang* deficiency of the Spleen and Lungs).

aetiological factors pertaining to the patterns therein. These accounts serve as quick summaries of the relevant TCM theory and highlight the most common causes. Each pattern is described in terms of its pathophysiology, its clinical features, principles of treatment, prescriptions, modifications to the primary formula(e) and variations. It is important to remember that this is a guide book, and subject to revision as our knowledge and experience grow, thus the patterns themselves and the way they manifest should not be regarded as fixed or in any way immutable. Different regions of the world, with different customs, diets and climates may have different patterns or variations that have not been described here. This is where the collected clinical experience of practitioners world wide can combine to make not only a fascinating account of TCM as it is practised in the West, but also contribute to the development of new directions of TCM.

Pathophysiology

The pathophysiology section describes the mechanism behind the principal 'disease' or main symptom. It also contains some information about the variability of certain patterns and interesting or unique aetiological features.

Clinical features

The clinical features are collections of signs and symptoms that define a particular pattern of disharmony. Much of the material in this book has been derived from original sources, although we have attempted where possible to introduce aspects of our experience. Some patterns described in the text are not found in Chinese texts, but have been consistently observed (and treated) in clinics here. Some of the patterns described are uncommon or only dealt with in hospital, so we have little or no experience with them.

Treatment principles

Defining the pattern of disharmony is the final step before selection of a principle of treatment and a prescription to treat the disorder. Clearly defined treatment principles are an essential prerequisite to accurate prescribing and good therapeutic results. Treatment principles usually describe a set of treatment priorities depending on the nature of a disorder. For example, two patients may be diagnosed with the pattern of Spleen *qi* deficiency. Even though they will both have signs and symptoms suggestive of Spleen *qi* deficiency, the main symptom of one may be diarrhoea and loss of appetite, the other heavy uterine bleeding. In both cases the primary treatment principle is to tonify Spleen *qi*. The secondary treatment principle refines the first by guiding the point or formula selection towards a specific treatment for Spleen deficient diarrhoea (like *Shen Ling Bai Zhu San*) or Spleen deficient bleeding (*Gui Pi Tang*).

The priority assigned to treatment principles varies, however, depending on the severity of the condition. In the case of Spleen deficient bleeding, for example, if the bleeding is particularly heavy, the main priority is to first stop the bleeding and only when the bleeding is under control treat the root cause, the Spleen deficiency. The first prescription then may be *Yun Nan Bai Yao* and/or acupuncture on Sp.1 (*yin bai*), Du.20 (*bai hui*) etc, with *Gui Pi Tang* following.

Herbal Prescriptions

The majority of formulae given in the text have been modified to focus on the particular problem being treated. As always in Chinese medicine, the application of formulae and their modifications should be flexible and varied to meet the precise needs of each individual.

In some cases several formulae are offered as possible prescriptions for a pattern. These formulae will all have similar therapeutic action but take into account minor variations in the clinical presentation.

The English names of the formulae are drawn from two main sources. First, when a widely available powdered form of a formula is available we have taken the name from Hong Yen-hsu's *Commonly Used Chinese Herbal Formulas*. We have selected these names because many practitioners nowadays use powdered herbal extracts because they are convenient, patient compliance is good and in general powders are manufactured to GMP standards ensuring consistency and quality.

Second, where a formula is not listed by Hsu we have drawn the name from Dan Bensky and Andrew Gamble's *Formulas and Strategies*. Where a formula is not found in either Hsu or Bensky, the translation spirit of *Formulas and Strategies* is retained.

The sources quoted with prescriptions refer to the text the prescription was sourced from. This applies mostly to modified formulae. When no doses were given in the original source text, Bensky and Barolet (1990), Bensky and Gamble (1993), *Practical Chinese Herbs* (1985) and *Practical Chinese Herbal Formulas* (1989) were consulted for standard doses. The doses given are by no means definitive and should be varied depending on the individual presentation.

Where a prescription includes an endangered species we have endeavoured to provide a reasonable alternative where possible. We have retained the original ingredients of prescriptions for historical accuracy, but we strongly urge substitution of these substances. Endangered species are marked with an open circle (°) and herbs with potentially toxic or other side effects are marked with an asterisk (*). Both are listed with details in Appendices at the end of the text (p.944-952). Other substances derived from animals (that are neither toxic nor endangered) are tagged with the following symbol (').

Modifications

The modifications section gives information about the addition or deletion of herbs from the primary prescription so as to tailor the prescription as closely as possible to the individual patient's needs.

Variations and additional prescriptions

This section provides information about variations to the main pattern and its presentation, and lists prescriptions which vary from the primary prescription or group of prescriptions.

Patent medicines

Information on patent medicines is drawn from the *Clinical Manual of Chinese Patent Medicines* (Maclean 2000) and Margaret Naeser's *Outline to Chinese Herbal Patent Medicines in Pill Form*. The English name of any patent medicine may vary from country to country depending on differences between factories and regional licencing regulations. Because there are so many variations, we have stayed with the *pin yin* name for the formula, the Chinese characters and one common English name. Be aware that formulae of the same name may have quite different compositions depending on the company of origin, so it is advisable to check the list of ingredients before use.

Some patent medicines listed in the text may contain endangered species, although it appears in most cases substitutions or deletions are commonly made (like dog bone for tiger bone), while retaining the original name of a formula. Recent tests performed by the forensic laboratory of the U.S Fish and Wildlife Service on a series of commonly available patent medicines found no evidence of endangered species in the medicine even though the packaging listed these substances as ingredients. While these medicines are included for the sake of completeness and accuracy, we strongly urge practitioners to avoid the use of patent medicines listing endangered species.

Many patent medicines have been shown to contain contaminants–either unlisted pharaceutical drugs or heavy metals. Consult the *Clincal Manual of Chinese Patent Medicines* for the most up to date information regarding those medicines registered by the Australian Therapeutic Goods Administration (TGA) and thus known to be clean.

Acupuncture

The points suggested for each pattern are sourced from standard works on acupuncture and are by no means exhaustive. A selection of points is given as a list rather than as a prescription. More points are usually suggested than should actually be treated in a single session. It is up to the practitioner to select points according to the normal rules of point selection and the requirements of each individual.

Key to the Symbols following Acupuncture Points
- \+ denotes a tonifying method (*bu fa* 补法)
- \- denotes a reducing method (*xie fa* 泻法)
- no symbol denotes an even method (*ping bu ping xie fa* 平补平泻法)
- ▲ denotes moxa, either stick, warm needle, rice grain or moxa box
- Ω denotes cupping
- ↓ indicates a point should be bled

Clinical notes
Clinical notes are an attempt to relate TCM patterns with possible Western medical diseases, and to give some general indication about prognosis, where known. For patterns with which we have little or no clinical experience, no prognosis is given. Where we have some experience, a general prognosis is given. Hopefully, as our collective experience in the West grows, we will be able to fill in some of the blanks with a degree of confidence.

In attempting to associate a certain pattern with a group of biomedically defined diseases, we are mindful of the traps involved, principally the temptation to equate a pattern and a disease directly. For example, hepatitis is sometimes described as being equivalent to Damp Heat in the Liver. This is of course incorrect, as patients with hepatitis may present with a number of patterns (Liver *qi* stagnation, *yin* deficiency etc.), depending on factors like constitution, the strength of the pathogen and the patient's environment. All of these factors influence the ultimate manifestation and pattern and, therefore, the diagnosis and treatment. There is an increasing trend in the current TCM literature towards differentiating biomedically defined diseases (for example using hepatitis rather than hypochondriac pain as the 'disease' category starting point). This approach can be useful as far as it goes, but ultimately it lacks the breadth of understanding and flexibility of application of the traditional approach.

Nevertheless, the reality of TCM practice in the West is that patients often arrive at the clinic with a biomedically defined disease name, and although correct TCM diagnosis proceeds in its own fashion, the medical diagnosis is often useful in terms of prognosis. For example, for two patients presenting with the TCM pattern of Wind Damp *bi* syndrome, one with osteo-arthritis and the other with Behçet's syndrome, the prognosis for the latter (at least in our experience) is often poorer. At the same time, TCM treatment of a pattern can be enhanced by an understanding of the biomedical and physiological basis of a disorder. For example, the treatment of chronic viral hepatitis is improved by the addition of herbs with a known liver protective and AST/ALT normalising effect, such as **wu wei zi** (Fructus Schizandrae Chinensis) 五味子. Similarly, treatment of benign prostatic hypertrophy is improved by the addition of herbs that soften hardness and disperse swelling, even when they are not specifically indicated by traditional diagnostic methods.

Limitations of the text

Traditional Chinese medicine is a fluid analytical model used to describe the interaction between pathogenic influence and the strength of the patient, and the influence of lifestyle, diet and emotional life on the actual manifestations of any particular disease. Its strengths are to take into account the responses of an individual to the various conditions that produce ill health, and to prescribe as closely as possible to the individual's needs.

Traditional Chinese medicine is primarily focused on identifying and rectifying functional disorders, and thus is at its best before structural or biochemical change has produced an identifiable pathology. The identification of a pattern or patterns, which is the final step in the diagnostic process, is the weaving together of numerous strands of observation and information. Since these strands include not only information about pathogenic influences but also constitution, emotions, diet and life circumstance, in short, a summary of all the influences to which an individual is subject, a comprehensive and unique picture can be constructed.

In the real world of course, things are often complicated. Patients frequently exhibit signs of multiple patterns, or contradictory signs and symptoms. The art and skill of the practitioner is reflected in his or her ability to weave the information into a meaningful diagnosis. The fact that real life and the pathologies derived from it are usually more complicated than that described in standard text books, creates a problem when presenting a work like this. In order to analyse common patterns, they need to be described discretely, whereas in reality they are not so discrete, and overlap more than the text would suggest.

To take the example of Liver *qi* stagnation, it can occur as an uncomplicated pattern on its own and often does, but more frequently it is accompanied by other patterns of disharmony, either as a result of the *qi* stagnation or independent of it. Liver *qi* stagnation can lead to Blood stagnation, Heat, Spleen deficiency with Dampness or Phlegm and Damp Heat, to name only a few potential complications. When there is Heat, *yin* deficiency may occur, when the Spleen is damaged *yang* deficiency may eventually develop and so on. The experienced practitioner gets a feel for these complications—the many undercurrents, tides and eddies of overlapping patterns—and unravelling these, to determine the logical starting point for treatment, eventually becomes second nature.

We hope this book can help the progress of practitioners who may still be new to the path—one which can be travelled for a lifetime and every day reveal finer nuances of the interplay between people and their inner and outer worlds. Once again, we would like to say that we welcome comments and contributions, particularly to the clinical notes sections. With time and future editions, we hope this handbook will come to represent the collected voice of TCM practitioners in the West.

Disorders of the Lung

1. Acute Exterior Disorders

Excess patterns
Wind Cold
Wind Heat
Summer Dampness
Autumn Dryness
Wind Cold with Interior Heat

With underlying deficiency
Qi deficiency
Yang deficiency
Yin deficiency
Blood deficiency

Appendix 1 – Warm Diseases (*wen bing* 温病)

Appendix 1 – Febrile Disease caused by Cold (*shang han* 伤寒)

1. ACUTE EXTERIOR DISORDERS
gan mao 感冒

The term *gan mao* refers to a variety of disorders characterised by symptoms like headache, nasal congestion, sneezing, sore throat, fever, chills and a floating pulse. In some varieties acute nausea, vomiting and diarrhoea occur. In healthy individuals they are generally mild and self limiting, and most people will experience *gan mao* once or twice every year. *Gan mao* disorders are usually diagnosed as the common cold, upper respiratory tract infections, viral gastroenteritis or influenza.

In Chinese medicine, *gan mao* disorders are due to invasion of the superficial layers of the body by pathogenic Wind, accompanied by Cold, Heat, Dampness or Dryness. In susceptible individuals the pathogen may penetrate to deeper levels of the body, affecting the internal organs. The potential for penetration of an external pathogen largely depends on the relative strength of the pathogen and the strength or weakness of the body's resistance.

In old China a great deal of attention was given to these seemingly mild conditions, with an emphasis on prompt treatment. The reason for this was that in the early stages *gan mao* disorders resemble their more serious counterparts, the *wen bing* (溫病) or Warm diseases. The theoretic description and understanding of Warm diseases reached its zenith in the 17th century with Ye Tian-shi and his *Wen Re Lun* (Discussion of Warmth and Heat, 1745). In contrast to the *gan mao* disorders the *wen bing* are generally not so easily resolved by the treatments applied to *gan mao* (like diaphoresis). Before the widespread availability of antibiotic therapy, *wen bing* disorders were a major cause of death. The *wen bing* category includes, for example pneumonia and bronchitis, infectious encephalitis and meningitis, and other acute febrile diseases that may progress rapidly to febrile rashes or convulsions. A summary of *wen bing* analysis is presented in appendix 1 at the end of this chapter.

Gan mao disorders are generally predictable in their outcome, and resolve quickly with correct treatment. The key to success is timing–the earlier the intervention the faster the resolution. However, if the incorrect treatment is applied or if the patient is frail or chooses to ignore the body's signals and 'soldier on' through illness, the pathogen may progress further into the body and lodge in the *shao yang* or *yang ming* level, as classified by Zhang Zhong-jing in the Han dynasty. This penetration is very commonly seen in clinic, and often expressed as the 'cold that never really went away'. A brief summary of Zhang's analysis is presented in appendix 2 at the end of this chapter.

AETIOLOGY

All the disorders described in this chapter are due to invasion of Wind, accompanied by Cold, Heat, Dampness or Dryness. They usually occur during the corresponding season (Wind Cold invasion during winter, Dampness during humid weather), although they can appear all year round.

In TCM, external Wind is the carrier that enables access to the body by other pathogens. Access

> **BOX 1.1 SOME BIOMEDICAL CAUSES OF ACUTE EXTERIOR DISORDERS**
> - the common cold
> - influenza
> - upper respiratory tract infections
> - acute gastroenteritis
> - food poisoning
> - sinusitis
> - rhinitis
> - early stage of measles
> - parotitis
> - early stage of encephalitis or meningitis

occurs when the *wei qi* is generally weak or temporarily dispersed, or because the invading pathogen is very strong. The term Wind also includes climatic wind and abrupt environmental changes, for example sudden weather changes or going from a climate-controlled building to the outside. This Wind can temporarily disperse *wei qi*, even if *zheng qi* is intact, allowing penetration particularly through the nose, mouth or the 'Wind gates' of the upper back and neck. *Wei qi* retreats from the surface to the interior of the body during sleep, leaving the surface undefended. This is why sleeping uncovered or next to an open window enables Wind to penetrate causing Wind Cold or Wind in the channels of the neck (causing problems like torticollis).

The response to invasion by external pathogens may reflect the state of the *zheng qi* of the individual. If the *zheng qi* is strong the defense mounted will be vigorous and will produce marked symptoms, for example, strong fever or strong chills. But the battle will generally be short lived, as the *zheng qi* (with or without the aid of correct treatment) drives out the pathogen rapidly. Where the *zheng qi* is not so strong symptoms may be milder since the defence mounted is less vigorous. However, the danger of the pathogen penetrating more deeply is greater. These cases describe those lingering subacute infections or post infection syndromes so commonly seen nowadays.

A very strong pathogen can enter regardless of the strength of *wei qi*, and is seen in epidemics of influenza where people of all constitutions can fall ill.

TREATMENT

The location of *gan mao* disorders is at the surface of the body, thus the primary therapy employed is diaphoresis–the induction of a sweat, and secondarily, promotion of the Lungs descending function. Depending on the nature of the pathogen, the herbs used will be acrid and dispersing, and warm (for Wind Cold), cool (for Wind Heat), moistening (for dryness) or aromatically drying (for Dampness). In general, once a sweat occurs, the pathogen is expelled and the patient recovers.

When patients with an obvious underlying deficiency catch a cold, the use of diaphoretic herbs has to be tempered with caution, as excessive sweating can disperse *qi* and damage fluids. This is particularly so in the case of the elderly and seriously debilitated (however do not make the mistake of assuming that all elderly patients are deficient and thus in need of tonification). In debilitated patients, diaphoretics are combined with herbs to supplement the underlying deficiency. Be aware that diagnosis can be difficult in patients with significant deficiency–if a patient's *qi* or *yang* is deficient to the point where it is unable to mount an adequate defence against an invading pathogen, the characteristic signs and symptoms may be muted or absent. Often patients in this situation only experience exacerbation of pre-existing symptoms.

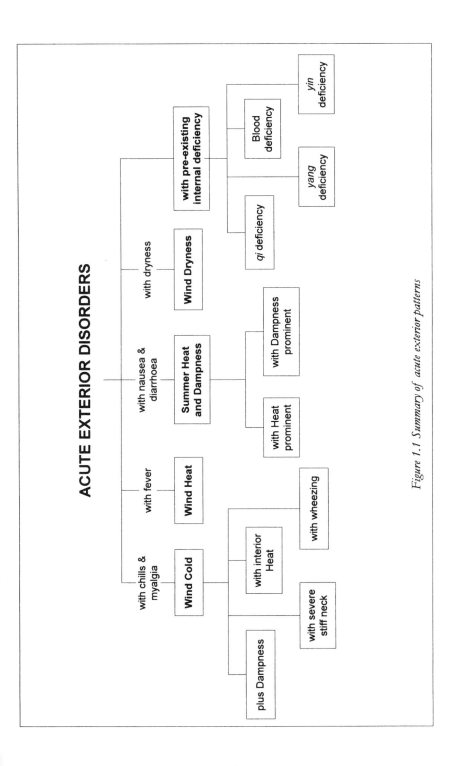

Figure 1.1 Summary of acute exterior patterns

1.1 WIND COLD

Pathophysiology
- In this pattern, Wind Cold enters through the pores, *tai yang* channels and Lungs. Because the nature of Cold is to 'freeze and constrict', it will shut the pores behind it, locking the Wind and Cold beneath the surface.

Clinical features
- acute simultaneous fever and chills, with the chills more prominent than the fever
- no sweating
- occipital headache
- muscle aches, neck stiffness
- nasal obstruction, or runny nose with thin watery mucus
- sneezing
- cough or wheezing with thin watery mucus

T normal or with a thin white coat
P floating, or floating and tight

Treatment principle
Expel Wind and Cold
Redirect Lung *qi* downward

Prescription

JING FANG BAI DU SAN 荆防败毒散
(*Schizonepeta and Ledebouriella Powder to Overcome Pathogenic Influences*)

jing jie (Herba seu Flos Schizonepetae Tenuifolia) 荆芥	10g
fang feng (Radix Ledebouriellae Divaricatae) 防风	10g
jie geng (Radix Platycodi Grandiflori) 桔梗	10g
qian hu (Radix Peucedani) 前胡	10g
qiang huo (Rhizoma et Radix Notopterygii) 羌活	10g
zhi ke (Fructus Citri Aurantii) 枳壳	10g
du huo (Radix Angelicae Pubescentis) 独活	6g
chuan xiong (Radix Ligustici Chuanxiong) 川芎	6g
chao xing ren* (dry fried Semen Pruni Armeniacae) 炒杏仁	6g
sheng jiang (Rhizoma Zingiberis Officinalis Recens) 生姜	3pce

Method: Decoction. The herbs should be gently simmered for no longer than 20 minutes. Take hot or follow with hot porridge to induce sweating. (Source: *Zhong Yi Nei Ke Lin Chuang Shou Ce*)

1. ACUTE EXTERIOR DISORDERS

Modifications
- With some mild internal Damp (fullness and distension in the chest and epigastrium, poor appetite and nausea), add **zhi xiang fu** (prepared Rhizoma Cyperi Rotundi) 制香附 10g, **zi su ye** (Folium Perillae Frutescentis) 紫苏叶 12g and **chen pi** (Pericarpium Citri Reticulatae) 陈皮 10g.

Variations and additional prescriptions

Wind Damp
- With Wind Dampness as well (headache or heavy headedness, aching and heaviness in the limbs, generalised muscle aches, thick white tongue coat), the correct treatment is to expel Wind and Damp with **QIANG HUO SHENG SHI TANG** (*Notopterygium Decoction to Overcome Dampness* 羌活胜湿汤).

    qiang huo (Rhizoma et Radix Notopterygii) 羌活 9g
    du huo (Radix Angelicae Pubescentis) 独活 9g
    gao ben (Rhizoma et Radix Ligustici) 藁本 6g
    fang feng (Radix Ledebouriellae Divaricatae) 防风 6g
    chuan xiong (Radix Ligustici Chuanxiong) 川芎 6g
    man jing zi (Fructus Viticis) 蔓荆子 6g
    zhi gan cao (honey fried Radix Glycyrrhizae Uralensis)
    炙甘草 3g
    Method: Decoction. (Source: *Formulas and Strategies*)

Neck and shoulder stiffness
- With neck and shoulder stiffness and occipital headache, add **ge gen** (Radix Puerariae) 葛根 12g, or use **GE GEN TANG** (*Pueraria Combination* 葛根汤).

    ge gen (Radix Puerariae) 葛根 9g
    ma huang* (Herba Ephedra) 麻黄 6g
    gui zhi (Ramulus Cinnamomi Cassiae) 桂枝 6g
    bai shao (Radix Paeoniae Lactiflora) 白芍 6g
    zhi gan cao (honey fried Radix Glycyrrhizae Uralensis)
    炙甘草 3g
    sheng jiang (Rhizoma Zingiberis Officinalis Recens)
    生姜 3pce
    da zao (Fructus Zizyphi Jujubae) 大枣 5pce
    Method: Decoction. (Source: *Shi Yong Zhong Yao Xue*)

Wheezing, asthma
- With significant wheezing and tightness in the chest, add **ma huang** (Herba Ephedra) 麻黄 10g and **su zi** (Fructus Perillae Fructescentis)

苏子 10g, or expel Wind Cold and redirect *qi* downwards with **MA HUANG TANG** (*Ma Huang Combination* 麻黄汤).

    ma huang* (Herba Ephedra) 麻黄 6-9g
    gui zhi (Ramulus Cinnamomi Cassiae) 桂枝 6-9g
    xing ren* (Semen Pruni Armeniacae) 杏仁 9-12g
    zhi gan cao (honey fried Radix Glycyrrhizae Uralensis)
        炙甘草 3g
    Method: Decoction. (Source: *Shi Yong Zhong Yao Xue*)

Headache

- If the headache is severe and the patient's main concern, the correct treatment is to disperse Wind cold and stop pain with **CHUAN XIONG CHA TIAO SAN** (*Cnidium and Thea Formula*).

    chuan xiong (Radix Ligustici Chuanxiong) 川芎 120g
    jing jie (Herba seu Flos Schizonepetae Tenuifolia) 荆芥 120g
    bo he (Herba Mentha Haplocalycis) 薄荷 240g
    bai zhi (Radix Angelicae Dahuricae) 白芷 60g
    qiang huo (Rhizoma et Radix Notopterygii) 羌活 60g
    gan cao (Radix Glycyrrhizae Uralensis) 甘草 60g
    fang feng (Radix Ledebouriellae Divaricatae) 防风 45g
    xi xin* (Herba cum Radice Asari) 细辛 30g
    Method: Grind the herbs to a powder and take six grams with hot water or ginger tea 2-3 times daily. May also be decocted with a 90 % reduction in dosage, in which case the formula is cooked for no longer than 15 minutes, and **bo he** (6g) is added at the end of cooking (*hou xia* 后下). (Source: *Shi Yong Fang Ji Xue*)

Patent medicines

Gan Mao Ling 感冒灵 (Gan Mao Ling)
Gan Mao Qing Re Chong Ji 感冒清热冲剂 (Colds and Flu Tea)
Chuan Xiong Cha Tiao Wan 川芎茶调丸 (Chuan Xiong Cha Tiao Wan)
   - with prominent headache

Acupuncture

LI.4 (*he gu* -), GB.20 (*feng chi* -), Bl.12 (*feng men* -Ω), Bl.13 (*fei shu* -Ω), Du.14 (*da zhui* -)
- with cough, add Lu.7 (*lie que* -)
- with significant wheezing, use *ding chuan* (M-BW-1)
- if the nose is congested or runny, add Du.23 (*shang xing*)
- with a weak pulse, add St.36 (*zu san li* +)

Clinical notes

- The kinds of biomedical conditions that may present as Wind Cold type *gan mao* include the common cold, influenza, gastric flu or upper

respiratory tract infections.
- Simple measures help to prevent colds, for example a scarf to cover the vulnerable neck area is particularly useful.
- Although mostly self limiting, colds can become a problem if the patient is run down or continues to work during the illness.
- For effective treatment, timing is important. If treated in the first 24 hours, resolution is usually quick. A useful treatment method in the early stage of a Wind Cold with *no* sweating, is to soak for 15 minutes in a very hot bath (with epsom salts or a fist sized chunk of root ginger added). Get out of the bath without drying, wrap in a robe and sweat for another 5-10 minutes. Have a warm shower and dry off.
- Acupuncture treatment can be applied 2-3 times daily in severe cases.

1.2 WIND HEAT

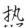

Pathophysiology
- Wind Heat enters through the nose or mouth, and as both Wind and Heat are *yang* pathogens, the symptoms tend to focus in the upper body. In contrast to the Wind Cold pattern, the herbs used here are cool in nature and are milder diaphoretics, as the pores are already open.

Clinical features
- acute fever with mild chills or no chills
- sore, dry or scratchy throat
- mild sweating
- headache (usually frontal)
- thirst
- cough with thick or sticky yellow mucus
- nasal obstruction, or a nasal discharge which is thick and yellow or green

T normal or red tipped with a thin yellow coat
P floating and rapid

Treatment principle
Expel Wind Heat
Clear Heat from the Lungs

Prescription

YIN QIAO SAN 银翘散
(*Lonicera and Forsythia Formula*)

jin yin hua (Flos Lonicerae Japonicae) 金银花	10-15g
lian qiao (Fructus Forsythia Suspensae) 连翘	10-15g
lu gen (Rhizoma Phragmitis Communis) 芦根	15g
dan zhu ye (Herba Lophatheri Gracilis) 淡竹叶	9g
jie geng (Radix Platycodi Grandiflori) 桔梗	9g
dan dou chi (Semen Sojae Preparatum) 淡豆豉	9g
niu bang zi (Fructus Arctii Lappae) 牛蒡子	9g
jing jie (Herba seu Flos Schizonepetae Tenuifolia) 荆芥	9g
bo he (Herba Mentha Haplocalycis) 薄荷	6g
gan cao (Radix Glycyrrhizae Uralensis) 甘草	3g

Method: Decoction. The herbs should be gently simmered for no longer than 20 minutes. **Bo he** is added at the end of cooking (*hou xia* 后下). Take cool or at room temperature. (Source: *Shi Yong Zhong Yao Xue*)

Modifications
- For severe headaches, add **sang ye** (Folium Mori Albae) 桑叶 10g, **ju hua** (Flos Chrysanthemi Morifolii) 菊花 15g and **man jing zi** (Fructus

Viticis) 蔓荆子 10g.
- For severe cough, add **qian hu** (Radix Peucedani) 前胡 10g, **chuan bei mu** (Bulbus Fritillariae Cirrhosae) 川贝母 10g and **quan gua lou** (Fructus Trichosanthis) 全括楼 15g.
- If the throat is red, very sore and swollen, add **shan dou gen** 山豆根 18g and **da qing ye** (Folium Daqingye) 大青叶 30g. See also Sore Throat, p.285.
- With high fever and severe thirst, add **sheng shi gao** (Gypsum) 生石膏 30g, **ban lan gen** (Radix Isatidis seu Baphicacanthi) 板蓝根 30g, **zhi mu** (Rhizoma Anemarrhenae Asphodeloides) 知母 10g and **tian hua fen** (Radix Trichosanthes Kirilowii) 天花粉 30g.
- With epistaxis, add **bai mao gen** (Rhizoma Imperatae Cylindricae) 白茅根 30g, **ou jie** (Nodus Nelumbinis Nuciferae) 藕节 10g. See also Epistaxis, p.168.

Patent medicines
Yin Qiao Jie Du Pian 银翘解毒片 (Yin Chiao Chieh Tu Pien)
Gan Mao Ling 感冒灵 (Gan Mao Ling)
Ban Lan Gen Chong Ji 板蓝根冲剂 (Ban Lan Gen Chong Ji)

Acupuncture
Du.14 (*da zhui* -Ω), Bl.12 (*feng men* -Ω), LI.11 (*qu chi* -), LI.4 (*he gu* -), SJ.5 (*wai guan* -)
- if the throat is very sore and swollen, add Lu.11 (*shao shang* ↓) and SI.17 (*tian rong* -)
- with cough add Lu.5 (*chi ze* -)

Clinical notes
- Biomedical conditions that may present as Wind Heat type *gan mao* include the common cold, tonsillitis, upper respiratory tract infection, acute bronchitis, and the early stage of measles, encephalitis or meningitis.
- In cases of severe Wind Heat see also *fei yong* (Lung Abscess), p.109.
- Responds well to correct and timely treatment. Acupuncture can be applied 2-3 times daily in severe cases. The treatment may need modification after 2-3 days if the patient has not improved.
- The patient should be advised to stay warm and well covered even though there is fever.

1.3 SUMMERHEAT AND DAMPNESS

Pathophysiology
- Summer Heat (or Summer Damp) patterns mostly occur during hot humid weather, often at the end of Summer and early Autumn. A common pattern in tropical and subtropical climates, Summer Heat/Dampness has a particular affinity for the Spleen so acute digestive symptoms are prominent.

Clinical features
- acute, relatively high fever which is unrelieved by sweating
- heaviness in the body
- nausea and vomiting
- diarrhoea
- woolly-headedness, like 'being wrapped in a damp towel'
- fatigue and lethargy
- thirst
- irritability and restlessness
- concentrated urine
- maybe a sore throat
- when there is sweating it is often of an oozing, sticky nature
- in general all symptoms are worse around mid afternoon

T greasy white or yellow coat
P soft, soggy, and possibly rapid

Treatment principle
Clear Summer Damp
Transform Dampness

Prescription

XIN JIA XIANG RU YIN 新加香薷饮
(*Newly Augmented Elsholtzia Combination*) modified

The focus of this prescription is on releasing the exterior, and is selected when the exterior and Heat signs (fever, thirst, urine) are prominent, and the digestive symptoms are relatively mild.

xiang ru (Herba Elsholtzia seu Moslae) 香薷	9g
jin yin hua (Flos Lonicerae Japonicae) 金银花	15g
bian dou (Semen Dolichos Lablab) 扁豆	15g
hua shi (Talcum) 滑石	12g
lian qiao (Fructus Forsythia Suspensae) 连翘	9g
hou po (Cortex Magnoliae Officinalis) 厚朴	9g
huo xiang (Herba Agastaches seu Pogostemi) 藿香	9g
pei lan (Herba Eupatorii Fortuneii) 佩兰	9g

he ye (Folium Nelumbinis Nuciferae) 荷叶 6g
gan cao (Radix Glycyrrhizae Uralensis) 甘草 3g

Method: Decoction. The herbs should be gently simmered for no longer than 20 minutes. This formula should be taken cool as **xiang ru** can cause vomiting when taken hot. (Source: *Zhong Yi Nei Ke Lin Chuang Shou Ce*)

HUO XIANG ZHENG QI SAN 藿香正气散
(Agastache Formula)

This prescription is selected when internal Dampness (with little Heat) is prominent and the exterior symptoms are relatively mild. It is also suitable for Wind Cold with concurrent or pre-existing Damp stagnation in the digestive tract.

huo xiang (Herba Agastaches seu Pogostemi) 藿香 12g
fu ling (Sclerotium Poriae Cocos) 茯苓 12g
zi su ye (Folium Perillae Frutescentis) 紫苏叶 9g
ban xia* (Rhizoma Pinelliae Ternatae) 半夏 9g
da fu pi (Pericarpium Arecae Catechu) 大服皮 9g
chao bai zhu (dry fried Rhizoma Atractylodes
  Macrocephalae) 炒白术 9g
chen pi (Pericarpium Citri Reticulatae) 陈皮 6g
bai zhi (Radix Angelicae Dahuricae) 白芷 6g
hou po (Cortex Magnoliae Officinalis) 厚朴 6g
jie geng (Radix Platycodi Grandiflori) 桔梗 6g
zhi gan cao (honey fried Radix Glycyrrhizae Uralensis)
  炙甘草 6g
sheng jiang (Rhizoma Zingiberis Officinalis Recens)
  生姜 3pce
da zao (Fructus Zizyphi Jujubae) 大枣 2pce

Method: Decoction. The herbs should be gently simmered for no longer than 20 minutes. (Source: *Shi Yong Zhong Yao Xue*)

SAN REN TANG 三仁汤
(Three Nut Decoction)

This formula is selected when Dampness and Heat lodge at the surface and *qi* level. The main features are aching and heaviness in the body, afternoon fever, a pale sallow complexion and a greasy tongue coat. This formula does not release the exterior, instead it opens up Lung *qi* and leaches Damp Heat out through the urine.

yi ren (Semen Coicis Lachryma-jobi) 苡仁 18-30g
hua shi (Talcum) 滑石 15g
xing ren* (Semen Pruni Armeniacae) 杏仁 12g
ban xia* (Rhizoma Pinelliae Ternatae) 半夏 9g

dan zhu ye (Herba Lophatheri Gracilis) 淡竹叶 9g
bai dou kou (Fructus Amomi Kravanh) 白豆蔻 6g
hou po (Cortex Magnoliae Officinalis) 厚朴 6g
tong cao Medulla Tetrapanacis Papyriferi) 通草 6g
Method: Decoction. (Source: *Shi Yong Fang Ji Xue*)

LIAN PO YIN 连朴饮
(*Coptis and Magnolia Bark Decoction*)

This formula is selected for Damp Heat invasion with Heat predominant. The main features are vomiting and diarrhoea, fullness in the chest and epigastrium, fever unrelieved by sweating, irritability and restlessness, greasy yellow tongue coat and dark urine. There may also be small, itchy, fluid filled vesicular eruptions on the neck and trunk (miliaria crystallina).

huang lian (Rhizoma Coptidis) 黄连 3g
hou po (Cortex Magnoliae Officinalis) 厚朴 6g
shan zhi zi (Fructus Gardeniae Jasminoidis) 山栀子 9g
dan dou chi (Semen Sojae Preparatum) 淡豆豉 9g
shi chang pu (Rhizoma Acori Graminei) 石菖蒲 3g
ban xia* (Rhizoma Pinelliae Ternatae) 半夏 3g
lu gen (Rhizoma Phragmitis Communis) 芦根 60g
Method: Decoction. (Source: *Shi Yong Fang Ji Xue*)

Patent medicines
Huo Xiang Zheng Qi Pian 藿香正气片 (Huo Hsiang Cheng Chi Pien)
Xing Jun San 行军散 (Marching Powder, Five Pagodas Brand)
Liu Shen Shui 六神水 (Liu Shen Shui)
Bao Ji Wan 保济丸 (Po Chai Pills)
Shen Qu Cha 神曲茶 (Shen Qu Cha)

Acupuncture
Lu.6 (*kong zui* -), LI.4 (*he gu* -), SJ.6 (*zhi gou* -), Sp.9 (*yin ling quan* -), Ren.12 (*zhong wan* -), St.36 (*zu san li* -)
- with high fever add Du.14 (*da zhui* -)
- with nausea add PC.6 (*nei guan*)
- with diarrhoea add *zhi xie* (N-CA-3), Bl.25 (*tian shu*)
- with myalgia add Sp.21 (*da bao*)

Clinical notes
- Biomedical conditions that may present as Summerheat and Dampness type *gan mao* include acute gastroenteritis, food poisoning, gastric flu and the early stage of glandular fever (infectious mononucleosis).

- Responds well to early treatment, but has a tendency to drag on or become recurrent if neglected. This appears in patients who return to work or activity before they are fully recovered and the Dampness completely cleared–they may continue to have relapses for up to several weeks.

1.4 WIND DRYNESS

Pathophysiology
- This pattern is usually due to an invasion of Wind and Dryness mostly during Autumn. It may also follow a Wind Heat attack which dries and damages body fluids. The Lung system is especially sensitive to dryness.

Clinical features
- dryness is the main feature, particularly in the nose, lips, mouth and throat
- cracked lips
- mild fever
- aversion to wind and cold
- headache
- slight sweating
- dry cough with little or no mucus

T unremarkable or dry, with a slightly red body and a thin white coat
P floating and wiry, maybe rapid

Treatment principle
Expel Wind and moisten Dryness
Nourish *yin*, soothe the Lungs

Prescription

SANG XING TANG 桑杏汤
(*Morus and Apricot Seed Combination*) modified

sang ye (Folium Mori Albae) 桑叶	12g
chao xing ren* (dry fried Semen Pruni Armeniacae) 炒杏仁	9g
nan sha shen (Radix Adenophorae seu Glehniae) 南沙参	24g
lu gen (Rhizoma Phragmitis Communis) 芦根	18g
chuan bei mu (Bulbus Fritillariae Cirrhosae) 川贝母	12g
jie geng (Radix Platycodi Grandiflori) 桔梗	9g
shan zhi zi (Fructus Gardeniae Jasminoidis) 山栀子	9g
dan dou chi (Semen Sojae Preparatum) 淡豆豉	9g
bo he (Herba Mentha Haplocalycis) 薄荷	6g

Method: Decoction. **Bo he** is added at the end of cooking (*hou xia* 后下). The herbs should be gently simmered for no longer than 20 minutes. (Source: *Zhong Yi Nei Ke Lin Chuang Shou Ce*)

Modifications
- For severe thirst, add **shi gao** (Gypsum) 石膏 15g and **tian hua fen** (Radix Trichosanthes Kirilowii) 天花粉 12g.
- If there is blood streaked mucus, add **bai mao gen** (Rhizoma Imperatae Cylindricae) 白茅根 30g and **ou jie** (Nodus Nelumbinis Nuciferae) 藕节 15g.

Patent medicines
Yin Qiao Jie Du Pian 银翘解毒片 (Yin Chiao Chieh Tu Pien)
Gan Mao Ling 感冒灵 (Gan Mao Ling)
Sang Ju Yin Pian 桑菊饮片 (Sang Chu Yin Pian)
African Sea Coconut Cough Syrup

Acupuncture
Du.14 (*da zhui* -), LI.11 (*qu chi* -), LI.4 (*he gu* -), Lu.5 (*chi ze* -), SJ.5 (*wai guan* -), Kid.6 (*zhao hai*), Sp.6 (*san yin jiao* +), Ren.22 (*tian tu*)

Clinical notes
- Biomedical conditions that may present as Wind Dryness type *gan mao* common cold, upper respiratory tract infection
- Quite a common pattern, even in relatively humid climates due to the prevalence of climate controlled buildings.
- Sipping pear juice is useful, especially for those individuals continually exposed to a dry climate.
- Responds well to correct herbal treatment, as herbs can directly moisturise dryness. Acupuncture is of only limited use in dry patterns.

1.5 WIND COLD WITH INTERIOR HEAT

Pathophysiology
- Wind Cold patterns with internal Heat occur in a constitutionally Hot individual or in someone with pre-existing internal Heat in the Lungs (often from a residual pathogen, or from smoking) who gets a Wind Cold attack.
- When a person with a hot constitution and strong *zheng qi* is invaded by strong Wind Cold the ensuing battle can be particularly vigorous, generating significant Heat to generate internal Heat while still having Cold on the exterior. The Heat may then affect the *yang ming* causing constipation and thirst (*tai yang-yang ming* overlap syndrome).

Clinical features
- high fever with severe chills or rigors
- loud cough with sticky yellow mucus
- no sweating
- generalised muscle aches
- nasal obstruction
- occipital headache
- strong thirst with desire for cold liquids
- sore throat
- irritability and restlessness
- dry stools or constipation

T red or with a red tip and edges, and a thin white or yellow coat
P floating and tight and possibly rapid

Treatment principle
Expel Wind and Cold
Clear internal Heat

Prescription

MA XING SHI GAN TANG 麻杏石甘汤
(*Ma Huang, Apricot Seed, Gypsum and Licorice Combination*) modified

sheng shi gao (Gypsum) 生石膏	15g
chao xing ren* (dry fried Semen Pruni Armeniacae) 炒杏仁	9g
gan cao (Radix Glycyrrhizae Uralensis) 甘草	6g
ma huang* (Herba Ephedrae) 麻黄	6g
pi pa ye (Folium Eriobotryae) 枇杷叶	12g
jing jie (Herba seu Flos Schizonepetae Tenuifolia) 荆芥	9g
fang feng (Radix Ledebouriellae Divaricatae) 防风	9g
sang bai pi (Cortex Mori Albae Radicis) 桑白皮	9g

qian hu (Radix Peucedani) 前胡	9g
shan zhi zi (Fructus Gardeniae Jasminoidis) 栀子	9g
huang qin (Radix Scutellariae Baicalensis) 黄芩	9g
jie geng (Radix Platycodi Grandiflori) 桔梗	9g

Method: Decoction. **Shi gao** should be cooked for 30 minutes prior to the other herbs (*xian jian* 先煎). After the other herbs are added, they should be gently simmered for no longer than 20 minutes. (Source: *Zhong Yi Nei Ke Lin Chuang Shou Ce*)

Modifications

- With severe muscle and bone aches, add **gui zhi** (Ramulus Cinnamomi Cassiae) 桂枝 10g and **zi su ye** (Folium Perillae Frutescentis) 紫苏叶 12g.
- With constipation, add **da huang** (Radix et Rhizoma Rhei) 大黄 3-6g.

Variations and additional prescriptions

DA QING LONG TANG 大青龙汤
(*Major Blue Dragon Combination*) see p.52

Patent medicines

Fang Feng Tong Sheng Wan 防风通圣丸 (Fang Feng Tong Sheng Wan)
Ma Xing Zhi Ke Pian 麻杏止咳片 (Ma Hsing Chih Ke Pian)
Zhi Sou Ding Chuan Wan 止嗽定喘丸 (Zhi Sou Ding Quan Wan)

Acupuncture

Du.14 (*da zhui* -Ω), Bl.12 (*feng men* -Ω), LI.11 (*qu chi* -), LI.4 (*he gu* -), Lu.5 (*chi ze* -), SJ.5 (*wai guan* -)
- If the throat is very sore and swollen, add Lu.11 (*shao shang* ↓) and SI.17 (*tian rong* -)
- with much internal Heat add SJ.2 (*ye men* -), Lu.10 (*yu ji* -)

Clinical notes

- Biomedical conditions that may present as Wind Cold with interior heat type *gan mao* include influenza, the common cold, upper respiratory tract infection, acute asthma, acute bronchitis, pneumonia, whooping cough, tonsillitis, pharyngitis, malaria and Dengue fever.
- Acupuncture can be applied 2-3 times daily in severe cases. Rapid result can usually be expected when treatment is timely.

1.6 ACUTE EXTERIOR DISORDER WITH DEFICIENCY

- In acute exterior disorders the general principle of treatment regardless of the condition of the patient is to first expel the pathogen using diaphoresis.
- There are some special cases, however, where simultaneous support of *zheng qi* and expulsion of pathogens is required. Patients in this category show obvious deficiency of *qi*, Blood, *yin*, or *yang*. The following patterns are seen more frequently in immunocompromised patients, the frail or the elderly and postpartum or pregnant women.

1.6.1 *QI* DEFICIENCY (AND EXTERNAL WIND)

Pathophysiology

- In this pattern the patient's *qi* is weakened. Because *zheng qi* is reduced, the body's defensive response to the pathogen is weak and thus the symptoms (which reflect the intensity of the struggle) are mild. Depending on the degree of deficiency the symptoms may range from mild to mid range. Even though the symptoms in this pattern frequently appear to be mild, this does not mean that the condition is not serious. In some patients, for example, the elderly a simple cold can easily and quickly lead to more severe and sometimes fatal complications.

Clinical features

- mild chills and fever
- headache
- sweating
- nasal obstruction
- cough with white or clear mucus
- recurrent mild sore throat and swollen cervical lymph nodes
- fatigue, lethargy and weakness
- low voice, reluctance to speak
- shortness of breath
- all symptoms are worse with exertion
- the cold tends to linger on, or is recurrent

T pale, with a thin white coat
P floating and weak

Treatment principle

Clear the exterior and support *qi*

Prescription

SHEN SU YIN 参苏饮
(*Ginseng and Perilla Combination*)

> **dang shen** (Radix Codonopsis Pilosulae) 党参 15g
> **zi su ye** (Fructus Perillae Frutescentis) 紫苏叶 10g
> **ge gen** (Radix Puerariae) 葛根 15g
> **qian hu** (Radix Peucedani) 前胡 10g
> **ban xia*** (Rhizoma Pinelliae Ternatae) 半夏 12g
> **fu ling** (Sclerotium Poriae Cocos) 茯苓 15g
> **chen pi** (Pericarpium Citri Reticulatae) 陈皮 10g
> **jie geng** (Radix Platycodi Grandiflori) 桔梗 10g
> **zhi ke** (Fructus Citri Aurantii) 枳壳 10g
> **mu xiang** (Radix Aucklandiae Lappae) 木香 6g
> **gan cao** (Radix Glycyrrhizae Uralensis) 甘草 6g
> **sheng jiang** (Rhizoma Zingiberis Officinalis Recens)
> 生姜 3pce
> **da zao** (Fructus Zizyphi Jujubae) 大枣 3pce
>
> Method: Decoction. The herbs should be gently simmered for no longer than 20 minutes. (Source: *Zhong Yi Nei Ke Lin Chuang Shou Ce*)

Variations and additional prescriptions

♦ In patients who are frequently ill with colds and flu and those who find it difficult to throw off colds or who experience mild exterior symptoms when fatigued or with exertion, the correct treatment is to bolster *wei qi* and strengthen the Spleen with **YU PING FENG SAN** (*Jade Screen Powder* 玉屏风散). This formula is used between acute cold episodes or in the post acute phase if the cold is difficult to throw off. It should not be used for an acute exterior disorder as **huang qi** can lock a pathogen in the body, aggravating the condition. In acute cases the previous formula is appropriate. This is an excellent formula to strengthen immunity in patients subject to frequent colds.

> **huang qi** (Radix Astragali Membranacei) 黄芪 30-120g
> **bai zhu** (Rhizoma Atractylodis Macrocephalae) 白术 60g
> **fang feng** (Radix Ledebouriellae Divaricatae) 防风 60g
>
> Method: Grind the herbs to a powder and take 6-9 grams twice daily with warm water. (Source: Formulas and Strategies)

Patent medicines

Shen Su Yin 参苏饮 (Ginseng and Perilla Combination)
Yu Ping Feng Wan 玉屏风丸 (Yu Ping Feng Wan)

Acupuncture
GB.20 (*feng chi* -), Lu.7 (*lie que* -), Bl.12 (*feng men* -Ω), LI.4 (*he gu* -), ST.36 (*zu san li* +), Ren.4 (*qi hai* +)
- In between colds, Du.14 (*da zhui* ▲) and ST.36 (*zu san li* ▲) may be used to strenthen *wei qi*.

Clinical notes
- Biomedical conditions that may present as esternal Wind with *qi* deficiency type *gan mao* include recurrent colds, chronic fatigue syndrome and general poor immunity.
- Unfortunately this is an increasingly common presentation in the modern day polluted environment. Susceptible individuals may experience damage to the immune system from the toxic overload of chemicals, ranging from potent pesticides used in agriculture, to the ubiquitous domestic chemicals found in paints, varnishes, carpet glues, particle board and many cleaning products. Over time, with appropriate treatment and avoidance of toxic chemicals, many of these individuals can rebuild their *zheng* and *wei qi* and be more able to fend off attack by external Wind.

1. ACUTE EXTERIOR DISORDERS

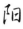

1.6.2 *YANG* DEFICIENCY (AND EXTERNAL WIND COLD)

Pathophysiology
- *Yang* deficiency with exterior Wind Cold occurs in patients with pre-existing *yang* deficiency, most often the elderly. Because *yang qi* is weak, *wei qi* will also be weak and Wind Cold can easily invade.
- In the clinic, the patient often presents not with the obvious Wind Cold symptoms, but with an otherwise unexplained aggravation of a pre-existing Kidney *yang* deficiency. In terms of *Shang Han Lun* analysis (p.46), this is a simultaneous *tai yang* and *shao yin* pattern facilitated by the Bladder (channel)–Kidney (channel) relationship.

Clinical features
- strong chills or shivering, possibly with mild feverishness
- chronic aversion to cold, with a desire to curl up
- exhaustion
- headache, general myalgia and aches in the bones
- either no sweating or spontaneous sweating; when there is sweating the aversion to cold is more pronounced
- low, soft voice with a reluctance to speak
- waxy pale complexion
- cold body and extremities
- there may be a history of exposure to wind or cold prior to the aggravation of symptoms

T pale and swollen, with a white coat
P deep and weak

Treatment principle
Support *yang*, clear the exterior

Prescription

SHEN FU ZAI ZAO WAN 参附再造丸
(*Ginseng and Aconite Pills for a New Lease on Life*) modified

This formula is selected when the *yang* deficiency is quite pronounced. It focuses primarily on tonifying *yang* and *qi*, and secondarily on dispersing Wind.

    ren shen (Radix Ginseng) 人参 9g
    zhi fu zi* (Radix Aconiti Carmichaeli Praeparata) 制附子 6g
    gui zhi (Ramulus Cinnamomi Cassiae) 桂枝 9g
    huang qi (Radix Astragali Membranacei) 黄芪 20g
    chuan xiong (Radix Ligustici Chuanxiong) 川芎 6g

fang feng (Radix Ledebouriellae Divaricatae) 防风 10g
qiang huo (Rhizoma et Radix Notopterygii) 羌活 8g
xi xin* (Herba cum Radice Asari) 细辛 3g
bai shao (Radix Paeoniae Lactiflora) 白芍 9g
sheng jiang (Rhizoma Zingiberis Officinalis Recens) 生姜 3g
da zao (Fructus Zizyphi Jujubae) 大枣 5g

Method: Decoction. **Zhi fu zi** should be cooked for 30 minutes prior to the other herbs (*xian jian* 先煎). The other herbs should be gently simmered for no longer than 20 minutes. (Source: *Zhong Yi Nei Ke Lin Chuang Shou Ce*)

MA HUANG FU ZI XI XIN TANG 麻黄附子细辛汤
(*Ma Huang, Asarum and Prepared Aconite Decoction*)

This formula is more dispersing than the primary formula. It is selected when the underlying *yang* deficiency is not too severe, and strong Cold is lodged in the surface, evidenced by the absence of sweating. In severe cases of *yang* deficiency, this formula is too dispersing and can lead to devastated *yang*.

ma huang* (Herba Ephedrae) 麻黄 6g
zhi fu zi* (Radix Aconiti Carmichaeli Praeparata) 制附子 9g
xi xin* (Herba cum Radice Asari) 细辛 6g

Method: Decoction. **Zhi fu zi** should be cooked for 30 minutes prior to the other herbs (*xian jian* 先煎). (Source: Formulas and Strategies)

Modifications
- If the stools are loose or watery add **rou gui** (Cortex Cinnamomi Cassiae) 肉桂 6g and **pao jiang** (roasted Rhizoma Zingiberis Officinalis) 炮姜 6g.

Patent medicines
Shen Fu Zai Zao Wan 参附再造丸 (Shen Fu Zai Zao Wan)

Acupuncture
GB.20 (*feng chi* -), Lu.7 (*lie que* -), Bl.12 (*feng men* -Ω), LI.4 (*he gu* -), ST.36 (*zu san li* +▲), Ren.4 (*qi hai* +▲), Du.14 (*da zhui* +▲)

Clinical notes
- Biomedical conditions that may present as *gan mao* with underlying *yang* deficiency include the common cold in frail or elderly patients with poor immune response.

1.6.3 BLOOD DEFICIENCY (AND EXTERNAL WIND)

Pathophysiology
- Blood deficiency with external Wind (and Cold or Heat) occurs in patients with pre-existing Blood deficiency, or following blood loss (traumatic, postpartum, post surgical haemorrhage). It can also occur during pregnancy.

Clinical features
- acute headache
- fever
- mild chills
- little or no sweating
- lustreless, sallow complexion
- pale nails and lips
- fatigue
- palpitations
- dizziness

T pale
P thready or floating, thready and weak

Treatment principle
Nourish Blood, clear the exterior

Prescription

CONG BAI QI WEI YIN 葱白七味饮
(*Shallot and Seven Herb Drink*) modified

cong bai (Bulbus Allii Fistulosi) 葱白	3pce
ge gen (Radix Puerariae) 葛根	18g
sheng di (Radix Rehmanniae Glutinosae) 生地	15g
mai dong (Tuber Ophiopogonis Japonici) 麦冬	15g
dan dou chi (Semen Sojae Preparatum) 淡豆豉	10g
jing jie (Herba seu Flos Schizonepetae Tenuifolia) 荆芥	10g
e jiaoˆ (Gelatinum Corii Asini) 阿胶	10g
sheng jiang (Rhizoma Zingiberis Officinalis Recens) 生姜	3g

Method: Decoction. The herbs should be gently simmered for no longer than 20 minutes. **Cong bai** is added towards the end of cooking (*hou xia* 后下), **e jiao** is melted before being added to the strained decoction (*yang hua* 烊化). (Source: *Zhong Yi Nei Ke Lin Chuang Shou Ce*)

Modifications
- With signs of Cold (aversion to cold and chills), add **zi su ye** (Fructus Perillae Frutescentis) 紫苏叶 9g and **fang feng** (Radix Ledebouriellae Divaricatae) 防风 9g.

- With signs of Heat (obvious fever, sore throat, rapid pulse), add **jin yin hua** (Flos Lonicerae Japonicae) 金银花 15g and **lian qiao** (Fructus Forsythia Suspensae) 连翘 15g.
- With continual bleeding (post-partum or menstrual), add **ou jie** (Nodus Nelumbinis Nuciferae) 藕节 10g, **san qi** (Radix Notoginseng) 三七 6g and **bai ji fen** (powdered Rhizoma Bletillae Striatae) 白芨粉 3g.
- With poor digestion, loss of appetite and abdominal distension, add **chen pi** (Pericarpium Citri Reticulatae) 陈皮 9g, **mai ya** (Fructus Hordei Vulgaris Germinantus) 麦芽 9g and **ji nei jin^** (Endothelium Corneum Gigeriae Galli) 鸡内金 9g.

Patent medicines
Gan Mao Ling 感冒灵 (Gan Mao Ling)
Shi San Tai Bao Wan 十三太保丸 (Shih San Tai Pao Wan)
Xiao Chai Hu Wan 小柴胡丸 (Xiao Chai Hu Wan) + *Si Wu Wan* 四物丸 (Si Wu Wan) 50:50

Acupuncture
GB.20 (*feng chi*), Lu.7 (*lie que*), Bl.12 (*feng men* Ω), LI.4 (*he gu*), ST.36 (*zu san li* +), Ren.4 (*qi hai* +), Du.14 (*da zhui* +)
- LI.4 (*he gu*) and Ren.4 (*qi hai* +) are contraindicated during pregnancy

Clinical notes
- Biomedical conditions that may present as *gan mao* with underlying Blood deficiency include pregnancy or post partum cold or flu and the early stage of puerperal fever.
- Only a very mild sweat is required and the herbs or acupuncture should be discontinued as soon as it occurs. If the treatment induces too much sweating there is the possibility of further damage to Blood and fluids.

1.6.4 *YIN* DEFICIENCY (AND EXTERNAL WIND)

Pathophysiology
- *Yin* deficiency with external Wind (and Cold or Heat) occurs in patients with pre-existing *yin* deficiency, most notably the elderly, and in those following a prolonged or debilitating illness.

Clinical features
- acute headache
- fever
- mild chills
- aversion to wind and cold
- little or no sweating or night sweats
- dizziness
- irritability and restlessness
- a sensation of heat in the palms and soles ('five hearts hot')
- thirst, dry mouth and throat
- dry cough with little or no mucus or blood streaked mucus

T red and dry, with little or no coat
P thready and rapid

Treatment principle
Nourish *yin*, clear the exterior

Prescription

JIA JIAN WEI RUI TANG 加减葳蕤汤
(Modified Yu Zhu Tang)

yu zhu (Rhizoma Polygonati Odorati) 玉竹	15g
cong bai (Bulbus Allii Fistulosi) 葱白	3pce
dan dou chi (Semen Sojae Preparatum) 淡豆豉	9g
jie geng (Radix Platycodi Grandiflori) 桔梗	9g
bai wei (Radix Cynanchi Baiwei) 白薇	9g
bo he (Herba Mentha Haplocalycis) 薄荷	6g
hong zao (Fructus Zizyphi Jujubae) 红枣	4pce
zhi gan cao (honey fried Radix Glycyrrhizae Uralensis) 炙甘草	6g

Method: Decoction. The herbs should be gently simmered for no longer than 20 minutes. **Bo he** is added towards the end of cooking (*hou xia* 后下). **Wei rui** is another name for **yu zhu**. (Source: *Zhong Yi Nei Ke Lin Chuang Shou Ce*)

Modifications
- If the fever, chills and headache are severe, add **jing jie** (Herba seu Flos Schizonepetae Tenuifolia) 荆芥 9g.

- If Heat, with irritability and thirst are prominent, add **dan zhu ye** (Herba Lophatheri Gracilis) 淡竹叶 9g, **tian hua fen** (Radix Trichosanthes Kirilowii) 天花粉 15g and **huang lian** (Rhizoma Coptidis) 黄连 6g.
- If the throat is dry, with a cough with sticky, hard to expectorate mucus, add **gua lou pi** (Pericarpium Trichosanthis) 瓜楼皮 12g, **she gan** (Rhizoma Belamacandae) 射干 9g and **niu bang zi** (Fructus Arctii Lappae) 牛蒡子 9g.
- If the cough causes chest pain and there are streaks of blood in the mucus, add **bai mao gen** (Rhizoma Imperatae Cylindricae) 白茅根 9g, **sheng pu huang** (unprocessed Pollen Typhae) 生蒲黄 9g and **ou jie** (Nodus Nelumbinis Nuciferae) 藕结 9g.

Patent medicines
Gan Mao Ling 感冒灵 (Gan Mao Ling)
Shi San Tai Bao Wan 十三太保丸 (Shih San Tai Pao Wan)

Acupuncture
GB.20 (*feng chi*), Lu.7 (*lie que* -), Bl.12 (*feng men* Ω), LI.4 (*he gu* -), Sp.6 (*san yin jiao* +), Kid.3 (*tai xi* +), Lu.9 (*tai yuan* +)
- LI.4 (*he gu*) is contraindicated during pregnancy

Clinical notes
- Biomedical conditions that may present as *yin* deficiency type *gan mao* include common colds in elderly, debilitated or otherwise *yin* deficient patients.
- Only a very mild sweat is required and treatment should be discontinued as soon as it occurs. If the treatment induces too much sweating there is the possibility of further damage to *yin* and fluids.

SUMMARY OF GUIDING FORMULAE FOR ACUTE EXTERIOR DISORDERS

Wind Cold - *Jing Fang Bai Du San* 荆防败毒散
- with Dampness - *Qiang Huo Sheng Shi Tang* 羌活胜湿汤
- with stiff neck - *Ge Gen Tang* 葛根汤
- with wheezing - *Ma Huang Tang* 麻黄汤

Wind Heat - *Yin Qiao San* 银翘散

Summer Heat and Dampness - *Xin Jia Xiang Ru Yin* 新加香薷饮
- with prominent Damp - *Huo Xiang Zheng Qi San* 藿香正气散
- Damp Heat - *San Ren Tang* 三仁汤 or *Lian Po Yin* 连朴饮

Wind Dryness - *Sang Xing Tang* 桑杏汤

Wind Cold with Internal Heat - *Ma Xing Shi Gan Tang* 麻杏石甘汤

Exterior disorder with internal deficiency
- *qi* deficiency - *Shen Su Yin* 参苏饮
- *yang* deficiency - *Shen Fu Zai Zao Wan* 参附再造丸
- Blood deficiency - *Cong Bai Qi Wei Yin* 葱白七味饮
- *yin* deficiency - *Jia Jian Wei Rui Tang* 加减葳蕤汤

Endnote

For more information regarding herbs marked with an asterisk*, an open circle° or a hatˆ, see the tables on pp.944-952.

Appendix 1.1
WARM DISEASES (*wen bing* 温病)

Wen bing are disorders that are due to pathogenic Wind and Heat. They are generally virulent and tend to be epidemic, affecting even robust individuals with intact *wei qi*. During the Ming 1368-1644 AD and Qing dynasties 1644-1911 AD, the theoretical (and practical) treatment protocols for *wen bing* reached their zentith. The main authors of *wen bing* theory, notably Ye Tian-shi, Xue Sheng-bai and Wu Ju-tong, postulated four levels through which a pathogen could move, each one successively more serious than the previous. The four levels are the *wei* (corresponding to the surface, an external disorder), *qi* (involving the Lungs, chest, Stomach and Intestines), *ying* (or nutritive) and Blood. By the time a pathogen has entered the *ying* and Blood levels, the disorder is characterised by febrile rashes, disordered consciousness and convulsions.

1. *WEI* LEVEL
The *wei* level is the surface. This disorder is the same as Wind Heat and is dealt with as described in the section on Acute Exterior Disorders.

2. *QI* LEVEL
Once the Heat has penetrated beyond the *wei* level it can develop in several ways, depending on the patient's constitution, predisposing lifestyle factors and the strength of the pathogen. *Qi* level disorders affect the chest and diaphragm, Lungs and digestive tract.

2.1 Heat in the Lungs
Clinical features
- cough and/or dyspnoea with sticky or hard to expectorate yellow or green mucus - in severe cases blood streaked mucus or rusty coloured mucus
- fever
- dry mouth and thirst
- sweating
- tightness or pain in the chest

T red tip with a yellow coat. If there is copious mucus the tongue coat is thick, yellow and greasy
P rapid and possibly slippery

Treatment principle
   Clear Heat from the Lungs, redirect Lung *qi* downwards

Prescription

MA XING SHI GAN TANG 麻杏石甘汤
(Ma Huang, Apricot Seed, Gypsum and Licorice Combination)

> **ma huang*** (Herba Ephedra) 麻黄 12g
> **shi gao** (Gypsum) 石膏 48g
> **xing ren*** (Semen Pruni Armeniacae) 杏仁 18g
> **zhi gan cao** (honey fried Radix Glycyrrhizae Uralensis)
> 炙甘草 6g
> Method: Decoction.

Modifications

- Today generally, and especially in cases of severe Heat, other Heat clearing herbs are added, typically herbs like **yu xing cao** (Herba Houttuyniae) 鱼腥草 24g, **huang qin** (Radix Scutellariae Baicalensis) 黄芩 15g, **jin yin hua** (Flos Lonicera Japonicae) 20g, **zhi mu** (Rhizoma Anemarrhenae Asphodeloides) 知母 12g, and **sang bai pi** (Cortex Mori Albae Radicis) 桑白皮 15g.
- With significant chest pain, add **tao ren** (Semen Persicae) 桃仁 9g and **yu jin** (Tuber Curcumae) 郁金 9g.
- With haemoptysis or blood streaked mucus, add **qian cao tan** (charred Radix Rubiae Cordifoliae) 茜草炭 12g, **bai mao gen** (Rhizoma Imperatae Cylindricae) 白茅根 9g and **ce bai ye tan** (charred Cacumen Biotae Orientalis) 侧柏叶炭 12g. See also Haemoptysis, p.193.
- If there is copious yellow mucus and dyspnoea with or without constipation, add **da huang** (Radix et Rhizoma Rhei) 大黄 6-9g and **gua lou ren** (Semen Trichosanthis) 栝楼仁 9g.

Patent medicines

Ma Xing Zhi Ke Pian 麻杏止咳片 (Ma Hsing Chih Ke Pien)
Qing Fei Yi Huo Pian 清肺抑火片 (Ching Fei Yi Huo Pien)
Niu Huang Jie Du Pian 牛黄解毒片 (Peking Niu Huang Chieh Tu Pien)

Acupuncture

Lu.5 (*chi ze* -), Lu.6 (*kong zui* -), Lu.1 (*zhong fu* -), Bl.13 (*fei shu* -), Lu.10 (*yu ji* -)

Clinical notes

- Biomedical conditions that may present as Heat in the Lungs include bronchitis, pneumonia, lobar pneumonia, whooping cough and epiglottitis.

2.2 Heat accumulating in the Stomach and Intestines

- This syndrome may present in a variety of ways, depending on its location and intensity, and other pathogens involved.

2.2a Heat in the *yang ming* channels

- In this case the Heat is thought to primarily affect the *yang ming* channels, and is 'formless' (i.e. without constipation). This is the classical pattern defined by the four 'bigs', i.e. big sweat, big thirst, big fever and big pulse.
- high fever with profuse sweating
- great thirst
- irritability
- red complexion
- frontal headache
- toothache
- bleeding gums

T dry yellow tongue coat
P flooding and rapid

Treatment principle

Clear and drain Heat from the *yang ming* channels

Prescription

BAI HU TANG 白虎汤
(*Anemarrhena and Gypsum Combination*)

The four 'bigs' have always been considered a prerequisite for the use of the formula, but they are not always all present in every patient. For example, in some cases fluids may be restrained by the Heat, so there is no sweating. As long as there is severe Heat in *yang ming* without constipation, this formula is applicable.

shi gao (Gypsum) 石膏	30g
zhi mu (Rhizoma Anemarrhenae Asphodeloides) 知母	9g
geng mi (Semen Oryzae) 梗米	9g
gan cao (Radix Glycyrrhizae Uralensis) 甘草	3g

Method: Decoction.

Modifications

- In cases with severe Heat, add **jin yin hua** (Flos Lonicera Japonicae) 金银花 15g, **lian qiao** (Fructus Forsythia Suspensae) 连翘 12g, **ban lan gen** (Radix Isatidis seu Baphicacanthi) 板蓝根 9g, and **da qing ye** (Folium Daqingye) 大青叶 12g.
- If fluids have been significantly damaged, add **shi hu** (Herba Dendrobii) 石斛 9g, **tian hua fen** (Radix Trichosanthes Kirilowii)

天花粉 9g and **lu gen** (Rhizoma Phragmitis Communis) 芦根 18g.
- With petechial haemorrhage, disorientation, irritability and restlessness associated with Toxic Heat, add **huang lian** (Rhizoma Coptidis) 黄连 6g, **huang qin** (Radix Scutellariae Baicalensis) 黄芩 9g, **huang bai** (Cortex Phellodendri) 黄柏 9g and **shan zhi zi** (Fructus Gardeniae Jasminoidis) 山栀子 9g.

Patent medicines
Dao Chi Pian 导赤片 (Tao Chih Pien)
Niu Huang Jie Du Pian 牛黄解毒片 (Peking Niu Huang Chieh Tu Pien)

Acupuncture
LI.11 (*qu chi* -), LI.4 (*he gu* -), St.37 (*shang ju xu* -), St. 39 (*xia ju xu* -), St.44 (*nei ting* -), St.25 (*tian shu* -), Bl.25 (*da chang shu*)

Clinical notes
- Biomedical conditions that may present as Heat in the *yang ming* channels include encephalitis, meningitis and heat stroke.

2.2b Heat and Phlegm in the chest and *yang ming*
- This condition is thought to be due to 'knotting' of Heat and Phlegm in the chest and epigastrium (*jie xiong* 结胸)
- focal chest or epigastric distension, fullness or pain which is worse for pressure
- red complexion
- heat in the body that may only be apparent with palpation
- thirst
- bitter taste in the mouth
- nausea
- constipation
- maybe cough with sticky yellow mucus

T greasy or dirty yellow tongue coat
P slippery and possibly floating or rapid

Treatment principle
Clear Heat, transform Phlegm
Open the chest and dissipate knotting

Prescription

XIAO XIAN XIONG TANG 小陷胸汤
(*Minor Sinking Into the Chest Decoction*)

> **gua lou** (Fructus Trichosanthis) 栝楼 24g
> **huang lian** (Rhizoma Coptidis) 黄连 3g
> **ban xia*** (Rhizoma Pinelliae Ternatae) 半夏 9g
> Method: Decoction.

Patent medicines

Qing Qi Hua Tan Wan 清气化痰丸 (Pinellia Expectorant Pills)
Qing Fei Yi Huo Pian 清肺抑火片 (Ching Fei Yi Huo Pien)

Acupuncture

St.40 (*feng long* -), St.37 (*shang ju xu* -), St.44 (*nei ting* -), LI.4 (*he gu* -), LI.11 (*qu chi* -), St.25 (*tian shu*), Bl.25 (*da chang shu* -), Lu.5 (*chi ze* -)

Clinical notes

- Biomedical conditions that may present as Heat and Phlegm in the chest and *yang ming* include pleurisy, bronchitis, gastritis and intercostal neuralgia.

2.2c Strong Heat in *yang ming* with constipation

- severe constipation or faecal impaction with watery diarrhoea
- painful and distended abdomen, which feels worse for pressure
- tense, firm abdomen
- tidal fever
- in severe cases confusion or disordered consciousness

T thick, yellow or brown and dry tongue coat
P deep and strong

Treatment principle

Purge Heat through the bowel

Prescription

DA CHENG QI TANG 大承气汤
(*Major Rhubarb Combination*)

> **da huang** (Radix et Rhizoma Rhei) 大黄 9g
> **mang xiao** (Mirabilitum) 芒硝 12g
> **zhi shi** (Fructus Immaturus Citri Aurantii) 枳实 9g
> **hou po** (Cortex Magnoliae Officinalis) 厚朴 12g
> Method: Decoction. For powerful purgation **da huang** is added a few minutes

towards the end of cooking (*hou xia* 后下). **Mang xiao** is dissolved in the strained decoction (*chong fu* 冲服).

Modifications
* If body fluids have been significantly damaged, delete **hou po** and **zhi shi**, and add **xuan shen** (Radix Scrophulariae Ningpoensis) 玄参 18g, **sheng di** (Radix Rehmanniae Glutinosae) 生地 12g and **mai dong** (Tuber Ophiopogonis Japonici) 麦冬 12g. This makes **ZENG YE CHENG QI TANG** (*Increase the Fluids and Order the Qi Decoction* 增液承气汤).
* With Heat affecting the Small Intestine (dysuria and frequency), add **chi shao** (Radix Paeoniae Rubrae) 赤芍 12g, **sheng di** (Radix Rehmanniae Glutinosae) 生地 12g, **huang bai** (Cortex Phellodendri) 黄柏 12g and **huang lian** (Rhizoma Coptidis) 黄连 6g.

Patent medicines
Niu Huang Qing Huo Wan 牛黄清火丸 (Niu Huang Qing Huo Wan)
Qing Fei Yi Huo Pian 清肺抑火片 (Ching Fei Yi Huo Pien)

Acupuncture
St.25 (*tian shu* -), Bl.25 (*da chang shu* -), SJ.6 (*zhi gou* -),
St.37 (*shang ju xu* -), LI.11 (*qu chi* -), LI.4 (*he gu* -), St.44 (*nei ting* -)

Clinical notes
* Biomedical conditions that may present as Heat in *yang ming* with constipation include acute appendicitis, cholecystitis, pancreatitis and intestinal obstruction.

2.2d Damp Heat in *yang ming*
* This is external Damp Heat that settles in *yang ming*, thought originally to be due to an inappropriate purge in the exterior stage of a pathogenic disorder.
* urgent, foul smelling, hot diarrhoea with a burning anus
* fever or afternoon fever which is unrelieved with sweating
* sweating that tends to come in waves and is worse in the afternoon
* restlessness and irritability
* thirst

T red with a yellow coat
P rapid

Treatment principle
Clear Damp Heat, stop diarrhoea

Prescription

GE GEN HUANG QIN HUANG LIAN TANG 葛根黄芩黄连汤
(Kudzu, Coptis and Scute Combination)

ge gen (Radix Puerariae) 葛根 15g
huang qin (Radix Scutellariae Baicalensis) 黄芩 9g
huang lian (Rhizoma Coptidis) 黄连 6g
zhi gan cao (honey fried Radix Glycyrrhizae Uralensis)
炙甘草 6g
Method: Decoction.

Patent medicines

Chuan Xin Lian Kang Yan Pian 穿心莲抗炎片
 (Chuan Xin Lian Antiphlogistic Tablets)
Huang Lian Jie Du Wan 黄连解毒丸 (Huang Lian Jie Du Wan)
Yu Dai Wan 愈带丸 (Yudai Wan [Leucorrhoea Pills])
Huang Lian Su Pian 黄连素片 (Tabellae Berberini)
Jia Wei Xiang Lian Pian 加味香连片 (Chiawei Hsianglienpian)

Acupuncture

LI.11 (*qu chi* -), LI.4 (*he gu* -), St.44 (*nei ting* -), St.37 (*shang ju xu* -), St.25 (*tian shu* -), *zhi xie* (N-CA-3)

Clinical notes

• Biomedical conditions that may present as Damp Heat in *yang ming* include acute gastroenteritis and bacillary or amoebic dysentery.

2.3 Heat lingering in the chest and diaphragm

Pathophysiology
- This condition corresponds to lingering Heat (in the chest and diaphragm) in the aftermath of a febrile disease or during a relapse.

Clinical features
- mild but lingering feverishness
- irritability and restlessness
- insomnia
- thirst, dry mouth and lips
- fullness and discomfort in the chest
- sore throat
- constipation

T slightly red with a thin yellow coat
P slightly rapid

Treatment principle
Vent and clear Heat, alleviate restlessness and irritability

Prescription

ZHI ZI DOU CHI TANG 栀子豆豉汤
(Gardenia and Soybean Combination)

    shan zhi zi (Fructus Gardeniae Jasminoidis) 山栀子 9g
    dan dou chi (Semen Sojae Preparatum) 淡豆豉 9g
    Method: Decoction. This formula is rarely used alone and is usually added to other prescriptions to specifically treat post-febrile irritability, restlessness and discomfort in the chest. It may also serve as the basis upon which to build a broader formula, depending on the accompanying pattern.

Modifications
- For severe irritability and restlessness, add **lian qiao** (Fructus Forsythia Suspensae) 连翘 12g, **bo he** (Herba Mentha Haplocalycis) 薄荷 6g, **dan zhu ye** (Herba Lophatheri Gracilis) 淡竹叶 9g and **huang qin** (Radix Scutellariae Baicalensis) 12g.
- With constipation, add **da huang** (Radix et Rhizoma Rhei) 大黄 3-6g and **zhi shi** (Fructus Immaturus Citri Aurantii) 枳实 9g.

Acupuncture
PC.7 *(da ling)*, PC.8 *(lao gong)*, Ren.17 *(shan zhong)*, St.37 *(shang ju xu -)*, St.44 *(nei ting -)*, LI.11 *(qu chi -)*

3. *YING* LEVEL
3.1 Heat entering the Pericardium
Clinical features
- high fever which is worse at night
- dry mouth but no great thirst
- irritability and restlessness
- insomnia
- disordered consciousness or delirium
- faint erythema and purpura

T deep red and dry
P thready and rapid

Treatment principle

Clear Heat from the *ying* level, support *yin*

Prescription

QING YING TANG 清营汤
(*Clear the Ying Decoction*)

xi jiao° (Cornu Rhinoceri) 犀角	3g
sheng di (Radix Rehmanniae Glutinosae) 生地	30g
xuan shen (Radix Scrophulariae Ningpoensis) 玄参	12g
mai dong (Tuber Ophiopogonis Japonici) 麦冬	12g
jin yin hua (Flos Lonicera Japonicae) 金银花	12g
lian qiao (Fructus Forsythia Suspensae) 连翘	9g
dan shen (Radix Salviae Miltiorrhizae) 丹参	9g
dan zhu ye (Herba Lophatheri Gracilis) 淡竹叶	6g
huang lian (Rhizoma Coptidis) 黄连	3g

Method: Decoction. **Shui niu jiao**^ (Cornu Bubali) 水牛角 is usually substituted for **xi jiao** with a 5-10 fold increase in dose. It should be powdered and decocted for 30 minute before the other herbs are added (*xian jian* 先煎).

Patent medicines

Zi Xue Dan 紫雪丹 (Tzuhsueh Tan)
An Gong Niu Huang Wan 安宫牛黄丸 (An Gong Niu Huang Wan)
 - these formulas are usually reserved for severe cases with mental confusion, delirium or convulsions

Acupuncture

PC.3 (*qu ze* ↓), Bl.40 (*wei zhong* ↓), PC.9 (*zhong chong* ↓), LI.11 (*qu chi* -), Du.26 (*ren zhong* -), PC.7 (*da ling*)

Clinical notes
- Biomedical conditions that may present as Heat entering the Pericardium include encephalitis, meningitis, septicaemia and acute leukaemia.
- Patients with this patttern may require hospitalisation.

3.2 Heat obstructing the Pericardium
Clinical features
- This is a progression from the previous syndrome where the intense Heat in the Pericardium has scorched fluids and formed Phlegm. The resulting Phlegm Heat gives rise to serious disturbances of consciousness and possibly unconsciousness.
- The symptoms are the same as previously, with an intensification in the delirium, cold extremities, convulsions and coma

T deep red, dry and retracted
P thready and rapid

Treatment principle
Clear Heat, restore consciousness

Prescription
QING YING TANG 清营汤 p.38
(*Clear the Ying Decoction*) plus either
AN GONG NIU HUANG WAN 安宫牛黄丸 p.914
(*Calm the Palace Pill with Cattle Gallstone*) or
ZHI BAO DAN 至宝丹 p.660
(*Greatest Treasure Special Pill*)

Method: In situations where the patient is delerious or comatose, the medicine may be administered via a nasogastric tube or enema.

Modifications
- If there are convulsions, add **gou teng** (Ramulus Uncariae) 钩藤 15g, **ling yang jiao**° (Cornu Antelopis) 羚羊角 3g, or use **ZI XUE DAN** (*Purple Snow Special Pill* 紫雪丹, p.707).
- With constipation, add **da huang** (Radix et Rhizoma Rhei) 大黄 6-9g and **mang xiao** (Mirabilitum) 芒硝 9g.

Patent medicines
Zhi Bao Dan 至宝丹 (Zhi Bao Dan)
Zi Xue Dan 紫雪丹 (Tzuhsueh Tan)
An Gong Niu Huang Wan 安宫牛黄丸 (An Gong Niu Huang Wan)

Acupuncture

PC.3 (*qu ze* ↓), Bl.40 (*wei zhong* ↓), PC.9 (*zhong chong* ↓), LI.11 (*qu chi* -), Du.26 (*ren zhong* -)
- with coma add *shi xuan* ↓ (M-UE-1)

Clinical notes

- Biomedical conditions that may present as Heat obstructing the Pericardium include encephalitis, meningitis, acute leukaemia and septicaemia.
- This condition should be managed in hospital.

4. BLOOD LEVEL
4.1 Heat causing the Blood to move recklessly
Clinical features
- The main differentiating feature here (compared to the *ying* level) is the appearance of febrile rashes and haemorrhaging.
- high fever with dense and obvious erythema or purpura covering a substantial portion of the body
- various types of bleeding (epistaxis, haemoptysis etc.)
- in severe cases there is delirium and/or convulsions

T deep red and dry with very raised papillae
P thready and rapid or minute and rapid

Treatment principle
Cool the Blood, dispel stagnant Blood

Prescription

XI JIAO DI HUANG TANG 犀角地黄汤
(*Rhinoceros Horn and Rehmannia Decoction*) modified

xi jiao° (Cornu Rhinoceri) 犀角	3g
sheng di (Radix Rehmanniae Glutinosae) 生地	30g
chi shao (Radix Paeoniae Rubrae) 赤芍	12g
mu dan pi (Cortex Moutan Radicis) 牡丹皮	9g

Method: Decoction. **Shui niu jiao**^ (Cornu Bubali) 水牛角 is usually substituted for **xi jiao** with a 5-10 fold increase in dose. It should be powdered and decocted for 30 minute before the other herbs are added (*xian jian* 先煎).

Modifications
- In severe cases (and probably in most cases at this stage) herbs like **da qing ye** (Folium Daqingye) 大青叶, **ban lan gen** (Radix Isatidis seu Baphicacanthi) 板蓝根 and **zi cao** (Radix Lithospermi) 紫草 are added to enhance the effect and relieve toxicity.
- With severe bleeding, add **qian cao gen tan** (charred Radix Rubiae Cordifoliae) 茜草根炭 12g, **bai mao gen** (Rhizoma Imperatae Cylindricae) 白茅根 9g and **xiao ji tan** (charred Herba Cephalanoplos) 小蓟炭 9g.
- With Blood stasis (purplish rash), add **tao ren** (Semen Persicae) 桃仁 9g and **dan shen** (Radix Salviae Miltiorrhizae) 丹参 12g.
- With convulsions, add **ling yang jiao**° (Cornu Antelopis) 羚羊角 3g and **gou teng** (Ramulus Uncariae) 钩藤 15g.
- With delirium, combine with **AN GONG NIU HUANG WAN** (*Calm the Palace Pill with Cattle Gallstone* 安宫牛黄丸, p.914).

Patent medicines
Zi Xue Dan 紫雪丹 (Tzuhsueh Tan)
An Gong Niu Huang Wan 安宫牛黄丸 (An Gong Niu Huang Wan)

Acupuncture
PC.3 (*qu ze* ↓), Bl.40 (*wei zhong* ↓), PC.9 (*zhong chong* ↓),
LI.11 (*qu chi* -), Du.26 (*ren zhong* -)
  • with coma add *shi xuan* ↓ (M-UE-1)

Clinical notes
  • Biomedical conditions that may present as Heat causing reckless movement of Blood include severe infection like meningococcal meningitis, encephalitis, leukaemic crisis and septicaemia.
  • This condition should be managed in hospital.

4.2 Hot Blood and Blood stasis
Clinical features
  • This condition occurs as Heat invades the lower *jiao* and 'evaporates' the Blood, causing stasis.
  • acute lower abdominal pain which is worse for pressure
  • fever which is worse at night
  • constipation or black tarry stools
  • in severe cases manic behaviour or delirium

T deep red or purple with purple spots
P deep and full

Treatment principle
Clear Heat and break up Blood stagnation

Prescription

TAO HE CHENG QI TANG 桃核承气汤
(*Persica and Rhubarb Combination*) modified

tao ren (Semen Persicae) 桃仁	12g
da huang (Radix et Rhizoma Rhei) 大黄	12g
dang gui (Radix Angelicae Sinensis) 当归	9g
chi shao (Radix Paeoniae Rubrae) 赤芍	9g
mu dan pi (Cortex Moutan Radicis) 牡丹皮	6g
gui zhi (Ramulus Cinnamomi Cassiae) 桂枝	6g
mang xiao (Mirabilitum) 芒硝	6g
zhi gan cao (honey fried Radix Glycyrrhizae Uralensis) 炙甘草	6g

Method: Decoction. **Mang xiao** is dissolved in the strained decoction (*chong fu* 冲服).

Patent medicines
Tao He Cheng Qi San 桃核承气散 (Persica and Rhubarb Combination)

Acupuncture
Sp.4 (*gong sun* -), Sp.10 (*xue hai* -), Sp.8 (*di ji* -), St.40 (*feng long* -), PC.9 (*zhong chong* ↓), *zi gong* (M-CA-18), Sp.6 (*san yin jiao*), Liv.2 (*xing jian* -)

Clinical notes
- Biomedical conditions that may present as Hot Blood with Blood stasis include pelvic inflammatory disease, acute endometritis, retained placenta, ruptured ectopic pregnancy and puerperal fever.

Table A1.1a Overview of Wen Bing patterns

Level	Depth	Pathology		Features	Guiding Formula
Wei	superficial, affects the exterior	Wind Heat surface level syndrome		fever & chills, sore throat, sweating, thirst, headache, floating pulse, red tipped tongue	YIN QIAO SAN
Qi	Internal, affecting the chest, Lungs and Intestines	Heat in the Lungs		cough or dyspnoea with sticky yellow sputum, fever, thirst, chest pain, rapid pulse, red tongue with a yellow coat	MA XING SHI GAN TANG
		Heat in the Stomach and Intestines	Heat in the yang ming channel	high fever, sweating, thirst, irritability, dry yellow tongue coat, flooding, rapid pulse	BAI HU TANG
			Heat & Phlegm in yang ming	focal chest or epigastric distension, thirst, nausea, bitter taste, constipation, slippery pulse, greasy yellow tongue coat	XIAO XIAN XIONG TANG
			Heat in yang ming organ	constipation, abdominal pain worse for pressure, tidal fever, thick dry yellow or brown tongue coat, deep strong pulse	DA CHENG QI TANG
			Damp Heat in yang ming	urgent foul diarrhoea, afternoon fever unrelieved by sweating, restlessness & irritability, red tongue with a yellow coat & rapid slippery pulse	GE GEN HUANG QIN HUANG LIAN TANG
		Heat lingering in the chest and diaphragm		mild lingering fever, irritability, insomnia, thirst & dryness following a febrile disease	ZHI ZI DOU CHI TANG

Appendix 1.1 – Summary of Warm Disease (*wen bing*) analysis

Table A1.1b Overview of Wen Bing patterns

Level	Depth	Pathology	Features	Guiding Formula
Ying	Deepest (and most dangerous) levels	Heat entering the Pericardium	high fever, insomnia, irritability & restlessness, delerium, faint erythema & purpura, deep red dry tongue, thready rapid pulse	QING YING TANG
		Heat obstructing the Pericardium	Same as the previous pattern with serious disturbance of consciousness and possibly loss of consciousness	QING YING TANG plus AN GONG NIU HUANG WAN
Blood		Heat causing Blood to move recklessly	Similar to the Heat in the ying level, with the addition of obvious rashes, bleeding and possibly convulsions	XI JIAO DI HUANG TANG
		Hot Blood & Blood stasis	acute lower abdominal pain worse for pressure, fever, constipation with tarry stools, deep red or purple tongue	TAO HE CHENG QI TANG

Appendix 1.2
FEBRILE DISEASES CAUSED BY COLD
(*Shang Han* 伤寒)

The *Shang Han Lun* (Treatise on Febrile Diseases caused by Cold), written by one of the great geniuses of Chinese medicine, Zhang Zhong-jing of the Han dynasty (220BC-200AD), was a remarkable achievement and remains a milestone of clinical medicine. It discusses numerous disease states and 108 prescriptions, most of which are still in use today. Henan Province, where Zhang Zhong-jing lived was a very cold area. Diseases there were mainly caused by cold which turned to fever. Legend has it that of the 200 odd members of Zhang's clan, 75% died from an epidemic disease, probably typhoid, which inspired him to study medicine.

The *Shang Han Lun* is an analysis of how Cold penetrates into the body and the disorders that result. It postulates that there are six levels that pathogenic influences can enter depending on the relative strength or weakness of the pathogen and the *zheng qi*. The six levels, in order of increasing depth, are:

- the *tai yang*–associated with Urinary Bladder and Small Intestine channels and organs
- the *shao yang*–associated with Gall Bladder and *san jiao* channels
- the *yang ming*–associated with Stomach and Large Intestine channels and organs
- the *tai yin*–associated with Lung and Spleen organs
- the *shao yin*–associated with Heart and Kidney organs
- the *jue yin*–associated with Liver and Pericardium organs

Manner of entry
Wind Cold first encounters the body at the *tai yang* level. If it is not expelled by the *zheng qi* or therapeutic intervention, it may then penetrate further into the body. Once Wind Cold has passed the first most superficial level, there are several ways that pathogenic Cold can enter the body and progress:

Sequential penetration
- Where a Wind Cold attack is not cleared at the *tai yang* level it may then progress through all six levels in order of depth - *tai yang* > *shao yang* > *yang ming* > *tai yin* > *shao yin* > *jue yin*.

Non sequential penetration
- Penetration from one level to another in a non-sequential fashion, and in a way not related to the connections between the various channels.

Internal external penetration
- If a patient has a pre-existing weakness in an organ system, a pathogen can pass from the external member of the *yin yang* pair to the internal partner. For example, if there is pre-existing Kidney weakness, then Wind Cold can penetrate straight from *tai yang* to *shao yin* as a result of the *yin yang* relationship between the Urinary Bladder and Kidney. For example, in a patient with Kidney *yang* deficiency who gets a Wind Cold attack, the Kidney deficiency symptoms may suddenly get worse rather than the typical Wind Cold symptoms appearing.

Direct penetration
- This occurs when there is deficiency in the more superficial levels. The pathogen goes straight into the *yin* levels, bypassing the *yang* levels altogether.

Overlapping
- Overlapping patterns occur when two (or more) levels (often *tai yang* and *yang ming* or *shao yang*) are involved at the same time.

The diagnostic system laid out in the *Shang Han Lun* is still widely used and remarkably relevant even after two millenia. Some adjustments were needed in the 16th and 17th centuries, probably in response to new forms of disease (the *wen bing*), but the efficacy of the prescriptions and the accuracy of Zhang's observation are astounding. The *Shang Han* model is particularly useful in the increasingly common post infection syndromes.

The summary described here is necessarily brief, and readers are encouraged to study the *Shang Han Lun* itself for more detail. Some good translations are available (see bibliography).

YANG LEVELS
1. *TAI YANG* SYNDROMES
1.1 *Tai yang* channel syndrome
Pathophysiology
- Wind Cold penetrates the *tai yang* channels (Urinary Bladder and Small Intestine) particularly where they traverse the neck and upper back. The symptoms and treatment principle are the same as for Wind Cold (p.6) but the prescription given here is the original one prescribed by Zhang Zhongjing in the *Shang Han Lun*.

Clinical features
- acute simultaneous fever and chills, with the chills more prominent than the fever
- no sweating; the absence of sweating is a key feature here, indicating an excess condition of the surface (i.e. the Cold has contracted and 'locked' the pores behind it)
- occipital headache
- muscle aches, neck stiffness
- nasal obstruction, or runny nose with thin watery mucus
- sneezing
- cough or wheezing with thin watery mucus

T normal or with a thin white coat
P floating, or floating and tight

Treatment principle
Disperse Wind Cold
Redirect Lung *qi* downward

Prescription

MA HUANG TANG 麻黄汤
(*Ma Huang Combination*)

ma huang* (Herba Ephedra) 麻黄	9g
xing ren* (Semen Pruni Armeniacae) 杏仁	9g
gui zhi (Ramulus Cinnamomi Cassiae) 桂枝	6g
gan cao (Radix Glycyrrhizae Uralensis) 甘草	3g

Method: Decoction.

Variations and additional prescriptions
External deficiency pattern
- If there is mild sweating, floating pulse, mild fever and chills, mild nasal congestion, indicating a weak exterior, the correct treatment is to expel

Wind Cold and regulate *ying wei* with **GUI ZHI TANG** (*Cinnamon Combination* 桂枝汤).

    gui zhi (Ramulus Cinnamomi Cassiae) 桂枝 9g
    bai shao (Radix Paeoniae Lactiflora) 白芍 9g
    zhi gan cao (honey fried Radix Glycyrrhizae Uralensis)
    炙甘草 6g
    sheng jiang (Rhizoma Zingiberis Officinalis Recens) 生姜 9g
    da zao (Fructus Ziziphi Jujubae) 大枣 4pce
    Method: Decoction.

Patent medicines
Gan Mao Ling 感冒灵 (Gan Mao Ling)
Xiao Qing Long Wan 小青龙丸 (Xiao Qing Long Wan)
Chuan Xiong Cha Tiao Wan 川芎茶调丸 (Chuan Xiong Cha Tiao Wan)
    - with prominent headache

Acupuncture
GB.20 (*feng chi* -), Bl.12 (*feng men* -Ω), Bl.13 (*fei shu* -Ω), Lu.7 (*lie que* -), LI.4 (*he gu* -)
- with wheezing, add *ding chuan* (M-BW-1)
- if the nose is congested or runny, add Du.23 (*shang xing*)
- the patient should have a mild sweat after a few minutes, although it may only be noticeable on the palms

Clinical notes
- Biomedical conditions that may present as *tai yang* channel syndrome include the common cold and acute asthma.

1.2 *Tai yang* organ (Urinary Bladder) syndrome
Pathophysiology
- Wind Cold may penetrate into the Urinary Bladder itself in some cases via the *tai yang* channel–this is *tai yang fu* syndrome. The presence of Cold disrupts the 'transformation of *qi* in the Urinary Bladder', that is, it disrupts fluid metabolism.

Clinical features
- the symptoms are those of the *tai yang* channel syndrome with additional symptoms of urinary difficulty:
    - urinary retention
    - dribbling urine or broken urinary stream
    - scanty urine, oedema
    - nausea with epigastric splash on palpation

- strong thirst with vomiting immediately after drinking

Treatment principle
Expel Cold from both *tai yang* channel and organ

Prescription

WU LING SAN 五苓散
(*Hoelen Five Formula*)

> **ze xie** (Rhizoma Alismatis Orientalis) 泽泻 15g
> **fu ling** (Sclerotium Poriae Cocos) 茯苓 12g
> **zhu ling** (Sclerotium Polypori Umbellati) 猪苓 12g
> **bai zhu** (Rhizoma Atractylodes Macrocephalae) 白术 12g
> **gui zhi** (Ramulus Cinnamomi Cassiae) 桂枝 6g
> Method: Decoction.

Acupuncture
BL.64 (*jing gu*), KI.3 (*tai xi*), SJ.3 (*zhong zhu*), BL.39 (*wei yang*), St.28 (*shui dao*), Bl.28 (*pang guang shu*), Ren.9 (*shui fen* ▲)

Clinical notes
- Biomedical conditions that may present as *tai yang* organ syndrome includeacute nephritis and gastroenteritis.

1.3 Wind Cold with retention of Phlegm Dampness
Pathophysiology
- This variation is the product of pre-existing Phlegm Damp in the Lungs which is stirred up by a Wind Cold pathogen. It occurs in patients with chronic fluid metabolism problems as a result of prior Lung and Spleen weakness. The main difference between this condition and an uncomplicated Wind Cold invasion is the quantity of mucus.

Clinical features
- simultaneous fever and chills, with chills predominant
- copious clear, watery mucus from the nose and lungs
- dyspnoea or orthopnoea in severe cases
- rattling cough
- fullness in the chest
- sneezing
- no sweating
- stiff neck and muscle aches
- occipital headache

T normal, or with a moist or greasy white coat

P floating and tight, or slightly slippery

Treatment principle
Expel Wind Cold and dry Dampness

Prescription

XIAO QING LONG TANG 小青龙汤
(*Minor Blue Dragon Combination*)

ma huang* (Herba Ephedra) 麻黄	9g
gui zhi (Ramulus Cinnamomi Cassiae) 桂枝	9g
gan jiang (Rhizoma Zingiberis Officinalis) 干姜	3g
xi xin* (Herba cum Radice Asari) 细辛	3g
wu wei zi (Fructus Schizandrae Chinensis) 五味子	9g
bai shao (Radix Paeoniae Lactiflora) 白芍	9g
ban xia* (Rhizoma Pinelliae Ternatae) 半夏	9g
zhi gan cao (honey fried Radix Glycyrrhizae Uralensis) 炙甘草	9g

Method: Decoction.

Patent medicines
Xiao Qing Long Wan 小青龙丸 (Xiao Qing Long Wan)

Acupuncture
Bl.12 (*feng men* - Ω), Bl.13 (*fei shu* - Ω), SP.3 (*tai bai* -), ST.40 (*feng long* -), SJ.5 (*wai guan*)

Clinical notes
- Biomedical conditions that may present as a Wind Cold with Phlegm Damp pattern include acute bronchitis, acute exacerbation of chronic bronchitis, common cold, influenza, asthma and hayfever.

1.4 Wind Cold with pre-existing internal Heat
Pathophysiology
- If there is pre-existing internal Heat, invasion by Wind Cold will result in a severe influenza like attack. The internal Heat is usually generated by a diet rich in heating foods, alcohol and coffee, or by smoking. It may also result from stress and emotional turmoil leading to chronic *qi* stagnation with stagnant Heat.
- In some cases the internal Heat can be the product of the intense struggle between the pathogen and the body's *wei qi*, especially when both are strong.

Clinical features
- high fever with severe chills or rigors
- loud cough with sticky yellow mucus
- no sweating
- severe occipital headache
- generalised muscle aches
- strong thirst with desire for cold drinks
- sore throat
- irritability and restlessness
- dry stools or constipation

T red or with a red tip and edges, and a thin white or yellow coat
P floating and tight and possibly rapid

Treatment principle
Expel Wind Cold
Clear internal Heat

Prescription

DA QING LONG TANG 大青龙汤
(Major Blue Dragon Combination)

shi gao (Gypsum) 石膏	15g
ma huang* (Herba Ephedra) 麻黄	9g
xing ren* (Semen Pruni Armeniacae) 杏仁	9g
sheng jiang (Rhizoma Zingiberis Officinalis Recens) 生姜	9g
gui zhi (Ramulus Cinnamomi Cassiae) 桂枝	6g
zhi gan cao (honey fried Radix Glycyrrhizae Uralensis) 炙甘草	6g
da zao (Fructus Zizyphi Jujubae) 大枣	3pce

Method: Decoction.

Patent medicines
Ma Xing Zhi Ke Pian 麻杏止咳片 (Ma Hsing Chih Ke Pian)
Zhi Sou Ding Chuan Wan 止嗽定喘丸 (Zhi Sou Ding Chuan Wan)

Acupuncture
Du.14 (*da zhui* - Ω), Bl.12 (*feng men* - Ω), LI.11 (*qu chi* -), Lu.10 (*yu ji* -) LI.4 (*he gu* -), Lu.5 (*chi ze* -), SJ.5 (*wai guan* -), SJ.2 (*ye men* -)
- If the throat is very sore and swollen add Lu.11 (*shao shang* ↓) and SI.17 (*tian rong* -).

Clinical notes
- Biomedical conditions that may present as Wind Cold with internal Heat patterns include influenza, upper respiratory tract infection, acute bronchitis, pneumonia and whooping cough.

2. *SHAO YANG* SYNDROME

Pathophysiology
- The *shao yang* level is neither internal nor external, but represents a transitional zone between the surface and the interior of the body. Pathogens can hide here and get locked away, sometimes for prolonged periods. The principle of treatment described by the *Shang Han Lun* is to harmonise the *shao yang*. In this context harmonisation means closing the space available to the pathogen. It also refers to the fact that because the disorder is no longer external and not yet internal diaphoresis and purging are inappropriate.

Clinical features
- alternating fever and chills
- nausea
- poor appetite
- hypochondriac pain, distension or tenderness
- fullness in the chest
- dizziness
- irritability
- bitter taste in the mouth

T often unremarkable, or coated only on the left side, or slightly red on the edges

P wiry

Treatment principle
Harmonise *shao yang*

Prescription

XIAO CHAI HU TANG 小柴胡汤
(*Minor Bupleurum Combination*)

chai hu (Radix Bupleuri) 柴胡	12g
huang qin (Radix Scutellariae Baicalensis) 黄芩	9g
ban xia* (Rhizoma Pinelliae Ternatae) 半夏	12g
sheng jiang (Rhizoma Zingiberis Officinalis Recens) 生姜	9g
ren shen (Radix Ginseng) 人参	9g
zhi gan cao (honey fried Radix Glycyrrhizae Uralensis) 炙甘草	6g
da zao (Fructus Zizyphi Jujubae) 大枣	4pce

Method: Decoction.

Patent medicines
Xiao Chai Hu Wan 小柴胡丸 (Xiao Chai Hu Wan)

Acupuncture
SJ.5 (*wai guan*), GB.39 (*xuan zhong*), GB.41 (*zu lin qi*), Bl.19 (*dan shu*)

Clinical notes
- Biomedical conditions that may present as *shao yang* syndrome include the post acute stage of upper respiratory tract infections, influenza, post viral syndrome, mastitis, malaria, chronic hepatitis, post partum fever and cholecystitis.
- *Shao yang* syndrome is a common presentation of post viral fatigue.

3. YANG MING SYNDROME
阳明证
- This syndrome is characterised by being fully internal, affecting the Stomach and Intestines. The symptoms and treatments are identical to those described in 'Heat in *yang ming*' syndrome of the *wen bing* analysis (see Appendix 1.1, p.32).

YIN LEVELS

At this stage the fight between the pathogen and the body's *zheng qi* has consumed considerable amounts of the body's resources. Typically the pathogen has 'burnt itself out' in the struggle, so these *yin* levels represent mostly deficient syndromes.

4. *TAI YIN* SYNDROME

Pathophysiology
- In *tai yin* syndrome, *qi* has been depleted and the *qi* producing organs are weakened. In Zhang's day, excessive purgation in the treatment of an exterior syndrome (which weakens the Spleen) was thought responsible for *tai yin* syndrome. This is still relevant today, as occasionally patients (particularly those with a hygienist tendency) attempt to treat colds and flu by purging or enemas.

Clinical features
- abdominal distension, especially after meals
- abdominal pain or discomfort which is relieved by warmth and pressure
- poor appetite
- vomiting of thin fluids
- diarrhoea or loose stools with undigested food
- no thirst
- fatigue and lethargy
- oedema (especially eyes and fingers)
- pale or sallow complexion
- a yellowish discolouration on the inner corner of eyelids
- cold extremities and abdomen
- weakness or heaviness in the limbs

T pale, wet and swollen
P deep and slow

Treatment principle
Warm and tonify Spleen *qi* and *yang*

Prescription

FU ZI LI ZHONG WAN 附子理中丸
(*Aconite, Ginseng and Ginger Formula*)

zhi fu zi* (Radix Aconiti Carmichaeli Praeparata) 制附子 90g
gan jiang (Rhizoma Zingiberis Officinalis) 干姜 90g
ren shen (Radix Ginseng) 人参 90g
bai zhu (Rhizoma Atractylodes Macrocephalae) 白术 90g

zhi gan cao (honey fried Radix Glycyrrhizae Uralensis)
炙甘草 90g
Method: Grind the herbs to a powder and form into 3-gram pills with honey. Take one pill 2-3 times daily. May also be decocted with a 90% reduction in dosage, in which case **zhi fu zi** is decocted for 30 minutes before the other herbs (*xian jian* 先煎).

Patent medicines
Fu Zi Li Zhong Wan 附子理中丸 (Li Chung Yuen Medical Pills)
Li Zhong Wan 理中丸 (Li Zhong Wan)

Acupuncture
Bl.20 (*pi shu* +▲), Ren.12 (*zhong wan* +▲), St.36 (*zu san li* +▲), Du.4 (*ming men* +▲), Ren.6 (*qi hai* +▲), Ren.4 (*guan yuan* +▲), Lu.9 (*tai yuan* +), Sp.6 (*san yin jiao* +)

Clinical notes
- Biomedical conditions that may present as *tai yin* syndrome include chronic gastritis, irritable bowel syndrome, chronic colitis, digestive weakness, leaky gut syndrome, chronic candidiasis, coeliac disease and food intolerances.
- This pattern generally responds well to correct and prolonged treatment.

5. *SHAO YIN* SYNDROMES

- This level involves the Heart and Kidneys. If there is pre-existing Heart or Kidney weakness, then external pathogens may penetrate to the *shao yin* level. If Wind Cold attacks the *tai yang* channels and there is pre-existing Kidney weakness, the main manifestation may simply be a worsening of the Kidney deficiency symptoms. The pattern can go towards either *yin* or *yang* deficiency, depending on the patient's constitution.
- The *yin* deficient pattern usually occurs in those of hot (or *yang*) constitution; the *yang* deficient pattern in those of a cold (or *yin*) constitution. Historically, excess diaphoresis in the treatment of *tai yang* syndrome was thought to lead to the *yin* deficient pattern, due to damage to fluids and *yin*.

5.1 Heart and Kidney *yin* deficiency
Clinical features
- low grade fever that rises in the afternoon or evening
- sensation of heat in the palms and soles ('five hearts hot')
- insomnia, excessive dreaming or nightmares
- lower back pain or weakness
- restlessness and agitation or panic attacks
- poor concentration and memory
- dry throat, mouth and skin
- scanty dark urine or mild dysuria
- tendency to constipation
- tinnitus
- palpitations
- night sweats
- facial flushing, malar flush
- mouth and tongue ulcers

T red with little or no coat
P thready and rapid

Treatment principle
Nourish Heart and Kidney *yin*
Calm the *shen*

Prescription

TIAN WANG BU XIN DAN 天王补心丹
(*Ginseng and Zizyphus Formula*)

sheng di (Radix Rehmanniae Glutinosae) 生地	120g
tian dong (Tuber Asparagi Cochinchinensis) 天冬	30g
mai dong (Tuber Ophiopogonis Japonici) 麦冬	30g

dang gui (Radix Angelicae Sinensis) 当归 30g
wu wei zi (Fructus Schizandrae Chinensis) 五味子 30g
bai zi ren (Semen Biotae Orientalis) 柏子仁 30g
suan zao ren (Semen Zizyphi Spinosae) 酸枣仁 30g
ren shen (Radix Ginseng) 人参 15g
xuan shen (Radix Scrophulariae Ningpoensis) 玄参 15g
dan shen (Radix Salviae Miltiorrhizae) 丹参 15g
fu ling (Sclerotium Poriae Cocos) 茯苓 15g
yuan zhi (Radix Polygalae Tenuifoliae) 远志 15g
jie geng (Radix Platycodi Grandiflori) 桔梗 15g
zhu sha* (Cinnabaris) 朱砂 5g

Method: Grind the herbs (except **zhu sha**) to a powder and form into 9-gram pills with honey. Coat the pills with the **zhu sha**. The dose is one pill 2-3 times daily.

Patent medicines
Tian Wang Bu Xin Dan 天王补心丹 (Tien Wang Pu Hsin Tan)
Bu Nao Wan 补脑丸 (Cerebral Tonic Pills)
Jian Nao Wan 健脑丸 (Healthy Brain Pills)

Acupuncture
Bl.15 (*xin shu* +), Bl.23 (*shen shu* +), Ht.7 (*shen men* +), PC.6 (*nei guan*), PC.7 (*da ling*), Sp.6 (*san yin jiao* +), Kid.3 (*tai xi* +)
- with palpitations add Ht.5 (*tong li*)
- with night sweats add Ht.6 (*yin xi*)
- with insomnia add *an mian* (N-HN-54)

Clinical notes
- Biomedical conditions that may present as Heart and Kidney *yin* deficiency include menopausal syndrome, chronic apthous ulcers, neuresthenia, sleep disorders and anxiety neurosis.
- This pattern generally responds well to correct treatment.

5.2 Heart and Kidney *yang* deficiency
Clinical features
- cold extremities, aversion to cold
- generalised oedema, with aching and heaviness in the extremities
- copious clear urination, nocturia or oliguria
- fatigue and constant sleepiness; sleeping with knees drawn up to the chest
- cough with thin watery mucus
- palpitations
- dizziness
- abdominal pain which is relieved by warmth and pressure

- lower back ache

T pale, swollen and wet, with a greasy white coat
P slow, deep and weak

Treatment principle

Warm and strengthen Heart and Kidney *yang*

Prescription

ZHEN WU TANG 真武汤
(*True Warrior Decoction*)

This formula is particulary good for the oedema and fluid metabolism disorders associated with this pattern.

zhi fu zi* (Radix Aconiti Carmichaeli Praeparata) 制附子 9g
bai zhu (Rhizoma Atractylodes Macrocephalae) 白术 6g
fu ling (Sclerotium Poriae Cocos) 茯苓 9g
sheng jiang (Rhizoma Zingiberis Officinalis Recens) 生姜 9g
bai shao (Radix Paeoniae Lactiflora) 白芍 9g

Method: Decoction. **Zhi fu zi** is cooked for 30 minutes before adding the other herbs (*xian jian* 先煎).

JIN KUI SHEN QI WAN 金匮肾气丸
(*Rehmannia Eight Formula*)

This is the representitive Kidney *yang* strengthening formula, and is excellent as a general *yang* tonic. It is is more tonifying to the Kidney than the previous formula, and is prefered for excessive urination and nocturia.

shu di (Radix Rehmanniae Glutinosae Conquitae) 熟地 240g
shan yao (Radix Dioscoreae Oppositae) 山药 120g
shan zhu yu (Fructus Corni Officinalis) 山茱萸 120g
fu ling (Sclerotium Poria Cocos) 茯苓 90g
ze xie (Rhizoma Alismatis Orientalis) 泽泻 90g
mu dan pi (Cortex Moutan Radicis) 牡丹皮 90g
zhi fu zi* (Radix Aconiti Carmichaeli Praeparata) 制附子 60g
rou gui (Cortex Cinnamomi Cassiae) 肉桂 40g

Method: Grind the herbs to powder and form into 9-gram pills with honey. The dose is 2-3 pills daily. May also be decocted with a 90% reduction in dosage. When decocted **zhi fu zi** is cooked for 30 minutes before adding the other herbs (*xian jian* 先煎). (Source: *Shi Yong Zhong Yi Nei Ke Xue*)

Variations and additional prescriptions

Collapse of yang
- If this condition progresses to the point where *yang* is on the point of collapse, with icy cold extremities, dulled sensorium, watery diarrhoea,

shortness of breath and imperceptible pulse, then the correct treatment is to rescue devastated *yang*, warm the middle *jiao* and stop diarrhoea with **SI NI TANG** (*Frigid Extremities Decoction* 四逆汤).

zhi fu zi* (Radix Aconiti Carmichaeli Praeparata) 制附子 6-9g
gan jiang (Rhizoma Zingiberis Officinalis) 干姜 6g
zhi gan cao (honey fried Radix Glycyrrhizae Uralensis)
炙甘草 6g

Method: Decoction. **Zhi fu zi** is cooked for 30 minutes before the other herbs (*xian jian* 先煎).

Patent medicines
Jin Kui Shen Qi Wan 金匮肾气丸 (Sexoton Pills)

Acupuncture
Bl.20 (*pi shu* +▲), Bl.23 (*shen shu* +▲), Ren.9 (*shui fen* ▲), Ren.6 (*qi hai* +▲), Kid.7 (*fu liu* -), Kid.3 (*tai xi* +), Sp.9 (*yin ling quan* -), Sp.6 (*san yin jiao* -), St.36 (*zu san li* +▲)

Clinical notes
- Biomedical conditions that may present as Heart and Kidney *yang* deficiency include congestive cardiac failure, chronic nephritis, chronic enteritis, hypothyroidism, primary hyperaldosteronism, chronic bronchitis, vomiting and diarrhoea due to acute or chronic gastroenteritis.
- Heart and Kidney *yang* deficiency symptoms generally respond well to correct treatment.

6. *JUE YIN* SYNDROMES

Pathophysiology
- A miscellaneous syndrome that includes signs of Heat and Cold and is often associated with internal parasites, historically roundworms. The classical presentation is the pattern that appears in the *Shang Han Lun*. It represents a complex and unusual pattern involving a mixture of Heat, Cold and *qi* deficiency.
- The second pattern, *jue yin* channel syndrome, is a common presentation of migraine type headaches.

6.1 Classical presentation
Clinical features
- intermittent abdominal pain
- intense thirst
- painful heat or burning sensation in chest
- a sensation of *qi* rising up and striking the heart
- hunger with no desire to eat
- icy cold extremities
- diarrhoea and vomiting (occasionally vomiting of roundworms)

T light yellow coat
P wiry and rapid

Treatment principle
Warm the organs and expel roundworms

Prescription

WU MEI WAN 乌梅丸
(*Mume Pill*)

This interesting formula, with its mix of very hot and very cold herbs, treats a variety or complex patterns characterised by Heat, Cold and *qi* deficiency. It may be used for chronic gastrointestinal conditions with apparent contradictory presentations, for example chronic dysentery with abdominal pain that is relieved by warmth in a patient with a red tongue.

wu mei (Fructus Pruni Mume) 乌梅	480 (24)g
huang lian (Rhizoma Coptidis) 黄连	480 (9)g
huang bai (Cortex Phellodendri) 黄柏	180 (9)g
gan jiang (Rhizoma Zingiberis Officinalis) 干姜	300 (9)g
dang gui (Radix Angelicae Sinensis) 当归	120 (9)g
ren shen (Radix Ginseng) 人参	180 (9)g
zhi fu zi* (Radix Aconiti Carmichaeli Praeparata) 制附子	180 (6)g
gui zhi (Ramulus Cinnamomi Cassiae) 桂枝	180 (6)g

chuan jiao (Pericarpium Zanthoxyli Bungeani) 川椒 .... 120 (3)g
xi xin* (Herba cum Radice Asari) 细辛 .... 180 (3)g
Method: Grind the herbs to a fine powder and form into 9-gram pills with honey. The dose is one pill 2-3 times daily. May also be decocted with the doses in brackets, in which case **zhi fu zi** is cooked for 30 minutes before adding the other herbs (*xian jian* 先煎).

Modifications
- With little evidence of Heat, delete or decrease the dose of **zhi fu zi** and **gui zhi**.
- With severe abdominal pain, add **chuan lian zi*** (Fructus Meliae Toosendan) 川楝子 9g and **mu xiang** (Radix Aucklandiae Lappae) 木香 9g.
- With constipation, add **bing lang** (Semen Arecae Catechu) 槟榔 9g and **zhi shi** (Fructus Immaturus Citri Aurantii) 枳实 6g.

Clinical notes
- Biomedical conditions that may present as *jue yin* syndrome include ascariasis and other parasitic gut infections, chronic gastroenteritis, chronic colitis and chronic dysentery.

6.2 *Jue yin* channel syndrome
This pattern reflects rebellious *qi* in the Liver and Stomach channels.

Clinical features
- headache, especially at the crown of the head, or migraine
- nausea, vomiting, dry retching
- cold extremities, cold intolerance (especially during episodes)

T greasy white coat
P thready, wiry and slow

Treatment principle
Warm the Liver and Stomach
Redirect *qi* downwards, stop vomiting

Prescription
WU ZHU YU TANG 吴茱萸汤
(*Evodia Combination*)

wu zhu yu (Fructus Evodiae Rutaecarpae) 吴茱萸 6g
dang shen (Radix Codonopsis Pilosulae) 党参 15g
sheng jiang (Rhizoma Zingiberis Officinalis Recens) 生姜 .. 10pce
da zao (Fructus Zizyphi Jujubae) 大枣 6pce
Method: Decoction.

Acupuncture
Liv.3 (*tai chong* -▲), PC.6 (*nei guan*), Du.20 (*bai hui* ▲),
St.36 (*zu san li* +▲), Ren.12 (*zhong wan* ▲)

Clinical notes
- Biomedical conditions that may present as *jue yin* channel syndrome includemigraine headaches, chronic gastritis, hypertension, trigeminal neuralgia and acute gastroenteritis.
- The *jue yin* channel pattern generally responds well to correct treatment.

Appendix 1.2 – Summary of *Shang Han Lun* analysis

Table A1.2a Overview of Shang Han Lun *patterns, yang levels*

Level	Depth	Pathology	Features	Guiding Formula
Tai yang (Urinary Bladder & Small Intestine)	external	Tai yang channel syndrome	chills, fever, no sweating, occipital headache, stiff neck, myalgia, runny nose with thin watery mucus, cough, floating tight pulse	MA HUANG TANG
		Tai yang organ syndrome	Same as above with urinary dysfunction; retention of urine, oedema, oliguria, nausea with epigastric splash	WU LING SAN
		Wind Cold with Phlegm Damp	Same as tai yang channel syndrome with dyspnoea, cough & copious thin watery mucus	XIAO QING LONG TANG
		Wind Cold with internal Heat	high fever with severe chills or rigors, cough with yellow sputum, no sweating, myalgia, sore throat, constipation, irritability, floating, tight & rapid pulse	DA QING LONG TANG
Shao yang (Gall Bladder & san jiao)	between the exterior & the interior	alternating fever & chills, nausea, anorexia, fatigue, bitter taste, hypochondriac pain, fullness in the chest, dizziness, irritability, wiry pulse		XIAO CHAI HU TANG
Yang ming (Stomach & Intestines)	internal	Heat in the yang ming channel	high fever, sweating, thirst, irritability, dry yellow tongue coat, flooding, rapid pulse	BAI HU TANG
		Heat in yang ming organ	constipation, abdominal pain worse for pressure, tidal fever, thick dry yellow or brown tongue coat, deep strong pulse	DA CHENG QI TANG

Table A1.2b Overview of Shang Han Lun *patterns,* yin *levels*

Level	Depth	Pathology	Features	Guiding Formula
Tai yin (Spleen & Lung)	internal		abdominal distension, abdominal pain better for warmth, anorexia, loose stools or diarrhoea, fatigue, oedema, pale complexion, cold extremities, weak limbs, pale swollen tongue, deep slow pulse	FU ZI LI ZHONG WAN
Shao yin (Heart & Kidney)		'Hot transformation' · Heart & Kidney yin deficiency	low grade afternoon fever, five hearts hot, insomnia, much dreaming, poor memory, dry mouth, palpitations, night sweats, anxiety, facial flushing, mouth ulcers, red dry tongue, thready, rapid pulse	TIAN WANG BU XIN DAN
		'Cold transformation' · Heart & Kidney yang deficiency	cold intolerance, cold extremities, generalised oedema, copious urination, nocturia, fatigue, sleepiness, palpitations, low back ache, pale swollen tongue, deep weak pulse	ZHEN WU TANG
Jue yin (Liver)		Jue yin syndrome	intense thirst, heat in the chest, qi rising up to strike the heart, hunger with no desire to eat, icy extremities, diarrhoea & vomiting, wiry, rapid pulse	WU MEI WAN
		Jue yin channel syndrome	headache, nausea, vomiting, dry retching, cold extremities, wiry thready pulse	WU ZHU YU TANG

Disorders of the Lung

2. Cough

Acute patterns
Wind Cold
Wind Heat
Warm Dryness
Cool Dryness
Lung Heat (Fire)

Chronic patterns
Lung *qi* deficiency
Lung *yin* deficiency
Spleen and Kidney *yang* deficiency
Phlegm Damp
Blood stagnation

Acute or Chronic patterns
Phlegm Heat
Liver Fire

Appendix – *fei yong* (Lung Abscess)

2 COUGH
ke sou 咳嗽

Coughing, in the language of TCM, is simply a failure of the natural descent of Lung *qi*, or a rebellion of Lung *qi* upwards. There are two general mechanisms: Lung *qi* which is too weak to descend, and simply 'floats' upward; or blockage of Lung *qi's* downward movement by a pathogen.

The first mechanism is one of deficiency, associated with weakness of Lung *qi* or *yin*. One aspect of healthy Lung function is the descent of Lung *qi* (and Fluids) to the Kidneys for reprocessing. When Lung *qi* is too weak to descend properly, it simply 'floats' upwards. *Yin* deficiency can cause cough by drying Lung Fluids and generating deficient Heat which rises, taking Lung *qi* with it.

The second mechanism is one of excess, and the result of obstruction to Lung *qi* by external pathogens like Wind, Cold or Heat, or by internally generated pathogens like Phlegm, Dampness, Heat, pathological fluids or stagnant *qi*. Excess cough may be acute or chronic. When associated with external pathogens the cough is usually acute, whereas Phlegm Damp coughs are often chronic. Excess type cough often has some deficiency at its root. For example the cough due to Spleen and Kidney *yang* deficiency occurs because of a failure of fluid metabolism–pathological fluids accumulate in the Lungs and obstruct Lung *qi*–a mixed excess and deficient pattern.

AETIOLOGY
External pathogens
Any of the external pathogens, but particularly Wind Cold, Heat and Dryness, can give rise to cough due to the relatively superficial and therefore vulnerable position of the Lungs. The Lungs are considered to be the 'delicate' organ, easily affected by environmental conditions. Entry to the Lungs may be through the nose and mouth, or through the skin (the Lungs and skin are closely related).

Lung deficiency
This refers to Lung *qi* or *yin* deficiency. The Lungs need a moist environment to function properly and are easily damaged by heat and dryness. Lung *qi* may be compromised by poor posture, shallow breathing and lack of exercise, or conversely by repeated or extreme physical overexertion. Prolonged or unexpressed grief or sadness can weaken Lung *qi*. If Spleen *qi* is deficient then Lung *qi* will not be supported via the generating (*sheng* 生) cycle.

Lung *yin* can be damaged by dry hot environments, inhalation of heating substances like tobacco, inhaled steroids and bronchodilators, and as a secondary result of Kidney *yin* deficiency.

Spleen *qi* deficiency and Phlegm

Overwork, excessive worry or mental activity, irregular dietary habits, excessive consumption of cold, raw, sweet or greasy foods or prolonged illness can weaken Spleen *qi*. Weakness of the Spleen can lead to the generation of Dampness which over time may congeal into Phlegm. Once Phlegm is present, it can accumulate in the Lungs. TCM classics describe the Spleen as "the creator of Phlegm, the Lungs are the storehouse of Phlegm". Similarly, a primary Spleen weakness can lead to Lung weakness (due to the five phase generating [*sheng* 生] cycle relationship). If the Lungs are chronically weak they may fail to send the appropriate fluid portion to the Kidneys. These congested fluids may become Phlegm over time.

> **BOX 2.1 SOME BIOMEDICAL CAUSES OF COUGH**
>
> **Respiratory**
> - upper respiratory tract infections
> - postnasal drip
> - acute and chronic bronchitis
> - pleurisy
> - bronchiectasis
> - severe infections (including whooping cough, pneumonia, pulmonary tuberculosislung abscess, HIV infection)
> - atelectasis
> - respiratory tumours
> - asthma[1]
> - pneumothorax
> - foreign body
> - cystic fibrosis
> - sarcoidosis
>
> **Cardiac**
> - congestive cardiac failure
> - mitral valve disease
>
> **Drugs**
> - ACE inhibitors
>
> **Other**
> - smoking
> - psychogenic

Liver invading the Lungs

The Liver and the Lungs have a close relationship. According to the controlling (*ke* 克) cycle of five phase theory (Fig 2.1), the Lungs restrain the Liver and prevent it from getting too 'strong'. When the Lungs are weak or the Liver too 'strong' (that is Liver *qi* is stagnant or there is some other excess pattern involving the Liver), then the controlling cycle breaks down and the pent up Liver energy rebels backwards - a reverse controlling cycle. The distinguishing feature of a Liver invading Lung cough is its relationship to stress or emotional disturbance.

Prolonged Liver *qi* stagnation can also contribute to the generation of Phlegm. This it does firstly by invading and weakening the Spleen which

---

1. Chronic coughs, particularly in children, are often diagnosed as asthma, and the treatment commonly applied (in children and adults) is inhaled steroids and bronchodilators. For a discussion of this topic see pp.157.

then produces Dampness and Phlegm, and secondly by retarding movement and distribution of fluids which over time congeal into Phlegm.

Kidney deficiency

Kidney function can influence respiration in several ways. The Kidney plays a role in respiration–it aids in the 'grasping' of *qi*. As Lung *qi* descends with a breath, the Kidney is said to anchor it. If the Kidney is weak this anchoring function is poor and the inspired *qi* floats upwards. Lung and Kidney *yin* have a close relationship. If Kidney *yin* is weak, or there is deficient Heat generated by *yin* deficiency, this can affect Lung *yin*–the Heat can dry up Lung *yin*, or the *yin* simply fails to be supported by the weakened Kidney.

Kidney (and Spleen) *yang* deficiency can give rise to cough by failing to move and process fluids - these fluids accumulate in the Lung and block the descent of Lung *qi*. Although this type of cough is based on a profound deficiency, the manifestation (i.e. the cough) is excess, and in some cases can be severe and even life threatening.

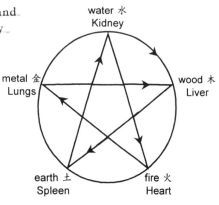

Fig 2.1. The star represents the controlling cycle (ke 克), the circle the generative cycle (sheng 生)

DIAGNOSIS

Those coughs characterised by the presence of a pathogen are excess by definition, those characterised by an absence of some physiological substance (usually *qi* or *yin*) are deficient. Excess coughs tend to be acute, and are generally loud and paroxysmal. Deficient coughs tend to be chronic and weak, and worse with exertion, at night or when fatigued.

The first step in diagnosis is to determine whether the cough is acute or chronic. Acute cough is of no more than a couple of weeks duration, and is usually due to external pathogens, although it may also be of internal origin, for example Liver invading the Lungs. Acute cough is always excess. Chronic cough is either deficient or excess, or more commonly, a mixture of both, and is defined by its recurrent and prolonged nature. In general a cough that persists longer than a few weeks is considered chronic.

TREATMENT

Most types of cough respond quite well to TCM treatment, especially those acute coughs due to invading exterior pathogens. Chronic and deficient types also generally respond well, however the possibility of a more sinister cause, like carcinoma should be kept in mind in those patients with persistent and unresponsive cough. A common type of cough, and one that needs no specific therapy other than avoidance of tobacco, is the smoker's cough. In the absence of any major damage to the Lung *yin*, simply stopping smoking will resolve the problem.

Acupuncture is the treatment of choice in the initial stages of an exterior attack - it is simple, quick and quite reliable, and the patient often leaves the clinic cured or feeling much better. For the chronic deficiencies (especially *yin* deficiency), herbs are generally better, although a combination of herbs and acupuncture may offer the best possible approach.

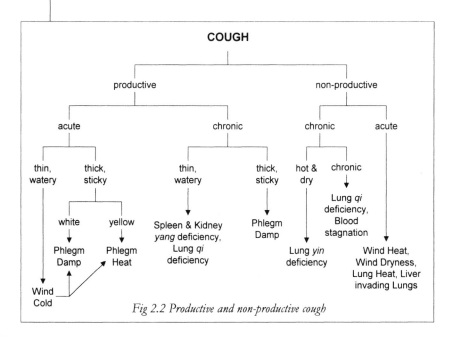

Fig 2.2 Productive and non-productive cough

BOX 2.2 KEY DIAGNOSTIC POINTS

Acute and chronic
- Acute cough is excess
- Chronic cough is deficient or excess or mixed

Aggravation
- worse with exertion or when tired - deficiency
- worse in the afternoon or evening - *yin* deficiency
- worse in the morning - Phlegm
- worse with emotional upset - rebellious Liver *qi* invading the Lungs

Mucus
- copious indicates the presence of Phlegm
    - and yellow or green - Phlegm Heat
    - and white - Phlegm Damp
    - thin and watery - Cold fluids
- no mucus - Heat, Dryness or *yin* deficiency
- blood streaked - Lung Heat, Fire or *yin* deficiency

Sound
- loud, hacking and barking - excess
- weak (and usually dry) - deficiency
- loose and rattling - Phlegm

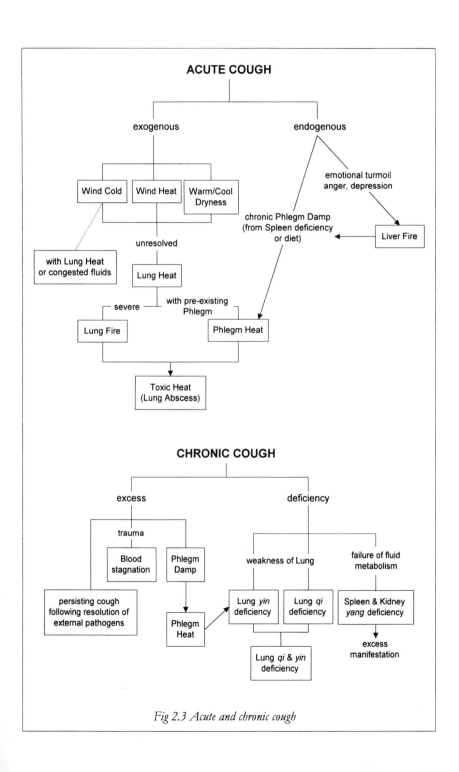

Fig 2.3 *Acute and chronic cough*

2.1 WIND COLD

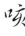

Pathophysiology
- Wind Cold enters through the pores, *tai yang* channels and Lungs, and obstructs the descent of Lung *qi*. Lung *qi* then accumulates and ascends causing cough. Because the nature of Cold is to 'freeze and constrict', it will shut the pores behind it, trapping the pathogen in the superficial layers of the body.

Clinical features
- Acute cough, which is frequent and loud with a moderate amount of thin clear or white mucus. Initially the cough may be non productive.
- simultaneous fever and chills, chills more prominent than the fever
- no sweating
- occipital or frontal headache
- muscle aches, neck stiffness
- nasal obstruction, or runny nose with thin watery mucus
- dyspnoea and wheezing
- sneezing

T normal or with a thin white coat
P floating, or floating and tight

Treatment principle
Expel Wind and Cold
Redirect Lung *qi* downward, stop cough

Prescription

HUA GAI SAN 华盖散
(*Canopy Powder*)

ma huang* (Herba Ephedra) 麻黄	9g
sang bai pi (Cortex Mori Albae Radicis) 桑白皮	9g
su zi (Fructus Perillae Fructescentis) 苏子	9g
xing ren* (Semen Pruni Armeniacae) 杏仁	9g
chi fu ling (Sclerotium Poriae Cocos Rubrae) 赤茯苓	9g
chen pi (Pericarpium Citri Reticulatae) 陈皮	9g
gan cao (Radix Glycyrrhizae Uralensis) 甘草	6g

Method: Decoction. (Source: *Formulas and Strategies*)

Modifications
- If Wind Cold exterior signs are severe (muscle aches, chills greater than fever) add **fang feng** (Radix Ledebouriellae Divaricatae) 防风 9g and **qiang huo** (Rhizoma et Radix Notopterygii) 羌活 9g.

- If the cough is severe and distressing, add **zi wan** (Radix Asteris Tatarici) 紫菀 9g and **kuan dong hua** (Flos Tussilagi Farfarae) 款冬花 9g.
- With frontal headache or severe nasal congestion add **bai zhi** (Radix Angelicae) 白芷 9g.
- If the cough is productive, with thick white mucus, fullness in the chest and epigastrium, a greasy white tongue coat and a soggy pulse add **cang zhu** (Rhizoma Atractylodis) 苍术 9g and **hou po** (Cortex Magnoliae Officinalis) 厚朴 9g.

Variations and additional prescriptions

With pre-existing thin Fluids in the Lungs
- When there are pre-existing thin fluids in the Lungs (usually due to underlying Spleen and Lung deficiency), they can be stirred up by a Wind Cold invasion. In addition to the Wind Cold pattern there is expectoration of copious thin watery mucus, copious thin watery nasal discharge and excessive lacrimation. The correct treatment is to disperse Wind Cold from the exterior, and warm and transform fluids with **XIAO QING LONG TANG** (*Minor Blue Dragon Combination* 小青龙汤)

ma huang* (Herba Ephedra) 麻黄	9g
bai shao (Radix Paeoniae Lactiflora) 白芍	9g
ban xia* (Rhizoma Pinelliae Ternatae) 半夏	9g
gui zhi (Ramulus Cinnamomi Cassiae) 桂枝	6g
gan jiang (Rhizoma Zingiberis Officinalis) 干姜	3g
xi xin* (Herba cum Radice Asari) 细辛	3g
wu wei zi (Fructus Schizandrae Chinensis) 五味子	3g
zhi gan cao (honey fried Radix Glycyrrhizae Uralensis) 炙甘草	3g

  Method: Decoction to be taken hot. (Source: *Shi Yong Zhong Yao Xue*)

With Heat in the Lungs
- If there is Heat in the Lungs combined with external Wind Cold (known as 'Cold wrapping up Fire'), there will be symptoms of loud cough with sticky yellow mucus, laboured breathing, fever and chills, no sweating, myalgia, nasal congestion or clear nasal discharge. The correct treatment is to dispel Wind Cold, clear Lung Heat and redirect *qi* downwards with **MA XING SHI GAN TANG** (*Ma Huang, Apricot Seed, Gypsum and Licorice Combination* 麻杏石甘汤 modified, see Lung Heat p.84).

With qi deficiency
- An alternative to the primary prescription, particularly useful in weak or rundown patients who contract a Wind Cold, and in those who are

unable to throw a cold off, is **SHEN SU YIN** (*Ginseng and Perilla Combination* 参苏饮 modified, p.21). Also useful for Wind Cold coughs in children.

Patent medicines
Gan Mao Ling 感冒灵 (Gan Mao Ling)
Gan Mao Qing Re Chong Ji 感冒清热冲剂 (Colds and Flu Tea)
Gan Mao Zhi Ke Chong Ji 感冒止咳冲剂 (Gan Mao Zhi Ke Chong Ji)
Chuan Xiong Cha Tiao Wan 川芎茶调丸 (Chuan Xiong Cha Tiao Wan)
 - with prominent headache

Acupuncture
LI.4 (*he gu* -), Lu.7 (*lie que* -), GB.20 (*feng chi* -), Bl.12 (*feng men* - Ω), Bl.13 (*fei shu* -Ω), Lu.5 (*chi ze* -), Ren.17 (*shan zhong* -), Ren.22 (*tian tu* -)
 • with wheezing add *ding chuan* (M-BW-1)
 • if the nose is congested or runny add Du.23 (*shang xing*)

Clinical notes
 • The cough in this pattern may be associated with biomedical conditions such as common cold, upper respiratory tract infection, influenza, acute asthma, croup or pharyngitis.
 • This pattern responds well to correct and timely treatment.

2.2 WIND HEAT

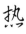

Pathophysiology
- This pattern is due to Wind Heat which invades the Lungs through the nose and mouth, or Wind Cold which transforms into Heat, blocking the descent of Lung *qi*.

Clinical features
- acute hacking, dry cough, or cough with sticky, yellow, difficult to expectorate mucus
- mild fever with little or no chills
- nasal obstruction, or a nasal discharge which is thick and yellow or green
- sore, dry or scratchy throat
- thirst
- mild sweating
- headache (usually frontal)

T normal or red tipped with a thin white or yellow coat
P floating and rapid

Treatment principle
Expel Wind and clear Heat
Redirect Lung *qi* downward, stop cough
Transform Phlegm

Prescription

SANG JU YIN 桑菊饮
(*Morus and Chrysanthemum Formula*) modified

sang ye (Folium Mori Albae) 桑叶	10g
ju hua (Flos Chrysanthemi Morifolii) 菊花	10g
lu gen (Rhizoma Phragmitis Communis) 芦根	30g
lian qiao (Fructus Forsythia Suspensae) 连翘	15g
chao xing ren* (dry fried Semen Pruni Armeniacae) 炒杏仁	10g
jie geng (Radix Platycodi Grandiflori) 桔梗	10g
qian hu (Radix Peucedani) 前胡	10g
niu bang zi (Fructus Arctii Lappae) 牛蒡子	10g
bo he (Herba Mentha Haplocalycis) 薄荷	6g
gan cao (Radix Glycyrrhizae Uralensis) 甘草	6g

Method: Decoction. Do not cook for more than 20 minutes. **Bo he** is added near the end of cooking (*hou xia* 后下). (Source: *Zhong Yi Nei Ke Lin Chuang Shou Ce*)

Modifications

- If the cough is severe, add **yu xing cao** (Herba Houttuyniae) 鱼腥草 15g and **zhi pi pa ye** (honey fried Folium Eriobotryae) 炙枇杷叶 9g.
- If the Heat is relatively severe, with high fever and strong thirst, add **huang qin** (Radix Scutellariae Baicalensis) 黄芩 9g, **zhi mu** (Rhizoma Anemarrhenae Asphodeloides) 知母 9g and **gua lou** (Fructus Trichosanthis) 瓜楼 12g to powerfully clear Lung Heat. See also Lung Heat, p.84 and *fei yong* (Lung Abscess), p.109.
- With sore throat add **she gan** (Rhizoma Belamacandae) 射干 9g. See also Sore Throat, p.285.
- If there is epistaxis or mild haemoptysis or blood streaked mucus, add **bai mao gen** (Rhizoma Imperatae Cylindricae) 白茅根 18g and **ou jie** (Nodus Nelumbinis Nuciferae) 藕节 9g.
- Nausea, vomiting, fullness in the epigastrium, loose stools or explosive diarrhoea with tenesmus indicate that Summer Heat is also involved – add **huo xiang** (Herba Agastaches seu Pogostei) 藿香 12g, **pei lan** (Herba Eupatorii Fortunei) 佩兰 9g and **xiang ru** (Herba Elsholtziae Splendentis) 香薷 9g.

Variations and additional prescriptions

Post Wind attack residual cough

- If Wind Cold and Wind Heat are indistinguishable, or if the cough lingers on after the exterior symptoms (either Hot or Cold) have been resolved, or if it relapses with itchy throat, hard to expectorate mucus and no exterior symptoms, use **ZHI SOU SAN** (*Stop Coughing Powder* 止嗽散).

jie geng (Radix Platycodi Grandiflori) 桔梗	9g
zi wan (Radix Asteris Tatarici) 紫菀	9g
bai bu* (Radix Stemonae) 百部	9g
bai qian (Radix et Rhizoma Cynanchi Baiqian) 白前	9g
jing jie (Herba seu Flos Schizonepetae Tenuifolia) 荆芥	6g
chen pi (Pericarpium Citri Reticulatae) 陈皮	6g
gan cao (Radix Glycyrrhizae Uralensis) 甘草	3g

  Method: Decoction. (Source: *Shi Yong Zhong Yao Xue*)

Post Wind attack residual cough with shaoyang *symptoms*

- Sometimes following resolution of acute symptoms a paroxysmal or dry cough develops. The cough is worse at night. This is the commonly encountered post infectious cough (less commonly whooping cough). It is often accompanied by loss of appetite, fatigue, dizziness and occasional mild alternating fever and chills. The treatment is to expel residual pathogens (from *shao yang*) and stop the cough with **XIAO CHAI HU TANG** (*Minor Bupleurum Combination* 小柴胡汤) modified.

chai hu (Radix Bupleuri) 柴胡 12g
ban xia* (Rhizoma Pinelliae Ternatae) 半夏 12g
qing hao (Herba Artemesiae Apiaceae) 青蒿 12g
huang qin (Radix Scutellariae Baicalensis) 黄芩 9g
sheng jiang (Rhizoma Zingiberis Officinalis Recens) 生姜 9g
ren shen (Radix Ginseng) 人参 9g
zi wan (Radix Asteris Tatarici) 紫菀 9g
bai bu* (Radix Stemonae) 百部 9g
bai qian (Radix et Rhizoma Cynanchi Baiqian) 白前 9g
zhi gan cao (honey fried Radix Glycyrrhizae Uralensis)
炙甘草 6g
da zao (Fructus Zizyphi Jujubae) 大枣 4pce
Method: Decoction.

Patent medicines
Yin Qiao Jie Du Pian 银翘解毒片 (Yin Chiao Chieh Tu Pien)
Gan Mao Ling 感冒灵 (Gan Mao Ling)
Ban Lan Gen Chong Ji 板蓝根冲剂 (Ban Lan Gen Chong Ji)
Chuan Bei Pi Pa Gao 川贝枇杷膏 (Nin Jiom Pei Pa Kao)
  - an excellent syrup for dry, irritating cough
African Sea Coconut Cough Syrup
Xiao Chai Hu Wan 小柴胡丸 (Xiao Chai Hu Wan)

Acupuncture
Du.14 (*da zhui* - Ω), Bl.12 (*feng men* - Ω), Bl.13 (*fei shu* - Ω),
LI.11 (*qu chi* -), LI.4 (*he gu* -), Lu.5 (*chi ze* -), SJ.5 (*wai guan* -)
  • If the throat is very sore and swollen, add Lu.11 (*shao shang* ↓) and SI.17 (*tian rong* -)

Clinical notes
  • The cough in this pattern may be associated with biomedical conditions such as common cold, tonsillitis, upper respiratory tract infection, tracheitis, laryngitis, whooping cough, croup, acute bronchitis or the early stage of measles.
  • This pattern responds well to correct and timely treatment. In cases of severe croup, however, medical attention or hospitalisation may be required.
  • Post acute or residual coughs may require longer treatment due to the deeper level of damage to *yin* and fluids that may ensue.

2.3 WIND AND DRYNESS

- Warm Dryness
- Cool Dryness

Pathophysiology
- Dryness patterns are due to pathogenic Wind and Dryness (with either Heat or Cold depending on the season) invading the Lungs. It usually occurs during dry seasons or periods of dry weather, which damage Lung fluids and obstruct the descent of Lung *qi*. Today, due to air conditioned and climate controlled buildings, this syndrome can occur at any time of the year.

2.3.1 Warm Dryness
Clinical features
- Dry hacking non-productive cough. The cough may cause chest pain. If there is any mucus present, it is usually scant, sticky, thick and hard to expectorate, and possibly blood streaked.
- dry throat, mouth, nose and lips
- headache
- mild fever or chills

T normal or with a red tip and a thin yellow dry coat
P thready and rapid

Treatment principle
Clear Heat from the Lungs, moisten Dryness
Redirect Lung *qi* downward, stop cough

Prescription

SANG XING TANG 桑杏汤
(*Morus and Apricot Seed Combination*) modified

sang ye (Folium Mori Albae) 桑叶	12g
chao xing ren* (dry fried Semen Pruni Armeniacae) 炒杏仁	12g
nan sha shen (Radix Adenophorae seu Glehniae) 南沙参	24g
lu gen (Rhizoma Phragmitis Communis) 芦根	18g
zhi pi pa ye (honey fried Folium Eriobotryae) 炙枇杷叶	15g
mai dong (Tuber Ophiopogonis Japonici) 麦冬	12g
quan gua lou (Fructus Trichosanthis) 全栝楼	12g
chuan bei mu (Bulbus Fritillariae Cirrhosae) 川贝母	12g
shan zhi zi (Fructus Gardeniae Jasminoidis) 山栀子	10g
dan dou chi (Semen Sojae Preparatum) 淡豆豉	10g
li pi (Fructus Pyri) 梨皮	6g

Method: Decoction. (Source: *Zhong Yi Nei Ke Lin Chuang Shou Ce*)

Modifications
- With severe Heat, add **zhi mu** (Rhizoma Anemarrhenae Asphodeloides) 知母 12g and **shi gao** (Gypsum) 石膏 18g.
- With severe headache and fever, add **bo he** (Herba Mentha Haplocalycis) 薄荷 6g, **lian qiao** (Fructus Forsythia Suspensae) 连翘 12g and **chan tui**^ (Periostracum Cicadae) 蝉蜕 9g.
- With a sore throat, add one or two of the following herbs: **xuan shen** (Radix Scrophulariae) 玄参 15g, **ma bo** (Fructificatio Lasiosphaerae seu Calvatiae) 马勃 3g or **she gan** (Rhizoma Belamcandae) 射干 9g.
- With epistaxis or blood streaked mucus, add **bai mao gen** (Rhizoma Imperatae Cylindricae) 白茅根 15g and **sheng di tan** (charred Radix Rehmanniae Glutinosae) 生地炭 15g.

Variations and additional prescriptions
- If Warm Dryness persists, or the Dryness is severe enough to damage Lung *yin*, this can give rise to a frequent hacking non-productive cough, fullness and pain in the chest and behind the sternum, headache, haemoptysis, parched throat, wheezing and a dry tongue without coat. The correct treatment is to moisten Dryness, clear Heat and nourish Lung *yin* with **QING ZAO JIU FEI TANG** (*Eriobotrya and Ophiopogon Combination* 清燥救肺汤).

    shi gao (Gypsum) 石膏 18-30g
    sang ye (Folium Mori Albae) 桑叶 9g
    xing ren* (Semen Pruni Armeniacae) 杏仁 9g
    mai dong (Tuber Ophiopogonis Japonici) 麦冬 9g
    hei zhi ma (Semen Sesami Indici) 黑芝麻 9g
    zhi pi pa ye (honey fried Folium Eriobotryae) 炙枇杷叶 9g
    nan sha shen (Radix Adenophorae seu Glehniae) 南沙参 9g
    e jiao^ (Gelatinum Corii Asini) 阿胶 6g
    gan cao (Radix Glycyrrhizae Uralensis) 甘草 3g
    Method: Decoction. **E jiao** is melted before being added to the strained decoction (*yang hua* 烊化).

Patent medicines
Yin Qiao Jie Du Pian 银翘解毒片 (Yin Chiao Chieh Tu Pien)
Gan Mao Ling 感冒灵 (Gan Mao Ling)
Sang Ju Yin Pian 桑菊饮片 (Sang Chu Yin Pian)
Zhi Sou Wan 止嗽丸 (Zhi Sou Wan)
Chuan Bei Pi Pa Gao 川贝枇杷膏 (Nin Jiom Pei Pa Kao)

凉燥

2.3.2 Cool Dryness

Clinical features
- cough with little or no mucus
- ticklish or itchy dry throat
- dry nose and lips
- mild headache
- chills, mild fever
- no sweating

T thin white dry coat
P floating and tight

Treatment principle
Clear the Lungs, moisten Dryness
Redirect Lung *qi* downward, stop cough

Prescription

XING SU SAN 杏苏散
(*Apricot Kernel and Perilla Leaf Powder*)

    chao xing ren* (dry fried Semen Pruni Armeniacae)
    炒杏仁 9g
    zi su ye (Fructus Perillae Frutescentis) 紫苏叶 6g
    fu ling (Sclerotium Poriae Cocos) 茯苓 6g
    qian hu (Radix Peucedani) 前胡 6g
    jie geng (Radix Platycodi Grandiflori) 桔梗 6g
    zhi ke (Fructus Citri Aurantii) 枳壳 6g
    chen pi (Pericarpium Citri Reticulatae) 陈皮 6g
    ban xia* (Rhizoma Pinelliae Ternatae) 半夏 6g
    sheng jiang (Rhizoma Zingiberis Officinalis Recens)
    生姜 3pce
    da zao (Fructus Zizyphi Jujubae) 大枣 2pce
    gan cao (Radix Glycyrrhizae Uralensis) 甘草 3g
    Method: Decoction. (Source: *Shi Yong Fang Ji Xue*)

Patent medicines
Gan Mao Ling 感冒灵 (Gan Mao Ling)
Zhi Sou Wan 止嗽丸 (Zhi Sou Wan)
Chuan Bei Pi Pa Gao 川贝枇杷膏 (Nin Jiom Pei Pa Kao)

Acupuncture (applicable to both Dryness patterns)
Bl.12 (*feng men* - Ω), Bl.13 (*fei shu* - Ω), Lu.5 (*chi ze* -), Lu.7 (*lie que* -),
Lu.9 (*tai yuan* +), Kid.7 (*fu liu* +), Kid.6 (*zhao hai* +)

- Acupuncture is excellent for expelling Wind and stopping cough, but is of limited value in moistening dryness.

Clinical notes (applicable to both patterns)
- The cough in these patterns may be associated with biomedical conditions such as common cold, upper respiratory tract infection, tonsillitis or bronchitis.
- This pattern responds well to correct treatment, however, herbs are better suited for moistening dryness than acupuncture. If the disorder is recurrent, the patient's environment (air conditioning, climate controled buildings etc.) may need to be assessed and modified if possible. Sipping pear juice is useful.

2.4 LUNG HEAT

Pathophysiology
* Lung Heat results from the penetration of a pathogen into the Lungs, usually Wind Heat, although Wind Cold may generate Heat once in the Lungs. By this stage, however, the Heat is internal and there are generally no exterior symptoms remaining.

Clinical features
* dry, hacking, painful cough with little or no mucus; if there is a small amount of mucus, it is sticky and hard to expectorate and may be blood streaked
* fever with or without sweating
* chest tightness and pain
* sensation of heat in the chest
* red complexion and nose
* dry mouth and thirst
* shortness of breath, laboured breathing or wheezing

T red or with a red tip and a yellow coat
P flooding and rapid, or wiry and rapid

Treatment principle
Clear Heat from the Lungs
Redirect Lung *qi* downwards, stop cough

Prescription

MA XING SHI GAN TANG 麻杏石甘汤
(*Ma Huang, Apricot Seed, Gypsum and Licorice Combination*) modified

zhi ma huang* (honey fried Herba Ephedra) 炙麻黄	9g
xing ren* (Semen Pruni Armeniacae) 杏仁	12g
shi gao (Gypsum) 石膏	30g
zhi gan cao (honey fried Radix Glycyrrhizae Uralensis) 炙甘草	6g
yu xing cao (Herba Houttuyniae) 鱼腥草	18g
huang qin (Radix Scutellariae Baicalensis) 黄芩	12g
jin yin hua (Flos Lonicera Japonicae) 金银花	12g
zhi sang bai pi (honey fried Cortex Mori Albae Radicis) 炙桑白皮	12g
zhi mu (Rhizoma Anemarrhenae Asphodeloides) 知母	9g

Method: Decoction.

Modifications

- If there are any signs of Wind Cold remaining, use unprocessed **ma huang** (Herba Ephedra) 麻黄.
- With chest pain, add **tao ren** (Semen Persicae) 桃仁 9g and **yu jin** (Tuber Curcumae) 郁金 9g.
- If the cough is severe, add **ma dou ling*** (Fructus Aristolchiae) 马兜铃 9g and **zhi pi pa ye** (honey fried Folium Eriobotryae) 炙枇杷叶 9g.
- With mild haemoptysis or blood streaked mucus, add **qian cao tan** (charred Radix Rubiae Cordifoliae) 茜草炭 12g, **bai mao gen** (Rhizoma Imperatae Cylindricae) 白茅根 9g and **ce bai ye tan** (charred Cacumen Biotae Orientalis) 侧柏叶炭 12g. See also Haemoptysis, p.193.
- With severe thirst, add **tian hua fen** (Radix Trichosanthis Kirilowii) 天花粉 9g.
- With sore throat, add 2 or 3 of the following herbs: **she gan** (Rhizoma Belamacandae) 射干 9g, **xuan shen** (Radix Scrophulariae) 玄参 15g, **jie geng** (Radix Platycodi Grandiflori) 桔梗 9g or **ma bo** (Fructificatio Lasiosphaerae seu Calvatiae) 马勃 3g. See also Sore Throat, p.289.
- With copious yellow mucus and dyspnoea with or without constipation, see Phlegm Heat, p.90.

Variations and additional prescriptions

Severe Heat ('Lung Fire')

- If the Heat is more severe and systemic (termed 'Lung Fire') with a loud, barking, painful cough, fever, concentrated urine, constipation, dry mouth and tongue with mouth ulcers, severe thirst, malaise and restlessness, the correct treatment is drain Fire downwards and unblock the bowels with **LIANG GE SAN** (*Cool the Diaphram Powder* 凉隔散).

    da huang (Radix et Rhizoma Rhei) 大黄 10g
    mang xiao (Mirabilitum) 芒硝 10g
    gan cao (Radix Glycyrrhizae Uralensis) 甘草 10g
    lian qiao (Fructus Forsythia Suspensae) 连翘 20g
    dan zhu ye (Herba Lophatheri Gracilis) 淡竹叶 10g
    huang qin (Radix Scutellariae Baicalensis) 黄芩 12g
    shan zhi zi (Fructus Gardeniae Jasminoidis) 山栀子 12g
    bo he (Herba Mentha Haplocalycis) 薄荷 6g

    Method: Decoction. **Bo he** is added near the end of cooking (*hou xia* 后下), **mang xiao** is dissolved in the strained decoction (*chong fu* 冲服). (Source: *Shi Yong Zhong Yi Nei Ke Xue*)

Patent medicines

Qing Fei Yi Huo Pian 清肺抑火片 (Ching Fei Yi Huo Pien)
Chuan Xin Lian Kang Yan Pian 穿心莲抗炎片
    (Chuan Xin Lian Antiphlogistic Tablets)

Ma Xing Zhi Ke Pian 麻杏止咳片 (Ma Hsing Chih Ke Pian)
Zhi Sou Ding Chuan Wan 止嗽定喘丸 (Zhi Sou Ding Quan Wan)
Niu Huan Qing Huo Wan 牛黄清火丸 (Niu Huang Qing Huo Wan)
- Lung Fire

Acupuncture

Lu.5 (*chi ze* -), Lu.6 (*kong zui* -), Lu.10 (*yu ji* -), Bl.13 (*fei shu* -), Ren.17 (*shan zhong*), LI.4 (*he gu* -), Du.14 (*da zhui* -), Lu.1 (*zhong fu* -)
- In severe cases, add Du.12 (*shen zhu* -) and Du.10 (*ling tai* -)

Clinical notes

- The cough in this pattern may be associated with biomedical conditions such as upper respiratory tract infection, pneumonia, bronchitis or tracheitis.
- This pattern generally responds well to correct treatment.

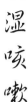

2.5 PHLEGM DAMP

Pathophysiology
- Phlegm Damp causes a chronic cough–the result of inappropriate diet or recurrent respiratory tract disease such as bronchitis, tonsillitis or sinusitis which has been treated with antibiotics (see p.131). It is especially common in children and those with a dairy rich diet. It is most often a mixed excess (Phlegm Damp) and deficiency (Spleen and Lung) condition. The correct treatment depends on ascertaining the mixture of deficiency and Phlegm. Because of its obstructing quality, Phlegm Damp may periodically become hot, causing acute Phlegm Heat cough or wheeze.

Clinical features
- chronic or recurrent cough with profuse thin or thick white or clear mucus; there is a noticeable rattle in the chest with coughing and it tends to be worse in the morning and after eating
- fullness and stuffiness in the chest and epigastrium
- poor appetite
- nausea or vomiting
- loose stools
- lethargy and weakness

T pale and swollen with toothmarks and a moist, greasy white coat
P soft and slippery

Treatment principle
Strengthen the Spleen, dry Damp
Transform Phlegm, stop cough

Prescription

ER CHEN TANG 二陈汤
(*Citrus and Pinellia Combination*) modified

ban xia* (Rhizoma Pinelliae Ternatae) 半夏	12g
fu ling (Sclerotium Poriae Cocos) 茯苓	15g
chao xing ren* (dry fried Semen Pruni Armeniacae) 炒杏仁	9g
chen pi (Pericarpium Citri Reticulatae) 陈皮	9g
zhe bei mu (Bulbus Fritillariae Thunbergii) 浙贝母	9g
cang zhu (Rhizoma Atractylodis) 苍术	9g
hou po (Cortex Magnoliae Officinalis) 厚朴	9g
zhi ke (Fructus Citri Aurantii) 枳壳	9g
jie geng (Radix Platycodi Grandiflori) 桔梗	9g
zi wan (Radix Asteris Tatarici) 紫菀	9g

kuan dong hua (Flos Tussilaginis Farfarae) 款冬花 9g
gan cao (Radix Glycyrrhizae Uralensis) 甘草 3g
Method: Decoction. (Source: *Shi Yong Zhong Yi Nei Ke Xue*)

Modifications

- With very copious mucus, loss of appetite, epigastric fullness and a thick tongue coat, add **bai jie zi** (Semen Sinapsis Albae) 白芥子 6g, **su zi** (Fructus Perillae Fructescentis) 苏子 6g and **lai fu zi** (Semen Raphani Sativi) 莱服子 6g.
- With Cold (aversion to cold, watery mucus, cold extremities, chilliness), add **xi xin*** (Herba cum Radice Asari) 细辛 3g and **gan jiang** (Rhizoma Zingiberis Officinalis) 干姜 6g.

Variations and additional prescriptions

Spleen and Lung qi *deficiency with Phlegm accumulation*

- If Spleen deficiency appears to be prominent the treatment should primarily strengthen the Spleen to resolve Phlegm. The guiding formula is **LIU JUN ZI TANG** (*Six Major Herbs Combination* 六君子汤).

    dang shen (Radix Codonopsis Pilosulae) 党参 12g
    fu ling (Sclerotium Poriae Cocos) 茯苓 12g
    chao bai zhu (dry fried Rhizoma Atractylodis Macrocephalae) 炒白术 9g
    ban xia* (Rhizoma Pinelliae Ternatae) 半夏 9g
    chen pi (Pericarpium Citri Reticulatae) 陈皮 6g
    gan cao (Radix Glycyrrhizae Uralensis) 甘草 6g
    sheng jiang (Rhizoma Zingiberis Officinalis Recens) 生姜 3pce
    da zao (Fructus Zizyphi Jujubae) 大枣 4pce
    Method: Decoction. (Source: *Shi Yong Zhong Yao Xue*)

Chronic and recurrent Cold Phlegm Damp in the Lungs

- In older patients and children with chronic wheezing (see appendix, p.157), Phlegm Damp, Cold and Kidney deficiency combine to produce a pattern that recurs every Winter. In this pattern, there are repeated attacks of productive cough with thin watery mucus, usually triggered by a Cold invasion during the Winter months. Wheezing, breathlessness and tightness in the chest are common, particularly at night and early in the morning. The mucus may also be scanty and tenacious. In severe cases there is orthopnoea. There may also be weakness and pain of the lower back and legs, fatigue and oedema of the extremities. The treatment is to redirect *qi* downward, stop cough and wheezing and warm and transform Cold Phlegm. The guiding prescription is **SU ZI JIANG QI TANG** (*Perilla Fruit Combination* 苏子降气汤).

su zi (Fructus Perillae Fructescentis) 苏子 9g
ban xia* (Rhizoma Pinelliae Ternatae) 半夏 9g
qian hu (Radix Peucedani) 前胡 9g
dang gui (Radix Angelicae Sinensis) 当归 6g
chen pi (Pericarpium Citri Reticulatae) 陈皮 6g
hou po (Cortex Magnoliae Officinalis) 厚朴 3g
zhi gan cao (honey fried Radix Glycyrrhizae Uralensis)
炙甘草 3g
rou gui (Cortex Cinnamomi Cassiae) 肉桂 3g
Method: Grind the herbs to a fine powder and take 6-grams as a draft, 2-3 times daily. May also be decocted, in which case powdered **rou gui** is added to the strained decoction (*chong fu* 冲服). (Source: *Shi Yong Zhong Yao Xue*)

Patent medicines
Su Zi Jiang Qi Wan 苏子降气丸 (Su Zi Jiang Qi Wan)
Er Chen Wan 二陈丸 (Er Chen Wan)
Tong Xuan Li Fei Pian 通宣理肺片 (Tung Hsuan Li Fei Pien)
Qi Guan Yan Ke Sou Tan Chuan Wan 气管炎咳嗽痰喘丸
  (Cough and Phlegm Pills)

Acupuncture
Bl.13 (*fei shu* ▲), Bl.43 (*gao huang shu* ▲), Bl.20 (*pi shu* ▲), Lu.5 (*chi ze* -), Lu.7 (*lie que* -), Lu.9 (*tai yuan* -), Liv.13 (*zhang men* +), Sp.3 (*tai bai* +), St.40 (*feng long* -), Sp.6 (*san yin jiao* +), St.36 (*zu san li* +)
- with wheezing add *ding chuan* (M-BW-1)
- with fullness in the chest add PC.5 (*jian shi*)

Clinical notes
- The cough in this pattern may be associated with biomedical conditions such as upper respiratory tract infection, chronic bronchitis, bronchiectasis, emphysema or asthma.
- This pattern generally responds well to correct treatment.
- Dietary modification, in particular reduction of dairy products, sugar, greasy foods and in some patients, wheat, is essential for good results. In elderly patients and children with recurrent Cold Phlegm, prolonged treatment is needed for satisfactory results.

LUNGS

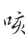

2.6 PHLEGM HEAT

Pathophysiology
- Phlegm Heat is related to Lung Heat and Phlegm Damp. Lung Heat can either dry or congeal Lung fluids. When congealed, fluids become Phlegm Heat. This usually follows a Wind Heat (or Cold) pathogenic invasion of the Lungs. See also *fei yong* (Lung Abscess), p.111.
- Phlegm Heat cough can also occur as an acute flareup in those with chronic Phlegm Damp in the Lungs, particularly where there is a pre-existing tendency to Heat as a result of overindulgence in heating substances like alcohol, spicy foods and tobacco.
- Phlegm Heat in the Lungs is mostly acute, however in some patients it can linger at a low level and become chronic, with consequent involvement of the Spleen. The key feature is the continued presence of yellow or green Phlegm. The accompanying symptoms are generally milder.

Clinical features
- hacking cough with profuse thick, yellow or green, hard to expectorate mucus; in some cases there may be blood streaked mucus
- fullness and stuffiness in the chest and epigastrium
- wheezing that tends to be worse at night and first thing in the morning
- poor appetite, nausea
- loose stools or constipation
- lethargy and weakness
- maybe a sore or congested throat
- bitter taste in the mouth

T thick, greasy, yellow coat, although maybe only on the root
P soft or slippery and rapid

Treatment principle
Expel Phlegm and clear Heat
Redirect Lung *qi* downward, stop cough

Prescription

QING JIN HUA TAN TANG 清金化痰汤
(*Clear Metal, Transform Phlegm Decoction*) modified

gua lou (Fructus Trichosanthis) 瓜楼	18g
sang bai pi (Cortex Mori Albae Radicis) 桑白皮	12g
zhe bei mu (Bulbus Fritillariae Thunbergii) 浙贝母	9g
zhi mu (Rhizoma Anemarrhenae Asphodeloides) 知母	9g
huang qin (Radix Scutellariae Baicalensis) 黄芩	9g
shan zhi zi (Fructus Gardeniae Jasminoidis) 山栀子	9g

chen pi (Pericarpium Citri Reticulatae) 陈皮 9g
jie geng (Radix Platycodi Grandiflori) 桔梗 9g
yu xing cao (Herba Houttuyniae) 鱼腥草 30g
gan cao (Radix Glycyrrhizae Uralensis) 甘草 6g
Method: Decoction. (Source: *Zhong Yi Nei Ke Lin Chuang Shou Ce*)

Modifications

- With streaks of blood in the mucus or haemoptysis, add **bai mao gen** (Rhizoma Imperatae Cylindricae) 白茅根 9g, **chao pu huang** (dry fried Pollen Typhae) 炒蒲黄 9g and **ou jie** (Nodus Nelumbinis Nuciferae) 藕节 9g. See also Haemoptysis, p.195.
- If there is vigorous Lung Heat with high fever, distressing cough, wheezing and severe thirst, delete **jie geng** and **chen pi** and add **jin yin hua** (Flos Lonicera Japonicae) 金银花 15g, **shi gao** (Gypsum) 石膏 20g and **ting li zi** (Semen Descurainiae seu Lepidii) 葶苈子 9g.
- With constipation, add **da huang** (Radix et Rhizoma Rhei) 大黄 6-9g.
- During the convalescent stage of this condition, the patient often has nightsweats, residual hard to expectorate mucus and fatigue due to the Heat damaging Lung *yin*. In this case, add **di gu pi** (Cortex Lycii Chinensis) 地骨皮 12g and **qing hao** (Herba Artemesiae Annuae) 青蒿 12g and more herbs to nourish Lung *yin*. See also *fei yong* (Lung Abscess), p.114.

Variations and additional prescriptions

- In cases where the mucus is yellow or green, purulent and foul smelling, **WEI JING TANG** (*Reed Decoction* 苇茎汤) modified, may be selected. Traditionally indicated for Lung abscess, it is appropriate for cases with significant Phlegm Heat and Toxic Heat (i.e. with pus in the mucus, like severe bronchitis or pneumonia). See also *fei yong* (Lung Abscess) p.111.

lu gen (Rhizoma Phragmitis Communis) 芦根 30g
yi ren (Semen Coicis Lachryma-jobi) 苡仁 30g
dong gua ren (Semen Benincasae Hispidae) 冬瓜仁 24g
tao ren (Semen Persicae) 桃仁 9g
yu xing cao (Herba Houttuyniae) 鱼腥草 30g
jin yin hua (Flos Lonicera Japonicae) 金银花 15g
huang qin (Radix Scutellariae Baicalensis) 黄芩 12g
jie geng (Radix Platycodi Grandiflori) 桔梗 9g
Method: Decoction.

Patent medicines

Qing Qi Hua Tan Wan 清气化痰丸 (Pinellia Expectorant Pills)
Qing Fei Yi Huo Pian 清肺抑火片 (Ching Fei Yi Huo Pien)
Chuan Ke Ling 喘咳灵 (Chuan Ke Ling)

She Dan Chuan Bei Ye 蛇胆川贝液 (She Dan Chuan Bei Ye)

Acupuncture
Lu.5 (*chi ze* -), St.40 (*feng long* -), Lu.1 (*zhong fu* -), Lu.6 (*kong zui* -), Lu.7 (*lie que* -), LI.11 (*qu chi* -), Bl.13 (*fei shu* -), Lu.10 (*yu ji* -), Ren.17 (*shan zhong*)
- with wheezing add *ding chuan* (M-BW-1)
- with fullness in the chest add PC.5 (*jian shi*)

Clinical notes
- The cough in this pattern may be associated with biomedical conditions such as acute and chronic bronchitis, bronchiectasis, pneumonia, whooping cough or lung abscess.
- Generally responds reasonably well to correct treatment, plus avoidance of heating foods and tobacco. In severe cases, and in the elderly, frail or debilitated, concurrent use of antibiotics may be necessary to quickly cool the Heat. Herbs and acupuncture support the swift action of the antibiotics, and finish the job by expelling the pathogen, clearing residual Phlegm, strengthening resistance and nourishing damaged *yin*.

肝火犯肺咳嗽

2.7 LIVER FIRE INVADING THE LUNGS

Pathophysiology
- Liver Fire invading the Lungs can be acute or chronic. Most commonly the episodes of coughing are acute and provoked by some intense emotional situation. The cough typically persists for several weeks then subsides, only to reoccur weeks or months later. Liver Fire invading the Lungs is an example of a reverse controlling (*ke* 克, p.70) cycle disorder. This usually occurs in someone with chronic Liver *qi* stagnation, so there is a large emotional component, and satisfactory long term treatment must deal with both the underlying Liver *qi* stagnation and acute manifestation of Fire. Once the acute episode is under control, the underlying *qi* stagnation needs to be dealt with so as to prevent recurrence.

Clinical features
- Paroxysmal, severe cough; the cough comes in bursts, and causes focal chest and hypochondriac pain. The cough is aggravated or provoked by stress, emotional turmoil and anger. There may be blood streaked mucus.
- During episodes of coughing, the patient may get hot, flushed and upset. The cough often drags on, or reoccurs fairly regularly and may become self perpetuating as anxiety and worry about the illness further complicates the existing emotional stress.
- red face and red sore eyes
- bitter taste in the mouth, thirst
- quick temper, irritability, restlessness, depression
- hypochondriac tension or discomfort
- dizziness, headaches
- on examination, acupuncture points like Liv.14 (*qi men*) and Liv.3 (*tai chong*) are very tender and reactive

T red and dry with a thick or thin yellow coat
P wiry or slippery and rapid

Treatment principle
Clear Liver Fire, moisten the Lungs and transform Phlegm

Prescription

> DAI GE SAN 黛蛤散
> (*Indigo and Conch Powder*) plus
> QING JIN HUA TAN TANG 清金化痰汤
> (*Clear Metal, Transform Phlegm Decoction*) modified

This formula is best for severe cases and for patients with concurrent Phlegm Heat.

dai ge san (see below) 黛蛤散 5g
shan zhi zi (Fructus Gardeniae Jasminoidis) 山栀子 10g
sang bai pi (Cortex Mori Albae Radicis) 桑白皮 12g
huang qin (Radix Scutellariae Baicalensis) 黄芩 10g
gua lou (Fructus Trichosanthis) 瓜楼 15g
zhe bei mu (Bulbus Fritillariae Thunbergii) 浙贝母 10g
zhi mu (Rhizoma Anemarrhenae Asphodeloides) 知母 10g
jie geng (Radix Platycodi Grandiflori) 桔梗 10g
di gu pi (Cortex Lycii Chinensis) 地骨皮 12g
mai dong (Tuber Ophiopogonis Japonici) 麦冬 15g
gan cao (Radix Glycyrrhizae Uralensis) 甘草 6g

Method: Decoction. **DAI GE SAN** is a prepared powder composed of **qing dai** (Pulverata Indigo) 青黛, **hai ge ke fen** (powdered Concha Cylinae Sinensis) 海蛤壳粉, and sometimes **pu huang** (Pollen Typae) 蒲黄. It is usually added to the strained decoction (*chong fu* 冲服). (Source: *Zhong Yi Nei Ke Lin Chuang Shou Ce*)

SANG DAN XIE BAI TANG 桑丹泻白汤
(*Mulberry Leaf and Moutan Decoction to Drain the White*)

This formula is not as cooling as the primary prescription and is more suitable for mild cases.

sang bai pi (Cortex Mori Albae Radicis) 桑白皮 12g
sang ye (Folium Mori Albae) 桑叶 9g
di gu pi (Cortex Lycii Chinensis) 地骨皮 15g
mu dan pi (Cortex Moutan Radicis) 牡丹皮 4.5g
zhu ru (Caulis Bambusae in Taeniis) 竹茹 6g
zhe bei mu (Bulbus Fritillariae Thunbergii) 浙贝母 9g
geng mi (Semen Oryzae) 粳米 9g
zhi gan cao (honey fried Radix Glycyrrhizae Uralensis) 炙甘草 1.8g
da zao (Fructus Zizyphi Jujubae) 大枣 2pce

Method: Decoction. (Source: *Formulas and Strategies*)

Modifications (apply to both prescriptions)

- If insomnia and restlessness are severe add **huang lian** (Rhizoma Coptidis) 黄连 6g and **dan zhu ye** (Herba Lophatheri Gracilis) 淡竹叶 10g.
- With blood streaked mucus, delete **jie geng** and **mai dong**, and add **mu dan pi** (Cortex Moutan Radicis) 牡丹皮 10g, **ou jie** (Nodus Nelumbinis Nuciferae) 藕节 10g, and **xian he cao** (Herba Agrimoniae Pilosae) 仙鹤草 30g.
- With constipation, add **da huang** (Radix et Rhizoma Rhei) 大黄 6-9g.
- With chest or flank pain, add **yu jin** (Tuber Curcumae) 郁金 9g and **chuan lian zi*** (Fructus Meliae Toosendan) 川楝子 9g.

♦ With severe Liver Heat, add **long dan cao** (Radix Gentianae Longdancao) 龙胆草 6-9g.

Follow up treatment
♦ For patients prone to this type of disorder, a *qi* regulating formula (in combination with relaxation and stress management) is indicated once the acute phase has settled. Appropriate *qi* moving formulae include **XIAO YAO SAN** (*Bupleurum and Dang Gui Formula* 逍遥散, p.139), **SI NI SAN** (*Frigid Extremities Powder* 四逆散, p.926), **YUE JU WAN** (*Escape Restraint Pill* 越鞠丸, p.567) and **CHAI HU SHU GAN SAN** (*Bupleurum and Cyperus Formula* 柴胡舒肝散, p.566).

Patent medicines
Qing Qi Hua Tan Wan 清气化痰丸 (Pinellia Expectorant Pills)
Long Dan Xie Gan Wan 龙胆泻肝丸 (Long Dan Xie Gan Wan)
Qing Fei Yi Huo Pian 清肺抑火片 (Ching Fei Yi Huo Pien)
Chuan Xin Lian Kang Yan Pian 穿心莲抗炎片
   (Chuan Xin Lian Antiphlogistic Tablets)

Acupuncture
Bl.13 (*fei shu* -), Lu.5 (*chi ze* -), Liv.2 (*xing jian* -), Liv.3 (*tai chong* -), GB.34 (*yang ling quan* -), Bl.18 (*gan shu* -), Liv.14 (*qi men* -), PC.6 (*nei guan*)
• with haemoptysis add Lu.6 (*kong zui* -)

Clinical notes
• The cough in this pattern may be associated with biomedical conditions such as pleurisy, upper respiratory tract infection, tonsillitis, bronchitis, pneumonia, tracheitis, whooping cough in adults, chronic chest infection or chronic bronchitis.
• The acute episode responds well to correct treatment, however the underlying *qi* stagnation often needs a comprehensive approach involving relaxation, stress management and removal (or amelioration of) the factors causing stress.
• In severe cases or in debilitated patients, concurrent use of antibiotics (especially if there is also Phlegm Heat) along with TCM treatment may be necessary to control the acute phase.

2.8 LUNG *YIN* DEFICIENCY

Pathophysiology
- When Lung *yin* is damaged by chronic or severe disease, febrile diseases, smoking, excessive use of bronchodilators, or prolonged exposure to hot or drying environments a chronic cough may develop. Lung *yin* deficiency can also follow Kidney *yin* deficiency.
- Lung *yin* deficiency can cause cough in two ways. Firstly as an expression of the weakness of the Lungs descending function, and secondly from the rising of any resultant *yin* deficient Heat.

Clinical features
- Chronic weak, dry cough, with little or no mucus. If mucus is present, it is hard to expectorate, sticky and may be blood streaked. There may be occasional haemoptysis in severe cases.
- dry mouth and throat
- low grade fever which rises in the afternoon or evening
- facial flushing or malar flushing
- night sweats
- a sensation of heat in the palms and soles ('five hearts hot')
- emaciation, fatigue

T red and dry, with little or no coat, or a peeled coat (mirror tongue)
P thready and rapid

Treatment principle
Nourish Lung *yin* to stop cough
Moisten the Lungs, transform Phlegm

Prescription

BAI HE GU JIN TANG 百合固金汤
(*Lily Combination*)

This formula is selected in milder cases, when Lung *yin* deficiency is primary.

bai he (Bulbus Lilii) 百合	24g
sheng di (Radix Rehmanniae Glutinosae) 生地	12g
shu di (Radix Rehmanniae Glutinosae Conquitae) 熟地	18g
mai dong (Tuber Ophiopogonis Japonici) 麦冬	15g
xuan shen (Radix Scrophulariae) 玄参	9g
chuan bei mu (Bulbus Fritillariae Cirrhosae) 川贝母	9g
jie geng (Radix Platycodi Grandiflori) 桔梗	9g
dang gui (Radix Angelicae Sinensis) 当归	9g
bai shao (Radix Paeoniae Lactiflora) 白芍	9g
gan cao (Radix Glycyrrhizae Uralensis) 甘草	3g

Method: Decoction. (Source: *Formulas and Strategies*)

YUE HUA WAN 月华丸
(*Moonlight Pill*) modified

This formula has a stronger tonifying action than the primary prescription and is used for more severe and chronic cases. It is commonly used for consumptive Lung disease.

sha shen (Radix Adenophorae seu Glehniae) 沙参	30g
mai dong (Tuber Ophiopogonis Japonici) 麦冬	30g
tian dong (Tuber Asparagi cochinchinensis) 天冬	30g
sheng di (Radix Rehmanniae Glutinosae) 生地	30g
shu di (Radix Rehmanniae Glutinosae Conquitae) 熟地	30g
bai bu* (Radix Stemonae) 百部	30g
shan yao (Radix Dioscoreae Oppositae) 山药	30g
e jiao^ (Gelatinum Corii Asini) 阿胶	30g
chuan bei mu (Bulbus Fritillariae Cirrhosae) 川贝母	30g
fu ling (Sclerotium Poriae Cocos) 茯苓	15g
san qi (Radix Notoginseng) 三七	15g
sang ye (Folium Mori Albae) 桑叶	60g
ju hua (Flos Chrysanthemi Morifolii) 菊花	60g

Method: Decoction or pills. When decocted the dose is reduced by 50-70%. To make pills, grind the herbs to a fine powder and form into 9-gram pills with honey. The dose is 3-5 pills daily. (Source: *Shi Yong Zhong Yi Nei Ke Xue*)

Modifications (where not already included)

- With haemoptysis, delete **jie geng** and add **ou jie** (Nodus Nelumbinis Nuciferae) 藕节 10g, **san qi fen** (powdered Radix Notoginseng) 三七粉 5g or **bai ji fen** (Rhizoma Bletillae Striatae) 白芨粉 5g, the last two to the strained decoction.
- With severe cough, add **bai bu*** (Radix Stemonae) 百部 9g, **zi wan** (Radix Asteris Tatarici) 紫菀 9g and **kuan dong hua** (Flos Tussilagi Farfarae) 款冬花 9g.
- If there is some sticky, deeply rooted mucus, add **hai ge ke fen**^ (powdered Concha Cyclinae Sinenesis) 海蛤壳粉 3g to the strained decoction.
- If there is prominent afternoon or tidal fever, add **yin chai hu** (Radix Stellariae Dichotomae) 银柴胡 10g, **di gu pi** (Cortex Lycii Chinensis) 地骨皮 15g and **huang qin** (Radix Scutellariae Baicalensis) 黄芩 9g.
- With copious mucus left over following an acute upper respiratory tract infection in a patient with pre-existing *yin* deficiency, the principle is to carefully clear the mucus first, before nourishing Lung *yin*.

Variations and additional prescriptions

Lung and Kidney yin *deficiency*
* With Lung and Kidney *yin* deficiency (signs of Lung *yin* deficiency with lower back, knee and heel pain, tinnitus, dizziness), the correct treatment is to nourish Lung and Kidney *yin* with **MAI WEI DI HUANG WAN** (*Ophiopogon, Schizandra and Rehmannia Formula* 麦味地黄丸, p.148) as guiding formula.

Heart yin *deficiency*
* With Heart *yin* deficiency (irritability, palpitations, insomnia and mouth ulcers), **XUAN MIAO SAN** (*Wonderful Scrophularia Powder* 玄妙散) may be used instead.

    xuan shen (Radix Scrophulariae) 玄参 9g
    dan shen (Radix Salviae Miltiorrhizae) 丹参 9g
    nan sha shen (Radix Adenophorae seu Glehniae) 南沙参 12g
    fu ling (Sclerotium Poriae Cocos Pararadicis) 茯神 12g
    bai zi ren (Semen Biotae Orientalis) 柏子仁 9g
    mai dong (Tuber Ophiopogonis Japonici) 麦冬 9g
    jie geng (Radix Platycodi Grandiflori) 桔梗 9g
    chuan bei mu (Bulbus Fritillariae Cirrhosae) 川贝母 9g
    xing ren* (Semen Pruni Armeniacae) 杏仁 9g
    he huan hua (Flos Albizziae Julibrissin) 合欢花 9g
    dan zhu ye (Herba Lophatheri Gracilis) 淡竹叶 3g
    deng xin cao (Medulla Junci Effusi) 灯心草 3g
    Method: Decoction. (Source: *Shi Yong Zhong Yi Nei Ke Xue*)

Lung yin *damage following a febrile illness*
* If the *yin* deficiency produces substantial Heat or follows a febrile disease which damages Lung *yin*, with a dry cough and wheeze, dry and parched throat and scanty or blood streaked mucus, **BU FEI E JIAO TANG** (*Tonify the Lungs Decoction with Ass-Hide Gelatin* 补肺阿胶汤) may be selected as the guiding formula.

    e jiao^ (Gelatinum Corii Asini) 阿胶 9g
    ma dou ling* (Fructus Aristolchiae) 马兜铃 6g
    xing ren* (Semen Pruni Armeniacae) 杏仁 9g
    niu bang zi (Fructus Arctii Lappae) 牛蒡子 6g
    nuo mi (Semen Oryzae) 糯米 12g
    gan cao (Radix Glycyrrhizae Uralensis) 甘草 3g
    Method: Decoction. **E jiao** is melted before being added to the strained decoction (*yang hua* 烊化). (Source: *Shi Yong Zhong Yao Xue*)

Patent medicines

Yang Yin Qing Fei Wan 养阴清肺丸 (Yang Yin Qing Fei Wan)

Ba Xian Chang Shou Wan 八仙长寿丸 (Ba Xian Chang Shou Wan)
Bai He Gu Jin Wan 百合固金丸 (Bai He Gu Jin Wan)
Luo Han Guo Chong Ji 罗汉果冲剂 (Luo Han Guo Beverage)
Chuan Bei Pi Pa Gao 川贝枇杷膏 (Nin Jiom Pei Pa Kao)

Acupuncture

Bl.13 (*fei shu* +), Bl.43 (*gao huang shu* +), Lu.9 (*tai yuan* +), Lu.5 (*chi ze* -), Lu.7 (*lie que*), Kid.6 (*zhao hai*), Bl.23 (*shen shu* +), Kid.3 (*tai xi* +),
 • with severe Heat add Lu.10 (*yu ji* -)

Clinical notes

- The cough in this pattern may be associated with biomedical conditions such as emphysema, chronic bronchitis, bronchiectasis, silicosis, pulmonary tuberculosis, pharyngitis, atmospheric pollution or long term medicated asthma.
- This pattern can be difficult to treat satisfactorily, and success is largely dependent on the degree of deficiency and the chronic nature of the disorder. Long term therapy is necessary. Many patients will need adjuvant medical treatment for some time. Many chronic and long term lung diseases fall into this category.
- When Lung *yin* is damaged following an acute febrile illness or Phlegm Heat, there is usually residual Phlegm in the Lungs that may persist for some time. This complicates treatment because *yin* tonics aggravate Phlegm, and Phlegm resolving herbs can damage *yin*. The general principle of treatment however, is to first clear the excess, then tonify. Clearing of residual Phlegm without damaging *yin* can usually be achieved with gentle patent medicines such as *She Dan Chuan Bei Kou Fu Ye* 蛇胆川贝液 (Snake Bile and Friltillaria Liquid).

肺气虚咳嗽

2.9 LUNG *QI* DEFICIENCY

Pathophysiology
- When Lung *qi* is weak, its descending function is impaired and a chronic cough results.

Clinical features
- Chronic, weak cough which tires the patient out, and which is aggravated or initiated by exertion, fatigue or exposure to wind. Mucus, if present, is thin and mostly clear, frothy or white.
- shortness of breath
- spontaneous sweating
- aversion to wind
- frequent colds
- weak low voice or a reluctance to speak
- fatigue

T pale with a thin white coat
P weak

Treatment principle
Tonify Lung *qi*, calm cough
Transform thin mucus

Prescription

BU FEI TANG 补肺汤
(*Tonify the Lungs Decoction*)

zhi huang qi (honey fried Radix Astragali Membranacei) 炙黄芪 18-30g
shu di (Radix Rehmanniae Glutinosae Conquitae) 熟地 18g
sang bai pi (Cortex Mori Albae Radicis) 桑白皮 12g
ren shen (Radix Ginseng) 人参 9g
zhi zi wan (honey fried Radix Asteris Tatarici) 炙紫菀 9g
wu wei zi (Fructus Schizandrae Chinensis) 五味子 6g
Method: Decoction. (Source: *Shi Yong Zhong Yi Nei Ke Xue*)

Modifications

- With thin mucus, delete **sang bai pi**, and add **bai zhu** (Rhizoma Atractylodis Macrocephalae) 白术 9g, **fu ling** (Sclerotium Poriae Cocos) 茯苓 12g, **gan jiang** (Rhizoma Zingiberis Officinale) 干姜 6g and **kuan dong hua** (Flos Tussilaginis Farfarae) 款冬花 9g.

- With spontaneous sweating, add **mu li^** (Concha Ostreae) 牡蛎 15g, **ma huang gen** (Radix Ephedrae) 麻黄根 9g, **fu xiao mai** (Semen Tritici Aestivi Levis) 浮小麦 12g.

Variations and additional prescriptions
Lung and Spleen qi *deficiency*
- With Spleen deficiency as well (loose stools, poor appetite, puffy eyelids, sallow complexion, abdominal distension, copious watery mucus), the correct treatment is to strengthen the Spleen to resolve Phlegm with **LIU JUN ZI TANG** (*Six Major Herbs Combination*) modified.

    ren shen (Radix Ginseng) 人参 9g
    bai zhu (Rhizoma Atractylodis Macrocephalae) 白术 12g
    fu ling (Sclerotium Poriae Cocos) 茯苓 12g
    gan cao (Radix Glycyrrhizae Uralensis) 甘草 6g
    ban xia* (Rhizoma Pinelliae Ternatae) 半夏 9g
    chen pi (Pericarpium Citri Reticulatae) 陈皮 6g
    hou po (Cortex Magnoliae Officinalis) 厚朴 9g
    xing ren* (Semen Pruni Armeniacae) 杏仁 9g
    Method: Decoction. (Source: *Shi Yong Zhong Yi Nei Ke Xue*)

Lung qi *and* yin deficiency
- Lung deficiency syndromes frequently overlap. The copious sweating of *qi* deficiency can damage *yin* and the chronic cough of *yin* deficiency can deplete Lung *qi*, so it is not uncommon to see Lung *qi* and *yin* deficiency together in the clinic. The manifestations are a combination of the syndromes—chronic cough with scant mucus that is hard to expectorate, shortness of breath, spontaneous sweating, a dry mouth and tongue, a pale or pink and swollen tongue with surface cracks and little coating, and a weak and thready pulse. The guiding formula for tonifying Lung *qi* and *yin* is **SHENG MAI SAN** (*Generate the Pulse Powder* 脉散).

    ren shen (Radix Ginseng) 人参 9-15g
    mai dong (Tuber Ophiopogonis Japonici) 麦冬 9-12g
    wu wei zi (Fructus Schizandrae Chinensis) 五味子 3-6g
    Method: Decoction. White ginseng (**bai ren shen** 白人参) is prefered here as it is less heating than the Korean variety.

Patent medicines
Bu Zhong Yi Qi Wan 补中益气丸 (Bu Zhong Yi Qi Wan)
Xiang Sha Liu Jun Zi Wan 香砂六君子丸 (Xiang Sha Liu Jun Wan)
Yu Ping Feng Wan 玉屏风丸 (Yu Ping Feng Wan)
Shen Qi Da Bu Wan 参芪大补丸 (Shen Qi Da Bu Wan)
Sheng Mai Wan 生脉丸 (Sheng Mai Wan)
Ren Shen Yang Ying Wan 人参养营丸 (Ginseng Tonic Pills)

Acupuncture
Bl.13 (*fei shu* +▲), Bl.43 (*gao huang shu* +▲), Lu.9 (*tai yuan* +),
Lu.7 (*lie que*), Du.14 (*da zhui* +▲), St.36 (*zu san li* +▲),

Ren.17 (*shan zhong*), Sp.6 (*san yin jiao* +), Ren.12 (*zhong wan* +), Bl.20 (*pi shu* +▲)
- with spontaneous sweating, add LI.4 (*he gu*) and Kid.7 (*fu liu*)
- with thin watery Phlegm, add St.40 (*feng long* -) and Sp.3 (*tai bai* +)

Clinical notes
- The cough in this pattern may be associated with biomedical conditions such as chronic bronchitis, asthma, weak immunity, emphysema or hayfever.
- Generally responds well to correct and prolonged treatment.

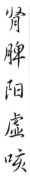

2.10 SPLEEN AND KIDNEY *YANG* DEFICIENCY

Pathophysiology
- This pattern is characterised by a failure of Spleen and Kidney *yang* to adequately process fluids. These fluids accumulate in the Lungs and obstruct the descent of Lung *qi*. The cough can be quite severe, especially when there is a lot of fluid in the Lungs, in which case removing the excess fluid through diuresis is the treatment priority. Once the condition has stabilised, appropriate treatment for strengthening Spleen and Kidney *yang* can be phased in.

Clinical features
- chronic, recurrent cough with thin watery mucus, usually with wheezing and dyspnoea; the cough is worse with exertion
- generalised oedema, possibly pitting oedema
- cold intolerance
- cold, heavy limbs
- spontaneous sweating
- nocturia or difficult urination
- dizziness and palpitations

T pale and swollen with a moist white coat
P deep and slippery

Treatment principle
Warm *yang*, disperse Cold
Transform *qi* to move fluids

Prescription

ZHEN WU TANG 真武汤
(*True Warrior Decoction*)

This formula has a powerful fluid mobilising and diuretic activity, and is used when there is fluid in the Lungs causing cough. Once the fluid has resolved, other *yang* strengthening formulae may be more appropriate (see variations).

zhi fu zi* (Radix Aconiti Carmichaeli Praeparata) 制附子 9g
fu ling (Sclerotium Poriae Cocos) 茯苓 9g
sheng jiang (Rhizoma Zingiberis Officinalis Recens) 生姜 9g
bai shao (Radix Paeoniae Lactiflora) 白芍 9g
bai zhu (Rhizoma Atractylodis Macrocephalae) 白术 6g
Method: Decoction. **Zhi fu zi** is cooked for 30 minutes prior to the other herbs (*xian jian* 先煎). (Source: *Shi Yong Zhong Yi Nei Ke Xue*)

Modifications
- For severe cough, add **gan jiang** (Rhizoma Zingiberis Officinale) 干姜 6g, **xi xin*** (Herba cum Radice Asari) 细辛 3g and **wu wei zi** (Fructus Schizandrae Chinensis) 五味子 6g.
- With severe fluid accumulation in the Lungs, add **ting li zi** (Semen Descurainiae seu Lepidii) 葶苈子 9g.
- If there is fullness in the chest and hypochondrium, add **bai jie zi** (Semen Sinapsis Albae) 白芥子 9g and **xuan fu hua** (Flos Inulae) 旋复花 9g.
- For severe shortness of breath, add **dang shen** (Radix Codonopsis Pilosulae) 党参 12g.
- With loose stools, add **gan jiang** (Rhizoma Zingiberis Officinale) 干姜 6g.

Variations and additional prescriptions
- Once the cough has stabilised and excess fluid drained from the Lungs, the treatment principle is to strengthen Spleen and Kidney *yang* with a formula like **JIN KUI SHEN QI WAN** (*Rehmannia Eight Formula* 金匮肾气丸, p.150).

Acupuncture
Bl.20 (*pi shu* +▲), Bl.23 (*shen shu* +▲), Ren.9 (*shui fen* ▲), Ren.6 (*qi hai* +▲), Kid.7 (*fu liu* -), Kid.3 (*tai xi* +), Sp.9 (*yin ling quan* -), Sp.6 (*san yin jiao* -), St.36 (*zu san li* +▲)
- with orthopnoea from fluid in the Lungs, add St.28 (*shui dao* - ▲) and Bl.28 (*pang guang shu* -)
- with nocturia, add Ren.4 (*guan yuan* +▲)

Clinical notes
- The cough in this pattern may be associated with biomedical conditions such as congestive cardiac failure, pulmonary oedema, chronic bronchitis or chronic asthma.
- This pattern can be tricky to treat satisfactorily, largely dependent on the degree of deficiency. Fluid metabolism, however, generally improves fairly quickly. Long term therapy is necessary to maintain the result.

2.11 BLOOD STAGNATION

血瘀咳嗽

Pathophysiology
- A Blood stagnation cough usually follows some sort of trauma to the chest wall, like contusions or fractures of the ribs. It may also reflect the late stage of a serious Lung disease, such as lung cancer.

Clinical features
- Recurrent, irritating cough (with a history of trauma or other chronic Lung disease), which tends to be worse at night. If there is mucus it is usually scanty, or may be blood streaked or may have dark patches of clotted blood. There may be pain around the site of the injury during coughing episodes.
- there may be cold extremities–a frequent sign of Blood stagnation in chronic Lung disease

T pale or purplish, with brown or purple stagnation spots
P wiry or thready and weak, depending on the duration of the condition

Treatment principle
Resolve stagnant Blood in the Lungs, stop cough

Prescription

XUE FU ZHU YU TANG 血府逐瘀汤
(*Achyranthes and Persica Combination*) modified

tao ren (Semen Persicae) 桃仁	12g
hong hua (Flos Carthami Tinctorii) 红花	9g
dang gui (Radix Angelicae Sinensis) 当归	9g
xing ren* (Semen Pruni Armeniacae) 杏仁	9g
chuan niu xi (Radix Cyathulae Officinalis) 川牛膝	9g
sheng di (Radix Rehmanniae Glutinosae) 生地	9g
chi shao (Radix Paeoniae Rubrae) 赤芍	6g
chuan xiong (Radix Ligustici Chuanxiong) 川芎	6g
jie geng (Radix Platycodi Grandiflori) 桔梗	6g
zhi ke (Fructus Citri Aurantii) 枳壳	6g
wu wei zi (Fructus Schizandrae Chinensis) 五味子	6g
chai hu (Radix Bupleuri) 柴胡	6g
gan cao (Radix Glycyrrhizae Uralensis) 甘草	3g

Method: Decoction. (Source: *Shi Yong Zhong Yi Nei Ke Xue*)

Modifications
- With blood streaked mucus or dark clotty material in the mucus, add **san qi fen** (powdered Radix Notoginseng) 三七粉 5g and **bai mao gen**

(Rhizoma Imperatae Cylindricae) 白茅根 9g.

Patent medicines
Xue Fu Zhu Yu Wan 血府逐瘀丸 (Xue Fu Zhu Yu Wan)
Dan Shen Pian 丹参片 (Dan Shen Pills)
Jian Kang Wan 健康丸 (Sunho Multi Ginseng Tablets)
Sheng Tian Qi Pian 生田七片 (Raw Tian Qi Ginseng Tablets)
Jin Gu Die Shang Wan 筋骨跌伤丸 (Chin Koo Tieh Shang Wan)
Nei Xiao Luo Li Wan 内消瘰疬丸 (Nei Xiao Luo Li Wan)
Fu Ke Wu Jin Wan 妇科乌金丸 (Woo Garm Yuen Medical Pills)

Acupuncture
Bl.17 (*ge shu* -), Bl.13 (*fei shu* -), Lu.5 (*chi ze* -), LI.4 (*he gu* -), Liv.3 (*tai chong* -), PC.6 (*nei guan*), Sp.10 (*xue hai* -)
- with haemoptysis, add Lu.6 (*kong zui* -)
- following trauma, add points of pain (*ah shi*)

Clinical notes
- The cough in this pattern may be associated with biomedical conditions such as traumatic chest injury, lung cancer, pulmonary tuberculosis, chronic obstructive airways disease (COAD), emphysema and chronic asthma.
- If due to a recent trauma to the chest wall, this pattern can respond quite well to correct treatment (following appropriate resetting of broken ribs etc.). However, late stage Lung disease (for example long term damage to Lung *yin* by smoking) is difficult to resolve with TCM alone.

Endnote

For more information regarding herbs marked with an asterisk*, an open circle° or a hat ˆ, see the tables on pp.944-952.

SUMMARY OF GUIDING FORMULAE FOR COUGH

Acute

Wind Cold - *Hua Gai San* 华盖散
- with congested fluids - *Xiao Qing Long Tang* 小青龙汤
- with internal Heat - *Ma Xing Shi Gan Tang* 麻杏石甘汤

Wind Heat - *Sang Ju Yin* 桑菊饮
- persistent cough after resolution of exterior symptoms - *Zhi Sou San* 止嗽散

Wind Dryness
- Warm Dryness - *Sang Xing Tang* 桑杏汤
  - with damage to *yin* - *Qing Zao Jiu Fei Tang* 清燥救肺汤
- Cool Dryness - *Xing Su San* 杏苏散

Lung Heat - *Ma Xing Shi Gan Tang* 麻杏石甘汤
- Lung Fire - *Liang Ge San* 凉隔散

Phlegm Heat - *Qing Jin Hua Tan Tang* 清金化痰汤
- with purulent mucus - *Wei Jing Tang* 苇茎汤

Liver Fire - *Dai Ge San* 黛蛤散 + *Qing Jin Hua Tan Tang* 清金化痰汤

Chronic

Phlegm Damp - *Er Chen Tang* 二陈汤
- with Spleen *qi* deficiency - *Liu Jun Zi Tang* 六君子汤
- recurrent, with Kidney deficiency - *Su Zi Jiang Qi Tang* 苏子降气汤

Phlegm Heat - *Qing Jin Hua Tan Tang* 清金化痰汤

Liver Fire - *Sang Dan Xie Bai Tang* 桑丹泻白汤

Lung *yin* deficiency - *Bai He Gu Jin Tang* 百合固金汤
- with Kidney *yin* deficiency - *Mai Wei Di Huang Wan* 麦味地黄丸
- with Heart *yin* deficiency - *Xuan Miao San* 玄妙散
- following a febrile disease - *Bu Fei E Jiao Tang* 补肺阿胶汤

Lung *qi* deficiency - *Bu Fei Tang* 补肺汤
- with *yin* deficiency - *Sheng Mai San* 生脉散
- with Spleen *qi* deficiency - *Liu Jun Zi Tang* 六君子汤

Spleen and Kidney *yang* deficiency - *Zhen Wu Tang* 真武汤
- after cough has stabilised - *Jin Kui Shen Qi Wan* 金匮肾气丸

Blood stagnation - *Xue Fu Zhu Yu Tang* 血府逐瘀汤

Appendix
FEI YONG 肺痈 (Lung abscess)

In TCM terms, *fei yong* can develop in those attacked by powerful pathogenic Wind Heat, which may combine with pre-existing Phlegm or Phlegm Heat to generate Toxins. The term Toxin (*du* 毒) is defined here as a highly concentrated focus of pathogenic energy that destroys tissue to create pus.

The direct translation of *fei yong* is Lung abscess which can be somewhat misleading. In TCM terms, *fei yong* includes any severe suppurative lung infection manifesting with malodorous, purulent, discoloured sputum. This includes diseases such as bronchitis, pneumonia, pulmonary gangrene, bronchiectasis, and, of course, lung abscess.

In China, the disease diagnosis of *fei yong* is frequently the starting point for the analysis and treatment of severe, acute, suppurative lung infection. At a particular level of severity, the clinical features are similar regardless of the individual patient, and the main feature of treatment is recognition of the correct stage. Three stages are discussed; early, middle (with obvious pus formation and severe systemic symptoms) and convalescent stage. The various stages are marked by a progression from exterior excess to internal excess, and ultimately to deficiency.

AETIOLOGY
Toxic Heat
The presence of Toxic Heat is a key feature defining this pattern. Toxic Heat is an intense and concentrated species of Heat (alone or with Dampness or Phlegm) that is usually external (and occasionally epidemic) in origin. Most frequently Wind Heat is the pathogen responsible, although Wind Cold can transmute into Heat once lodged in the Lungs. When an area affected by Heat is constrained and the Heat unable to dissipate, destruction of the local tissue occurs, forming pus.

DIAGNOSIS

In the early stages *fei yong* resembles a straightforward Wind Heat attack, and indeed the initial prescription is very similar. The difference becomes apparent after a day or two as the condition progresses. The severity of the fever, rigors, cough with purulent sputum and general malaise provide clues as to the presence of Toxic Heat.

2. COUGH – Appendix: *fei yong* (Lung Abscess)

痈前期之肺痈

1. EARLY STAGE

Pathophysiology
- This stage of *fei yong* is due to simple invasion of a strong Wind Heat (or transmuted Wind Cold) pathogen. Alternatively, pre-existing Phlegm Damp can be inflamed by Wind Heat to create the early stage of *fei yong*. The body seals off a portion of the Heat which then intensifies, generating a locus of Toxic Heat. At this stage, the pattern (usually) resembles a Wind Heat attack with severe systemic symptoms.

Clinical features
- acute fever and chills or rigors
- chest pain which is worse when coughing
- cough with scant, sticky white or yellowish sputum
- painful or wheezy and difficult respiration
- dry throat, mouth, nose and lips
- lethargy, malaise, weakness, poor appetite

T red tip with a thin yellow coat
P floating, rapid or slippery

Treatment principle
Expel Wind and Heat
Clear Heat from the Lungs and transform Phlegm

Prescription

YIN QIAO SAN 银翘散
(*Lonicera and Forsythia Formula*) modified

jin yin hua (Flos Lonicerae Japonicae) 金银花	30g
lian qiao (Fructus Forsythia Suspensae) 连翘	30g
yu xing cao (Herba cum Radice Houttuyniae Cordatae) 鱼腥草	30g
bai mao gen (Rhizoma Imperatae Cylindricae) 白茅根	30g
lu gen (Rhizoma Phragmitis Communis) 芦根	30g
pu gong ying (Herba Taraxaci Mongolici) 蒲公英	18g
gua lou (Fructus Trichosanthis) 栝楼	12g
niu bang zi (Fructus Arctii Lappae) 牛蒡子	12g
jie geng (Radix Platycodi Grandiflori) 桔梗	12g
zhu ye (Herba Lophatheri Gracilis) 竹叶	10g
huang qin (Radix Scutellaria Baicalensis) 黄芩	10g
gan cao (Radix Glycyrrhizae Uralensis) 甘草	6g

Method: Decoction. Cook no longer than 30 minutes. (Source: *Zhong Yi Nei Ke Lin Chuang Shou Ce*)

Modifications

- With headache, add **ju hua** (Flos Chrysanthemi Morifolii) 菊花 12g, **sang ye** (Folium Mori Albae) 桑叶 10g and **man jing zi** (Fructus Viticis) 蔓荆子 10g.
- For a severe, distressing cough, add **xing ren*** (Semen Pruni Armeniacae) 杏仁 10g and **chuan bei mu** (Bulbus Fritillariae Cirrhosae) 川贝母 10g.
- With severe thirst for cold drinks, add **sha shen** (Radix Adenophorae seu Glehniae) 沙参 15g, **mai dong** (Tuber Ophiopogonis Japonici) 麦冬 10g, **tian dong** (Tuber Asparagi Cochinchinensis) 天冬 10g and **tian hua fen** (Radix Trichosanthes Kirilowii) 天花粉 15g.
- With chest pain, add **yu jin** (Tuber Curcumae) 郁金 10g and **tao ren** (Semen Persicae) 桃仁 10g.
- With severe wheezing, combine with **MA XING SHI GAN TANG** (*Ma Huang, Apricot Seed, Gypsum and Licorice Combination* 麻杏石甘汤, p.31).

Patent medicines

Qing Fei Yi Huo Pian 清肺抑火片 (Ching Fei Yi Huo Pien)
Chuan Xin Lian Kang Yan Pian 穿心莲抗炎片
  (Chuan Xin Lian Antiphlogistic Tablets)
Ma Xing Zhi Ke Pian 麻杏止咳片 (Ma Hsing Chih Ke Pien)
Niu Huang Jie Du Pian 牛黄解毒片 (Niu Huang Chieh Tu Pien)

Acupuncture

Du.14 (*da zhui* -), Du.12 (*shen zhu* -), Du.10 (*ling tai* -), BL.13 (*fei shu* -), Lu.5 (*chi ze* -), Lu.7 (*lie que* -), LI.4 (*he gu* -), LI.11 (*qu chi* -), SJ.5 (*wai guan* -), Lu.10 (*yu ji* -)

Clinical notes

- This pattern may be diagnosed as bronchitis, pneumonia, bronchiectasis, upper respiratory tract infection, asthmatic bronchitis and the early stage of lung abscess.
- This pattern can respond well to correct and timely treatment. This is usually a fairly serious infection and concurrent use of antibiotics may be necessary in some patients to quickly cool the Heat. Herbs and acupuncture can support the swift action of the antibiotics, to finish the job by expelling the pathogen, clearing residual Phlegm, strengthening resistance and nourishing damaged *yin*. In the latter stages of *fei yong*, i.e. when aiding the discharge of pus, stopping night sweats and aiding convalescence, TCM treatment excels.
- Acupuncture can be applied 2-3 times daily in severe cases.

2. MIDDLE STAGE (SUPPURATION, RUPTURE STAGE)

Pathophysiology
- At this stage the Heat and Toxins have intensified and damaged portions of Lung tissue, creating pus and Blood stasis.

Clinical features
- high fever with or without rigors
- the cough is hacking and painful, with expectoration of copious purulent malodorous mucus; the mucus may be streaked with blood
- restricted movement of chest, laboured breathing
- sweating
- dry mouth and throat
- irritability, restlessness, lethargy, malaise
- a chest X-ray at this stage may show a space occupying lesion

T red with a greasy yellow coat
P slippery and rapid, or flooding and rapid

Treatment principle
Clear Heat and Toxins
Disperse accumulation of pus and Blood stasis

Prescription

QIAN JIN WEI JING TANG 千金苇茎汤
(*Reed Decoction*) plus
JIE GENG TANG 桔梗汤
(*Platycodon Decoction*) modified

lu gen (Rhizoma Phragmitis Communis) 芦根	30g
yi ren (Semen Coicis Lachryma-jobi) 苡仁	30g
tao ren (Semen Persicae) 桃仁	10g
dong gua ren (Semen Benincasae Hispidae) 冬瓜仁	30g
yu xing cao (Herba cum Radice Houttuyniae Cordatae) 鱼腥草	30g
jin yin hua (Flos Lonicerae Japonicae) 金银花	30g
lian qiao (Fructus Forsythia Suspensae) 连翘	20g
jie geng (Radix Platycodi Grandiflori) 桔梗	10g
huang qin (Radix Scutellariae Baicalensis) 黄芩	10g
zhe bei mu (Bulbus Fritillariae Thunbergii) 浙贝母	10g
chi shao (Radix Paeoniae Rubrae) 赤芍	10g
huang lian (Rhizoma Coptidis) 黄连	6g

Method: Decoction. Cook no longer than 30 minutes. (Source: *Zhong Yi Nei Ke Lin Chuang Shou Ce*)

Modifications

- With severe Heat and thirst, add **shi gao** (Gypsum) 石膏 30g cooked for 30 minutes prior to the other herbs, **zhi mu** (Rhizoma Anemarrhenae Asphodeloides) 知母 12g and **shan zhi zi** (Fructus Gardeniae Jasminoidis) 山栀子 15g.
- With severe Toxic Heat, add **ban zhi lian** (Herba Scutellariae Barbatae) 半枝莲 15g, **ban bian lian** (Herba Lobeliae Chinensis) 半边莲 15g and **zi hua di ding** (Herba cum Radice Violae Yedoensitis) 紫花地丁 30g.
- For fullness in the chest and wheezing with copious sputum, add **ting li zi** (Semen Descurainiae seu Lepidii) 葶苈子 10g, **sang bai pi** (Cortex Mori Albae Radicis) 桑白皮 15g and **gua lou** (Fructus Trichosanthis) 栝楼 15g.
- With chest pain, add **yu jin** (Tuber Curcumae) 郁金 15g and **yan hu suo** (Rhizoma Corydalis Yanhusuo) 延胡索 9g.
- With constipation, add **da huang** (Radix et Rhizoma Rhei) 大黄 9g and **zhi shi** (Fructus Citri Aurantii Immaturus) 枳实 10g.
- With blood streaked sputum, delete **jie geng, tao ren** and **chi shao**, and add **bai mao gen** (Rhizoma Imperatae Cylindricae) 30g, **ou jie** (Nodus Nelumbinis Nuciferae Rhizomatis) 藕节 15g, **bai ji** (Rhizoma Bletillae Striatae) 白芨 15g, and **mu dan pi** (Cortex Moutan Radicis) 12g, or add **YUN NAN BAI YAO** (*Yun Nan White Powder* 云南白药) to the strained decoction.
- If the Heat has damaged the *yin*, with relapsing afternoon and evening fever, restlessness, insomnia and nightsweats, add **di gu pi** (Cortex Lycii Radicis) 地骨皮 9g, **qing hao** (Herba Artemesiae Annuae) 青蒿 15g and **bie jia**° (Carapax Amydae Sinensis) 鳖甲 15g. See also Convalescent stage, p.114.

Patent medicines

Qing Fei Yi Huo Pian 清肺抑火片 (Ching Fei Yi Huo Pien)
Qing Qi Hua Tan Wan 清气化痰丸 (Pinellia Expectorant Pills)
Chuan Xin Lian Kang Yan Pian 穿心莲抗炎片
    (Chuan Xin Lian Antiphlogistic Tablets)
Huang Lian Su Pian 黄连素片 (Tabellae Berberini)
Niu Huan Qing Huo Wan 牛黄清火丸 (Niu Huang Qing Huo Wan)
Ma Xing Zhi Ke Pian 麻杏止咳片 (Ma Hsing Chih Ke Pien)
Niu Huang Jie Du Pian 牛黄解毒片 (Peking Niu Huang Chieh Tu Pien)

Acupuncture

Lu.5 (*chi ze* -), Lu.1 (*zhong fu* -), St.40 (*feng long* -), Bl.13 (*fei shu* -), Du.14 (*da zhui* -), Du.12 (*shen zhu* -), Du.10 (*ling tai* -), Lu.6 (*kong zui* -), Ren.17 (*shan zhong* -), SJ.6 (*zhi gou* -), PC.7 (*da ling*)

- with severe Heat, bleed Lu.11 (*shao shang* ↓) and LI.1 (*shang yang* ↓)

Clinical notes
- Biomedical conditions that may be diagnosed as middle (or suppurative) stage *fei yong* include bronchitis, pneumonia, bronchiectasis, upper respiratory tract infection, asthmatic bronchitis and ruptured lung abscess.
- This pattern can respond well to correct treatment. See also clinical notes, p.110.

恢复期

3. CONVALESCENT STAGE

Pathophysiology
- At this stage, the patient is recovering and the pathogen has subsided. *Zheng qi* has been damaged and is weak. Following a strong Heat pathogenic disorder Lung *yin* and fluids are damaged, and the general pattern shifts from an excess Heat to a deficient Heat. The main features at this stage are drenching night sweats, weakness and marked irritability.

Clinical features
- lingering low fever which tends to rise in the afternoon and evening
- easing cough with small quantities of sputum, which may still contain some purulent material
- spontaneous sweating, drenching night sweats
- weakness and fatigue
- mild chest pain
- shortness of breath
- poor appetite
- dry mouth and throat
- irritability and restlessness
- insomnia

T red with a thin yellow coat
P thready, rapid and weak

Treatment principle
Strengthen and tonify *qi* and *yin*
Clear any remaining Toxins

Prescription

SHA SHEN MAI MEN DONG TANG 沙参麦门冬汤
(*Adenophora and Ophiopogon Combination*) modified

sha shen (Radix Adenophorae seu Glehniae) 沙参	15g
mai dong (Tuber Ophiopogonis Japonici) 麦冬	15g
sheng di (Radix Rehmanniae Glutinosae) 生地	15g
chao yi ren (dry fried Semen Coicis Lachryma-jobi) 炒苡仁	15g
huang qi (Radix Astragali Membranacei) 黄芪	15g
jin yin hua (Flos Lonicerae Japonicae) 金银花	15g
tai zi shen (Radix Pseudostellariae Heterophyllae) 太子参	12g
he huan pi (Cortex Albizziae Julibrissin) 合欢皮	24g
bai ji fen (powdered Rhizoma Bletillae Striatae) 白芨粉	9g
jie geng (Radix Platycodi Grandiflori) 桔梗	9g
gan cao (Radix Glycyrrhizae Uralensis) 甘草	6g

yu xing cao (Herba cum Radice Houttuyniae Cordatae)
鱼腥草 15g

Method: Decoction. Cook no longer than 30 minutes. **Bai ji fen** is added to the strained decoction (*chong fu* 冲服). (Source: *Zhong Yi Nei Ke Lin Chuang Shou Ce*)

Modifications

- For persistent low fever, add **di gu pi** (Cortex Lycii Radicis) 地骨皮 9g, **bai wei** (Radix Cynanchi Baiwei) 白薇 9g and **qing hao** (Herba Artemesiae Annuae) 青蒿 15g.
- For severe drenching night sweats, add **qing hao** (Herba Artemesiae Annuae) 青蒿 15g, **di gu pi** (Cortex Lycii Radicis) 地骨皮 9g, **mu li** (Concha Ostreae) 牡蛎 15g and **ma huang gen** (Radix Ephedrae) 麻黄根 9g.
- If the Spleen has been weakened, with poor appetite, indigestion and abdominal distension, delete **sheng di** and add **dang shen** (Radix Codonopsis Pilosulae) 党参 15g, **bai zhu** (Rhizoma Atractylodis Macrocephalae) 白术 9g and **fu ling** (Sclerotium Poriae Cocos) 茯苓 15g.
- For persistent cough, add **gua lou** (Fructus Trichosanthis) 栝楼 15g, **pi pa ye** (Folium Eriobotryae Japonicae) 枇杷叶 10g and **chuan bei mu** (Bulbus Fritillariae Cirrhosae) 川贝母 10g.
- If there is persistent bloody sputum, add **san qi fen** (powdered Radix Notoginseng) 三七粉 6g and **bai mao gen** (Rhizoma Imperatae Cylindricae) 白茅根 12g, or combine with **YUN NAN BAI YAO** (*Yun Nan White Powder* 云南白药).

Patent medicines

Sheng Mai Wan 生脉丸 (Sheng Mai Wan)
Yang Yin Qing Fei Wan 养阴清肺丸 (Yang Yin Qing Fei Wan)
Luo Han Guo Chong Ji 罗汉果冲剂 (Luo Han Guo Beverage)
Bai He Gu Jin Wan 百合固金丸 (Bai He Gu Jin Wan)
She Dan Chuan Bei Ye 蛇胆川贝液 (She Dan Chuan Bei Ye)
  - excellent for difficult to expectorate residual sputum
Qing Qi Hua Tan Wan 清气化痰丸 (Pinellia Expectorant Pills)
  - add a small dose of the latter patent medicine if there is residual Phlegm Heat

Acupuncture

Lu.1 (*zhong fu* -), Ren.17 (*shan zhong* -), LI.11 (*qu chi* -), Bl.13 (*fei shu*), Du.14 (*da zhui*), St.36 (*zu san li* +), Kid.3 (*tai xi* +), Lu.9 (*tai yuan* +)
  - with severe night sweats, add Ht.6 (*yin xi*) and SI.3 (*hou xi*)
  - for irritability add Ht.7 (*shen men*) and Liv.8 (*qu quan*)

Clinical notes

- This pattern occurs in the convalescent stage of disorders such as bronchitis, pneumonia, bronchiectasis, upper respiratory tract infection and asthmatic bronchitis.
- Ongoing treatment at this stage can produce good results. The nightsweats and residual fever usually improve rapidly.

Disorders of the Lung

3. Wheezing

Excess patterns
Wind Cold
Wind Cold with congested fluids
Wind Cold with internal Heat
Wind Heat
Phlegm Damp
Phlegm Heat
Qi stagnation

Deficient patterns
Lung *qi* and *yin* deficiency
Lung and Spleen *qi* deficiency
Lung and Kidney *yin* deficiency
Kidney *yang* deficiency

Appendix 1 – Asthma
Appendix 2 – Paediatric asthma

3 | WHEEZING
xiao chuan 哮喘

In Chinese medicine, wheezing refers to a sense of tightness, congestion, breathlessness or constriction in the chest with difficult inspiration. The term asthma is commonly used when referring to this condition, however true asthma is only one of a number of biomedical diagnoses that may fall into the TCM category of wheezing, hence the adage of Western medicine, 'All that wheezes is not asthma, however a lot of it is'. Because asthma is diagnosed so frequently, a separate discussion is warranted (appendix 1 and 2, pp.155, 157).

In TCM terms, wheezing is due to failure of Lung *qi* to descend as it naturally should. There are two primary mechanisms, excess and deficient. Excess wheezing is due to obstruction to Lung *qi* by an external pathogen (Wind plus Heat or Cold) or internally generated pathogens (Phlegm, Heat or *qi* stagnation). Deficient wheezing occurs when Lung *qi* is too weak to descend under its own steam, or Kidney *qi* is unable to grasp *qi* and aid the Lungs. In either case, the end result is accumulation of *qi* in the chest, leading to a sense of fullness, tightness or constriction.

Wheezing may be acute or chronic, and in many cases acute episodes occur on a background of chronic disease. In severe cases, the breathing difficulty may be serious enough to cause severe distress, and perhaps precipitate collapse, anoxia and even death. This is a medical emergency requiring immediate hospitalisation.

AETIOLOGY
External pathogens
Any of the external pathogens can give rise to wheezing due to the relatively superficial and therefore vulnerable position of the Lungs. Most frequently implicated are Wind Cold (as Cold constricts the bronchi, narrowing the airway) and Wind Heat. The Lungs are considered to be the 'delicate' organ and easily affected by the environment. Entry to the Lungs may be through the nose and mouth, or the skin (the Lungs and skin are closely related). In most cases there will also be an underlying deficiency, allowing Wind (plus Cold or Heat) to enter.

Spleen deficiency
Spleen deficiency can contribute to wheezing by leading to weakness of Lung *qi* and by generating Phlegm. Spleen deficiency is frequently implicated in the chronic wheezing of children. Overwork, excessive worry or mental activity, irregular dietary habits, excessive consumption of cold, raw or sweet

foods, or prolonged illness can weaken Spleen *qi* or *yang*. Long term or frequent use of antibiotics can weaken the Spleen and encourage the generation of Dampness and Phlegm.

Phlegm Damp, Phlegm Heat

Phlegm is frequently implicated in wheezing. It can be the result of several factors. In the Western world, diet is a common cause of Phlegm accumulation. Overeating generally, which stresses the digestive system leading to inefficient digestion and buildup of Dampness and Phlegm, is common. Similarly, a high average consumption of dairy foods, sugar, meat and fatty foods, commonplace in the developed world, is a significant contributing factor to the manufacture and accumulation of Phlegm and Dampness.

Phlegm Heat may accumulate if too much rich food is consumed or if pre-existing Heat in the body congeals Fluids into Phlegm.

Prolonged Liver *qi* stagnation may damage the Spleen and retard the movement of fluids which congeal into Phlegm. A tendency to Phlegm problems may also be constitutional.

Yang deficiency (affecting any or all of the Kidneys, Spleen or Heart) can cause impaired fluid metabolism and retard movement of Fluids, with consequent accumulation of Phlegm Fluids.

Once Phlegm is present it can gather in the Lungs (the Lungs are the 'storehouse' of Phlegm). In the Lungs, Phlegm may be obvious (as an ongoing rattle, cough or throat clearing) or latent. If the Phlegm is latent (or hidden), it may only appear when an external pathogen flushes it out.

Liver *qi* stagnation

The Liver system is the one most affected (and easily obstructed) by stress, frustration, anger and repressed emotion. It strongly affects the chest because

---

BOX 3.1 SOME BIOMEDICAL CAUSES OF WHEEZING

Respiratory
- asthma
- acute and chronic bronchitis, bronchiolitis
- emphysema
- carcinoma
- cystic fibrosis
- pulmonary tuberculosis
- foreign body
- pneumothorax
- atelectasis
- pleural effusion
- epiglottitis
- aspergillosis

Cardiovascular
- cardiac asthma
- cor pulmonale
- left ventricular failure
- pulmonary embolism
- cardiomyopathy

Gastrointestinal
- reflux oesophagitis

Other
- anxiety
- high altitude
- obesity
- anaemia
- lack of fitness
- hypoparathyroidism

of the pathway of the channel, and the position of the Liver organ itself, directly beneath the diaphragm. Once the circulation of Liver *qi* is disrupted, *qi* can accumulate in the chest causing a sensation of tightness, stuffiness, distension and, particularly, difficulty getting a deep breath.

Complications of *qi* stagnation can also contribute to wheezing. Liver *qi* stagnation can damage the Spleen and retard fluid movement, causing buildup of Dampness and congealing of fluids into Phlegm. Prolonged *qi* stagnation can also generate Heat. The common feature of all varieties of Liver *qi* stagnation type wheezing is provocation with emotional turmoil and stress.

Lung deficiency

This refers to Lung *qi* or *yin* deficiency. When the Lungs are weak, Lung *qi* may not be able to follow its correct trajectory, and ascends or simply accumulates in the chest instead of descending. Lung *qi* may be compromised by poor posture, shallow breathing and lack of exercise, or conversely by repeated or extreme physical overexertion. Prolonged, excessive or unexpressed grief or sadness can weaken Lung *qi*. Lung *qi* deficiency can also lead to Phlegm accumulation, as the fluids that should be sent to the Kidney for reprocessing accumulate and congeal in the Lungs. If Spleen *qi* is deficient then Lung *qi* will not be supported via the generating (*sheng* 生) cycle, p.70.

Lung *yin* can be damaged by dry hot environments, febrile diseases, smoking and as a secondary result of Kidney *yin* deficiency. Lung *qi* and *yin* may also be dispersed by the use of some bronchodilating medications.

Kidney deficiency

Kidney *qi* aids the Lungs in the grasping of *qi*. As Lung *qi* descends with a breath, the Kidney anchors it. If the Kidney is weak this anchoring function is inadequate and the inspired *qi* is not drawn down completely.

TREATMENT

The majority of patients presenting with wheezing disorders are already medicated and their symptoms generally controlled. They will have inhalant medications to control their acute attacks, usually drugs like salbutamol, theophylline or beclamethasone.

The main aim of TCM treatment, therefore, is to improve Lung function and gradually decrease the reliance on drugs. The long term side effects of bronchodilators (Box 1, p.155) warrant persistent efforts to reduce the reliance on the drugs if possible.

TCM is also effective during acute episodes, or during periods of frequent or uncontrolled attacks. During an episode, the main principle of treatment is to first stop the wheezing, and then when the patient is more comfortable,

deal with the root. There are therefore two distinct phases of treatment:
- **treatment during an acute episode of wheezing**
- **treatment in between episodes**

TCM treatment can have the most far reaching effect in the phase between acute episodes with the aim of strengthening lung function and reducing or eliminating attacks. In general, the longer a patient has been medicated, the more treatment the patient will require (this is especially true for adults, children are generally more responsive), and the enduring results come from regular and persistent treatment. In very chronic cases, one or two years of treatment may be required. The main point is that results in long term wheezing disorders are slow, and patients often get discouraged. As well as good quality treatment, lots of reassurance and positive encouragement are necessary when treating these chronic patterns.

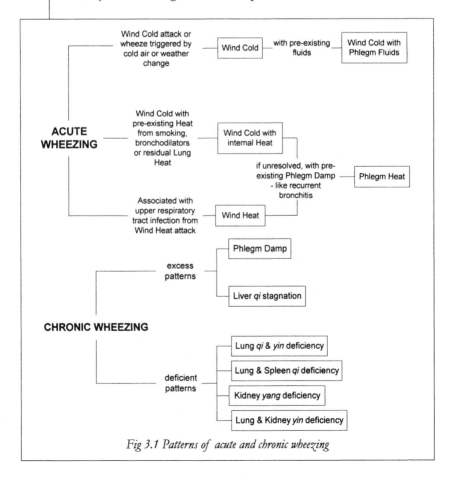

Fig 3.1 Patterns of acute and chronic wheezing

3.1 WIND COLD

风寒束肺哮喘

Pathophysiology
- Wind Cold invades the Lungs, blocking the descent of Lung *qi*, causing accumulation of *qi*, constriction of the chest and wheezing. This pattern generally occurs as an acute episode or an acute exacerbation of a chronic condition.
- The exterior symptoms noted below may not be present in every case— Wind Cold may simply penetrate the Lungs, constricting the bronchi. This corresponds to an acute attack of wheezing triggered by cold air or weather change.

Clinical features
- acute wheezing and tightness in the chest which may be triggered by cold air, cold drinks or weather changes
- cough with thin watery or frothy mucus
- simultaneous fever and chills, chills more prominent than the fever
- no sweating
- occipital or frontal headache, muscle aches, neck stiffness
- nasal obstruction, or runny nose with thin watery mucous, sneezing

T normal or with a thin white coat
P floating, or floating and tight

Treatment principle
Dispel Wind and Cold
Redirect Lung *qi* downwards, stop wheezing

Prescription

MA HUANG TANG 麻黄汤
(*Ma Huang Combination*)

This prescription is for wheezing with clear exterior signs. Generally once sweating occurs the wheezing will subside.

    ma huang* (Herba Ephedrae) 麻黄 9g
    gui zhi (Ramulus Cinnamomi Cassiae) 桂枝 6g
    chao xing ren* (dry fried Semen Pruni Armeniacae) 炒杏仁 9g
    gan cao (Radix Glycyrrhizae Uralensis) 甘草 3g
    Method: Decoction. (Source: *Shi Yong Zhong Yi Nei Ke Xue*)

Modifications
- With no clear exterior signs, delete **gui zhi** and use **zhi ma huang*** (honey fried Herba Ephedrae) 炙麻黄.
- For severe wheezing, add **su zi** (Fructus Perillae Frutescentis) 苏子 9g

and **qian hu** (Radix Peucedani) 前胡 9g.
* With copious mucus, add two or three of the following herbs: **ban xia*** (Rhizoma Pinelliae Ternatae) 半夏 9g, **chen pi** (Pericarpium Citri Reticulatae) 陈皮 6g, **tian nan xing*** (Rhizoma Arisaematis) 天南星 6g or **bai jie zi** (Semen Sinapsis Albae) 白芥子 6g.
* With severe fullness and stuffiness in the chest, add **jie geng** (Radix Platycodi Grandiflori) 桔梗 9g, **zhi ke** (Fructus Citri Aurantii) 枳壳 9g and **zi su geng** (Ramulus Perillae Frutescentis) 紫苏梗 9g.

Variations and additional prescriptions
* If the wheezing is not relieved following sweating, use **GUI ZHI JIA HOU PO XING REN TANG** (*Cinnamon, Magnolia and Apricot Seed Combination* 桂枝厚朴杏仁汤) to harmonise *ying wei*, redirect *qi* downwards and alleviate wheezing.

  gui zhi (Ramulus Cinnamomi Cassiae) 桂枝 6g
  bai shao (Radix Paeoniae Lactiflora) 白芍 12g
  chao xing ren* (dry fried Semen Pruni Armeniacae) 炒杏仁 ... 10g
  hou po (Cortex Magnoliae Officinalis) 厚朴 9g
  sheng jiang (Rhizoma Zingiberis Officinalis Recens) 生姜 3g
  da zao (Fructus Zizyphi Jujubae) 大枣 3g
  zhi gan cao (honey fried Radix Glycyrrhizae Uralensis) 炙甘草 3g
  Method: Decoction. (Source: *Shi Yong Zhong Yi Nei Ke Xue*)

* In patients with significant *qi* deficiency, **ma huang** and **gui zhi** may be too dispersing. An alternative prescription that supports *qi* is **SHEN SU YIN** (*Ginseng and Perilla Combination* 参苏饮, p.21).

Patent medicines
Xiao Qing Long Wan 小青龙丸 (Xiao Qing Long Wan)
Gan Mao Qing Re Chong Ji 感冒清热冲剂 (Gan Mao Qing Re Chong Ji)
Gan Mao Zhi Ke Chong Ji 感冒止咳冲剂 (Gan Mao Zhi Ke Chong Ji)

Acupuncture
ding chuan (M-BW-1), LI.4 (*he gu* -), Lu.7 (*lie que* -),Bl.12 (*feng men* -Ω), Bl.13 (*fei shu* -Ω), GB.20 (*feng chi* -), Lu.5 (*chi ze* -), Ren.22 (*tian tu* -), Ren.17 (*shan zhong* -)
  • If the nose is congested or runny add Du.23 (*shang xing*)

Clinical notes
• See 3.2 Wind Cold with Phlegm Fluids, p.125.

3.2 WIND COLD WITH PHLEGM FLUIDS

Pathophysiology
- In this pattern Wind Cold invades the Lungs and stirs up chronic pre-existing Phlegm in the chest. The Wind Cold and Phlegm block the descent of Lung *qi*, which accumulates in the chest, causing wheezing. This pattern is generally an acute episode, or an acute exacerbation of a chronic condition.

Clinical features
In addition to the symptoms listed for the Wind Cold pattern (p.122) there are additional symptoms of:
- wheezing with expectoration of copious thin watery or stringy mucus
- orthopnoea
- cough
- copious thin watery nasal discharge
- excessive lacrimation

Treatment principle
Warm the Lungs and disperse Cold
Warm and transform Phlegm Fluids, stop wheezing

Prescription

XIAO QING LONG TANG 小青龙汤
(*Minor Blue Dragon Combination*)

ma huang* (Herba Ephedra) 麻黄	9g
gui zhi (Ramulus Cinnamomi Cassiae) 桂枝	9g
wu wei zi (Fructus Schizandrae Chinensis) 五味子	9g
bai shao (Radix Paeoniae Lactiflora) 白芍	9g
ban xia* (Rhizoma Pinelliae Ternatae) 半夏	9g
zhi gan cao (honey fried Radix Glycyrrhizae Uralensis) 炙甘草	9g
gan jiang (Rhizoma Zingiberis Officinalis) 干姜	3g
xi xin* (Herba cum Radice Asari) 细辛	3g

Method: Decoction to be taken hot. (Source: *Shi Yong Zhong Yi Nei Ke Xue*)

Modifications
- With severe wheezing, add **xing ren*** (Semen Pruni Armeniacae) 杏仁 9g, **she gan** (Rhizoma Belamcandae) 射干 9g, **qian hu** (Radix Peucedani) 前胡 9g and **zi wan** (Radix Asteris Tatarici) 紫菀 9g.
- With Heat, add **shi gao** (Gypsum) 石膏 18g and **lu gen** (Rhizoma Phragmitis Communis) 芦根 18g.
- If Phlegm Fluids are very copious, with marked congestion and

orthopnoea, combine with **TING LI DA ZAO XIE FEI TANG** (*Descurainia and Jujube Decoction to Drain the Lungs* 葶苈大枣泻肺汤).
   ting li zi (Semen Descurainiae seu Lepidii) 葶苈子 9-12g
   da zao (Fructus Zizyphi Jujubae) 大枣 12pce
   Method: Decoction. (Source: *Shi Yong Zhong Yi Nei Ke Xue*)

Variations and additional prescriptions

♦ Phlegm Fluids may accumulate due to a failure of Spleen and Kidney *yang* to transform fluids. After the acute phase has resolved, formulae to strengthen the Spleen and Kidneys and transform fluids, such as **LING GUI ZHU GAN TANG** (*Atractylodes and Hoelen Combination* 苓桂术甘汤, p.818), **LIU JUN ZI TANG** (*Six Major Herbs Combination* 六君子汤, p.88), **JIN KUI SHEN QI WAN** (*Rehmannia Eight Formula* 金匮肾气丸, p.150), should be used to consolidate the treatment.

With Heart and Kidney yang *deficiency*

♦ When Heart and Kidney *yang* deficiency give rise to Phlegm Fluids, causing pulmonary oedema with wheezing, orthopnoea and frothy mucus, the correct treatment is to warm *yang* and promote urination with **ZHEN WU TANG** (*True Warrior Decoction* 真武汤, p.103).

Patent medicines

Xiao Qing Long Wan 小青龙丸 (Xiao Qing Long Wan)
Gan Mao Qing Re Chong Ji 感冒清热冲剂 (Gan Mao Qing Re Chong Ji)
Gan Mao Zhi Ke Chong Ji 感冒止咳冲剂 (Gan Mao Zhi Ke Chong Ji)

Acupuncture

ding quan (M-BW-1), Bl.12 (*feng men* -Ω), Bl.13 (*fei shu* -Ω), SP.3 (*tai bai* -), ST.40 (*feng long* -), Lu.7 (*lie que* -), Lu.6 (*kong zui* -), PC.6 (*nei guan*), Ren.17 (*shan zhong*)
   • with orthopnoea from fluid in the Lungs, add St.28 (*shui dao* - ▲) and Ren.9 (*shui fen* ▲)

Clinical notes

• The wheezing in Wind Cold patterns may be diagnosed as biomedical conditions such as acute bronchitis, acute exacerbation of chronic bronchitis, asthmatic bronchitis, common cold, influenza, hayfever or congestive cardiac failure.
• The acute symptoms respond well to correct and timely treatment. Depending on the reason for the accumulated Phlegm Fluids (Spleen, Kidney or Heart *yang* deficiency), treatment of the root may be prolonged, but generally responds well.

3.3 WIND COLD WITH INTERNAL HEAT

外寒里热哮喘

Pathophysiology
- If a Wind Cold attack occurs in someone with a pre-existing internal Heat (whether from *yang* excess, *yin* deficiency, Phlegm accumulation or smoking), then wheezing and chest constriction can occur with accompanying signs of Heat. This pattern may progress to a Phlegm Heat pattern in patients with pre-existing Phlegm.
- In some cases, although there is no obvious pre-existing internal Heat, it can be generated by the intense struggle between a strong pathogen and robust *zheng qi*. This produces pronounced and severe symptoms.

Clinical features
- acute wheezing with fullness or tightness in the chest
- fever and chills (or even rigors)
- loud cough with sticky yellow mucus
- no sweating or mild sweating
- muscle aches
- nasal obstruction
- occipital headache
- thirst with desire for cold liquids
- sore throat
- irritability and restlessness
- dry stools or constipation

T red or with a red tip and edges, and a thin white or yellow coat
P floating and tight, and possibly rapid

Treatment principle
Redirect Lung *qi* downward, stop wheezing
Dispel external Cold, clear internal Heat, transform Phlegm

Prescription
DING CHUAN TANG 定喘汤
(*Stop Wheezing Decoction*)

bai guo* (Semen Ginko Bilobae) 白果	12g
zhi ma huang* (honey fried Herba Ephedrae) 炙麻黄	9g
su zi (Fructus Perillae Frutescentis) 苏子	9g
ban xia* (Rhizoma Pinelliae Ternatae) 半夏	9g
kuan dong hua (Flos Tussilaginis Farfarae) 款冬花	9g
chao xing ren* (dry fried Semen Pruni Armeniacae) 炒杏仁	9g
sang bai pi (Cortex Mori Albae Radicis) 桑白皮	9g
huang qin (Radix Scutellariae Baicalensis) 黄芩	6g

jie geng (Radix Platycodi Grandiflori) 桔梗 3g
Method: Decoction. (Source: *Shi Yong Zhong Yao Xue*)

Modifications
♦ If there is no sweating (i.e. Wind Cold locking the pores shut), use unprocessed (*sheng* 生) **ma huang**.*

Patent medicines
Ding Chuan Wan 定喘丸 (Ding Chuan Wan)
Ma Xing Zhi Ke Pian 麻杏止咳片 (Ma Hsing Chih Ke Pien)
Chuan Ke Ling 喘咳灵 (Chuan Ke Ling)

Acupuncture
Du.14 (*da zhui* -Ω), ding chuan (M-BW-1), Bl.12 (*feng men* -Ω), LI.11 (*qu chi* -), LI.4 (*he gu* -), Lu.5 (*chi ze* -), SJ.5 (*wai guan* -), Ren.17 (*shan zhong*),
• If the throat is very sore and swollen add Lu.11 (*shao shang* ↓) and SI.17 (*tian rong* -)
• with much internal Heat add SJ.2 (*ye men* -), Lu.10 (*yu ji* -)

Clinical notes
• The wheezing in Wind Cold with internal Heat patterns may be diagnosed as biomedical conditions such as common cold, upper respiratory tract infection, acute asthma, acute bronchitis, pneumonia and whooping cough.
• The acute symptoms respond well to prompt and correct treatment.

3.4 WIND HEAT

风热犯肺哮喘

Pathophysiology
- Wind Heat invades the Lungs blocking the descent of Lung *qi*, causing acute wheezing and chest tightness. It commonly progresses to the Phlegm Heat type (an interior pattern, p.135), particularly when there is pre-existing Phlegm Damp.

Clinical features
- acute wheezing and cough with scant, sticky yellow, hard to expectorate mucus
- fullness or tightness in the chest
- mild fever with little or no chills
- thirst
- nasal obstruction, or a thick and yellow or green nasal discharge
- sore, dry or scratchy throat
- mild sweating
- headache (usually frontal)

T normal or red tipped with a thin white or yellow coat
P floating and rapid

Treatment principle
Expel Wind and Heat, clear Lung Heat
Redirect Lung *qi* downwards, stop wheezing

Prescription

SANG JU YIN 桑菊饮
(*Morus and Chrysanthemum Formula*) modified

This prescription is suitable for milder wheezing with more signs of Wind Heat.

sang ye (Folium Mori Albae) 桑叶	12g
ju hua (Flos Chrysanthemi Morifolii) 菊花	9g
lu gen (Rhizoma Phragmitis Communis) 芦根	15g
jin yin hua (Flos Lonicerae Japonicae) 金银花	12g
lian qiao (Fructus Forsythia Suspensae) 连翘	9g
chao xing ren* (dry fried Semen Pruni Armeniacae) 炒杏仁	9g
jie geng (Radix Platycodi Grandiflori) 桔梗	9g
ban lan gen (Radix Isatidis seu Baphicacanthi) 板蓝根	9g
sang bai pi (Cortex Mori Albae Radicis) 桑白皮	9g
bo he (Herba Mentha Haplocalycis) 薄荷	6g
huang qin (Radix Scutellariae Baicalensis) 黄芩	6g

gan cao (Radix Glycyrrhizae Uralensis) 甘草 3g
Method: Decoction. Cook for 20 minutes only. **Bo he** is added near the end of cooking (*hou xia* 后下). (Source: *Shi Yong Zhong Yi Nei Ke Xue*)

MA XING SHI GAN TANG 麻杏石甘汤
(*Ma Huang, Apricot Seed, Gypsum and Licorice Combination*) modified

This prescription is used when wheezing is more severe and there are fewer signs of Wind, and more of Lung Heat.

zhi ma huang* (honey fried Herba Ephedrae) 炙麻黄 9g
chao xing ren* (dry fried Semen Pruni Armeniacae)
炒杏仁 9g
shi gao (Gypsum) 石膏 30g
gan cao (Radix Glycyrrhizae Uralensis) 甘草 3g
sang ye (Folium Mori Albae) 桑叶 15g
gua lou (Fructus Trichosanthis) 瓜楼 15g
ju hua (Flos Chrysanthemi Morifolii) 菊花 12g
ma dou ling* (Fructus Aristolochiae) 马兜铃 12g
huang qin (Radix Scutellariae Baicalensis) 黄芩 9g
Method: Decoction. **Shi gao** is cooked for 30 minutes before the other herbs (*xian jian* 先煎). (Source: *Zhong Yi Nei Ke Lin Chuang Shou Ce*)

QING ZAO JIU FEI TANG 清燥救肺汤
(*Eriobotrya and Ophiopogon Combination*)

If the Heat is severe enough to dry out the Lungs and damage Lung *yin*, this can give rise to wheezing, a frequent hacking non-productive cough, fullness and pain in the chest and behind the sternum, headache, haemoptysis, parched throat, and a dry tongue without coat. This formula moistens Dryness, clears Heat and nourishes Lung *yin*.

shi gao (Gypsum) 石膏 18-30g
sang ye (Folium Mori Albae) 桑叶 9g
xing ren* (Semen Pruni Armeniacae) 杏仁 9g
mai dong (Tuber Ophiopogonis Japonici) 麦冬 9g
hei zhi ma (Semen Sesami Indici) 黑芝麻 9g
zhi pi pa ye (honey fried Folium Eriobotryae) 炙枇杷叶 9g
nan sha shen (Radix Adenophorae seu Glehniae) 南沙参 9g
e jiao^ (Gelatinum Corii Asini) 阿胶 6g
gan cao (Radix Glycyrrhizae Uralensis) 甘草 3g
Method: Decoction. **E jiao** is is melted before being added to the strained decoction (*yang hua* 烊化). Source: *Shi Yong Zhong Yao Xue*)

Modifications
♦ With sore throat, add **she gan** (Rhizoma Belamcandae) 射干 9g.

- With epistaxis, mild haemoptysis or blood streaked mucus add **bai mao gen** (Rhizoma Imperatae Cylindricae) 白茅根 12g and **ou jie** (Nodus Nelumbinis Nuciferae) 藕节 9g. See also Haemoptysis, p.187.
- With constipation, add **da huang** (Radix et Rhizoma Rhei) 大黄 3-6g.

Patent medicines
Ding Chuan Wan 定喘丸 (Ding Chuan Wan)
Yin Qiao Jie Du Pian 银翘解毒片 (Yin Chiao Chieh Tu Pien)
Qing Fei Yi Huo Pian 清肺抑火片 (Ching Fei Yi Huo Pien)
Chuan Xin Lian Kang Yan Pian 穿心莲抗炎片
   (Chuan Xin Lian Antiphlogistic Tablets)
Qing Qi Hua Tan Wan 清气化痰丸 (Pinellia Expectorant Pills)
Ma Xing Zhi Ke Pian 麻杏止咳片 (Ma Hsing Chih Ke Pien)

Acupuncture
ding quan (M-BW-1), Du.14 (*da zhui* - Ω), Bl.12 (*feng men* - Ω), Lu.1 (*zhong fu* -), Ren.17 (*shan zhong* -), LI.11 (*qu chi* -), LI.4 (*he gu* -), Lu.5 (*chi ze* -), SJ.5 (*wai guan* -)
- If the throat is very sore and swollen add Lu.11 (*shao shang* ↓) and SI.17 (*tian rong* -)

Clinical notes
- The wheezing in Wind Heat patterns may be diagnosed as biomedical conditions such as bronchitis, acute asthma, upper respiratory tract infection, bronchitis, asthmatic bronchitis, pneumonia and whooping cough.
- This pattern responds well to correct treatment (especially in the early stages).

3.5 PHLEGM DAMP

痰湿壅肺哮喘

Pathophysiology
- Phlegm Damp wheezing is a chronic pattern usually associated with inappropriate diet and/or recurrent respiratory tract infections.
- Infections like bronchitis, sinusitis and tonsillitis are usually treated with multiple courses of antibiotics. Antibiotics, which are very Cold in nature, are good at cooling Heat (and killing microbes), but they damage Spleen *yang* and do disperse all the pathogenic factors. Therefore, pathogenic Phlegm remains in the Lungs, a situation which is then aggravated by the now impaired Spleen function. This sets the stage for further respiratory infections and courses of antibiotics creating a self-perpetuating cycle.
- A Phlegm generating diet (especially one rich in dairy products) can also predispose to Phlegm Damp type of wheezing.
- This pattern is not uncommon in children with a modern diet of take away food and too much ice cream. It is often these same children who suffer frequent upper respiratory tract or ear infections and take many courses of antibiotics.
- In general, this is a mixed excess (Phlegm Damp) and deficiency (Spleen and Lung) pattern. The long term success of treatment depends on ascertaining their relative balance.
- Because of its obstructing quality, Phlegm Damp may periodically generate Heat, causing acute Phlegm Heat wheeze (p.135).

Clinical features
- wheezing and cough with copious thick, sticky, hard to expectorate white or clear mucus; there is a noticeable rattle in the chest with the wheeze and it tends to be worse in the morning and after eating
- fullness, tightness and stuffiness in the chest
- poor appetite
- nausea or vomiting
- loose stools
- lethargy and weakness

T pale and swollen with toothmarks and a thick, moist, greasy white coat
P soft and slippery

Treatment principle
Transform Phlegm, stop wheeze
Strengthen the Spleen, dry Damp

Prescription

SAN ZI YANG QIN TANG 三子养亲汤
(*Three Seed Decoction to Nourish One's Parents*) plus
ER CHEN TANG 二陈汤
(*Citrus and Pinellia Combination*) modified

su zi (Fructus Perillae Frutescentis) 苏子	12g
bai jie zi (Semen Sinapsis Albae) 白芥子	10g
lai fu zi (Semen Raphani Sativi) 莱服子	10g
ban xia* (Rhizoma Pinelliae Ternatae) 半夏	15g
chen pi (Pericarpium Citri Reticulatae) 陈皮	10g
fu ling (Sclerotium Poriae Cocos) 茯苓	15g
cang zhu (Rhizoma Atractylodis) 苍术	10g
hou po (Cortex Magnoliae Officinalis) 厚朴	10g

Method: Decoction. (Source: *Shi Yong Zhong Yi Nei Ke Xue*)

Modifications

- With very copious Phlegm and severe wheezing causing the patient difficulty with lying flat (orthopnoea), add **ting li zi** (Semen Descurainiae seu Lepidii) 葶苈子 10g and **da huang** (Radix et Rhizoma Rhei) 大黄 6g.
- With Cold (aversion to cold, watery mucus, cold extremities, chilliness) add **xi xin*** (Herba cum Radice Asari) 细辛 3g and **gan jiang** (Rhizoma Zingiberis Officinalis) 干姜 6g.
- With mild Heat, add one or two of the following herbs: **huang qin** (Radix Scutellariae Baicalensis) 黄芩 6g, **gua lou ren** (Semen Trichosanthis) 瓜楼仁 12g, **sang bai pi** (Cortex Mori Albae Radicis) 桑白皮 9g, **dan nan xing*** (Pulvis Arisaemae cum Felle Bovis) 胆南星 6g or **hai ge ke**ˆ (Concha Cyclinae Sinensis) 海蛤壳 6g.
- With mild signs of Spleen deficiency, add **dang shen** (Radix Codonopsis Pilosulae) 党参 15g, **yi ren** (Semen Coicis Lachryma-jobi) 苡仁 20g and **bai zhu** (Rhizoma Atractylodis Macrocephalae) 白术 9g.

Variations and additional prescriptions

Lung and Spleen qi *deficiency with Phlegm Damp*
- If the Spleen deficiency appears to be primary (i.e. with significant digestive weakness, and thus the source of the ongoing Phlegm) the emphasis of treatment is first to strengthen the Spleen and second to resolve Phlegm. The formula is **LIU JUN ZI TANG** (*Six Major Herbs Combination* 六君子汤) modified.

ren shen (Radix Ginseng) 人参	9g
bai zhu (Rhizoma Atractylodis Macrocephalae) 白术	12g
fu ling (Sclerotium Poriae Cocos) 茯苓	12g

gan cao (Radix Glycyrrhizae Uralensis) 甘草 6g
ban xia* (Rhizoma Pinelliae Ternatae) 半夏 9g
chen pi (Pericarpium Citri Reticulatae) 陈皮 6g
cang zhu (Rhizoma Atractylodis) 苍术 9g
hou po (Cortex Magnoliae Officinalis) 厚朴 9g
su zi (Fructus Perillae Fructescentis) 苏子 9g
Method: Decoction. (Source: *Shi Yong Zhong Yi Nei Ke Xue*)

Chronic or recurrent Cold Phlegm Damp accumulation
- In older patients and children with chronic 'asthma' (see also appendix, p157), Phlegm Damp, Cold and Kidney deficiency combine to produce a pattern that recurs every Winter. In this pattern, there are repeated attacks of productive cough with thin watery mucus, usually triggered by a Cold invasion during the Winter months. Wheezing, breathlessness and tightness in the chest are common, particularly at night and early in the morning. The mucus may also be scanty and tenacious. In severe cases there is orthopnoea. There may also be lower back and leg pain and weakness, fatigue, and oedema of the extremities. The treatment is to redirect *qi* downward, stop cough and wheezing, and warm and transform Cold Phlegm. The guiding formula is **SU ZI JIANG QI TANG** (*Perilla Fruit Combination* 苏子降气汤).

su zi (Fructus Perillae Fructescentis) 苏子 12g
ban xia* (Rhizoma Pinelliae Ternatae) 半夏 9g
dang gui (Radix Angelicae Sinensis) 当归 9g
zhi gan cao (honey fried Radix Glycyrrhizae Uralensis)
炙甘草 3g
hou po (Cortex Magnoliae Officinalis) 厚朴 6g
chen pi (Pericarpium Citri Reticulatae) 陈皮 6g
qian hu (Radix Peucedani) 前胡 9g
rou gui (Cortex Cinnamomi Cassiae) 肉桂 3g
sheng jiang (Rhizoma Zingiberis Officinalis Recens) 生姜 6g
da zao (Fructus Zizyphi Jujubae) 大枣 3pce
Method: Grind the herbs to a fine powder and take 6-grams as a draft, 2-3 times daily. May also be decocted, in which case powdered **rou gui** is added to the strained decoction (*chong fu* 冲服). (Source: *Formulas and Strategies*)

Patent medicines
Su Zi Jiang Qi Wan 苏子降气丸 (Su Zi Jiang Qi Wan)
Er Chen Wan 二陈丸 (Er Chen Wan)
Qi Guan Yan Ke Sou Tan Chuan Wan 气管炎咳嗽痰喘丸
  (Cough and Phlegm Pills)
Ping Wei San 平胃散 (Ping Wei San)
She Dan Chuan Bei Ye 蛇胆川贝液 (She Dan Chuan Bei Ye)

Acupuncture

Bl.13 (*fei shu* ▲), Bl.20 (*pi shu* ▲), Lu.9 (*tai yuan* -), Sp.3 (*tai bai* +), St.40 (*feng long* -), *ding chuan* (M-BW-1), Lu.1 (*zhong fu* -), Ren.17 (*shan zhong* -), Lu.7 (*lie que* -), Ren.12 (*zhong wan* -), Ren.22 (*tian tu* -)

- with fullness in the chest, add PC.5 (*jian shi*)

Clinical notes

- The wheezing in Phlegm Damp patterns may be diagnosed as biomedical conditions such as chronic bronchitis, bronchiectasis, emphysema and asthma.
- This pattern generally responds well to correct and prolonged treatment.
- Dietary modification, in particular reduction of dairy products, sugar, greasy rich foods and in some people, wheat, is essential for good results. In elderly patients and children with recurrent Cold Phlegm, prolonged treatment is needed for satisfactory results.

3.6 PHLEGM HEAT

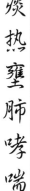

Pathophysiology
- Phlegm Heat can accumulate in the Lungs after invasion by Wind Heat (or Cold) which dries and congeals Lung Fluids.
- It may also develop from a chronic Phlegm Damp Lung condition, especially in those with a hot constitution or after excess consumption of heat inducing substances.
- Phlegm Heat in the Lungs is usualy an acute condition, but occasionally some residual Phlegm Heat will linger, causing low grade chronic wheezing with persistent coloured mucus. In such cases, in addition to clearing the Phlegm Heat, the Spleen and Lung may need to be strengthened.

Clinical features
- wheezing and cough that tends to be worse at night and first thing in the morning, with profuse thick, yellow or green, hard to expectorate mucus; in some cases there may be blood streaked mucus
- fullness, tightness, stuffiness and burning in the chest
- red complexion
- bitter taste in the mouth, dry mouth
- nausea, loss of appetite
- loose stools or constipation
- lethargy and weakness
- maybe a sore or congested throat

T thick, greasy, yellow coat, although maybe only on the root
P soft or slippery and rapid

Treatment principle
Expel Phlegm and clear Heat
Redirect Lung *qi* downward, stop wheezing

Prescription

MA XING SHI GAN TANG 麻杏石甘汤
(Ma Huang, Apricot Seed, Gypsum and Licorice Combination) modified

zhi ma huang* (honey fried Herba Ephedrae) 炙麻黄	9g
chao xing ren* (dry fried Semen Pruni Armeniacae) 炒杏仁	9g
shi gao (Gypsum) 石膏	30g
gan cao (Radix Glycyrrhizae Uralensis) 甘草	3g
yi ren (Semen Coicis Lachryma-jobi) 苡仁	15g
dong gua ren (Semen Benincasae Hispidae) 冬瓜仁	15g
lu gen (Rhizoma Phragmitis Communis) 芦根	15g

di long^ (Lumbricus) 地龙 6g

Method: Decoction. **Shi gao** is cooked for 30 minutes before the other herbs (*xian jian* 先煎). (Source: *Shi Yong Zhong Yi Nei Ke Xue*)

Modifications

- When Heat is severe, add two or three of the following herbs: **huang qin** (Radix Scutellariae Baicalensis) 黄芩 12g, **da qing ye** (Folium Daqingye) 大青叶 12g, **ban lan gen** (Radix Isatidis seu Baphicacanthi) 板蓝根 12g or **huang lian** (Rhizoma Coptidis) 黄连 6g.
- With severe wheezing and profuse mucus, add **she gan** (Rhizoma Belamacandae) 射干 9g, **sang bai pi** (Cortex Mori Albae Radicis) 桑白皮 12g and **ting li zi** (Semen Descurainiae seu Lepidii) 葶苈子 9g.
- With constipation, add **da huang** (Radix et Rhizoma Rhei) 大黄 3-6g and **gua lou ren** (Semen Trichosanthis) 瓜楼仁 12g. In this condition it is very important to keep the bowels open.
- During the convalescent stage of this condition, the patient often has considerable nightsweats, residual hard-to-expectorate mucus and fatigue due to the Heat damaging Lung *yin*. In this case add **di gu pi** (Cortex Lycii Chinensis) 地骨皮 12g and **qing hao** (Herba Artemesiae Apiaceae) 青蒿 12g. See also *fei yong* (Lung Abscess), p.114.

Variations and additional prescriptions

Chronic Phlegm Heat

- In chronic cases, the Phlegm Heat is persistent and the systemic symptoms are generally mild or absent. The main features are frequent expectoration of yellow mucus, throat clearing and clearly audible rattles and rales with breathing. There may be digestive or bowel disturbances, depending on the degree of Spleen involvement. The treatment principle is to root out residual Phlegm Heat with the following formula **ER CHEN TANG** (*Citrus and Pinellia Combination* 二陈汤) modified.

ban xia* (Rhizoma Pinelliae Ternatae) 半夏 9g
chen pi (Pericarpium Citri Reticulatae) 陈皮 9g
fu ling (Sclerotium Poriae Cocos) 茯苓 12g
gan cao (Radix Glycyrrhizae Uralensis) 甘草 6g
gua lou (Fructus Trichosanthis) 瓜楼 18g
zhu ru (Caulis Bambusae in Taeniis) 竹茹 9g
huang qin (Radix Scutellariae Baicalensis) 黄芩 9g

Method: Decoction. Once the Phlegm is resolved, a Spleen strengthening formula such as **LIU JUN ZI TANG** (*Six Major Herbs Combination*, p.88), can be used to consolidate the effect. (Source: *Shi Yong Fang Ji Xue*)

Wheezing associated with food stagnation or food intolerances
- In some patients wheezing may be induced by overeating or by certain foods. The wheezing in these cases is associated with obstruction to the natural descent of both Stomach and Lung *qi*, and typically the patient will have obvious digestive symptoms (especially bloating or constipation) associated with wheezing episodes. When wheezing is related to food stagnation or Phlegm Heat in the Stomach the correct treatment is to redirect Lung and Stomach *qi* downward, transform Phlegm and stop wheezing with **BAO HE WAN** (*Citrus and Crategus Formula* 保和丸) modified.

    chao shan zha (dry fried Fructus Crategi) 炒山楂 180g
    shen qu (massa Fermentata) 神曲 60g
    ban xia* (Rhizoma Pinelliae Ternatae) 半夏 90g
    fu ling (Sclerotium Poriae Cocos) 茯苓 90g
    chen pi (Pericarpium Citri Reticulatae) 陈皮 30g
    lai fu zi (Semen Raphani Sativi) 莱服子 30g
    lian qiao (Fructus Forsythia Suspensae) 连翘 30g
    da huang (Radix et Rhizoma Rhei) 大黄 20g

    Method: Grind the herbs to a powder and form into 9-gram pills with honey. Take one pill 2-3 times daily. (Source: *Shi Yong Zhong Yao Xue*)

Patent medicines
Qing Qi Hua Tan Wan 清气化痰丸 (Pinellia Expectorant Pills)
Qing Fei Yi Huo Pian 清肺抑火片 (Ching Fei Yi Huo Pien)
Ding Chuan Wan 定喘丸 (Ding Chuan Wan)
She Dan Chuan Bei Ye 蛇胆川贝液 (She Dan Chuan Bei Ye)

Acupuncture
Lu.5 (*chi ze* -), *ding chuan* (M-BW-1), St.40 (*feng long* -), Lu.6 (*kong zui* -), Lu.1 (*zhong fu* -), LI.11 (*qu chi* -), Bl.13 (*fei shu* -), Lu.10 (*yu ji* -), Ren.17 (*shan zhong*)
- with fullness in the chest add PC.5 (*jian shi*)

Clinical notes
- The wheezing in Phlegm Heat patterns may be diagnosed as biomedical conditions such as acute and chronic bronchitis, bronchiectasis, pneumonia, whooping cough, asthma, food allergy
- This pattern generally responds well to correct treatment, plus avoidance of heating foods and tobacco. In severe cases, especially in the elderly, frail or debilitated, concurrent use of antibiotics may be necessary to quickly cool the Heat. Herbs and acupuncture support the swift action of the antibiotics, and finish the job by clearing residual Phlegm, strengthening resistance and nourishing damaged *yin*.

3.7 LIVER *QI* STAGNATION DAMAGING THE LUNGS

肝气犯肺哮喘

Pathophysiology
- When *qi* stagnates in the Liver it can rebel backwards along the controlling (*ke* 克, p.70) cycle and disrupt the descent of Lung *qi*. Lung *qi* accumulates and the breath becomes shallow. In addition, the stagnation of *qi* in the Liver channel (which traverses the chest) and organ (which lies directly beneath the diaphragm) causes a sensation of tightness in the chest and difficulty in drawing a full breath.

Clinical features
- Tightness in the chest, dyspnoea, wheezing, shortness of breath, difficulty getting a deep and satisfying breath, with little or no mucus, clearly related to emotion. The sensation is generally described as 'tightness' or 'fullness' in the chest. During an episode the patient is often panicky or emotional.
- frequent sighing
- plum stone throat
- poor appetite
- insomnia
- palpitations
- vague chest pain
- premenstrual syndrome, irregular menstruation, breast tenderness

T unremarkable, or with brown or purplish stasis spots on the edges and a thin white coat
P wiry

Treatment principle
Move Liver *qi*, redirect Lung *qi* downwards, stop wheezing

Prescription

WU MO YIN ZI 五磨饮子
(*Five Milled Herb Decoction*)

This formula is good for acute episodes of chest tightness due to stagnant Liver *qi* in robust patients.

wu yao (Radix Linderae Strychnifoliae) 乌药 9g
zhi shi (Fructus Citri Aurantii Immaturus) 枳实 9g
bing lang (Semen Arecae Catechu) 槟榔 9g
mu xiang (Radix Aucklandiae Lappae) 木香 6g
chen xiang (Lignum Aquilariae) 沉香 6g

Method: Grind the herbs to a powder and take a tablespoon as a draft with warm water 2-3 times daily. May also be decocted. (Source: *Zhong Yi Nei Ke Lin Chuang Shou Ce*)

Modifications

- If the patient's constitution is weak, delete **mu xiang** and **zhi shi** and add **ren shen** (Panax Ginseng) 人参 9g.
- With insomnia and palpitations, add **suan zao ren** (Semen Zizyphi Spinosae) 酸枣仁 15g, **yuan zhi** (Radix Polygalae Tenuifoliae) 远志 6g and **bai zi ren** (Semen Biotae Orientalis) 柏子仁 12g.
- If the chest and hypochondriac region are distended and full, or painful and aching, add **chai hu** (Radix Bupleuri) 柴胡 10g and **zhi xiang fu** (prepared Rhizoma Cyperi Rotundi) 制香附 10g.
- If there are elements of hysterical wheezing, add **GAN MAI DA ZAO TANG** (*Licorice and Jujube Combination* 甘麦大枣汤), which consists of **xiao mai** (Semen Triticum) 小麦 60g, **gan cao** (Radix Glycyrrhizae Uralensis) 甘草 10g and **da zao** (Fructus Zizyphi Jujubae) 大枣 6g. This is a common formula for mental and emotional disorders.

XIAO YAO SAN 逍遥散
(*Bupleurum and Dang Gui Formula*)

This formula is suitable for recurrent mild episodes, and for those with Blood deficiency. A good formula for soothing Liver *qi* generally, and particularly in between episodes.

    chai hu (Radix Bupleuri) 柴胡 9g
    dang gui (Radix Angelicae Sinensis) 当归 9g
    bai shao (Radix Paeoniae Lactiflorae) 白芍 9g
    bai zhu (Rhizoma Atractylodis Macrocephalae) 白术 9g
    fu ling (Sclerotium Poria Cocos) 茯苓 9g
    zhi gan cao (honey fried Radix Glycyrrhizae Uralensis) 炙甘草 6g
    wei jiang (roasted Rhizoma Zingiberis Officinalis) 煨姜 6g
    bo he (Herba Mentha Haplocalycis) 薄荷 3g

Method: Decoction or pills. In decoction, **bo he** is added a few minutes before the end of cooking (*hou xia* 后下).

Variations and additional prescriptions

Liver qi *stagnation with Heat or Fire*

- If *qi* stagnation generates Heat or Fire with wheezing or chest tightness brought on by emotions, as well as symptoms such as thirst, bitter taste in the mouth, temporal headaches, feeling hot during episodes, irritability, constipation, concentrated urine, red edges on the tongue and a rapid pulse, the correct treatment is to clear Liver Heat (Fire) and redirect Lung *qi* downwards. In severe cases (i.e. Fire), the appropriate formula is **LONG DAN XIE GAN TANG** (*Gentiana Combination* 龙胆泻肝汤, p.365). For milder cases (i.e. stagnant Heat) the correct

formula is **DAN ZHI XIAO YAO SAN** (*Bupleurum and Paeonia Formula* 丹栀逍遥散)
    chai hu (Radix Bupleuri) 柴胡 12g
    bai shao (Radix Paeoniae Lactiflora) 白芍 12g
    fu ling (Sclerotium Poriae Cocos) 茯苓 12g
    shan zhi zi (Fructus Gardeniae Jasminoidis) 山栀子 12g
    dang gui (Radix Angelicae Sinensis) 当归 10g
    bai zhi (Radix Angelicae Dahuricae) 白芷 10g
    mu dan pi (Cortex Moutan Radicis) 牡丹皮 10g
    zhi gan cao (honey fried Radix Glycyrrhizae Uralensis) 炙甘草 6g
    wei jiang (roasted Rhizoma Zingiberis Officinalis) 煨姜 6g
    bo he (Herba Mentha Haplocalycis) 薄荷 6g
    Method: Decoction or as powder. When decocted **Bo he** is added towards the end of cooking (*hou xia* 后下). Both formulae may be modified by the addition of herbs to redirect *qi* downwards and clear Lung Heat, like **sang bai pi** (Cortex Mori Albae Radicis) 桑白皮 12g and **di gu pi** (Cortex Lycii Chinensis) 地骨皮 12g.

Liver qi *and Phlegm stagnation*
* Tightness and fullness in the chest, associated with 'plum stone throat', difficulty swallowing, anxiety, a greasy white tongue coat and a slippery wiry pulse indicate Phlegm Damp and *qi* stagnation in the throat and chest. The correct treatment is to promote movement of *qi*, transform Phlegm and redirect *qi* downwards with **BAN XIA HOU PO TANG** (*Pinellia and Magnolia Combination* 半夏厚朴汤)
    ban xia* (Rhizoma Pinelliae Ternatae) 半夏 12g
    hou po (Cortex Magnoliae Officinalis) 厚朴 9g
    fu ling (Sclerotium Poriae Cocos) 茯苓 12g
    sheng jiang (Rhizoma Zingiberis Officinalis Recens) 生姜 5pce
    zi su ye (Folium Perillae Frutescentis) 紫苏叶 6g
    Method: Decoction. (Source: *Shi Yong Fang Ji Xue*)

Patent medicines
Chai Hu Shu Gan Wan 柴胡舒肝丸 (Chai Hu Shu Gan Wan)
Xiao Yao Wan 逍遥丸 (Xiao Yao Wan)
Jia Wei Xiao Yao Wan 加味逍遥丸 (Jia Wei Xiao Yao Wan)
Shu Gan Wan 舒肝丸 (Shu Gan Wan)

Acupuncture
yin tang (M-HN-3), PC.5 (*jian shi*), P.6 (*nei guan*), Liv.14 (*qi men*), Liv.5 (*li gou*), Liv.3 (*tai chong*), LI.4 (*he gu*), Ren.17 (*shan zhong*), Ren.11 (*jian li*), Bl.18 (*gan shu*), Bl.15 (*xin shu*), Bl.13 (*fei shu*)

Clinical notes

- The wheezing in Liver *qi* invading the Lungs, or Liver Heat patterns may be diagnosed as biomedical conditions such as anxiety neurosis, stress related breathing difficulties and hysteria.
- Episodes respond well to correct treatment and relaxation. Long term results require an appropriate management plan with relaxation, exercise and stress management.

肺气阴虚哮喘

3.8 LUNG *QI* AND *YIN* DEFICIENCY

Pathophysiology
- Lung *qi* and *yin* deficiency describes a chronic condition, which is the result of either long term Lung disease or the extended use of asthma medications. There are elements of Lung *qi* deficiency, i.e. *qi* which cannot descend, and *yin* deficiency, i.e. Heat. Depending on the relative balance of *qi* and *yin* deficiency, the actual presentation can vary considerably.

Clinical features
- wheezing, panting, shortness of breath–all worse with exertion
- weak cough with little or no mucus
- soft voice with little desire to talk
- spontaneous sweating
- aversion to wind, frequent colds and flu
- dry mouth
- malar or facial flushing
- occasional sore dry throat

T pale red and dry, swollen and often extensively cracked with little or no coat
P weak and soft, possibly extending up the thenar eminence

Treatment principle
Tonify and nourish Lung *qi* and *yin*
Redirect Lung *qi* downward, stop wheezing

Prescription

SHENG MAI SAN 生脉散
(*Generate the Pulse Powder*) modified

ren shen (Radix Ginseng) 人参	9g
mai dong (Tuber Ophiopogonis Japonici) 麦冬	12g
wu wei zi (Fructus Schizandrae Chinensis) 五味子	6g
sha shen (Radix Adenophorae seu Glehniae) 沙参	15g
yu zhu (Rhizoma Polygonati Odorati) 玉竹	10g
chuan bei mu (Bulbus Fritillariae Cirrhosae) 川贝母	10g
chen pi (Pericarpium Citri Reticulatae) 陈皮	10g
qian hu (Radix Peucedani) 前胡	10g
gan cao (Radix Glycyrrhizae Uralensis) 甘草	6g

Method: Grind the herbs to a powder and form into 9-gram pills with honey. Take one pill 2-3 times daily. May also be decocted. (Source: *Zhong Yi Nei Ke Lin Chuang Shou Ce*)

Modifications

- If the patient tends toward *qi* deficiency with thin watery mucus and fewer if any hot symptoms, reduce the dose of **mai dong**, **sha shen** and **yu zhu** by half, and add **huang qi** (Radix Astragali Membranacei) 黄芪 30g, **gan jiang** (Rhizoma Zingiberis Officinalis) 干姜 5g and **zhi kuan dong hua** (honey fried Flos Tussilaginis Farfarae) 炙款冬花 10g.
- If the patient tends towards *yin* deficiency, replace **ren shen** with **xi yang shen** (Panax Quinquefolium) 9g and add **huang jing** (Rhizoma Polygonati) 黄精 12g.
- For irritability and insomnia or restless fitful sleep, add **suan zao ren** (Semen Zizyphi Jujubae) 酸枣仁 10g and **he huan pi** (Cortex Albizziae Julibrissin) 合欢皮 10g.
- In atopic patients (see modifications p.151), add two or three of the following herbs: **tu si zi** (Semen Cuscutae Chinensis) 菟丝子 12g, **du zhong** (Cortex Eucommiae Ulmoidis) 杜仲 12g, **hu tao ren** (Semen Juglandis Regiae) 胡桃仁 9g and **bu gu zhi** (Fructus Psoraleae Corylifoliae) 补股脂 12g.

Patent medicines

Sheng Mai Wan 生脉丸 (Sheng Mai Wan)
Ba Xian Chang Shou Wan 八仙长寿丸 (Ba Xian Chang Shou Wan)
Bai He Gu Jin Wan 百合固金丸 (Bai He Gu Jin Wan)

Acupuncture

Bl.13 (*fei shu* +), Bl.43 (*gao huang shu* +), Lu.9 (*tai yuan* +), Lu.7 (*lie que*), Kid.6 (*zhao hai*), Bl.23 (*shen shu* +), Kid.3 (*tai xi* +), Lu.5 (*chi ze* -), St.36 (*zu san li* +)
- with severe Heat add Lu.10 (*yu ji* -) and Kid.2 (*ran gu*)

Scarring plasters

- In between episodes, a sticking plaster with a small amount of irritant herbs like **da suan** (Bulbus Alli Sativi) 大蒜 and **xi xin*** (Herba cum Radice Asari) 细辛 may be placed over points such as Du.14 (*da zhui*) or Bl.43 (*gao huang shu*) for 1-2 days, until a blister forms. This method strengthens the Lungs and *wei qi*, and is useful in chronic wheezing.

Clinical notes

- The wheezing in this pattern may be diagnosed as chronic asthma, chronic obstructive airways disease, emphysema or tuberculosis.
- This pattern often follows years of medication with bronchodilators and steroid drugs. Prolonged therapy (more than one year) while gradually reducing medication is generally necessary for a satisfactory result.

肺脾气虚哮喘

3.9 LUNG AND SPLEEN *QI* DEFICIENCY

Pathophysiology
- Lung and Spleen *qi* deficiency type wheezing is particularly common in those who have suffered repeated upper respiratory tract, ear or other infections, and who have been treated with numerous courses of antibiotics (see Phlegm Damp, p.131). It also occurs in patients with an inherited weak constitution (deficient *qi*). Such patients are often diagnosed as 'asthmatic' during an upper respiratory tract infection when their lung capacity is reduced, then medicated with bronchodilators. These medications disperse Lung *qi* relieving bronchospasm, but over time deplete Lung *qi*. When Lung *qi* is thus weakened, it will not descend properly leading to wheezing and shortness of breath.

Clinical features
- wheezing and shortness of breath that are provoked by exercise and exertion, or that occur during colds and flu; if there is coughing it is usually weak, with thin white mucus
- frequent colds
- lethargic and easily fatigued
- pale complexion
- spontaneous sweating
- soft voice or reluctance to speak
- depending on the degree of Spleen involvement there may be loose stools, poor appetite, copious mucus, 'food allergies', abdominal distension and (in children) failure to thrive

T pale with a thin to thick white coat (depending on mucus)
P thready and weak

Treatment principle
Strengthen Lung and Spleen *qi*
Consolidate *wei qi*, stop wheezing

Prescription

BU ZHONG YI QI TANG 补中益气汤
(*Ginseng and Astragalus Combination*) modified

zhi huang qi (honey fried Radix Astragali Membranacei) 炙黄芪	12g
chao bai zhu (dry fried Rhizoma Atractylodis Macrocephalae) 炒白术	9g
mai dong (Tuber Ophiopogonis Japonici) 麦冬	9g
ren shen (Radix Ginseng) 人参	6g

zhi gan cao (honey fried Radix Glycyrrhizae Uralensis)
炙甘草 6g
chen pi (Pericarpium Citri Reticulatae) 陈皮 6g
dang gui (Radix Angelicae Sinensis) 当归 6g
sheng ma (Rhizoma Cimicifugae) 升麻 6g
chai hu (Radix Bupleuri) 柴胡 6g
wu wei zi (Fructus Schizandrae Chinensis) 五味子 6g
sheng jiang (Rhizoma Zingiberis Officinalis Recens) 生姜 3pce
da zao (Fructus Zizyphi Jujubae) 大枣 3pce
Method: Decoction or powder. When powdered the dose is 5-grams three times daily. (Source: *Shi Yong Zhong Yi Nei Ke Xue*)

Modifications

- With cold extemities, delete **mai dong** and add **gan jiang** (Rhizoma Zingiberis Officinalis) 干姜 6g.
- With copious thin watery mucus, add **gan jiang** (Rhizoma Zingiberis Officinalis) 干姜 6g, **ban xia*** (Rhizoma Pinelliae Ternatae) 半夏 9g and **hou po** (Cortex Magnoliae Officinalis) 厚朴 6g.
- With spontaneous sweating, add **mu li^** (Concha Ostreae) 牡蛎 15g, **ma huang gen** (Radix Ephedrae) 麻黄根 9g and **fu xiao mai** (Semen Tritici Aestivi Levis) 浮小麦 12g.
- In atopic patients (see modifications p.151), add two or three of the following herbs: **tu si zi** (Semen Cuscutae Chinensis) 菟丝子 12g, **du zhong** (Cortex Eucommiae Ulmoidis) 杜仲 12g, **hu tao ren** (Semen Juglandis Regiae) 胡桃仁 9g or **bu gu zhi** (Fructus Psoraleae Corylifoliae) 补骨脂 12g.

Variations and additional prescriptions
Spleen deficiency with Phlegm Damp
- For obvious Spleen deficiency signs, particularly if there is copious mucus, use **LIU JUN ZI TANG** (*Six Major Herbs Combination* 六君子汤, p.88), with the addition of **gan jiang** (Rhizoma Zingiberis Officinalis) 干姜 6g, **xi xin*** (Herba cum Radice Asari) 细辛 3g and **wu wei zi** (Fructus Schizandrae Chinensis) 五味子 6g.

With Blood deficiency
- If the dyspnoea and shortness of breath occur post-partum, after menstruation or following haemorrhage, the main treatment is to first powerfully tonify *qi* and Blood with **SHI QUAN DA BU TANG** (*Ginseng and Dang Gui Ten Combination* 十全大补汤, p.529) or **DANG GUI BU XUE TANG** (*Dang Gui Blood Tonic Decoction* 当归补血汤, p.555).

Patent medicines

Bu Zhong Yi Qi Wan 补中益气丸 (Bu Zhong Yi Qi Wan)
Xiang Sha Liu Jun Zi Wan 香砂六君子丸 (Xiang Sha Liu Jun Wan)
Shen Qi Da Bu Wan 参芪大补丸 (Shen Qi Da Bu Wan)
Shi Quan Da Bu Wan 十全大补丸 (Shi Quan Da Bu Wan)
 - with Blood deficiency

Acupuncture

Bl.13 (*fei shu* +▲), Bl.43 (*gao huang shu* +▲), Lu.9 (*tai yuan* +),
Ren.6 (*qi hai* +▲), Bl.20 (*pi shu* +▲), St.36 (*zu san li* +▲),
Ren.12 (*zhong wan* +▲), Sp.6 (*san yin jiao* +)

- The points of the upper back may also be gently cupped. This method is especially useful for children and those who have difficulty with moxa smoke.

Scarring plasters

- In between episodes, a sticking plaster with a small amount of irritant herbs like **da suan** (Bulbus Alli Sativi) 大蒜 and **xi xin*** (Herba cum Radice Asari) 细辛 may be placed over points such as Du.14 (*da zhui*) or Bl.43 (*gao huang shu*) for 1-2 days, until a blister forms. This method strengthens the Lungs and *wei qi*, and is useful in chronic wheezing.

Clinical notes

- The wheezing associated with Spleen and Lung *qi* deficiency may be diagnosed as childhood asthma, immune deficiency, chronic bronchitis or emphysema.
- A common type of asthma in children, but also occurs in adults. The wheezing in this pattern may be associated with digestive or food intolerance.
- Generally responds well to correct treatment, particularly when combined with appropriate dietary changes (see p.157).

3.10 LUNG AND KIDNEY *YIN* DEFICIENCY

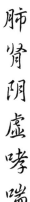

Pathophysiology
- Lung and Kidney *yin* deficiency wheezing is usually the result of chronic Lung disease, smoking or many years of medication for asthma, particularly steroids. When the Lungs and Kidneys are so damaged, the force for pulling the breath in and expelling it again is very weak and there is chronic or constant difficulty in breathing.

Clinical features
- Chronic wheezing that is often severe and may in some cases be constant, requiring ever increasing levels of medication. Typically, patients with this pattern are often hospitalised with severe attacks. There is little if any mucus and the wheezing tends to be worse at night. The accessory muscles are often well developed causing a barrel chest and thick neck.
- tightness and fullness in the chest
- malar or facial flushing
- night sweats
- heat intolerance
- warm dry skin
- dry mouth and throat
- chronic sore throat
- finger clubbing
- large red skin reaction to needles or finger pressure
- may be kyphosis of the upper back due to collapse of osteoporotic vertebrae as a result of years of oral steroids
- in patients medicated with oral steroids during childhood, there may be small stature

T red and dry with no coat. It may be so denuded of papillae as to look like fresh liver (a mirror tongue)

P thready and rapid (although steroids may make it feel fuller), extending up the thenar eminence

Treatment principle
Nourish and moisten Lung *yin*
Clear Heat, stop wheezing

Prescription

BAI HE GU JIN TANG 百合固金汤
(*Lily Combination*)

This formua is selected when Lung *yin* deficiency is primary.
bai he (Bulbus Lilii) 百合 12-24g

shu di (Radix Rehmanniae Glutinosae Conquitae) 熟地 15g
sheng di (Radix Rehmanniae Glutinosae) 生地 12g
mai dong (Tuber Ophiopogonis Japonici) 麦冬 9g
xuan shen (Radix Scrophulariae Ningpoensis) 玄参 9g
chuan bei mu (Bulbus Fritillariae Cirrhosae) 川贝母 6g
jie geng (Radix Platycodi Grandiflori) 桔梗 6g
dang gui (Radix Angelicae Sinensis) 当归 6-9g
bai shao (Radix Paeonia Lactiflorae) 白芍 6-9g
gan cao (Radix Glycrrhizae Uralensis) 甘草 6g

Method: Grind the herbs to powder and form into 9-gram pills with honey. The dose is 2-3 pills daily. May also be decocted with the doses as shown. (Source: *Formulas and Strategies*)

MAI WEI DI HUANG WAN 麦味地黄丸
(Ophiopogon, Schizandra and Rehmannia Formula)

This formula is selected when Kidney *yin* deficiency is significant (tidal fevers, frequent night sweats, concentrated urine, low back ache, tinnitus, recurrent afternoon sore throat).

shu di (Radix Rehmanniae Glutinosae Conquitae) 熟地 240g
shan yao (Radix Dioscoreae Oppositae) 山药 120g
shan zhu yu (Fructus Corni Officinalis) 山茱萸 120g
fu ling (Sclerotium Poria Cocos) 茯苓 90g
ze xie (Rhizoma Alismatis Orientalis) 泽泻 90g
mu dan pi (Cortex Moutan Radicis) 牡丹皮 90g
mai dong (Tuber Ophiopogonis Japonici) 麦冬 90g
wu wei zi (Fructus Schizandrae Chinensis) 五味子 60g

Method: Grind the herbs to powder and form into 9-gram pills with honey. The dose is 2-3 pills daily. May also be decocted with a 90% reduction in dosage. (Source: *Shi Yong Zhong Yi Nei Ke Xue*)

Modifications

- The effect of both primary prescriptions is improved by combining with the patent medicine **HE CHE DA ZAO WAN** (*Placenta Great Creation Pills* 河车大造丸, p.920) or **GE JIE SAN** (*Gecko Powder* 蛤蚧散).
- With significant spontaneous sweating or night sweats, add **huang qi** (Radix Astragali Membranacei) 黄芪 15g, **mu li** (Concha Ostreae) 牡蛎 15g, **ma huang gen** (Radix Ephedrae) 麻黄根 9g and **fu xiao mai** (Semen Tritici Aestivi Levis) 浮小麦 12g.
- In atopic patients (see modifications p.151), add small doses of one or two of the following herbs: **tu si zi** (Semen Cuscutae Chinensis) 菟丝子 6g, **du zhong** (Cortex Eucommiae Ulmoidis) 杜仲 3g, **hu tao ren** (Semen Juglandis Regiae) 胡桃仁 3g or **bu gu zhi** (Fructus Psoraleae Corylifoliae) 补骨脂 3g.

Patent medicines
Yang Yin Qing Fei Wan 养阴清肺丸 (Yang Yin Qing Fei Wan)
Ba Xian Chang Shou Wan 八仙长寿丸 (Ba Xian Chang Shou Wan)
Bai He Gu Jin Wan 百合固金丸 (Bai He Gu Jin Wan)
Luo Han Guo Chong Ji 罗汉果冲剂 (Luo Han Guo Beverage)
Chuan Bei Pi Pa Gao 川贝枇杷膏 (Nin Jiom Pei Pa Kao)

Acupuncture
Bl.13 (*fei shu* +), Bl.43 (*gao huang shu* +), Lu.9 (*tai yuan* +), Lu.1 (*zhong fu* +), Lu.7 (*lie que*), Kid.6 (*zhao hai*), Kid.27 (*shu fu*), Bl.23 (*shen shu* +), Kid.3 (*tai xi* +), Lu.5 (*chi ze* -), Kid.1 (*yong quan*)
- with severe Heat add Lu.10 (*yu ji* -)
- The points of the upper back and chest should be needled very carefully and superficially as patients with this pattern will often have hyperinflated lungs.

Scarring plasters
- In between episodes, a sticking plaster with a small amount of irritant herbs like **da suan** (Bulbus Alli Sativi) 大蒜 and **xi xin*** (Herba cum Radice Asari) 细辛 may be placed over points such as Du.14 (*da zhui*) or Bl.43 (*gao huang shu*) for 1-2 days, until a blister forms. This method strengthens the Lungs and *wei qi*, and is useful in chronic wheezing.

Clinical notes
- Wheezing associated with Lung and Kidney *yin* deficiency may be diagnosed as chronic asthma, chronic obstructive airways disease, pulmonary tuberculosis or silicosis.
- This can be a difficult condition to treat and requires great persistence to achieve a satisfactory result. Prolonged therapy (more than one year) while gradually reducing medication is generally necessary.

3.11 KIDNEY *YANG* DEFICIENCY

Pathophysiology
Kidney *yang* has a very important function in respiration. When Kidney *yang* is weak wheezing results for the following reasons:
- First, one of the fundamental fuctions of the Kidney is to anchor the *qi* upon inhalation. If it fails, Lung *qi* rises and accumulates in the chest.
- Second, Kidney *yang* is the basis for *zheng* and *wei qi* of the body. If Kidney *yang* is weak, the body is more vulnerable to external pathogens invading and obstructing Lung *qi*, causing wheezing.
- Third, Kidney *yang* is responsible for overseeing the fluid metabolism of the body. A failure in this function can lead to an accumulation of fluids in the Lung causing severe wheezing, orthopnoea and in serious cases, a sense that the patient is drowning.

Clinical features
- chronic wheezing, with inhalation more difficult than exhalation; the wheeze is worse for physical exertion, when fatigued or cold and following sex
- lethargy and listlessness
- spontaneous sweating
- frequent colds
- pale or cyanosed complexion, dark rings under the eyes and facial puffiness
- pitting oedema with scanty urination, or nocturia and urinary frequency
- lower back soreness or weakness, sore legs and knees
- cold extremities

T swollen and pale or purplish/bluish with a thin white coat
P deep, thready and slow or imperceptible or large, deficient and without root

Treatment principle
Strengthen Kidney *yang* to aid grasping of *qi*
Support *wei qi*

Prescription

JIN KUI SHEN QI WAN 金匱肾气丸
(*Rehmannia Eight Formula*)

shu di (Radix Rehmanniae Glutinosae Conquitae) 熟地	240g
shan yao (Radix Dioscoreae Oppositae) 山药	120g
shan zhu yu (Fructus Corni Officinalis) 山茱萸	120g
fu ling (Sclerotium Poriae Cocos) 茯苓	90g

mu dan pi (Cortex Moutan Radicis) 牡丹皮 90g
ze xie (Rhizoma Alismatis Orientalis) 泽泻 90g
rou gui (Cortex Cinnamomi Cassiae) 肉桂 60g
zhi fu zi* (Radix Aconiti Carmichaeli Preparata) 制附子 60g
Method: Grind the herbs to a fine powder and form into 9-gram pills with honey. The dose is one pill, 2-3 times daily. May also be decocted with a 90% reduction in dosage. In decoction, **zhi fu zi** is cooked for 30 minutes prior to the other herbs (*xian jian* 先煎). (Source: *Shi Yong Zhong Yao Xue*)

Modifications

- Giovanni Maciocia[1] speculates that allergic or atopic asthma (usually of juvenile onset) is associated with an inherited deficiency of the 'Lungs and Kidney defensive *qi* system'–*wei qi* and Kidney *yang*–which enables stubborn Wind to linger in the Lungs. On the basis of this theory, while utilising the appropriate constitutional formula in each case, he typically adds herbs to tonify this system. Usually only a few herbs are added, depending on the relative mix of Lung and Kidney weakness. These herbs are usually *yang* tonics, like **tu si zi** (Semen Cuscutae Chinensis) 菟丝子, **du zhong** (Cortex Eucommiae Ulmoidis) 杜仲, **hu tao ren** (Semen Juglandis Regiae) 胡桃仁 and **bu gu zhi** (Fructus Psoraleae Corylifoliae) 补骨脂. Smaller amounts of *yang* tonic herbs may be (cautiously) added in cases of *yin* deficiency.

- With copious tenacious mucus, add two or three of the following herbs: **su zi** (Fructus Perillae Frutescentis) 苏子 9g, **qian hu** (Radix Peucedani) 前胡 9g, **hai ge ke**ˆ (Concha Cyclinae Sinensis) 海蛤壳 9g, **xing ren*** (Semen Pruni Armeniacae) 杏仁 9g, **chen pi** (Pericarpium Citri Reticulatae) 陈皮 6g or **che qian zi** (Semen Plantaginis) 车前子 12g.

- If oedema is severe add **ting li zi** (Semen Descurainiae seu Lepidii) 葶苈子 9g and **chao bai zhu** (dry fried Rhizoma Atractylodes Macrocephalae) 炒白术 12g.

- In severe cases add **ren shen** (Radix Ginseng) 3-6g, **dong chong xia cao**ˆ (Cordyceps Sinensis) 10g, **wu wei zi** (Fructus Schizandrae Chinensis) 五味子 6g, **bu gu zhi** (Fructus Psoraleae Corylifoliae) 补骨脂 6g, **hu tao ren** (Semen Juglandis Regiae) 胡桃仁 10g or combine with **REN SHEN GE JIE SAN** (*Ginseng and Gecko Powder* 人参蛤蚧散).

    ren shen (Radix Ginseng) 人参
    ge jieˆ (Gecko) 蛤蚧
    Method: Grind equal quantities of both ingredients to a fine powder. The dose is 3-grams twice daily.

---

1. Maciocia G (1994) *The Practice of Chinese Medicine*, Churchill Livingstone, Edinburgh

Variations and additional prescriptions
Heart and Kidney yang *deficiency*
* Kidney and Heart *yang* deficiency can lead to significant generalised pitting and pulmonary oedema (as in congestive cardiac failure), severe wheezing, dyspnoea, orthopnoea and frothy mucus. The correct treatment is to warm the *yang* and promote urination with **ZHEN WU TANG** (*True Warrior Decoction* 真武汤) modified, until fluid balance is controlled. When fluids are moving the original prescription or other suitable tonifying prescription should be selected.

    zhi fu zi* (Radix Aconiti Carmichaeli Praeparata) 制附子 9g
    chao bai zhu (dry fried Rhizoma Atractylodis Macrocephalae) 炒白术 9g
    sheng jiang (Rhizoma Zingiberis Officinalis) 生姜 9g
    bai shao (Radix Paeoniae Lactiflora) 白芍 12g
    fu ling (Sclerotium Poriae Cocos) 茯苓 12g
    che qian zi (Semen Plantaginis) 车前子 12g
    ze xie (Rhizoma Alismatis Orientalis) 泽泻 12g
    Method: Decoction. **Zhi fu zi** is decocted for 30 minutes before the other herbs (*xian jian* 先煎), **che qian zi** is cooked in a muslin bag (*bao jian* 包煎).

Collapse of Heart yang
* If Heart *yang* is collapsing (with severe dyspnoea, icy extremities, copious sweating and an imperceptible pulse) immediate action to restore *yang*, strongly tonify *yuan qi* and prevent collapse, is required. Suitable formulae include **SI NI JIA REN SHEN TANG** (*Frigid Extremities Decoction plus Ginseng* 四逆加人参汤, p.926), **HEI XI DAN** (*Lead Special Pill* 黑锡丹, p.920) or **SHEN FU TANG** (*Ginseng and Prepared Aconite Decoction* 参附汤, p.665).

Patent medicines
Jin Kui Shen Qi Wan 金匮肾气丸 (Sexoton Pills)
Fu Zi Li Zhong Wan 附子理中丸 (Li Chung Yuen Medical Pills)
Ren Shen Lu Rong Wan 人参鹿茸丸 (Jen Shen Lu Yung Wan)
Ge Jie Bu Shen Wan 蛤蚧补肾丸 (Gejie Nourishing Kidney Pills)

Acupuncture
Bl.13 (*fei shu* +▲), Lu.9 (*tai yuan* +), Bl.23 (*shen shu* +▲), Kid.3 (*tai xi* +), Ren.6 (*qi hai* +▲), Ren.4 (*guan yuan* +▲)
* with congested fluids add Ren.9 (*shui fen* p), Kid.7 (*fu liu* -), Sp.9 (*yin ling quan* -), Sp.6 (*san yin jiao* -), St.28 (*shui dao* -)
* The points of the upper back and chest should be needled very carefully and superficially as patients with this pattern will often have hyperinflated lungs.

Scarring plasters

- In between episodes, a sticking plaster with a small amount of irritant herbs like **da suan** (Bulbus Alli Sativi) 大蒜 and **xi xin*** (Herba cum Radice Asari) 细辛 may be placed over points such as Du.14 (*da zhui*) or Bl.43 (*gao huang shu*) for 1-2 days, until a blister forms. This method strengthens the Lungs and *wei qi*, and is useful in chronic wheezing.

Clinical notes

- Wheezing associated with Kidney *yang* deficiency may be diagnosed as chronic asthma, pulmonary oedema, congestive cardiac failure, cardiac asthma, cor pulmonale
- Mild cases of Kidney *yang* deficiency can respond well to correct and prolonged treatment. In severe cases it can be difficult to treat, especially patients presenting with Kidney *yang* wheezing complicated by pulmonary oedema, or Heart and Kidney *yang* deficiency. These patients are usually on the maximum dose of conventional medicine.

SUMMARY OF GUIDING FORMULAE FOR WHEEZING

Acute patterns
Wind Cold - *Ma Huang Tang* 麻黄汤
- with congested fluids - *Xiao Qing Long Tang* 小青龙汤
- with internal Heat - *Ding Chuan Tang* 定喘汤

Wind Heat - *Sang Ju Yin* 桑菊饮
- more wheezing and Lung Heat - *Ma Xing Shi Gan Tang* 麻杏石甘汤
- with Lung *yin* deficiency - *Qing Zao Jiu Fei Tang* 清燥救肺汤

Chronic patterns
Phlegm Damp - *San Zi Yang Qin Tang* 三子养亲汤 + *Er Chen Tang* 二陈汤
- with significant Spleen deficiency - *Liu Jun Zi Tang* 六君子汤
- in elderly patients with recurrent wheezing in Winter and Kidney deficiency - *Su Zi Jiang Qi Tang* 苏子降气汤

Lung *qi* and *yin* deficiency - *Sheng Mai San* 生脉散

Lung and Spleen *qi* deficiency - *Bu Zhong Yi Qi Tang* 补中益气汤
- postpartum wheezing - *Shi Quan Da Bu Tang* 十全大补汤 or *Dang Gui Bu Xue Tang* 当归补血汤

Lung and Kidney *yin* deficiency - *Bai He Gu Jin Tang* 百合固金汤

Kidney *yang* deficiency - *Jin Kui Shen Qi Wan* 金匮肾气丸
- with severe congested Lung fluids - *Zhen Wu Tang* 真武汤

Acute or Chronic patterns
Phlegm Heat - *Ma Xing Shi Gan Tang* 麻杏石甘汤
- chronic Phlegm Heat - *Er Chen Tang* 二陈汤

Liver *qi* stagnation - *Wu Mo Yin Zi* 五磨饮子
- with hysteria - the above formula plus *Gan Mai Da Zao Tang* 甘麦大枣汤
- between episodes - *Xiao Yao San* 逍遥散
- with stagnant Heat - *Dan Zhi Xiao Yao San* 丹栀逍遥散
- with Liver Fire - *Long Dan Xie Gan Tang* 龙胆泻肝汤

Endnote

For more information regarding herbs marked with an asterisk*, an open circle° or a hat ˆ, see the tables on pp.944-952.

Appendix 3.1
ASTHMA (*qi chuan* 气喘)

In modern clinical practice, wheezing disorders (or those presenting with a reduced lung capacity) are frequently diagnosed as asthma, and whether this is correct or not, a discussion of asthma is warranted as it is expected that many practitioners will use this chapter for the analysis of asthma.

Asthma has become in the last few decades a very common disorder in developed nations. For example, 1 in 4 children and 1 in 10 adults are diagnosed with asthma in Australia. The precise reason for such a huge increase in atopic conditions like asthma has not yet been adequately explained, but we may suppose that aspects of our modern lifestyle and environment contribute a significant part of the picture.

Exposure to environmental airborne pollutants, especially fine particulate matter, appears to either directly cause inflammation in the bronchi, or exacerbate it. At the same time that atmospheric pollution has increased so has the number of chemicals (pesticides, preservatives etc.) in our food. While these may not be so directly involved in the aetiology of asthma, it is possible they play a role in over-sensitising or derailing parts of the immune system, thus producing abnormal responses to various external stimuli. One of these external stimuli, which has been strongly implicated as a trigger (or cause if exposure happens early in life) of asthma, is the excreta of dust mites.

SIDE EFFECTS OF ASTHMA MEDICATION ACCORDING TO TCM

- **Salbutamol** (Ventolin, Asmol): A b_2-adrenergic agent, salbutamol temporarily disperses accumulated *zong* and Lung *qi*, giving some relief from wheezing and chest tightness. Prolonged use significantly weakens the Lungs and depletes *zong qi*, ultimately creating a dependence on the medication as the Lungs become truly weak and cannot function properly without help. The depletion of *zong qi* is evident from the side effects, which include tachycardia, arrhythmias, hand tremors and insomnia.
- **Corticosteroids** (inhaled as Becotide or Becloforte, or orally as Prednisolone): Corticosteroids are warm, acrid and dispersing, and powerfully disperse Lung *qi* and *yin* by activating Kidney *yang*, in a similar way to **fu zi** (Radix Aconiti Carmichaeli Preparata) 附子. Overstimulation of *yang* eventually depletes *yin*. Chronic use of steroids in the treatment of asthma usually leads to the development of Lung and Kidney *yin* deficiency, which is difficult to treat satisfactorily. Patients on steroid therapy also seem to be slower to respond to TCM treatment.

In addition to the increase in pollutants and allergens in the environment, a marked change in behaviour and diet has occurred, particularly in children. More time spent watching television and less spent in physical activity combined with a Phlegm generating diet (sweets, ice cream, dairy) can lead to reduced lung capacity and vitality, and therefore increased vulnerability to Lung disorders.

Asthma has also long been known to have a genetic component. While the observed increase in incidence cannot be explained in terms of simple genetic inheritance, the decline in the quality of gametes can perhaps be considered a factor. TCM places great store in the quality of *jing* (gametes) in producing offspring with strong *qi*. It is now well recognised that sperm quality is affected by many environmental pollutants and that egg quality diminishes rapidly in women by their late 30s, an age when an increasing number of women have children.

The analysis of asthma in TCM can be made using the categories found in both the wheezing and cough sections of this book, according to the prominent symptoms. In many cases where medication has suppressed all symptoms, diagnosis will need to be made on constitutional and auxiliary signs and symptoms–still using the categories in this and the last chapter as a guide. The TCM effects of bronchodilating medications are summarised in Box 1.

It should be noted that TCM texts by Chinese authors describe asthma (not wheezing) as a disorder of Wind Cold, Kidney deficiency and Phlegm accumulation. The way chronic asthma presents in our clinics in the West does not, however, always fit these patterns. The picture may be complicated by the widespread use of medication, often from an early age. Sometimes there is little evidence of Phlegm accumulation (but see p.157) and few or no Kidney signs and symptoms.

The patterns described in this book are appropriate for the symptom of wheezing, which includes asthma amongst other disorders. There is a special exception associated with allergy, elucidated by Maciocia.[1] He has proposed an aetiology for allergic (or atopic) asthma based on an inherited deficiency of Lung and Kidney defensive *qi* (see also p.151). This deficiency allows Wind to settle and lodge in the bronchi causing chronic respiratory distress. In addition to the factors outlined above which affect the quality of *jing*, he thinks immunisations may play a part in the heightened sensitivity response of the atopic individual.

---

1. Maciocia G (1994) *The Practice of Chinese Medicine*, Churchill Livingstone, Edinburgh

Appendix 3.2
PAEDIATRIC ASTHMA (*Xiao Er Qi Chuan* 小儿气喘)

Asthma is a more prevalent disease in childhood than in adulthood and warrants separate mention here not only for this reason, but because children are generally treated differently to adults. TCM recognises that children have unique physiological characteristics and cannot be considered as minature adults. One of the features of paediatric physiology that is pertinent to our discussion of asthma is the immaturity of the digestive system. This inherent digestive weakness predisposes to incomplete breakdown of food and the accumulation of Phlegm. Fatty and cold foods, unfortunately the mainstay of many a modern child's diet, are especially dangerous in this regard. Phlegm is very clearly a key component of all types of paediatric asthma.

Asthma in children, even in its more severe forms, is amenable to TCM treatment providing very persistent treatment is applied between episodes, sometimes through several seasons or years. If the treatment is consistently kept ahead of the disease, that is, it is applied before acute episodes and when the child is generally stronger and more healthy (often during the Summer months), and lifestyle and diet changes (see below) are firmly adhered to, then if not a cure, it can significantly reduce attacks and morbidity.

Specifically, all children with asthma (no matter which category) need to be on a diet that reduces Phlegm. This means restricting foods that produce congestion of mucous membranes (for example peanut butter and dairy foods, such as ice cream), and foods that impair the Spleen's ability to breakdown food (excessive raw or cold foods and sugar). Aspects of lifestyle and behaviour that require attention are those that deplete *qi* and do not encourage its efficient production and movement. Many children spend far too many hours in front of the television and computer screen. Not only is the lack of movement not beneficial for the *qi* of the body, but the nature of the sometimes mindless absorbtion and focus on the screen is seen to deplete *qi*. At the other end of the spectrum, but also common in modern-day children, is the plethora of after school activities and the expectations of parents that their child, for example, should not only train in swimming, dance and gymnastics, but also play the violin! Such relentless pursuit of achievements in so many fields not only exhausts the child's *qi*, but leaves very little room for the valuable dreaming time of childhood.

As for adults, asthma is differentiated into acute and chronic categories. Acute episodes are best treated with Western medication or a combination of Chinese medicine and Western drugs. Acupuncture can be very helpful.

PATTERNS AND TREATMENT

Weekly acupuncture treatments are strongly advised and generally well tolerated in all but the Kidney *yang* deficient child who is quite phobic and easily traumatised. Children with Kidney *yang* deficiency patterns may respond to laser acupuncture. Practitioners experienced in treating childhood asthma have warned that it is important to approach the removal of Phlegm from the Lungs slowly, so as not to overwhelm Lung *qi* and cause obstruction. Often the use of points like Ren.22 (*tian tu*) will begin to clear the upper reaches of the Lungs, while points like St.40 (*feng long*) can be brought in a little later to start clearing deeper levels of Phlegm.

ACUTE ASTHMA ATTACK

During an attack, the only distinction that needs to be made is between Cold and Hot types. As noted previously, Phlegm is common to all patterns and lies dormant until stirred up by a pathogenic invasion or some other trigger.

Cold type
- This is an excess pattern, and while described as Cold it is really the absence of Heat that defines it. It may be triggered by changes in weather, exposure to cold or an upper resiratory tract infection, but may also be due to overeating, stress, or exposure to allergens such as animal fur, pollen and certain foods.
- wheezing and cough, often worse or more frequent during winter
- frothy clear or white tenacious sputum
- body and/or extremities are normal temperature, or cold
- pale or ashen complexion

T thin white or greasy white coat
P floating, tight or slippery

Hot type
- This type is associated with Heat, usually Wind Heat or Phlegm Heat, and is closely associated with an upper respiratory tract infection such as flu or bronchitis.
- wheezing and cough
- the cough may be unproductive, or with yellow sputum
- fever or feels hot to the touch
- sweating
- red complexion
- thirst
- constipation

T thin yellow or greasy yellow coat
P slippery and rapid

Kidney *yang* deficiency
* wheezing and cough in a frail child
* ashen complexion
* cold body and extremities
* general lack of vitality, soft voice, low spirits
* cold clammy sweat, especially on the head
* enuresis, frequent urination

T pale
P weak

Treatment of the acute episode
Most children will be taking some form of inhaled bronchodilating medication, and from a convenient and practical point of view, this is the treatment of choice for acute episodes. Herbs and acupuncture can also be effective for acute attacks, however, and are summarised below. The general principle is to expel pathogens, redirect Lung *qi* downward and calm asthma. Keep in mind that a small child with an acute attack is usually very frightened and lots of needles don't help.

Acupuncture [2]
Main points
   ding chuan (M-BW-1), Lu.7 (*lie que*), Ren.22 (*tian tu*), PC.6 (*nei guan*), Ren.17 (*shan zhong*), Bl.13 (*fei shu*).
   * In very frightened children, *ding chuan* retained and Lu.7 (*lie que*) not retained is often enough to settle them, after which other points may be added as appropriate. The fewer needles the better. Cupping on the upper back points can be useful in the Cold and Hot types. Kidney deficient children are often so phobic that needling is impossible, however they can usually tolerate laser acupuncture treatment.

Additional points for different patterns
   * for Cold type add St.36 (*zu san li* p), Ren.12 (*zhong wan* ▲), Bl.20 (*pi shu*), St.40 (*feng long*)
   * for Hot type add Lu.5 (*chi ze*), Du.14 (*da zhui*) and LI.11 (*qu chi*)
   * with emotional disturbance add Liv.3 (*tai chong*), LI.4 (*he gu*) and Ht.7 (*shen men*)
   * for Kidney deficiency, Lu.9 (*tai yuan*), Bl.20 (*pi shu*), Bl.23 (*shen shu*), Ren.4 (*guan yuan*), Kid.7 (*fu liu*), Kid.3 (*tai xi*), Sp.6 (*san yin jiao*). Moxa may be used.

---

2. From Scott J P (1991) *Acupuncture in the Treatment of Children*, Eastland Press, Seattle

Prescriptions

The herbal prescriptions for acute attacks are the same as for adults bit in a reduced dose. The formula may be concentrated and administered with an eyedropper. Select one only, depending on accompanying symptoms.

Cold type
MA HUANG TANG 麻黄汤
(*Ma Huang Combination*) p.122 - wheezing triggered by a cold
XIAO QING LONG TANG 小青龙汤
(*Minor Blue Dragon Combination*) p.124 - wheezing triggered by cold with copious watery mucus

Hot type
DING CHUAN TANG 定喘汤
(*Stop Wheezing Decoction*) p.126
BAO YING DAN 保婴丹
(*Protect the Child Special Pill*) - a popular paediatric patent medicine

CHRONIC PATTERNS OF ASTHMA

In practice, usually all of the following patterns are present to a greater or lesser extent. The key is to decide which is prominent and thus which pattern to start with.

Phlegm Damp
- cough with lots of mucus
- constant runny nose
- may occur in an otherwise robust child, and is often associated with accumulation disorder in infants–red cheeks, abdominal fullness, irregular bowel habits

Lung and Spleen deficiency
- weak child, possibly small for their age
- frequent colds, takes a long time to recover
- poor appetite, or very picky eater
- pale complexion
- general lack of vitality (or, paradoxically, hyperactivity)
- weak low voice

Lingering pathogenic factor
- swollen glands (usually in the neck) that are hard
- history of repeated infections treated with antibiotics
- loud cough

Kidney *yang* deficiency
• long history of asthma (often since birth)
• weak pale child, possibly small for their age
• enuresis
• cold extremities
• pale tongue

Treatment between episodes
Treatment at this stage focuses on the underlying pattern. Both acupuncture and herbs (in conjuction with diet) are effective *when given regularly*. A piecemeal approach is almost worse than nothing, causing the child to resist treatment and the parents to despair.

Acupuncture
Acupuncture treatment is generally very simple and the number of points kept to a minimum.
• For infants, the main points are the *si feng* (M-UE-9) points. These points can be needled with a fine gauge filiform needle. Needle all points on both hands at each treatment. It usually takes 4-5 days to get the full effect of the *si feng* points, so one weekly treatment is generally sufficient. These points are not suitable for Kidney *yang* deficiency, which should be gently warmed and tonified with moxa and cups.
• For children, the main points are selected from the Lung and Bladder channels, typically Lu.9 (*tai yuan*), Lu.5 (*chi ze*) and Bl.13 (*fei shu*). Gentle cupping may be applied to the upper back. Cupping and massage techniques can also be taught to the parents.

Herbal prescriptions
Lung and Spleen deficiency and Phlegm Damp types
Use LIU JUN ZI TANG (*Six Major Herbs Combination* 六君子汤, p.88) and add more Phlegm cutting herbs if necessary. It has been noticed by practitioners here that the addition of Phlegm removing herbs often provokes the coughing up of significant quantities of mucus, even though there had been little symptomatic evidence of mucus. As mentioned above, care does need to be taken when mobilising Phlegm from the Lungs; Lung *qi* must be strong enough to deal with the Phlegm as it is being dredged from the deeper and further reaching bronchioles. Also useful, for this and for patterns with a lingering pathogenic factor, especially in children under three years old, is the patent medicine BAO YING DAN (*Protect the Child Special Pill* 保婴丹). This medicine is particularly good if the Phlegm is associated with accumulation disorder.
Children over the age of three can take adult medicines at appropriately

reduced doseages. For those who catch cold frequently, combine LIU JUN ZI TANG with YU PING FENG SAN (*Jade Screen Powder* 玉屏风散, p.21). If they tend to have lots of watery mucous, SU ZI JIANG QI TANG (*Perilla Fruit Combination* 苏子降气汤, p.133) is useful. This formula is also good for children with Kidney *yang* deficiency.

Lingering Pathogenic Factors

'GUNGY GLAND MIX[3]'. This formula is applied in all cases where the glands in the neck are swollen or hardened and can be repeated until the glands have shrunk and softened. It may be boiled down to a very concentrated mix and squirted down the throat in small amounts, or it can be administered in ground powder form or granulated form. As always add or remove individual herbs according to the presentation.

xia ku cao (Spica Prunella Vulgaris) 夏枯草 15g
pu gong ying (Herba Taraxaci Mongolici cum Radice)
蒲公英 15g
xuan shen (Radix Scrophulariae Ningpoensis) 玄参 12g
jin yin hua (Flos Lonicerae Japonicae) 金银花 10g
lian qiao (Fructus Forsythia Suspensae) 连翘 10g
zhe bei mu (Bulbus Fritillariae Thunbergii) 浙贝母 10g
niu bang zi (Fructus Arctii Lappae) 牛蒡子 10g
cang er zi* (Fructus Xanthii Sibirici) 苍耳子 10g

Kidney *yang* deficiency

For children with asthma from birth, or early after birth, the congenital component needs to be addressed. This can be achieved with YOU GUI WAN (*Eucommia and Rehmannia Formula* 右归丸, p.256), JIN KUI SHEN QI WAN (*Rehmannia Eight Formula* 金匮肾气丸, p.150), or the patent medicines GE JIE BU SHEN WAN (*Gejie Nourishing Kidney Pills* 蛤蚧补肾丸) or HA CHIEH TING KAT WAN 蛤蚧定咳丸. Also useful is SU ZI JIANG QI TANG (*Perilla Fruit Combination* 苏子降气汤, p.133).

---

3. Courtesy of Helen Gordon, TCM paediatric specialist, Sydney, Australia.

Disorders of the Lung

4. Epistaxis

Excess patterns
Wind Heat
Toxic Heat
Stomach Heat
Liver Fire

Deficient patterns
Liver and Kidney *yin* deficiency
Spleen *qi* deficiency

4 EPISTAXIS
bi nü 鼻衄

Epistaxis is defined as bleeding from the nose from a cause other than physical trauma. The most common cause of epistaxis is trauma, however, from a TCM viewpoint, most cases due to trauma need little treatment other than first aid. This chapter deals with epistaxis related to an underlying physiological dysfunction.

Epistaxis can vary from mild spotting to severe and potentially dangerous bleeding. In TCM, the nose is closely associated with the Lungs and is traversed by the *yang ming* (Stomach and Large Intestine) channels. Epistaxis, therefore, is most commonly due to dysfunction of the Lungs and Stomach, particularly those associated with Heat. Liver Fire, *yin* deficiency, and Spleen deficiency failing to hold Blood in the vessels may also give rise to epistaxis.

Epistaxis can be differentiated into excess and deficient patterns. The excess patterns are associated with Heat in the Lungs, Stomach and Liver. The bleeding is often copious and acute, and there are signs of systemic Heat. In deficient patterns, the bleeding is generally mild and recurrent.

AETIOLOGY
Wind Heat, Lung Heat
External Wind Heat usually invades the Lung through the nose or mouth, and can affect any (or all) of the structures of the respiratory system (nose, sinuses, throat, pharynx, skin and lung). The Wind Heat can dry the nasal mucous membranes damaging the local *luo mai*, causing bleeding.

Toxic Heat
Toxic Heat is an intense and virulent species of Wind Heat or Damp Heat, which invades the Lung system through the nose or mouth. In this context Toxic Heat may be considered a particularly powerful variant of Wind Heat, such as that seen in epidemics where symptoms develop rapidly and affect the whole body. In this pattern it is the Heat that causes the bleeding by quickening Blood and forcing it from the vessels.

Stomach Heat
Simple overeating or overconsumption of heating foods (spicy hot foods and alcohol) can cause Stomach Heat directly. Any pre-existing Heat in the body, from Liver *qi* stagnation, *yin* deficiency or external invasion can do the same. If stagnant Liver *qi* invades the Stomach via the controlling (*ke* 克, p.70) cycle repeatedly, it can damage Stomach *yin* giving rise to Heat. Finally, external Cold or Heat can penetrate the Stomach and Intestines directly (the

yang ming level). The bleeding in this pattern is usually from the gums but may occasionally be from the nose, especially if the Lungs become involved.

Liver Fire

Frustration, anger, hatred, bitterness, repressed emotion and stress can all disrupt the circulation of Liver *qi*. When *qi* stagnates for any length of time, the resulting pressure can generate Heat. Depending on the severity of the stagnation (and to some extent the intensity of the aetiological conditions) this can cause stagnant Heat or the more severe Fire, the latter being exacerbated by a diet of heating foods and alcohol. Because one of the functions of the Liver is to store Blood, pathological Heat affecting the Liver is easily transferred to the Blood. Therefore, in addition to the Fire directly rising to the head and damaging the nasal passages, the Blood can be heated and forced from the vessels.

> **BOX 4.1 SOME BIOMEDICAL CAUSES OF EPISTAXIS**
>
> • dryness or erosion of the nasal mucous membranes
> • trauma
> • foreign body
> • nasal infection
> • thrombocytopoenia
> • haemophilia
> • hypertension
> • nasopharyngeal cancer
> • thromboembolism
> • anticoagulants
> • blood dyscrasia
> • epidemic haemorrhagic diseases

Liver and Kidney *yin* deficiency

When Liver and Kidney *yin* become damaged (from illness, overwork or taking drugs), the resultant Heat can dry the mucous membranes of the Lungs and nose, causing bleeding. Also, there is the tendency for *yang* to rise when *yin* is deficient. At a critical point of deficiency, Liver *yang* suddenly slips its mooring and surges towards the head, causing abrupt bleeding. Uncontrolled rising *yang*, as a result of *yin* deficiency, can increase the pressure in the Blood vessels of the head, damage the *luo mai* and cause nosebleed and scleral haemorrhage.

Spleen *qi* deficiency

Overwork, excessive worry, irregular or poor dietary habits or prolonged illness weaken Spleen *qi*. One of the main functions of Spleen *qi* is to exert an external pressure on the vessels preventing the leakage of Blood and when this aspect is weak, Blood 'oozes' out. Bleeding is generally mild, chronic and prolonged. This is in contrast to most other types of epistaxis in which the Blood is heated and quickened, and forced from the vessels.

> **BOX 4.2 FIRST AID TO STOP BLEEDING**
>
> **1. Cold compress**
> - to the bridge of the nose while pinching the soft part of the nose between the thumb and forefinger. This is best performed with the patient reclining.
> - applied to the neck (around Du.15 *ya men*). An ice cube applied to Du.15 may also be useful. The neck is where the *yang* channels meet, and cold applied here can restrain *yang*, redirect Fire downwards and cool the Blood. Suitable in excess patterns of epistaxis.
>
> **2. Haemostatic powder**
> - insert a ball of cotton wool coated with **YUN NAN BAI YAO** (云南白药) or **san qi** (Radix Notoginseng 三七) powder into the nose, and press the soft part of the nose between thumb and forefinger.
> - In recurrent cases, **YUN NAN BAI YAO** powder can be blown in the nose with a straw several times daily.
>
> **3. Moxibustion or counterirritant therapy**
> - for recurrent bleeding due to Heat (usually deficient Heat), direct or indirect moxibustion can be applied to Kid.1 (*yong quan*). Similarly, garlic paste, or powdered **wu zhu yu** (Fructus Evodiae Rutaecarpae) 吴茱萸 can be used on the same point. The feet can also by dipped in very hot water. All these methods lead Heat downward.
>
> **4. SI.3 (*hou xi*) - LI.4 (*he gu*) compression method**
> - this method is derived from martial arts first aid and is primarily employed in traumatic epistaxis. A piece of string or rubber band is tied around the open hand covering both points. The patient then closes the hand into a fist, increasing the pressure on both points.

DIAGNOSIS

The diagnosis of epistaxis is usually straightforward, but it can occasionally be confused with other TCM disease categories in which mucus and blood are expelled together. Epistaxis is diagnosed when only blood is lost through the nose, or the volume of blood is greater than mucus. In cases where the volume of mucus is greater, or it is simply streaked with blood, the disease diagnosis is usually naso-sinusitis (*bi yuan* 鼻渊). Diagnosis can be difficult when blood drains from the nose into the pharynx and is swallowed or coughed up. In such cases, where the bleeding is generally mild and comes from the posterior nasal cavity, the patient may present with coughing or vomiting blood. Any chronic case of epistaxis needs examination by rhinoscopy.

Epistaxis also occurs in very dry climates due to simple drying and cracking of the mucous membranes—this usually does not require specific treatment other than topical protection with an emollient substance like lanolin.

TREATMENT

In general, there are several steps to consider when treating any bleeding disorder. The first, and most important step, is to stop the bleeding. When the bleeding is severe, the initial focus of treatment is to use first aid or herbs to quickly staunch the bleeding. This can usually be acheived with a styptic formulae, or with the use of the patent medicine *Yun Nan Bai Yao* 云南白药 (Yunnan Paiyao).

Once bleeding has ceased, or is under control, the underlying pattern can be dealt with more fully. There are two additional aspects to consider. Any residual Blood outside the vessels is stagnant Blood, which must be moved as it may become pathological if allowed to remain. Thus, herbs to gently invigorate or regulate Blood are incorporated into the appropriate formula. This is especially important in Heat types of bleeding, as the herbs used to stop bleeding will likely be cold natured and astringent. These herbs congeal Blood. Finally, any *qi* or Blood deficiency that exists as a direct result of Blood loss should be supplemented.

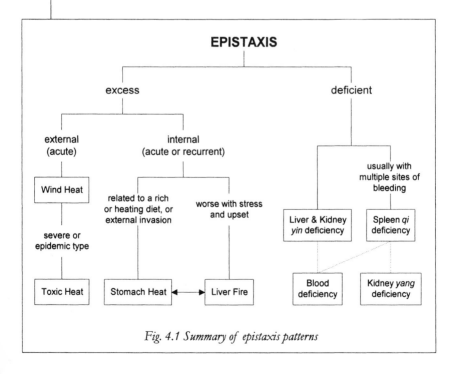

Fig. 4.1 Summary of epistaxis patterns

风
热
犯
肺
鼻
衄

4.1 WIND HEAT, LUNG HEAT

Pathophysiology
- Pathogenic Heat invades the Lungs through the mouth and nose, drying the nasal mucous membranes and damaging nasal capillaries, causing bleeding. This pattern is acute and usually not recurrent.

Clinical features
- nosebleed with fresh red blood, generally not copious
- dry nostrils, nasal obstruction
- fever, mild chills
- headache
- dry, sore throat, thirst
- cough

T normal or red tipped with a thin dry white or yellow coat
P floating and rapid

Treatment principle
Expel Wind and Heat
Cool Blood, stop bleeding

Prescription

SANG JU YIN 桑菊饮
(*Morus and Chrysanthemum Formula*) modified

This formula is selected when exterior signs and Wind Heat are primary.

sang ye (Folium Mori Albae) 桑叶	12g
ju hua (Flos Chrysanthemi Morifolii) 菊花	9g
bai mao gen (Rhizoma Imperatae Cylindricae) 白茅根	18g
lu gen (Rhizoma Phragmitis Communis) 芦根	15g
mu dan pi (Cortex Moutan Radicis) 牡丹皮	12g
shan zhi zi tan (charred Fructus Gardeniae Jasminoidis) 山栀子炭	12g
xing ren* (Semen Pruni Armeniacae) 杏仁	9g
lian qiao (Fructus Forsythia Suspensae) 连翘	9g
jie geng (Radix Platycodi Grandiflori) 桔梗	9g
bo he (Herba Mentha Haplocalycis) 薄荷	6g
gan cao (Radix Glycyrrhizae Uralensis) 甘草	3g

Method: Decoction. Do not cook longer than 20 minutes. **Bo he** is added near the end of cooking (*hou xia* 后下). (Source: *Shi Yong Zhong Yao Xue*)

Modifications
- If the exterior signs are severe (fever, chills, headache, sore throat), add **jing jie** (Herba seu Flos Schizonepetae Tenuifolia) 荆芥 10g and **fang**

feng (Radix Ledebouriellae Divaricatae) 防风 10g.
* With severe thirst, add **tian hua fen** (Radix Trichosanthes Kirilowii) 天花粉 12g and **mai dong** (Tuber Ophiopogonis Japonici) 麦冬 12g.
* If the throat is very sore, add **xuan shen** (Radix Scrophulariae Ningpoensis) 玄参 18g and **ma bo** (Fructificatio Lasiosphaerae seu Calvatiae) 马勃 3g.
* If cough is severe, add **chuan bei mu** (Bulbus Fritillariae Cirrhosae) 川贝母 9g, **dong gua ren** (Semen Benincasae Hispidae) 冬瓜仁 and **gua lou ren** (Semen Trichosanthis) 瓜楼仁 12g.
* With constipation, add **da huang** (Radix et Rhizoma Rhei) 大黄 6-9g and **gua lou ren** (Semen Trichosanthis) 瓜楼仁 9g.

MA XING SHI GAN TANG 麻杏石甘汤, p.193
(*Ma Huang, Apricot Seed, Gypsum and Licorice Combination*) modified

This formula is selected when Lung Heat is primary. There are no exterior symptoms remaining, but there is a dry hacking, painful cough, thirst, laboured breathing or wheezing and a flooding rapid pulse. The treatment is to clear Heat from the Lungs, cool the Blood and stop bleeding.

Patent medicines

Qing Fei Yi Huo Pian 清肺抑火片 (Ching Fei Yi Huo Pien)
Ma Xing Zhi Ke Pian 麻杏止咳片 (Ma Hsing Chih Ke Pien)
Yun Nan Bai Yao 云南白药 (Yunnan Paiyao)
- this medicine can be taken internally and/or blown into the nose with a straw. It is used in addition to the main formula. The red pill that accompanies the powder is only used in severe cases.

Acupuncture

LI.4 (*he gu* -), SJ.5 (*wai guan* -), Lu.11 (*shao shang* ↓), GB.20 (*feng chi* -), LI.20 (*ying xiang*), Bl.13 (*fei shu* -)
* if fever is severe add LI.11 (*qu chi* -)
* if cough is severe add Lu.5 (*chi ze* -)

Clinical notes

* The biomedical conditions that may present as Wind Heat or Lung Heat epistaxis include the common cold, tonsillitis, upper respiratory tract infection, acute bronchitis, pneumonia, early stage of measles and sinusitis.
* Responds well to correct and timely treatment.

4.2 TOXIC HEAT

Pathophysiology
- Toxic Heat type nosebleed accompanies symptoms of severe systemic Heat and distress. It occurs after a particularly virulent or epidemic pathogen invades the Lungs and body forcing Blood from the vessels. This pattern shares some characteristics with the Heat affecting the Blood pattern of the *wen bing* (see p.41)

Clinical features
- nosebleed, usually profuse and perhaps also with other sites of bleeding (gums, skin etc.)
- high fever
- malaise, irritability, restlessness
- dry mouth and throat, thirst
- insomnia
- concentrated urine
- in severe cases delirium

T red with a yellow coat
P forceful and rapid

Treatment principle
Purge Fire and eliminate Toxins
Cool the Blood and stop bleeding

Prescription

HUANG LIAN JIE DU TANG 黄连解毒汤
(*Coptis and Scute Combination*) modified

huang lian (Rhizoma Coptidis) 黄连	3g
huang qin (Radix Scutellariae Baicalensis) 黄芩	9g
huang bai (Cortex Phellodendri) 黄柏	6g
shan zhi zi (Fructus Gardeniae Jasminoidis) 山栀子	9g
sheng di (Radix Rehmanniae Glutinosae) 生地	12g
ce bai ye (Cacumen Biotae Orientalis) 侧柏叶	12g
ou jie (Nodus Nelumbinis Nuciferae Rhizomatis) 藕节	12g
qing dai (Indigo Pulverata Levis) 青黛	3g

Method: Decoction. **Qing dai** is added to the strained decoction (*chong fu* 冲服)
(Source: *Shi Yong Zhong Yi Nei Ke Xue*)

Modifications
- With severe dryness and thirst, add **shi hu** (Herba Dendrobii) 石斛 12g and **tian hua fen** (Radix Trichosanthis Kirilowii) 天花粉 12g.

- With constipation, add **da huang** (Radix et Rhizoma Rhei) 大黄 6-9g.
- If the throat is sore, add **xuan shen** (Radix Scrophulariae Ningpoensis) 玄参 18g and **ma bo** (Fructificatio Lasiosphaerae seu Calvatiae) 马勃 3g.

Variations and additional prescriptions
- When Toxic Heat enters the Blood affecting the *shen* and causing disordered consciousness, the correct treatment is to clear Toxic Heat, cool Blood and clear *ying* with **XI JIAO DI HUANG TANG** (*Rhinoceros Horn and Rehmannia Decoction* 犀角地黄汤 p.41) or **QING YING TANG** (*Clear the Ying Decoction* 清营汤 p.38).
- When there is delirium, a resucitation formula like **AN GONG NIU HUANG WAN** (*Calm the Palace Pill with Cattle Gallstone* 安宫牛黄丸, p.914), **ZHI BAO DAN** (*Greatest Treasure Special Pill* 至宝丹, p.660) or **ZI XUE DAN** (*Purple Snow Special Pill* 紫雪丹, p.707) is appropriate.

Patent medicines
Huang Lian Jie Du Wan 黄连解毒丸 (Huang Lian Jie Du Wan)
Qing Fei Yi Huo Pian 清肺抑火片 (Ching Fei Yi Huo Pien)
An Gong Niu Huang Wan 安宫牛黄丸 (An Gong Niu Huang Wan)
  - with delirium
Yun Nan Bai Yao 云南白药 (Yunnan Paiyao)
  - this medicine can be taken internally and/or blown into the nose with a straw. It is used in addition to the main formula. The red pill that accompanies the powder is only used in severe cases.

Acupuncture
PC.3 (*qu ze* ↓), Bl.40 (*wei zhong* ↓), Lu.11 (*shao shang* ↓), LI.11 (*qu chi* -), Du.26 (*ren zhong* -)
- with coma add PC.9 (*zhong chong* ↓) and *shi xuan* ↓ (M-UE-1)

Clinical notes
- Epistaxis associated with Toxic Heat may be diagnosed as biomedical conditions such as septicaemia, pneumonia, encephalitis, meningitis and sinusitis.
- This pattern should be managed in hospital.

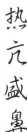

4.3 STOMACH HEAT

Pathophysiology
- The *yang ming* (Stomach and Large Intestine) channels strongly influence the nose. When Heat accumulates in the Stomach, it disrupts the natural descent of Stomach *qi*. The Heat rebels up through the Stomach channel to the nose, causing bleeding. This pattern can be acute, as the result of an exceptional episode of overindulgence, or an invasion of external Heat into the Stomach and Intestines (*yang ming*), but more commonly is chronic and recurrent.

Clinical features
- nosebleed with copious fresh red blood
- swollen, ulcerated or bleeding gums
- irritability
- frontal headache
- thirst with desire for cold drinks
- indeterminate gnawing hunger
- acid reflux
- bad breath
- constipation
- concentrated urine
- red swollen face and nose, bags under the eyes (if chronic)

T red with a yellow coat
P slippery and rapid

Treatment principle
Clear Heat from the Stomach
Cool the Blood, stop bleeding

Prescription

YU NU JIAN 玉女煎
(*Jade Woman Decoction*) modified

shi gao (Gypsum) 石膏	18-30g
sheng di (Radix Rehmanniae Glutinosae) 生地	18-30g
mai dong (Tuber Ophiopogonis Japonici) 麦冬	9g
zhi mu (Rhizoma Anemarrhenae Asphodeloides) 知母	9g
niu xi (Radix Achyranthis Bidentatae) 牛膝	9g
shan zhi zi (Fructus Gardeniae Jasminoidis) 山栀子	9g
mu dan pi (Cortex Moutan Radicis) 牡丹皮	9g

Method: Decoction. (Source: *Shi Yong Zhong Yi Nei Ke Xue*)

Modifications
- With severe bleeding, add **bai mao gen** (Rhizoma Imperatae Cylindricae) 白茅根 18g and **qian cao gen** (Radix Rubiae Cordifoliae) 茜草根 9g.
- With severe thirst, add **tian hua fen** (Radix Trichosanthes Kirilowii) 天花粉 12g and **shi hu** (Herba Dendrobii) 石斛 12g.
- If this pattern is usually related to overindulgence (typically of alcohol or spicy food), herbs to relieve food stagnation can be added, like **shan zha** (Fructus Crataegi) 山楂 9g, **chao shen qu** (dry fried Massa Fermentata) 炒神曲 12g and **ji nei jin^** (Endothelium Corneum Gigeriae Galli) 鸡内金 6g.
- With constipation, add **da huang** (Radix et Rhizoma Rhei) 大黄 6-9g and **gua lou ren** (Semen Trichosanthis) 瓜楼仁 12g.

Variations and additional prescriptions
- When nosebleed follows a pathogenic invasion into the Stomach and Intestines (*yang ming* syndrome) and is accompanied by high fever, sweating, thirst and a flooding pulse, the correct treatment is to clear Heat from *yang ming* with **BAI HU TANG** (*Anemarrhena and Gypsum Combination* 白虎汤, p.32), modified appropriately.

Patent medicines
Huang Lian Jie Du Wan 黄连解毒丸 (Huang Lian Jie Du Wan)
Qing Fei Yi Huo Pian 清肺抑火片 (Ching Fei Yi Huo Pien)
Niu Huang Jie Du Pian 牛黄解毒片 (Peking Niu Huang Chieh Tu Pien)
Niu Huang Qing Huo Wan 牛黄清火丸 (Niu Huang Qing Huo Wan)
Yun Nan Bai Yao 云南白药 (Yunnan Paiyao)
  - this medicine can be taken internally and/or blown into the nose with a straw. It is used in addition to the main formula. The red pill that accompanies the powder is only used in severe cases.

Acupuncture
Du.23 (*shang xing* -), St.3 (*ju liao* -), LI.2 (*er jian* -), St.44 (*nei ting* -), St.45 (*li dui* ↓), LI.4 (*he gu* -), LI.11 (*qu chi* -)

Clinical notes
- Epistaxis associated with Stomach Heat may be diagnosed as biomedical conditions such as alcoholism, overindulgence, gastritis, reflux oesophagitis, gingivitis, meningitis or encephalitis.
- This pattern can respond well to correct treatment combined with dietary and lifestyle modification, particularly limiting hot and spicy foods, alcohol and overeating.

肝火内动鼻衄

4.4 LIVER FIRE

Pathophysiology
- When Liver Fire causes nosebleed the Blood is quickened and forced from the vessels of the upper body. The key to this pattern is the relationship of the symptoms to emotional stress, and there will often be a history of emotional tension or high stress. In addition, there are frequently elements of Stomach Heat in this pattern, as the development of Liver Fire is aided by overindulgence in heating foods and beverages.

Clinical features
- nosebleed with copious fresh red blood, which is initiated by emotional turmoil; in some cases there may also be scleral haemorrhage
- bitter taste in the mouth, dry mouth
- hypochondriac tension or discomfort
- irritability, short temper
- temporal headache
- dizziness, tinnitus
- insomnia
- red, sore eyes; facial flushing
- in chronic cases the nose may be swollen and red with orange peel like skin, and spider naevi may be evident on the cheeks

T red with a thick yellow coat
P wiry, forceful and rapid

Treatment principle
Clear Liver Fire
Cool the Blood, stop bleeding

Prescription

LONG DAN XIE GAN TANG 龙胆泻肝汤
(*Gentiana Combination*) modified

long dan cao (Radix Gentianae Longdancao) 龙胆草	9g
sheng di (Radix Rehmanniae Glutinosae) 生地	15g
shan zhi zi (Fructus Gardeniae Jasminoidis) 山栀子	12g
ce bai ye (Cacumen Biotae Orientalis) 侧柏叶	12g
chuan niu xi (Radix Cyathulae Officinalis) 川牛膝	9g
ze xie (Rhizoma Alismatis Orientalis) 泽泻	9g
che qian zi (Semen Plantaginis) 车前子	6g
huang qin (Radix Scutellariae Baicalensis) 黄芩	6g
mu tong (Caulis Mutong) 木通	6g
dang gui (Radix Angelicae Sinensis) 当归	3g

gan cao (Radix Glycyrrhizae Uralensis) 甘草 3g
Method: Decoction. **Che qian zi** is usually cooked in a cloth bag (*bao jian*).

Modifications
- With severe bleeding, add **qian cao gen** (Radix Rubiae Cordifoliae) 茜草根 9g, **xian he cao** (Herba Agrimoniae Pilosae) 仙鹤草 12g and **bai mao gen** (Rhizoma Imperatae Cylindricae) 白茅根 18g.
- With severe Heat, add **huang lian** (Rhizoma Coptidis) 黄连 6g, **ling yang jiao fen°** (powdered Cornu Antelopis) 羚羊角粉 3g.
- With dryness, delete **che qian zi** and **ze xie**, and add **mai dong** (Tuber Ophiopogonis Japonici) 麦冬 12g, **xuan shen** (Radix Scrophulariae Ningpoensis) 18g and **zhi mu** (Rhizoma Anemarrhenae Asphodeloides) 知母 12g.

Variations and additional prescriptions
- Nosebleeds that occurs premenstrually are often associated with Heat in the Liver affecting the Blood. Accompanying symptoms include irritability, thirst, dizziness and a shortened cycle. In extreme cases, the period is scanty or even absent. The correct treatment is to clear Heat from the Liver, redirect *qi* and Blood downwards, and stop bleeding with **SI WU TANG** (*Dang Gui Four Combination* 四物汤) modified.

  sheng di (Radix Rehmanniae Glutinosae) 生地 30g
  bai mao gen (Rhizoma Imperatae Cylindricae) 白茅根 30g
  bai shao (Radix Paeoniae Lactiflorae) 白芍 15g
  chuan niu xi (Radix Cyathulae Officinalis) 川牛膝 15g
  yu jin (Tuber Curcumae) 郁金 9g
  dang gui (Radix Angelicae Sinensis) 当归 9g
  e jiao^ (Gelatinum Corii Asini) 阿胶 9g
  mu dan pi (Cortex Moutan Radicis) 牡丹皮 9g
  huang qin (Radix Scutellariae Baicalensis) 黄芩 9g
  chuan lian zi* (Fructus Meliae Toosendan) 川楝子 9g
  gan cao (Radix Glycyrrhizae Uralensis) 甘草 5g
  Method: Decoction. **E jiao** is melted before being added to the strained decoction (*yang hua* 烊化). (Source: *Shi Yong Zhong Yi Fu Ke Xue*)

Patent medicines
Long Dan Xie Gan Wan 龙胆泻肝丸 (Long Dan Xie Gan Wan)
Yun Nan Bai Yao 云南白药 (Yunnan Paiyao)
  - this medicine can be taken internally and/or blown into the nose with a straw. It is used in addition to the main formula. The red pill that accompanies the powder is only used in severe cases.

Acupuncture
Bl.13 (*fei shu* -), Lu.5 (*chi ze* -), Liv.2 (*xing jian* -), GB.20 (*feng chi* -), GB.18 (*cheng ling* -), GB.34 (*yang ling quan* -), Liv.3 (*tai chong* -), Bl.18 (*gan shu* -), LI.11 (*qu chi* -)

Clinical notes
- Epistaxis associated with Liver Fire may be diagnosed as biomedical conditions such as hypertension, alcoholism, hepatitis and bleeding diathesis.
- Episodes generally respond satisfactorily to correct treatment. Long term results require an appropriate management plan with lifestyle modification, relaxation, exercise and stress management.

4. EPISTAXIS

肝
肾
阴
虚
鼻
衄

4.5 LIVER AND KIDNEY *YIN* DEFICIENCY

Pathophysiology
- Liver and Kidney *yin* deficiency epistaxis has two aspects to it. The first is the background Liver and Kidney *yin* deficiency, the drying effect of which on the Lungs gives rise to the occasional weak bleeding. The second is the tendency for *yang* to rise when *yin* is deficient. Uncontrolled rising *yang* as a result of *yin* deficiency can increase the pressure in the vessels of the head, damaging the delicate *luo mai*, causing nosebleed and scleral haemorrhage.

Clinical features
- intermittent nosebleeds, usually with only small amounts of blood
- loose teeth, atrophy of the gums
- dizziness, tinnitus, blurred vision, poor memory
- malar or facial flushing, night sweats
- sensation of heat in the palms and soles ('five hearts hot')
- lower back ache

T red and dry with little or no coat
P thready and rapid

Treatment principle
Nourish *yin*, clear Heat
Cool the Blood, stop bleeding

Prescription

ZHI BAI BA WEI WAN 知柏八味丸
(*Anemarrhena, Phellodendron and Rehmannia Formula*)

shu di (Radix Rehmanniae Glutinosae Conquitae) 熟地	24g
shan yao (Radix Dioscoreae Oppositae) 山药	12g
shan zhu yu (Fructus Corni Officinalis) 山茱萸	12g
fu ling (Sclerotium Poria Cocos) 茯苓	9g
mu dan pi (Cortex Moutan Radicis) 牡丹皮	9g
ze xie (Rhizoma Alismatis Orientalis) 泽泻	9g
zhi mu (Rhizoma Anemarrhenae Asphodeloidis) 知母	9g
yan huang bai (salt fried Cortex Phellodendri) 盐黄柏	9g

Method: Grind the herbs to powder and form into 9-gram pills with honey. The dose is 2-3 pills daily. May also be decocted with the doses as shown. (Source: *Shi Yong Fang Ji Xue*)

Modifications
- If the bleeding is more than just a small amount, add **han lian cao** (Herba Ecliptae Prostratae) 旱莲草 12g, **ou jie** (Nodus Nelumbinis Nuciferae Rhizomatis) 藕节 12g and **e jiao**^ (Gelatinum Corii Asini) 阿胶 9g.

- With prominent deficient Heat, add **bie jia**° (Carapax Amydae Sinensis) 鳖甲 12g and **qing hao** (Herba Artemesiae Annuae) 青蒿 15g.
- If the Spleen is weak, double the dose of **shan yao** (Radix Dioscoreae Oppositae) 山药 and add **chen pi** (Pericarpium Citri Reticulatae) 陈皮 6g and **bai zhu** (Rhizoma Atractylodis Macrocephalae) 白术 12g.

Variations and additional prescriptions

With Liver yang rising
- In patients with hypertension, recurrent nosebleeds, dizziness and headaches, rising *yang* is predominant. The correct treatment is to nourish *yin*, sedate the Liver, anchor *yang* with **ZHEN GAN XI FENG TANG** (*Sedate the Liver and Extinguish Wind Decoction* 镇肝熄风汤, p.545).

With Blood deficiency
- In very chronic cases with persistent or severe bleeding, Blood deficiency may occur. The correct treatment is to focus on stopping the bleeding, and nourish Blood with **JIAO AI TANG** (*Ass-Hide Gelatin and Mugwort Decoction* 胶艾汤).

    e jiao^ (Gelatinum Corii Asini) 阿胶 9g
    ai ye* (Folium Artemisiae Argyi) 艾叶 9g
    shu di (Radix Rehmanniae Glutinosae Conquitae) 熟地 18g
    dang gui (Radix Angelicae Sinensis) 当归 9g
    bai shao (Radix Paeoniae Lactiflorae) 白芍 9g
    chuan xiong (Radix Ligustici Chuanxiong) 川芎 6g
    zhi gan cao (honey fried Radix Glycyrrhizae Uralensis)
        炙甘草 6g

Method: Decoction. **E jiao** is melted before being added to the strained decoction (*yang hua* 烊化). (Source: *Shi Yong Fang Ji Xue*)

Patent medicines

Zhi Bai Ba Wei Wan 知柏八味丸 (Zhi Bai Ba Wei Wan)
Qi Ju Di Huang Wan 杞菊地黄丸 (Lycium-Rehmannia Pills)
Tian Ma Gou Teng Wan 天麻钩藤丸 (Tian Ma Gou Teng Wan)
Yang Yin Jiang Ya Wan 养阴降压丸 (Yang Yin Jiang Ya Wan)
Yun Nan Bai Yao 云南白药 (Yunnan Paiyao)
   - this medicine can be taken internally and/or blown into the nose with a straw. It is used in addition to the main formula. The red pill that accompanies the powder is only used in severe cases.

Acupuncture

Bl.23 (*shen shu* +), Bl.18 (*gan shu* +), Kid.3 (*tai xi* +), Liv.3 (*tai chong*), Bl.7 (*tong tian*), Kid.1 (*yong quan*), Sp.1 (*yin bai* ▲), Sp.6 (*san yin jiao*)

Clinical notes
- Epistaxis associated with Liver and Kidney *yin* deficiency may be diagnosed as biomedical conditions such as hypertension, menopausal syndrome, leukaemia and Hodgkin's disease.

4.6 SPLEEN *QI* DEFICIENCY

Pathophysiology
- In contrast to the Heat patterns, a Spleen *qi* deficiency type nose bleed drips rather than pours as the deficient Spleen *qi* allows slow leakage of Blood from the vessels.

Clinical features
- occasional dripping nosebleed with pale pink blood; the quantity is usually small, but may occasionally be copious, maybe accompanied by other sites of bleeding–easy bruising, bleeding gums, heavy menstrual period, uterine bleeding
- pale complexion
- abdominal distension
- poor appetite
- loose stools
- fatigue
- postural dizziness

T pale with thin white coat
P thready and weak, or hollow if there has been significant blood loss

Treatment principle
Strengthen the Spleen, tonify *qi* and Blood
Stop bleeding

Prescription

GUI PI TANG 归脾汤
(*Ginseng and Longan Combination*) modified

huang qi (Radix Astragali Membranacei) 黄芪	30g
dang shen (Radix Codonopsis Pilosulae) 党参	15g
fu ling (Sclerotium Poriae Cocos) 茯苓	18g
suan zao ren (Semen Zizyphi Spinosae) 酸枣仁	15g
long yan rou (Arillus Euphoriae Longanae) 龙眼肉	15g
yuan zhi (Radix Polygalae Tenuifoliae) 远志	9g
mu xiang (Radix Aucklandiae Lappae) 木香	6g
gan cao (Radix Glycyrrhizae Uralensis) 甘草	6g
ce bai ye (Cacumen Biotae Orientalis) 侧柏叶	12g
di yu tan (charred Radix Sanguisorbae Officinalis) 地榆炭	12g
e jiao^ (Gelatinum Corii Asini) 阿胶	6g

Method: Decoction. **E jiao** is melted before being added to the strained decoction (*yang hua* 烊化). (Source: *Zhong Yi Er Bi Hou Ke Xue*)

Modifications

- If the bleeding persists, other astringent styptic herbs like **xian he cao** (Herba Agrimoniae Pilosae) 仙鹤草 12g, **chao pu huang** (dry fried Pollen Typhae) 炒蒲黄 9g and **han lian cao** (Herba Ecliptae Prostratae) 旱连草 12g can be added, or consider **JIAO AI TANG** (*Ass-Hide Gelatin and Mugwort Decoction* 胶艾汤, p.178).
- With Cold or *yang* deficiency, add two or three of the following herbs: **zhi fu zi*** (Radix Aconiti Carmichaeli Praeparata) 制附子 6g, **gan jiang** (Rhizoma Zingiberis Officinalis) 干姜 6g, **rou gui** (Cortex Cinnamomi Cassiae) 肉桂 3g, **xian ling pi** (Herba Epimedii) 仙灵脾 12g or **ba ji tian** (Radix Morindae Officinalis) 巴戟天 9g.

Variations and additional prescriptions

Spleen and Kidney yang *deficiency*

- If Spleen and Kidney *yang* are deficient, the correct treatment is to warm and tonify Spleen and Kidney *yang* with a guiding formula such as **YOU GUI WAN** (*Eucommia and Rehmannia Formula* 右归丸, p.256), or **JIN KUI SHEN QI WAN** (*Rehmannia Eight Formula* 金匮肾气丸, p.150) with the addition of herbs like **huang qi** (Radix Astragali Membranacei) 黄芪 and **dang shen** (Radix Codonopsis Pilosulae) 党参.

Patent medicines

Gui Pi Wan 归脾丸 (Gui Pi Wan)
Jin Kui Shen Qi Wan 金匮肾气丸 (Sexoton Pills)
 - *yang* deficiency
Yun Nan Bai Yao 云南白药 (Yunnan Paiyao)
 - this medicine can be taken internally and/or blown into the nose with a straw. It is used in addition to the main formula. The red pill that accompanies the powder is only used in severe cases.

Acupuncture

Sp.6 (*san yi jiao* +▲), Bl.20 (*pi shu* +▲), St.36 (*zu san li* +▲), Du.20 (*bai hui* +▲), Ren.6 (*qi hai* +▲), Sp.1 (*yin bai* ▲)

Clinical notes

- Epistaxis associated with *qi* deficiency may be diagnosed as biomedical conditions such as thrombocytopoenia, haemophilia, idiopathic thrombocytopoenic purpura and anaemia.
- This pattern generally responds well to correct treatment, although genetic bleeding disorders are difficult.

SUMMARY OF GUIDING FORMULAE FOR EPISTAXIS

Excess patterns

Wind Heat - *Sang Ju Yin* 桑菊饮

Toxic Heat - *Huang Lian Jie Du Tang* 黄连解毒汤
- with disordered consciousness - plus *Xi Jiao Di Huang Tang* 犀角地黄汤 or *Qing Ying Tang* 清营汤
- with delirium - *Zhi Bao Dan* 至宝丹, *An Gong Niu Huang Wan* 安宫牛黄丸

Stomach Heat - *Yu Nü Jian* 玉女煎
- with external invasion into *yang ming* - *Bai Hu Tang* 白虎汤

Liver Fire - *Long Dan Xie Gan Tang* 龙胆泻肝汤

Deficient patterns

Lung and Kidney *yin* deficiency - *Zhi Bai Ba Wei Wan* 知柏八味丸
- with *yang* rising - *Zhen Gan Xi Feng Tang* 镇肝熄风汤
- with Blood deficiency - *Jiao Ai Tang* 胶艾汤

Spleen *qi* deficiency - *Gui Pi Tang* 归脾汤
- with Kidney *yang* deficiency - *You Gui Wan* 右归丸, or *Jin Kui Shen Qi Wan* 金匮肾气丸

Endnote

For more information regarding herbs marked with an asterisk*, an open circle° or a hat^, see the tables on pp.944-952.

Disorders of the Lung

5. Haemoptysis

Wind Heat
Dryness affecting the Lungs
Wind Cold
Lung Heat
Phlegm Heat
Liver Fire invading the Lungs
Lung and Kidney *yin* deficiency with Fire
Spleen *qi* deficiency

5 HAEMOPTYSIS
ke xue 咳血

Haemoptysis is the coughing up or spitting of blood originating in the lungs. The blood may appear as fresh blood, blood clots or blood streaked mucus. Clinically, haemoptysis is less common as a primary presentation than as a subsidiary symptom of other TCM respiratory 'diseases', like cough or *fei yong* (Lung abscess). It often accompanies severe Heat patterns involving the Lungs, but in these cases (unless the bleeding is copious) the TCM diagnosis is more likely to be cough or *fei yong*. When haemoptysis is the primary presentation, it is usually a serious condition requiring investigation.

AETIOLOGY
Cough
A chronic or severe cough, from any cause, can result in haemoptysis. Repeated coughing can mechanically disrupt the delicate lining of the lungs, rupturing superficial vessels. If the cough causing the haemoptysis is simply a response to an inhaled irritant, then identification and removal of the irritant is the only treatment required.

Heat
Heat is the most common cause of haemoptysis. When there is Heat in the body it can influence the Blood, quickening it and forcing it from the vessels. The Heat may be excess or deficient in origin. Heat also dries and damages the lining of the Lungs, causing rupture of superficial vessels.

Excess Heat is either external, or internally generated. External Heat is due to Wind Heat or Wind Cold that turns hot once in the body. If *zheng qi* is weak or the pathogen strong the pathogen can penetrate further into the body, leading to Lung Heat or Phlegm Heat (when there is pre-existing Phlegm). Heat of external origin is probably the most common cause of haemoptysis.

Internal Heat can be the product of prolonged Liver *qi* stagnation (see Liver Fire), or excessive consumption of heating foods and tobacco. The presence of pre-existing internal Heat, derived from the aforementioned factors, can predispose patients to increased damage by external Heat. Once affected by Heat, chest fluids and *yin* can be dried out and damaged. This can cause thickening of fluids into Phlegm or an increase in the viscosity of Blood leading to sluggish and stagnant of Blood.

Deficient Heat is generated by *yin* deficiency. Lung *yin* is damaged by other chronic or severe hot Lung diseases, like recurrent Phlegm Heat. Smoking, living in very dry environments, use of bronchodilating medications and inhaled steroids or *yin* deficiency of other *zang* can contribute to Lung *yin* deficiency. A hot and spicy diet may also contribute by continually dispersing Lung *qi* and *yin*.

Dryness

Dryness easily damages the Lungs. The dryness may be external and associated with Wind and Heat or Cold, or may simply be the result of living in a very dry environment. Any of the Heat pathogens may dry the Lungs, including the Heat generated by *yin* deficiency. As well as generating Heat, *yin* deficiency fails to adequately moisten the Lungs.

Liver Fire

Emotions like frustration, resentment and anger can disrupt the circulation of Liver *qi*, which can over time generate sufficient Heat to be redefined as Fire. The Liver and the Lungs have a close relationship. According to five phase (*wu xing* 五行) theory, the Lungs restrain the Liver, and prevent it from getting too 'strong'. When the Lungs are weak or the Liver too 'strong' (that is, Liver *qi* is stagnant or there is some other excess pattern involving the Liver), then the controlling (*ke* 克, p.70) cycle breaks down and the pent up Liver *qi* or Fire rebels backwards along the controlling cycle. When Liver Fire damages the Lungs (via the reverse *ke* cycle) haemoptysis is the result. In contrast, when Liver *qi* stagnation follows the same path to affect the Lungs, the result is (usually) cough.

Spleen *qi* deficiency

Overwork, excessive worry, irregular dietary habits, excessive consumption of cold, raw foods or prolonged illness weaken Spleen *qi*. One of the main functions of Spleen *qi* is to exert an external pressure on the vessels preventing the leakage of Blood and when this aspect is weak Blood 'oozes' out. Bleeding of this type is generally mild, chronic and prolonged. This is in contrast to most other types of haemoptysis in which the Blood is heated and quickened and forced from the vessels. This is an uncommon type of haemoptysis as deficiency bleeding generally affects the lower body and skin.

BOX 5.1 SOME BIOMEDICAL CAUSES OF HAEMOPTYSIS

- acute infections (bronchitis, lobar pneumonia, URTI)
- chronic bronchitis
- bronchiectasis
- tuberculosis
- lung and laryngeal tumours
- pulmonary infarction
- HIV
- foreign body
- thromboembolism
- lung abscess
- anticoagulants
- trauma
- blood dyscrasia
- epidemic haemorrhagic diseases
- thrombocytopoenia
- mitral stenosis
- Goodpasture's syndrome
- roundworm or hookworm infestation

BOX 5.2 DIAGNOSIS OF HAEMOPTYSIS

Haemoptysis is frequently accompanied by other respiratory symptoms like a cough. The TCM diagnosis of haemoptysis is based on the relative quantities of blood and mucus (if present). When the volume of blood is larger than that of mucus, or the patient coughs only blood, then the diagnosis is obviously haemoptysis. If there is a cough with copious mucus with streaks of blood, then the most appropriate TCM disease diagnosis is probably cough.

Differential diagnosis
Haemoptysis should be distinguished from the following:
- **Haematemesis**: vomiting or spitting blood originating from the stomach. It can sometimes be tricky to determine the origin of blood expelled from the mouth, however expulsion of blood associated with stomach pain, blood that is dark or like coffee grounds or mixed with food or sour gastric juice is usually of gastric origin. If there is bleeding in the stomach the stools are usually dark and sticky. If the bleeding is in the lower oesophagus it is usually fresh and copious and occurs in patients with portal hypertension, particularly alcoholics.
- **Bleeding from the oral cavity**: If the blood originates from the gums, throat, nasal cavity or cheeks there is usually no cough, not much blood and it is fresh or mixed with saliva.
- ***fei yong***: In *fei yong* there may be coughing of blood mixed with malodorous purulent mucus. There is usually focal chest pain, fever, thirst and malaise. *Fei yong* represents a significant lung infection.

TREATMENT

In general there are several steps to consider when treating any bleeding disorder. The first, and most important step, is to stop the bleeding. When the bleeding is severe, the initial focus of treatment is to use first aid or herbs to quickly staunch the bleeding. This can usually be acheived with a styptic formula or with the use of the patent medicine *Yun Nan Bai Yao* 云南白药 (Yunnan Paiyao).

Once bleeding has ceased or is under control, the underlying pattern can be dealt with more fully. There are two additional aspects to consider. Any residual Blood outside the vessels is stagnant Blood, which must be moved as it may become pathological if allowed to remain. Thus, herbs to gently invigorate or regulate Blood are incorporated into the appropriate formula. This is especially important in Heat types of bleeding, as the herbs used to stop bleeding will likely be cold natured and astringent. These herbs congeal Blood. Finally, any *qi* or Blood deficiency that exists as a direct result of Blood loss should be supplemented.

5. HAEMOPTYSIS

5.1 WIND HEAT

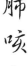

Pathophysiology
- Wind Heat invades the Lungs through the mouth and nose. Once lodged in the Lungs, Heat damages and dries the surface of the Lungs and the delicate *luo mai* causing bleeding.

Clinical features
- acute cough with yellow blood streaked mucus. The blood is fresh red. Depending on the degree of Heat, there may be only small amounts of sticky mucus with larger quantities of blood. (When there is more mucus than blood, or simply streaks of blood on the mucus, the TCM disease diagnosis of cough may be more appropriate, see p.77)
- sore throat
- fever, mild chills
- thirst
- headache
- sweating

T normal or red tip with a thin yellow coat
P floating and rapid

Treatment principle
Disperse Wind and clear Heat from the Lungs
Cool Blood and stop bleeding

Prescription

YIN QIAO SAN 银翘散
(*Lonicera and Forsythia Formula*) modified

jin yin hua (Flos Lonicerae Japonicae) 金银花	12-15g
lian qiao (Fructus Forsythia Suspensae) 连翘	12-15g
lu gen (Rhizoma Phragmitis Communis) 芦根	15g
dan zhu ye (Herba Lophatheri Gracilis) 淡竹叶	9g
niu bang zi (Fructus Arctii Lappae) 牛蒡子	9g
jing jie (Herba seu Flos Schizonepetae Tenuifolia) 荆芥	6g
bo he (Herba Mentha Haplocalycis) 薄荷	6g
chuan bei mu (Bulbus Fritillariae Cirrhosae) 川贝母	6g
xing ren* (Semen Pruni Armeniacae) 杏仁	6g
han lian cao (Herba Ecliptae Prostratae) 旱莲草	9g
bai mao gen (Rhizoma Imperatae Cylindricae) 白茅根	12g
ou jie (Nodus Nelumbinis Nuciferae Rhizomatis) 藕节	12g
qian cao gen (Radix Rubiae Cordifoliae) 茜草根	12g

Method: Decoction. Do not cook for more than 20 minutes. **Bo he** is added near the end of cooking (*hou xia* 后下). **Jie geng**, which appears in the original formula, has an ascending action and is unsuitable for haemoptysis. (Source: *Shi Yong Zhong Yi Nei Ke Xue*)

Modifications
- If the haemoptysis is severe, add **YUN NAN BAI YAO** (*Yunnan White Powder* 云南白药) or **san qi fen** (powdered Radix Notoginseng) 三七粉 3g to the cooked decoction (*chong fu* 冲服).
- With some Phlegm Heat (copious sticky yellow mucus, a greasy tongue coat and a slippery pulse), add **huang qin** (Radix Scutellariae Baicalensis) 黄芩 12g and **yu xing cao** (Herba Houttuyniae) 鱼腥草 15g.
- If following the resolution of the exterior symptoms, there is damage to body fluids, with a persistent dry cough, little or no mucus and a red dry tongue, delete **jing jie** and **bo he** and add **tian dong** (Tuber Asparagi Cochinchinensis) 天冬 9g, **mai dong** (Tuber Ophiopogonis Japonici) 麦冬 12g, **xuan shen** (Radix Scrophulariae Ningpoensis) 玄参 15g and **tian hua fen** (Radix Trichosanthes Kirilowii) 天花粉 9g.

Patent medicines
Yin Qiao Jie Du Pian 银翘解毒片 (Yin Chiao Chieh Tu Pien)
Qing Fei Yi Huo Pian 清肺抑火片 (Ching Fei Yi Huo Pien)
  - for more severe Heat
Yun Nan Bai Yao 云南白药 (Yunnan Paiyao)
  - this medicine can be taken in addition to the main formula selected. The red pill that accompanies the powder is only used in severe cases.

Acupuncture
Lu.6 (*kong zui* -), Lu.10 (*yu ji* -), Bl.13 (*fei shu* -), LI.4 (*he gu* -), SJ.5 (*wai guan* -), LI.16 (*ju gu* -)
- if fever is severe add LI.11 (*qu chi* -)
- if cough is severe add Lu.5 (*chi ze* -)
- sore swollen throat, add Lu.11 (*shao shang* ↓) and SI.17 (*tian rong* -)

Clinical notes
- The haemoptysis in this pattern may be associated with biomedical conditions such as the common cold, tonsillitis, upper respiratory tract infection, acute bronchitis, pneumonia, early stage of measles, encephalitis or meningitis.
- Generally responds well to correct and timely treatment.

5. HAEMOPTYSIS

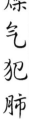
燥气犯肺咳血

5.2 DRYNESS AFFECTING THE LUNGS

Pathophysiology
- Seasonal dryness or depletion of normal fluids due to dry Heat, Wind or smoking can lead to dryness of the Lungs, damage to the delicate *luo mai* and consequent bleeding. This pattern is common in Autumn in China when very dry winds blow off the Gobi desert. This is not a common pattern in humid or damp climates, although widespread indoor climate control may influence this.

Clinical features
- dry, hacking cough with blood or scant, blood streaked mucus
- dry throat, lips, nose and mouth
- mild fever
- aversion to wind
- thirst
- irritability

T thin, dry, white coat
P floating and possibly rapid

Treatment principle
Clear and moisten the Lungs
Calm the cough and stop bleeding

Prescription

QING ZAO JIU FEI TANG 清燥救肺汤
(*Eriobotrya and Ophiopogon Combination*) modified

xing ren* (Semen Pruni Armeniacae) 杏仁	9g
sang ye (Folium Mori Albae) 桑叶	9g
sha shen (Radix Adenophorae seu Glehniae) 沙参	9g
zhi pi pa ye (honey fried Folium Eriobotryae Japonicae) 炙枇杷叶	9g
shi gao (Gypsum) 石膏	12g
mai dong (Tuber Ophiopogonis Japonici) 麦冬	9g
hei zhi ma (Semen Sesami Indici) 黑芝麻	9g
e jiao^ (Gelatinum Corii Asini) 阿胶	6g
sheng di tan (charred Radix Rehmanniae Glutinosae) 生地炭	12g
ce bai ye (Cacumen Biotae Orientalis) 侧柏叶	12g
gan cao (Radix Glycyrrhizae Uralensis) 甘草	3g

Method: Decoction. **E jiao** is melted before being added to the strained decoction (*yang hua* 烊化). (Source: *Shi Yong Zhong Yi Nei Ke Xue*)

Modifications
- With severe bleeding, add **qian cao gen** (Radix Rubiae Cordifoliae) 茜草根 9g, **xian he cao** (Herba Agrimoniae Pilosae) 仙鹤草 12g and **bai mao gen** (Rhizoma Imperatae Cylindricae) 白茅根 18g, or combine with **YUN NAN BAI YAO** (*Yunnan White Powder* 云南白药).
- With constipation, add **tao ren** (Semen Persicae) 桃仁 9g and **huo ma ren** (Semen Cannabis Sativae) 火麻仁 9g.

Patent medicines
Luo Han Guo Chong Ji 罗汉果冲剂 (Luo Han Guo Beverage)
Yang Yin Qing Fei Wan 养阴清肺丸 (Yang Yin Qing Fei Wan)
Chuan Bei Pi Pa Gao 川贝枇杷膏 (Nin Jiom Pei Pa Kao)
Yun Nan Bai Yao 云南白药 (Yunnan Paiyao)
   - this medicine can be taken in addition to the main formula selected. The red pill that accompanies the powder is only used in severe cases.

Acupuncture
Lu.6 (*kong zui* -), Lu.10 (*yu ji* -), Bl.13 (*fei shu* -), LI.4 (*he gu* -), SJ.5 (*wai guan* -), LI.16 (*ju gu* -), Kid.6 (*zhao hai* +), Lu.7 (*lie que*)
- with fever add LI.11 (*qu chi* -)
- if cough is severe add Lu.5 (*chi ze* -)

Clinical notes
- The haemoptysis in this pattern may be associated with biomedical conditions such as upper respiratory tract infection, influenza, acute and chronic bronchitis, pneumonia and whooping cough.
- Generally responds well to correct treatment.

5.3 WIND COLD

Pathophysiology
- Invasion of Wind Cold disrupts the circulaton of Lung *qi* and leads to coughing which can damage the *luo mai* of the Lungs. This is an uncommon cause of haemoptysis, except in those with pre-existing Lung disease and chronic cough.

Clinical features
- cough with thin watery mucus mixed with a small quantity of blood
- chill and mild fever or aversion to cold
- occipital headache
- stiff neck, myalgia
- nasal obstruction or runny nose with clear watery mucus

T usually unremarkable, with a thin white coat
P floating and tight

Treatment principle
Dispel Wind and Cold
Soothe the Lungs and stop bleeding

Prescription

JIN FEI CAO SAN 金沸草散
(*Inula Powder*) modified

jin fei cao (Herba Inulae) 金沸草	9g
qian hu (Radix Peucedani) 前胡	9g
jing jie (Herba seu Flos Schizonepetae Tenuifolia) 荆芥	6g
fu ling (Sclerotium Poria Cocos) 茯苓	9g
ban xia* (Rhizoma Pinelliae Ternatae) 半夏	9g
xi xin* (Herba cum Radice Asari) 细辛	3g
gan cao (Radix Glycyrrhizae Uralensis) 甘草	3g
sheng jiang (Rhizoma Zingiberis Officinalis Recens) 生姜	3pce
xian he cao (Herba Agrimoniae Pilosae) 仙鹤草	12g
bai mao gen (Rhizoma Imperatae Cylindricae) 白茅根	12g
chao pu huang (dry fried Pollen Typhae) 炒蒲黄	9g

Method: Decoction. (Source: *Shi Yong Zhong Yi Nei Ke Xue*)

Modifications
- If the bleeding is severe, combine with **YUN NAN BAI YAO** (*Yunnan White Powder* 云南白药).

Variations and additional prescriptions
- If, following the dispersal of the Wind and Cold, the cough and blood streaked mucus persists, use **ZHI SOU SAN** (*Stop Coughing Powder* 止嗽散) modified.
    jing jie (Herba seu Flos Schizonepetae Tenuifolia) 荆芥 9g
    zi wan (Radix Asteris Tatarici) 紫菀 9g
    bai bu* (Radix Stemonae) 百部 9g
    bai qian (Radix et Rhizoma Cynanchi Baiqian) 白前 9g
    chen pi (Pericarpium Citri Reticulatae) 陈皮 6g
    gan cao (Radix Glycyrrhizae Uralensis) 甘草 3g
    bai mao gen (Rhizoma Imperatae Cylindricae) 白茅根 12g
    xian he cao (Herba Agrimoniae Pilosae) 仙鹤草 12g
    Method: Decoction. (Source: *Shi Yong Zhong Yi Nei Ke Xue*)

Patent medicines
Gan Mao Ling 感冒灵 (Gan Mao Ling)
Gan Mao Qing Re Chong Ji 感冒清热冲剂 (Gan Mao Qing Re Chong Ji)
Gan Mao Zhi Ke Chong Ji 感冒止咳冲剂 (Gan Mao Zhi Ke Chong Ji)
Zhi Sou Wan 止嗽丸 (Zhi Sou Wan)
Chuan Xiong Cha Tiao Wan 川芎茶调丸 (Chuan Xiong Cha Tiao Wan)
 - with prominent headache
Yun Nan Bai Yao 云南白药 (Yunnan Paiyao)
 - this medicine can be taken in addition to the main formula selected. The red pill that accompanies the powder is only used in severe cases.

Acupuncture
LI.4 (*he gu* -), Lu.7 (*lie que* -), Lu.6 (*kong zui* -), Bl.12 (*feng men* -Ω), Bl.13 (*fei shu* -Ω), Du.14 (*da zhui* -)
- If there is significant wheezing use *ding chuan* (M-BW-1)
- If the nose is congested or runny add Du.23 (*shang xing*)

Clinical notes
- The haemoptysis in this pattern may be associated with biomedical conditions such as the common cold, influenza and upper respiratory tract infection.
- Generally responds well to correct treatment.

肺热咳血

5.4 LUNG HEAT

Pathophysiology
- Lung Heat results from the penetration of Wind Heat (or Wind Cold which turns hot) into the Lungs. Once lodged internally, Heat easily dries and damages the delicate Lung *luo mai* and may quicken the Blood, causing it to spill from the vessels. This pattern often follows unresolved Wind Heat.

Clinical features
- dry, hacking painful cough with blood and little or no mucus; if there is a small amount of mucus it is sticky, hard to expectorate and may be blood streaked
- fever with or without sweating
- shortness of breath, laboured breathing or wheezing
- chest tightness and pain
- sensation of heat in the chest
- dry mouth and thirst
- red face

T red or with a red tip and a yellow coat
P flooding and rapid, or wiry and rapid

Treatment principle
Clear Heat from the Lungs
Cool Blood and stop bleeding

Prescription

MA XING SHI GAN TANG 麻杏石甘汤
(*Ma Huang, Apricot Seed, Gypsum and Licorice Combination*) modified

zhi ma huang* (honey fried Herba Ephedra) 炙麻黄	9g
shi gao (Gypsum) 石膏	30g
xing ren* (Semen Pruni Armeniacae) 杏仁	9g
zhi gan cao (honey fried Radix Glycyrrhizae Uralensis) 炙甘草	6g
yu xing cao (Herba Houttuyniae) 鱼腥草	18g
sang bai pi (Cortex Mori Albae Radicis) 桑白皮	12g
huang qin (Radix Scutellariae Baicalensis) 黄芩	12g
qian cao gen (Radix Rubiae Cordifoliae) 茜草根	12g
bai mao gen (Rhizoma Imperatae Cylindricae) 白茅根	18g
ce bai ye (Cacumen Biotae Orientalis) 侧柏叶	12g

Method: Decoction.

Modifications

- If the bleeding is severe or resistant, combine with **YUN NAN BAI YAO** (*Yunnan White Powder* 云南白药)or add **san qi fen** (powdered Radix Notoginseng) 三七粉 to the cooked decoction (*chong fu* 冲服).
- With chest pain, add **tao ren** (Semen Persicae) 桃仁 9g and **yu jin** (Tuber Curcumae) 郁金 9g.
- If the cough is severe, add **ma dou ling*** (Fructus Aristolchiae) 马兜铃 9g and **zhi pi pa ye** (honey fried Folium Eriobotryae) 炙枇杷叶 9g.
- With severe thirst, add **tian hua fen** (Radix Trichosanthis Kirilowii) 天花粉 9g
- If the throat is very sore, add **she gan** (Rhizoma Belamacandae) 射干 9g, **xuan shen** (Radix Scrophulariae) 玄参 15g or **ma bo** (Fructificatio Lasiosphaerae seu Calvatiae) 马勃 9g.

Patent medicines

Qing Fei Yi Huo Pian 清肺抑火片 (Ching Fei Yi Huo Pien)
Chuan Xin Lian Kang Yan Pian 穿心莲抗炎片
  (Chuan Xin Lian Antiphlogistic Tablets)
Niu Huang Qing Huo Wan 牛黄清火丸 (Niu Huang Qing Huo Wan)
  - with constipation and severe Heat
Yun Nan Bai Yao 云南白药 (Yunnan Paiyao)
  - this medicine can be taken in addition to the main formula selected. The red pill that accompanies the powder is only used in severe cases.

Acupuncture

Lu.5 (*chi ze* -), Lu.6 (*kong zui* -), Lu.10 (*yu ji* -), Bl.13 (*fei shu* -), Ren.17 (*shan zhong*), LI.4 (*he gu* -)
- with fever add LI.11 (*qu chi* -)
- if cough is severe add Lu.5 (*chi ze* -)
- sore swollen throat, add SI.17 (*tian rong* -) and Lu.9 (*shao shang* ↓)

Clinical notes

- The haemoptysis in this pattern may be associated with biomedical conditions such as the common cold, upper respiratory tract infection, tonsillitis, bronchitis and tracheitis.

5.5 PHLEGM HEAT

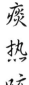

Pathophysiology
- Phlegm Heat is related to Lung Heat and Phlegm Damp. Lung Heat can dry or congeal Lung Fluids to become Phlegm Heat. This usually follows a Wind Heat (or Cold) invasion that penetrates into the Lungs.
- It also occurs as an acute flareup in those with chronic Phlegm Damp in the Lungs, particularly where there is a pre-existing tendency to Heat as a result of overindulgence in heating foods, alcohol and tobacco. See also *fei yong* (Lung Abscess) p.111.

Clinical features
- hacking or rattling cough with blood and/or profuse foul smelling, sticky yellow or green, blood streaked or rust-like mucus
- fever which may rise in the afternoon and evening
- fullness and stuffiness or mild pain in the chest
- wheezing that tends to be worse at night and first thing in the morning
- sore or congested throat
- bitter taste in the mouth
- loose stools or constipation
- lethargy, malaise
- loss of appetite, nausea
- abdominal distension

T thick, greasy yellow coat, maybe only on the root
P soft or slippery and rapid

Treatment principle
Expel Phlegm and clear Heat
Cool the Blood and stop bleeding

Prescription

WEI JING TANG 苇茎汤
(*Reed Decoction*) modified

lu gen (Rhizoma Phragmitis Communis) 芦根	30g
yi ren (Semen Coicis Lachryma-jobi) 苡仁	30g
yu xing cao (Herba Houttuyniae) 鱼腥草	30g
dong gua ren (Semen Benincasae Hispidae) 冬瓜仁	24g
bai mao gen (Rhizoma Imperatae Cylindricae) 白茅根	18g
ou jie (Nodus Nelumbinis Nuciferae Rhizomatis) 藕节	18g
huang qin (Radix Scutellariae Baicalensis) 黄芩	12g
xian he cao (Herba Agrimoniae Pilosae) 仙鹤草	12g
tao ren (Semen Persicae) 桃仁	9g

Method: Decoction. (Source: *Shi Yong Zhong Yi Nei Ke Xue*)

Modifications
- If the bleeding is severe or resistant, combine with **YUN NAN BAI YAO** (*Yunnan White Powder* 云南白药), or add **san qi fen** (powdered Radix Notoginseng) 三七粉 to the cooked decoction (*chong fu* 冲服).
- With severe cough and dyspnoea, add **zhi ma huang*** (honey fried Herba Ephedra) 炙麻黄 9g and **su zi** (Fructus Perillae Frutescentis) 苏子 9g.
- With constipation, add **da huang** (Radix et Rhizoma Rhei) 大黄 3-6g and **gua lou ren** (Semen Trichosanthis) 瓜楼仁 9g.
- During the convalescent stage of this condition, the patient often has nightsweats, residual hard to expectorate mucus and fatigue due to the Heat damaging Lung *yin*. In this case add **di gu pi** (Cortex Lycii Chinensis) 地骨皮 12g and **qing hao** (Herba Artemesiae Apiaceae) 青蒿 12g. See also p.114.

Patent medicines
Qing Qi Hua Tan Wan 清气化痰丸 (Pinellia Expectorant Pills)
Qing Fei Yi Huo Pian 清肺抑火片 (Ching Fei Yi Huo Pien)
Niu Huang Qing Huo Wan 牛黄清火丸 (Niu Huang Qing Huo Wan)
  - with constipation
Yun Nan Bai Yao 云南白药 (Yunnan Paiyao)
  - this medicine can be taken in addition to the main formula selected. The red pill included with the medicine is only used in severe cases.

Acupuncture
Lu.5 (*chi ze* -), St.40 (*feng long* -), Lu.6 (*kong zui* -), Lu.1 (*zhong fu* -), LI.11 (*qu chi* -), Bl.13 (*fei shu* -), Lu.10 (*yu ji* -), Ren.17 (*shan zhong*)
- with wheezing add *ding chuan* (M-BW-1)
- with fullness in the chest add PC.5 (*jian shi*)

Clinical notes
- The haemoptysis in this pattern may be associated with biomedical conditions such as acute and chronic bronchitis, bronchiectasis, pneumonia, whooping cough and lung abscess.
- Generally responds reasonably well to correct treatment, plus avoidance of heating foods and tobacco. In severe cases, the elderly, frail or debilitated, concurrent use of antibiotics may be necessary to quickly cool the Heat. Herbs and acupuncture support the swift action of the antibiotics, and finish the job by expelling the pathogen, clearing residual Phlegm, strengthening resistance and nourishing damaged *yin*.

5.6 LIVER FIRE

肝火犯肺咳血

Pathophysiology
- Long term stagnation of *qi* can generate Fire which can damage the Lungs via the (*ke* 克, p.70) cycle. In addition, Blood may be heated by contact with the hot Liver (the Liver stores Blood) and spill from the vessels. This process is exacerbated by excessive consumption of Liver heating substances. The Lungs are more vulnerable to Liver Fire when their *qi* is deficient.

Clinical features
- Paroxysmal intense cough which comes in bursts with blood streaked mucus or coughing of fresh red blood. The quantity of blood may be large or small. The cough may be initiated or aggravated by emotional upset or stress.
- during coughing episodes the patient is flushed, hot and upset
- focal chest or hypochondriac distension or pain
- temporal headache
- dizziness
- irritability and anger outbursts
- dry mouth and thirst
- bitter taste in the mouth
- red, sore eyes

T red with a yellow coat
P wiry and rapid

Treatment principle
Clear Heat from the Liver and Lungs
Cool the Blood and stop bleeding

Prescription

XIE BAI SAN 泻白散
(*Morus and Lycium Formula*) plus
DAI GE SAN 黛蛤散
(*Indigo and Conch Powder*) modified

chao sang bai pi (dry fried Cortex Mori Albae Radicis) 炒桑白皮	30g
di gu pi (Cortex Lycii Radicis) 地骨皮	30g
geng mi (Semen Oryzae) 粳米	15g
zhi gan cao (honey fried Radix Glycyrrhizae Uralensis) 炙甘草	3g
huang qin (Radix Scutellariae Baicalensis) 黄芩	9g

> **qing dai** (Indigo Pulverata Levis) 青黛 5g
> **hai ge ke fen** (powdered Concha Cyclinae Sinensis)
> 海蛤壳粉 5g
> **chao pu huang** (dry fried Pollen Typhae) 炒蒲黄 9g
> **bai mao gen** (Rhizoma Imperatae Cylindricae) 白茅根 18g
> **ou jie** (Nodus Nelumbinis Nuciferae Rhizomatis) 藕节 12g
> **qian cao gen** (Radix Rubiae Cordifoliae) 茜草根 12g
> Method: Decoction. **Qing dai** is cooked in a muslin bag (*bao jian* 包煎). (Source: *Shi Yong Zhong Yi Nei Ke Xue*)

KE XUE FANG 咳血方
(*Coughing of Blood Formula*)

This formula is suitable for chronic or recurrent haemoptysis due to Liver Fire. It is not as strong as the primary prescription, and is suited to prolonged use.

> **qing dai** (Indigo Pulverata Levis) 青黛 9g
> **shan zhi zi** (Fructus Gardeniae Jasminoidis) 山栀子 9g
> **fu hai shi** (Pumice) 浮海石 9g
> **gua lou ren** (Semen Trichosanthis) 瓜楼仁 9g
> **he zi** (Fructus Terminaliae Chebulae) 诃子 9g
> Method: Grind the herbs to a fine powder and form into 1.5-gram pills with honey. The dose is one pill, several times daily. May also be decocted, in which case **qing dai** is cooked in a muslin bag (*bao jian* 包煎). (Source: *Shi Yong Fang Ji Xue*)

Modifications

- With severe bleeding add **YUN NAN BAI YAO** (*Yunnan White Powder* 云南白药) or **san qi fen** (powdered Radix Notoginseng) 三七粉 3g to the cooked decoction (*chong fu* 冲服).
- With severe Liver Heat (dizziness, flushing and red, sore eyes), add **long dan cao** (Radix Gentianae Longdancao) 龙胆草 9g and **dai zhe shi** (Haematitum) 代赭石 12g.

Variations and additional prescriptions

- If the Heat is severe enough to affect the Blood, affecting the *shen* and causing disordered consciousness, the correct treatment is to first clear Toxic Heat, cool Blood and clear *ying* with a rescusitation formula like **AN GONG NIU HUANG WAN** (*Calm the Palace Pill with Cattle Gallstone* 安宫牛黄丸, p.914), **ZHI BAO DAN** (*Greatest Treasure Special Pill* 至宝丹, p.660), **ZI XUE DAN** (*Purple Snow Special Pill* 紫雪丹, p.707), **XI JIAO DI HUANG TANG** (*Rhinoceros Horn and Rehmannia Decoction* 犀角地黄汤, p.41) or **QING YING TANG** (*Clear the Ying Decoction* 清营汤, p.38).

Patent medicines

Long Dan Xie Gan Wan 龙胆泻肝丸 (Long Dan Xie Gan Wan)
Qing Fei Yi Huo Pian 清肺抑火片 (Ching Fei Yi Huo Pien)
Yun Nan Bai Yao 云南白药 (Yunnan Paiyao)
- this medicine can be taken in addition to the main formula selected. The red pill included with the medicine is only used in severe cases.

Acupuncture

Liv.2 (*xing jian* -), Bl.13 (*fei shu* -), Lu.6 (*kong zui* -), Lu.5 (*chi ze* -), GB.34 (*yang ling quan* -), Liv.3 (*tai chong* -), Bl.18 (*gan shu* -), Sp.10 (*xue hai* -)

Clinical notes

- The haemoptysis in this pattern may be associated with biomedical conditions such as pleurisy, upper respiratory tract infection, tonsillitis, bronchitis, pneumonia, tracheitis, bronchiectasis, hypertension, whooping cough in adults and lung cancer.
- Episodes generally respond satisfactorily to correct treatment. Long term resolution of recurrent Liver Fire patterns requires an appropriate management plan that includes lifestyle and dietary modification, relaxation, exercise and stress management.

Table 5.1 Comparison of excess Heat haemoptysis patterns

Pattern	Features	Tongue & Pulse	Guiding Formula
Wind Heat	acute cough with blood & scant blood streaked sputum, sore throat, fever, mild chills, thirst, sweating, headache	T: normal or red tip & thin yellow coat P: floating & rapid	YIN QIAO SAN
Lung Heat	dry, hacking cough with blood & little or no sputum, fever, chest tightness & pain, red face, shortness of breath, thirst	T: red or red tip & yellow coat P: flooding & rapid, or wiry & rapid	MA XING SHI GAN TANG
Phlegm Heat	hacking or rattling cough with sticky, yellow, blood streaked or rusty sputum, fullness in the chest, wheezing, loose stools or constipation, anorexia, nausea	T: thick, greasy yellow coat P: soft or slippery & rapid	WEI JING TANG
Liver Fire	intense paroxysmal cough with fresh blood, aggravated by emotion, chest & hypochondriac pain, irritability, pounding headache, bitter taste, red eyes, thirst	T: red with a thick or thin yellow coat P: wiry & rapid	XIE BAI SAN + DAI GE SAN

5.7 LUNG AND KIDNEY *YIN* DEFICIENCY WITH HEAT

阴虚火旺咳血

Pathophysiology
- Lung and Kidney *yin* deficiency leads to dryness in the Lungs and damages their delicate *luo mai*. The *yin* deficiency also generates Heat that aggravates the dryness and can cause the Blood to move recklessly. The result is a generally mild but persistent haemoptysis.

Clinical features
- dry weak cough with spots of fresh red blood, usually with little or no mucus, or mucus mixed with fresh red blood; the cough and haemoptysis are chronic and recurrent
- malar or facial flushing, afternoon or bone steaming fever, night sweats
- sensation of heat in the palms, soles and chest ('five hearts hot')
- insomnia
- dry mouth and throat
- dull pain in the chest
- dry and burning sensation in the skin
- lower back pain
- tinnitus, dizziness

T red with little or no coat
P thready and rapid

Treatment principle
Nourish *yin* and clear Heat
Cool the Blood and stop bleeding

Prescription

BAI HE GU JIN TANG 百合固金汤
(*Lily Combination*) modified

bai he (Bulbus Lilii) 百合	24g
shu di (Radix Rehmanniae Glutinosae Conquitae) 熟地	18g
sheng di (Radix Rehmanniae Glutinosae) 生地	15g
mai dong (Tuber Ophiopogonis Japonici) 麦冬	15g
xuan shen (Radix Scrophulariae) 玄参	9g
chuan bei mu (Bulbus Fritillariae Cirrhosae) 川贝母	9g
dang gui (Radix Angelicae Sinensis) 当归	9g
bai shao (Radix Paeoniae Lactiflora) 白芍	9g
gan cao (Radix Glycyrrhizae Uralensis) 甘草	3g
bai mao gen (Rhizoma Imperatae Cylindricae) 白茅根	18g
ou jie (Nodus Nelumbinis Nuciferae Rhizomatis) 藕节	12g
han lian cao (Herba Ecliptae Prostratae) 旱莲草	9g

ce bai ye (Cacumen Biotae Orientalis) 侧柏叶 12g
Method: Decoction. (Source: *Shi Yong Zhong Yi Nei Ke Xue*)

YUE HUA WAN 月华丸
(*Moonlight Pill*) modified

This formula has a stronger tonifying action than the primary prescription and is used for more severe and chronic *yin* deficiency. It is commonly used for consumptive Lung disease.

sha shen (Radix Adenophorae seu Glehniae) 沙参 30g
mai dong (Tuber Ophiopogonis Japonici) 麦冬 30g
tian dong (Tuber Asparagi cochinchinensis) 天冬 30g
sheng di (Radix Rehmanniae Glutinosae) 生地 30g
shu di (Radix Rehmanniae Glutinosae Conquitae) 熟地 30g
bai bu (Radix Stemonae) 百部 30g
shan yao (Radix Dioscoreae Oppositae) 山药 30g
e jiao (Gelatinum Corii Asini) 阿胶 30g
chuan bei mu (Bulbus Fritillariae Cirrhosae) 川贝母 30g
fu ling (Sclerotium Poriae Cocos) 茯苓 15g
san qi (Radix Notoginseng) 三七 15g
sang ye (Folium Mori Albae) 桑叶 60g
ju hua (Flos Chrysanthemi Morifolii) 菊花 60g

Method: Grind the herbs to a fine powder and form into 9-gram pills with honey. The dose is 3-5 pills daily. (Source: *Shi Yong Zhong Yi Nei Ke Xue*)

ZHENG YIN LI LAO TANG 拯阴理劳汤
(*Rescue yin, Manage Exhaustion Decoction*) modified

This formula is selected when deficient Heat is mild, and there are more signs of *qi* deficiency (shortness of breath, fatigue, light red blood, and a pink or reddish, swollen tongue with tooth marks).

bai ren shen (Panax Ginseng) 白人参 9g
mai dong (Tuber Ophiopogonis Japonici) 麦冬 9g
wu wei zi (Fructus Schizandrae Chinensis) 五味子 6g
dang gui (Radix Angelicae Sinensis) 当归 6g
bai shao (Radix Paeoniae Lactiflora) 白芍 6g
sheng di (Radix Rehmanniae Glutinosae) 生地 9g
mu dan pi (Cortex Moutan Radicis) 牡丹皮 6g
yi ren (Semen Coicis Lachryma-jobi) 苡仁 12g
lian zi (Semen Nelumbinis Nuciferae) 莲子 6g
chen pi (Pericarpium Citri Reticulatae) 陈皮 6g
xian he cao (Herba Agrimoniae Pilosae) 仙鹤草 9g
bai ji (Rhizoma Bletillae Striatae) 白芨 9g
ce bai ye (Cacumen Biotae Orientalis) 侧柏叶 9g

e jiao^ (Gelatinum Corii Asini) 阿胶 6g
gan cao (Radix Glycyrrhizae Uralensis) 甘草 3g

Method: Decoction. E jiao is melted before being added to the strained decoction (*yang hua* 烊化). (Source: *Shi Yong Zhong Yi Nei Ke Xue*)

Modifications

- If the bleeding persists, add **YUN NAN BAI YAO** (*Yunnan White Powder* 云南白药) or **san qi fen** (powdered Radix Notoginseng) 三七粉 3g to the cooked decoction (*chong fu* 冲服).
- With afternoon fever or bone steaming fever, add **di gu pi** (Cortex Lycii Radicis) 地骨皮 12g, **bai wei** (Radix Cynanchi Baiwei) 白薇 9g and **qing hao** (Herba Artemesiae Annuae) 青蒿 15g.
- With severe night sweats, add **mu li^** (Concha Ostreae) 牡蛎 30g, **fu xiao mai** (Semen Tritici Aestivi Levis) 浮小麦 12g and **ma huang gen** (Radix Ephedrae) 麻黄根 9g.
- With significant flushing, add **zhi mu** (Rhizoma Anemarrhenae Asphodeloides) 知母 12g and **huang bai** (Cortex Phellodendri) 黄柏 12g.

Patent medicines

Bai He Gu Jin Wan 百合固金丸 (Bai He Gu Jin Wan)
Yang Yin Qing Fei Wan 养阴清肺丸 (Yang Yin Qing Fei Wan)
Ba Xian Chang Shou Wan 八仙长寿丸 (Ba Xian Chang Shou Wan)
  - Lung and Kidney *yin* deficiency
Yun Nan Bai Yao 云南白药 (Yunnan Paiyao)
  - this medicine can be taken in addition to the main formula selected. The red pill included with the medicine is only used in severe cases.

Acupuncture

Lu.5 (*chi ze* +), Bl.13 (*fei shu* +), Bl.43 (*gao huang shu* +), Kid. 2 (*ran gu* -), Bl.23 (*shen shu* +), Kid.3 (*tai xi* +), Lu.9 (*tai yuan* +), Lu.1 (*zhong fu*)
  - with severe haemoptysis add Lu.6 (*kong zui*)
  - with severe Heat add Lu.10 (*yu ji* -)

Clinical notes

- The haemoptysis in this pattern may be associated with biomedical conditions such as lung cancer, pulmonary tuberculosis, chronic bronchitis, bronchiectasis, silicosis, asbestosis and bleeding diathesis.
- This pattern can be difficult to treat well, and generally requires prolonged therapy, often combined with Western medicine for satisfactory results.

5.8 SPLEEN *QI* DEFICIENCY

Pathophysiology
- Spleen *qi* deficiency gives rise to a relatively uncommon type of haemoptysis, as bleeding from deficient Spleen *qi* usually occurs in the lower part of the body. However, if Spleen *qi* is unable to maintain the integrity of Blood vessels, leakage of Blood into the skin and Lungs may occur.

Clinical features
- Coughing or spitting of blood or expectorating blood streaked mucus. There may also be bleeding from other parts of the body, typically the uterus, rectum or skin.
- pale lustreless or sallow complexion
- fatigue and lethargy
- dizziness, tinnitus
- palpitations
- poor appetite
- loose stools
- abdominal distension

T pale and swollen
P thready and weak or hollow

Treatment principle
Tonify *qi* to restrain Blood
Strengthen the Spleen, nourish Blood

Prescription

ZHENG YANG LI LAO TANG 拯阳理劳汤
(*Rescue yang, Manage Exhaustion Decoction*) modified

huang qi (Radix Astragali Membranacei) 黄芪	15g
bai zhu (Rhizoma Atractylodis Macrocephalae) 白术	12g
xian he cao (Herba Agrimoniae Pilosae) 仙鹤草	12g
ren shen (Panax Ginseng) 人参	9g
dang gui (Radix Angelicae Sinensis) 当归	6g
chen pi (Pericarpium Citri Reticulatae) 陈皮	6g
wu wei zi (Fructus Schizandrae Chinensis) 五味子	6g
e jiao^ (Gelatinum Corii Asini) 阿胶	6g
rou gui (Cortex Cinnamomi Cassiae) 肉桂	3g
gan cao (Radix Glycyrrhizae Uralensis) 甘草	3g

Method: Decoction. **E jiao** is melted before being added to the strained decoction (*yang hua* 烊化). (Source: *Shi Yong Zhong Yi Nei Ke Xue*)

GUI PI TANG 归脾汤, p.180
(*Ginseng and Longan Combination*) modified

This formula is selected when *shen* disturbance is obvious, with insomnia, anxiety or palpitations.

Modifications

- If the bleeding persists, add **YUN NAN BAI YAO** (*Yunnan White Powder* 云南白药) or **san qi fen** (powdered Radix Notoginseng) 三七粉 3g to the cooked decoction (*chong fu* 冲服), and consider **JIAO AI TANG** (*Ass-Hide Gelatin and Mugwort Decoction* 胶艾汤, p.178).
- Without Cold, delete **rou gui**, and add **shu di** (Radix Rehmanniae Glutinosae Conquitae) 熟地 15g.

Patent medicines

Gui Pi Wan 归脾丸 (Gui Pi Wan)
Ge Jie Da Bu Wan 蛤蚧大补丸 (Gejie Da Bu Wan)
Ren Shen Yang Ying Wan 人参养营丸 (Ginseng Tonic Pills)
Yun Nan Bai Yao 云南白药 (Yunnan Paiyao)
  - this medicine can be taken in addition to the main formula selected. The red pill included with the medicine is only used in severe cases.

Acupuncture

Sp.6 (*san yi jiao* +▲), Bl.20 (*pi shu* +▲), St.36 (*zu san li* +▲), Bl.23 (*shen shu* +▲), Ren.6 (*qi hai* +▲), Sp.1 (*yin bai* ▲)

Clinical notes

- The haemoptysis in this pattern may be associated with biomedical conditions such as thrombocytopoenia, haemophilia, AIDS related illness, lung cancer, pulmonary oedema and mitral stenosis.
- *Qi* deficiency symptoms can respond well to correct treatment, depending on the duration and depth of the disease. For *qi* deficiency patterns associated with HIV infection, tumours or other severe chronic or structural disorder, the outlook is poorer.

SUMMARY OF GUIDING FORMULAE FOR HAEMOPTYSIS

Excess patterns
Wind Heat - *Yin Qiao San* 银翘散

Wind Dryness - *Qing Zao Jiu Fei Tang* 清燥救肺汤

Wind Cold - *Jin Fei Cao San* 金沸草散
- persistent cough and haemoptysis after resolution of exterior symptoms - *Zhi Sou San* 止嗽散

Lung Heat - *Ma Xing Shi Gan Tang* 麻杏石甘汤

Phlegm Heat - *Wei Jing Tang* 苇茎汤

Liver Fire - *Xie Bai San* 泻白散 + *Dai Ge San* 黛蛤散

Deficient patterns
Lung and Kidney *yin* deficiency - *Bai He Gu Jin Tang* 百合固金汤
- with *qi* deficiency - *Zheng Yin Li Lao Tang* 拯阴理劳汤

Spleen *qi* deficiency - *Zheng Yang Li Lao Tang* 拯阳理劳汤

Endnote

For more information regarding herbs marked with an asterisk*, an open circle° or a hat^, see the tables on pp.944-952.

Disorders of the Lung

6. Loss of Voice and Hoarse Voice

Acute patterns
Wind Cold
Wind Heat
Lung Dryness
Phlegm Heat
Liver *qi* stagnation

Chronic patterns
Lung and Spleen *qi* deficiency
Lung and Kidney *yin* deficiency
Qi, Blood and Phlegm stagnation

6 | LOSS OF VOICE (HOARSE VOICE)
shi yin 失音

This condition is characterised by acute or chronic hoarseness, raspiness or complete loss of voice. Disorders of the voice are mostly due to disorders of the larynx and vocal cords, which in turn are related to the Lungs, Liver, Kidneys and Stomach. The larynx and vocal cords are part of the Lung system, and thus strongly influenced by the same factors that affect the Lungs–Wind, *yin* and *qi* deficiency and Phlegm. The Liver and Kidneys influence the throat through their internal channel pathways. The Stomach influences the throat through the channel pathway and because of its close anatomical relationship with the throat. The Stomach is prone to Heat disorders, and Heat tends to rise through the oesophagus to the throat.

In cases of persistent hoarseness, referral to a specialist for laryngoscopy to exclude neoplasm is advised.

AETIOLOGY
External pathogens
The Lungs are considered to be the 'delicate' organ–they are relatively superficial and therefore vulnerable to Wind Heat and Wind Cold. Wind and associated pathogens gain access to the vocal cords through the nose and mouth. Pathogens are most likely to lodge at the level of the throat where there is an underlying weakness, for example in patients with a history of repeated tonsillitis, smoking, or voice overuse.

Phlegm Heat
Dampness or Phlegm accumulating as a result of Spleen weakness may over time become Phlegm Heat. Alternatively, Phlegm Heat can accumulate if too many rich foods are consumed, or if pre-existing Heat in the body congeals Fluids into Phlegm.

Pre-existing Phlegm Heat can be stirred up Wind causing acute hoarseness or loss of voice. Heavy tobacco smoking which dries and congeals Lung Fluids is a common aggravating feature of this pattern. Chronic Phlegm Heat may lead to the formation of polyps or nodules on the vocal cords.

Liver *qi* stagnation
Frustration, anger and unexpressed emotion can disrupt the circulation of Liver *qi*. Because the Liver channel passes through the throat, the *qi* stagnation can affect the larynx and vocal cords. In extreme cases, for example outrage, the stagnation can completely obstruct the vocal cords so that speech is impossible or there is severe stuttering–the person chokes on his or her

own words. There are other interesting psychological aspects to this pattern. If emotions or feelings are unexpressed (due to lack of confidence, social constraint or embarassment) they can get caught in the throat, manifesting as a sensation of something lodged there–known in TCM as 'plum stone *qi*'. Long term emotional repression can eventually lead to Blood (and Phlegm) stagnation and structural changes in the throat (see *qi*, Blood and Phlegm stagnation below).

> **BOX 6.1 SOME BIOMEDICAL CAUSES OF HOARSE VOICE OR LOSS OF VOICE**
>
> **Intrapharyngeal**
> - acute and chronic laryngitis
> - tuberculous laryngitis
> - vocal cord polyps
> - smoking
>
> **Extrapharyngeal**
> - thyroid disorders
> - lesions of the neck
> - acromegaly
>
> **Paralysis of the vagus or recurrent laryngeal nerves**
> - traumatic injury to the throat
> - post surgical nerve damage

Lung deficiency

The strength and projection of the voice is dependent on Lung *qi*, the moisture and suppleness of the vocal cords on Lung *yin*. Weak *qi* and *yin*, by failing to support the vocal cords, lead to lack of force behind the voice, and chronic dryness, hoarseness or complete loss of voice.

Lung *qi* may be compromised by poor posture, shallow breathing and lack of exercise, or conversely by repeated or extreme physical overexertion. Prolonged or excessive grief or sadness can weaken Lung *qi*. If Spleen *qi* is deficient, then Lung *qi* will not be supported via the generating (*sheng* 生, p.70) cycle.

Lung *yin* is damaged by hot dry environments, febrile disease, smoking and as a secondary result of Kidney *yin* deficiency. Lung *qi* and *yin* can be damaged by overuse of the voice and some medications (like salbutamol and prednisone for asthma).

Kidney *yin* deficiency

Kidney *yin* deficiency generates Heat, which rises up to the throat through the Kidney channel, causing recurrent dryness, soreness or hoarseness, usually in the afternoon. Lung and Kidney *yin* have a close relationship. On the one hand, Kidney *yin* is the basis of Lung *yin*, and on the other hand Heat from Kidney *yin* deficiency will dry Lung Fluids. Kidney *yin* is weakened by overexertion, insufficient sleep, stimulant drug use, febrile illness, insufficient hydration and ageing.

Qi, Blood and Phlegm stagnation

Qi, Blood and Phlegm can accumulate and stagnate in the throat and vocal

> **BOX 6.2 KEY DIAGNOSTIC POINTS**
>
> **Aggravation**
> - in the afternoon - *yin* deficiency
> - in the morning - *qi* deficiency
> - with emotional upset - Liver *qi* stagnation
> - when fatigued and with overuse of the voice - *qi* and/or *yin* deficiency
>
> **Amelioration**
> - with rest - *qi* deficiency
>
> **Appearance of vocal cords**
> - red - excess Heat
> - pale and flaccid - *qi* deficiency
> - pale red - *yin* deficiency
> - nodular and lumpy - *qi*, Blood or Phlegm stagnation

cords as the result of other chronic pathology. Chronic Liver *qi* stagnation, Phlegm Heat and Lung weakness are all predisposing factors. The end result is structural changes in the throat or vocal cords, typically polyps or nodules.

Overuse

Overuse of the voice, amongst people like singers, teachers, race callers and actors can lead to hoarseness or loss of voice. The mechanism here is related to weakening of Lung *qi*.

6. LOSS OF VOICE and HOARSE VOICE   211

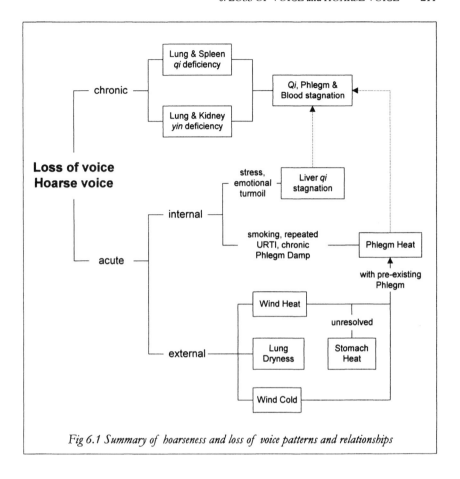

Fig 6.1 *Summary of hoarseness and loss of voice patterns and relationships*

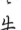

6.1 WIND COLD

Pathophysiology
- Wind Cold invades the Lungs and lodges in the throat, obstructing the free movement of Lung *qi*, thereby preventing full expression of the voice.

Clinical features
- sudden weakness, hoarseness or loss of the voice; the throat is mildly red and swollen and the vocal cords look normal or pale
- fever and chills, with chills predominant
- itchy or slightly sore throat
- occipital headache
- no sweating
- muscle aches, neck stiffness
- nasal obstruction, or runny nose with thin watery mucus
- sneezing
- cough or wheezing with thin watery mucus

T normal or with a thin white coat
P floating, or floating and tight

Treatment principle
Disperse Wind and Cold
Aid the descent of Lung *qi*

Prescription

LIU WEI TANG 六味汤
(*Six Flavour Decoction*)

jie geng (Radix Platycodi Grandiflori) 桔梗	12g
gan cao (Radix Glycyrrhizae Uralensis) 甘草	10g
jing jie (Herba seu Flos Schizonepetae Tenuifolia) 荆芥	10g
fang feng (Radix Ledebouriellae Divaricatae) 防风	10g
jiang can^ (Bombyx Batryticatus) 僵蚕	10g
chan tui^ (Periostracum Cicadae) 蝉蜕	10g
zi su ye (Fructus Perillae Frutescentis) 紫苏叶	10g
qian hu (Radix Peucedani) 前胡	10g
xing ren* (Semen Pruni Armeniacae) 杏仁	10g
sheng jiang (Rhizoma Zingiberis Officinalis Recens) 生姜	3pce
bo he (Herba Mentha Haplocalycis) 薄荷	6g

Method: Decoction. **Bo he** is added at the end of cooking (*hou xia* 后下).
(Source: *Zhong Yi Nei Ke Lin Chuang Shou Ce*)

Modifications
◆ With a productive cough, add **ban xia*** (Rhizoma Pinelliae Ternatae) 半夏 10g and **bai qian** (Radix et Rhizoma Cynanchi Baiqian) 白前 10g.

Variations and additional prescriptions
With internal Heat
◆ With a Wind Cold invasion on top of pre-existing internal Heat, the symptoms are those described above, plus thirst, sore throat, irritability, constipation and a yellow tongue coat. The correct treatment is to dispel Wind Cold and clear internal Heat with **DA QING LONG TANG** (*Major Blue Dragon Combination* 大青龙汤, p.52).

Patent medicines
Gan Mao Ling 感冒灵 (Gan Mao Ling)
Gan Mao Qing Re Chong Ji 感冒清热冲剂 (Colds and Flu Tea)
Chuan Xiong Cha Tiao Wan 川芎茶调丸 (Chuan Xiong Cha Tiao Wan)
- with prominent headache

Gargle
◆ Decoct equal amounts of **huo xiang** (Herba Agastaches seu Pogostemi) 藿香, **pei lan** (Herba Eupatorii Fortuneii) 佩兰, **zi su ye** (Fructus Perillae Frutescentis) 紫苏叶 and **cong bai** (Bulbus Allii Fistulosi) 葱白, and gargle warm as often as practical.

Acupuncture
L.I.4 (*he gu* -), Lu.7 (*lie que* -), GB.20 (*feng chi* -), Bl.12 (*feng men* - Ω), Bl.13 (*fei shu* - Ω), Ren.22 (*tian tu*), *bai lao* (M-HN-30)
• If there is significant wheezing use *ding chuan* (M-BW-1)
• If the nose is congested or runny add Du.23 (*shang xing*)

Clinical notes
• Wind Cold type hoarse voice or loss of voice may be associated with biomedical conditions such as the common cold, influenza, upper respiratory tract infection and laryngitis.
• This pattern responds well to correct treatment.

6.2 WIND HEAT

Pathophysiology
- Wind Heat, or Wind Cold which turns hot, penetrates and lodges in the throat and larynx causing redness, swelling, inflammation and pain, thereby making speech difficult.

Clinical features
- Sudden weakness, hoarseness or loss of voice. The throat and vocal cords are red and swollen and there may be a white or yellow exudate on their surfaces. In severe cases swelling significantly narrows the throat causing difficulty with swallowing.
- sore throat
- fever and chills, with predominant fever
- headache
- nasal obstruction
- fatigue, poor appetite, malaise
- productive cough

T slightly red tip and edges with a thin yellow or white coat
P floating and rapid

Treatment principle
Expel Wind and Heat
Moisten and benefit the throat

Prescription

SHU FENG QING RE TANG 疏风清热汤
(*Dispel Wind, Clear Heat Decoction*) modified

jin yin hua (Flos Lonicerae Japonicae) 金银花	30g
lian qiao (Fructus Forsythia Suspensae) 连翘	15g
xuan shen (Radix Scrophulariae Ningpoensis) 玄参	15g
sang bai pi (Cortex Mori Albae Radicis) 桑白皮	12g
jie geng (Radix Platycodi Grandiflori) 桔梗	12g
jing jie (Herba seu Flos Schizonepetae Tenuifolia) 荆芥	10g
fang feng (Radix Ledebouriellae Divaricatae) 防风	10g
niu bang zi (Fructus Arctii Lappae) 牛蒡子	10g
chan tuiˆ (Periostracum Cicadae) 蝉蜕	10g
pang da hai (Semen Sterculiae Scaphigerae) 胖大海	10g
bo he (Herba Mentha Haplocalycis) 薄荷	6g
gan cao (Radix Glycyrrhizae Uralensis) 甘草	6g

Method: Decoction. **Bo he** is added at the end of cooking (*hou xia* 后下).
(Source: *Zhong Yi Nei Ke Lin Chuang Shou Ce*)

QING YAN LI GE TANG 清咽利膈汤
(*Clear the Throat, Benefit the Diaphram Decoction*) modified

This formula is selected when the Heat pathogen penetrates further, lodges at the *yang ming* level and causes Stomach Heat. The symptoms are severe redness and swelling of the throat and vocal cords, yellow exudate, difficulty swallowing, high fever, thirst, constipation, bad breath, a thick dry yellow coat and flooding rapid pulse. The correct treatment is to clear Heat and Toxins and benefit the throat.

    lian qiao (Fructus Forsythia Suspensae) 连翘 30g
    shan zhi zi (Fructus Gardeniae Jasminoidis) 山栀子 10g
    huang qin (Radix Scutellariae Baicalensis) 黄芩 10g
    bo he (Herba Mentha Haplocalycis) 薄荷 9g
    mang xiao (Mirabilitum) 芒硝 9g
    da huang (Radix et Rhizoma Rhei) 大黄 9g
    gan cao (Radix Glycyrrhizae Uralensis) 甘草 9g
    jie geng (Radix Platycodi Grandiflori) 桔梗 15g
    huang lian (Rhizoma Coptidis) 黄连 9g
    jing jie (Herba seu Flos Schizonepetae Tenuifolia) 荆芥 6g
    fang feng (Radix Ledebouriellae Divaricatae) 防风 6g
Method: Decoction. **Mang xiao** is dissolved in the strained decoction (*chong fu* 冲服). (Source: *Zhong Yi Nei Ke Lin Chuang Shou Ce*)

Modifications
- When Wind Heat is complicated by pre-existing Phlegm Heat, add **gua lou** (Fructus Trichosanthis) 瓜楼 18g, **zhe bei mu** (Bulbus Fritillariae Thunbergii) 浙贝母 9g and **zhu ru** (Caulis Bambusae in Taeniis) 竹茹 9g.
- If the exterior symptoms have resolved but the heat and hoarseness persists, delete **jing jie** and **fang feng**.

Patent medicines
Yin Qiao Jie Du Pian 银翘解毒片 (Yin Chiao Chieh Tu Pien)
Qing Yin Wan 清音丸 (Qing Yin Wan)
Shuang Liao Hou Feng San 双料喉风散 (Superior Sore Throat Powder)
  - for topical use
Xi Gua Shuang 西瓜霜 (Watermelon Frost)
  - for topical use

Powders
- see Wind Heat sore throat, p.286-287

Gargle
- Decoct equal portions of **jin yin hua** (Flos Lonicerae Japonicae)

金银花, **jie geng** (Radix Platycodi Grandiflori) 桔梗 and **lian qiao** (Fructus Forsythia Suspensae) 连翘 and gargle warm as often as practical.

Acupuncture
Ren.22 (*tian tu* -), SJ.6 (*zhi gou* -), LI.4 (*he gu* -), LI.18 (*fu tu* -), Lu.6 (*kong zui* -), Lu.10 (*yu ji* -), LI.11 (*qu chi* -), *bai lao* (M-HN-30)
- If the throat is very sore and swollen add Lu.11 (*shao shang* ↓) and SI.17 (*tian rong* -)

Clinical notes
- Biomedical conditions that may present as Wind Heat type loss of voice or hoarse voice include tonsillitis, laryngitis, pharyngitis, upper respiratory tract infection and bronchitis.

Table 6.1 *Comparison of acute patterns of Hoarseness and Loss of Voice*

Pattern	Symptoms	Signs	Guiding Formula
Wind Cold	sudden weakness, hoarseness, or loss of voice, fever & chills, occipital headache, no sweating, myalgia, nasal obstruction or thin watery mucus	slightly red & swollen, pale or pink vocal cords T: normal or thin white coat P: floating & tight	LIU WEI TANG
Wind Heat	sudden weakness, hoarseness, or loss of voice, fever, mild chills, headache, sweating, malaise, cough with sticky yellow mucus	red, inflamed throat, red vocal cords with yellow or white exudate T: red tip with thin yellow coat P: floating & rapid	SHU FENG QING RE TANG
Phlegm Heat	husky, raspy, hoarse voice, throat clearing, expectoration of thick yellow sputum, cough, low fever, bitter taste	red throat with possible swellings of the vocal cords T: greasy yellow coat P: slippery, rapid	QING YAN NING FEI TANG
Liver *qi* stagnation	sudden loss of voice associated with emotion, 'plum stone' throat, irritability, depression	no inflammation or swelling T: normal or dark with a thin coat P: wiry	XIAO JIANG QI TANG

肺燥津伤失音

6.3 LUNG DRYNESS

Pathophysiology
- Lung Dryness is due to pathogenic Wind and Dryness (with either Heat or Cold depending on the season) invading the Lungs. It usually occurs during dry seasons (or periods of dry weather), damaging Lung fluids which are then unable to nourish and moisten the larynx and throat. Today, due to climate controlled buildings, this syndrome can occur in any season.

Clinical features
- hoarse, husky or raspy voice
- sore, dry, ticklish throat
- dry mouth, nose and lips
- dry, hacking, non-productive cough

T dry and normal or red with a thin coat
P slightly rapid

Treatment principle
Clear and moisten the Lungs
Benefit the throat

Prescription

SANG XING TANG 桑杏汤
(*Morus and Apricot Seed Combination*) modified

- **sang ye** (Folium Mori Albae) 桑叶 12g
- **chao xing ren*** (dry fried Semen Pruni Armeniacae) 炒杏仁 9g
- **nan sha shen** (Radix Adenophorae seu Glehniae) 南沙参 24g
- **zhi pi pa ye** (honey fried Folium Eriobotryae) 炙枇杷叶 15g
- **mai dong** (Tuber Ophiopogonis Japonici) 麦冬 12g
- **zhe bei mu** (Bulbus Fritillariae Thunbergii) 浙贝母 12g
- **shan zhi zi** (Fructus Gardeniae Jasminoidis) 山栀子 9g
- **jie geng** (Radix Platycodi Grandiflori) 桔梗 9g
- **mu hu die** (Semen Oroxyli Indici) 木蝴蝶 9g
- **li pi** (Fructus Pyri) 梨皮 6g

Method: Decoction. (Source: *Shi Yong Zhong Yi Nei Ke Xue*)

Modifications
- With Heat, add **zhi mu** (Rhizoma Anemarrhenae Asphodeloides) 知母 12g and **shi gao** (Gypsum) 石膏 18g.
- With headache and fever, add **bo he** (Herba Mentha Haplocalycis) 薄荷 6g, **lian qiao** (Fructus Forsythia Suspensae) 连翘 12g and **chan tui** (Periostracum Cicadae) 蝉蜕 9g.

- With exterior symptoms, add **jing jie** (Herba seu Flos Schizonepetae Tenuifolia) 荆芥 9g and **bo he** (Herba Mentha Haplocalycis) 薄荷 6g.
- With severe or painful cough, add **sang bai pi** (Cortex Mori Albae Radicis) 桑白皮 12g and **ma dou ling*** (Fructus Aristolochiae) 马兜铃 9g.
- With severe dryness, add **tian dong** (Tuber Asparagi Cochinchinensis) 天冬 9g and **tian hua fen** (Radix Trichosanthes Kirilowii) 天花粉 12g.
- If the throat is sore, add **xuan shen** (Radix Scrophulariae) 玄参 15g, **ma bo** (Fructificatio Lasiosphaerae seu Calvatiae) 马勃 3g, or **she gan** (Rhizoma Belamcandae) 射干 9g.
- With epistaxis or blood streaked mucus, add **bai mao gen** (Rhizoma Imperatae Cylindricae) 白茅根 18g and **sheng di tan** (charred Radix Rehmanniae Glutinosae) 生地炭 12g.

Variations and additional prescriptions
With Lung yin damage
- If the dryness is severe enough to damage Lung *yin*, this can give rise to severe hoarseness or total loss of voice, a frequent hacking non-productive cough, fullness and pain in the chest and behind the sternum, headache, haemoptysis, parched throat, wheezing and a dry tongue without coat. The correct treatment is to moisten Dryness, clear Heat and nourish Lung *yin* with **QING ZAO JIU FEI TANG** (*Eriobotria and Ophiopogon Combination* 清燥救肺汤) modified.

>   shi gao (Gypsum) 石膏 18g
>   sang ye (Folium Mori Albae) 桑叶 9g
>   xing ren* (Semen Pruni Armeniacae) 杏仁 9g
>   mai dong (Tuber Ophiopogonis Japonici) 麦冬 9g
>   hei zhi ma (Semen Sesami Indici) 黑芝麻 9g
>   zhi pi pa ye (honey fried Folium Eriobotryae) 炙枇杷叶 9g
>   nan sha shen (Radix Adenophorae seu Glehniae) 南沙参 9g
>   mu hu die (Semen Oroxyli Indici) 木蝴蝶 9g
>   e jiao^ (Gelatinum Corii Asini) 阿胶 6g
>   gan cao (Radix Glycyrrhizae Uralensis) 甘草 3g
>   Method: Decoction. **E jiao** is melted before being added to the strained decoction (*yang hua* 烊化). (Source: *Shi Yong Zhong Yi Nei Ke Xue*)

Patent medicines
Yang Yin Qing Fei Wan 养阴清肺丸 (Yang Yin Qing Fei Wan)
Qing Yin Wan 清音丸 (Qing Yin Wan)
Luo Han Guo Chong Ji 罗汉果冲剂 (Luo Han Guo Beverage)
Chuan Bei Pi Pa Gao 川贝枇杷膏 (Nin Jiom Pei Pa Kao)

Acupuncture
Ren.22 (*tian tu*), Lu.5 (*chi ze* -), Lu.10 (*yu ji* -), Kid.3 (*tai xi* +), Lu.7 (*lie que*), Kid.6 (*zhao hai*)
- acupuncture is of only limited use in Dryness patterns

Clinical notes
- Biomedical conditions that may present as Lung Dryness type loss of voice or hoarse voice include environmental dryness, overuse syndrome, smokers throat, pharyngitis, upper respiratory tract infection and bronchitis.

6.4 PHLEGM HEAT

Pathophysiology
There are two presentations of Phlegm Heat voice disorders:
- The first is acute, triggered by a Wind (Heat) invasion in a patient with pre-existing Phlegm accumulation. Heat and Phlegm mix and block the channels of the throat obstructing Lung *qi* and the larynx (see p.214-215).
- The second pattern is internally generated and can persist at a subacute level for prolonged periods. It occurs in heavy smokers. The pattern presented below is of this type.

Clinical features
- husky, raspy or hoarse voice, throat clearing and expectoration of thick yellow mucus, possibly worse in the morning, worse with smoking and prolonged use
- dry, sore, red or congested throat
- dry mouth with a bitter taste
- possible low fever
- cough with yellow mucus

T greasy yellow coat
P slippery, possibly rapid

Treatment principle
Clear the Lungs and resolve Phlegm
Clear Heat, benefit the throat

Prescription

QING YAN NING FEI TANG 清咽宁肺汤
(*Clear the Throat and Calm the Lungs Decoction*) modified

sang bai pi (Cortex Mori Albae Radicis) 桑白皮	15g
qian hu (Radix Peucedani) 前胡	10g
gan cao (Radix Glycyrrhizae Uralensis) 甘草	10g
jie geng (Radix Platycodi Grandiflori) 桔梗	10g
zhi mu (Rhizoma Anemarrhenae Asphodeloides) 知母	10g
zhe bei mu (Bulbus Fritillariae Thunbergii) 浙贝母	10g
huang qin (Radix Scutellariae Baicalensis) 黄芩	10g
shan zhi zi (Fructus Gardeniae Jasminoidis) 山栀子	10g
gua lou pi (Pericarpium Trichosanthis) 瓜楼皮	10g
chan tui^ (Periostracum Cicadae) 蝉蜕	10g
pang da hai (Semen Sterculiae Scaphigerae) 胖大海	10g
mu hu die (Semen Oroxyli Indici) 木蝴蝶	10g

Method: Decoction. (Source: *Zhong Yi Nei Ke Lin Chuang Shou Ce*)

Modifications
- With a very sore and congested throat, add **she gan** (Rhizoma Belamacandae) 射干 9g.
- With severe Heat, add **shi gao** (Gypsum) 石膏 15g.
- With *yin* and fluid damage, add **xuan shen** (Radix Scrophulariae Ningpoensis) 玄参 15g and **tian hua fen** (Radix Trichosanthes Kirilowii) 天花粉 12g.
- If the Phlegm Heat is severe, with thick malodorous mucus, cough, wheeze and more systemic symptoms, see Cough p.90 or *fei yong* (Lung Abscess), p.111.
- If there are nodules or polyps on the vocal cords, add the herbs suggested in *qi*, Blood and Phlegm stagnation, p.230.

Patent medicines
Qing Qi Hua Tan Wan 清气化痰丸 (Pinellia Expectorant Pills)
Qing Yin Wan 清音丸 (Qing Yin Wan)

Gargle
- see Wind Heat, p.215-216

Acupuncture
Ren.22 (*tian tu* -), Lu.7 (*lie que* -), St.40 (*feng long* -), LI.18 (*fu tu* -)
Lu.5 (*chi ze* -), Lu.1 (*zhong fu* -), Lu.6 (*kong zui* -), Lu.7 (*lie que* -),
LI.11 (*qu chi* -), Bl.13 (*fei shu* -), Lu.10 (*yu ji* -), Ren.17 (*shan zhong*)
- with wheezing add **ding chuan** (M-BW-1)
- with fullness in the chest add PC.5 (*jian shi*)

Clinical notes
- Biomedical conditions that may present as Phlegm Heat type loss of voice or hoarse voice include bronchitis, tonsillitis, laryngitis, pharyngitis, upper respiratory tract infection and smokers throat.
- Generally responds reasonably well to correct treatment, plus avoidance of heating foods and tobacco. For patients with severe cases (with obvious fever and systemic symptoms), and the elderly, frail or debilitated, concurrent use of antibiotics may be necessary to quickly cool the Heat. Herbs and acupuncture support the swift action of the antibiotics, and finish the job by expelling the pathogen, clearing residual Phlegm, strengthening resistance and nourishing damaged *yin*.

肝气郁滞失音

6.5 LIVER *QI* STAGNATION

Pathophysiology
- Liver *qi* stagnation represents a 'hysterical' or stress induced aphonia. Liver *qi* becomes so severely obstructed in the throat that a lump may be felt there and the vocal cords may shut down.

Clinical features
- sudden loss of voice brought on by depression, anger, worry, emotional turmoil or sudden upset
- 'plum stone' throat, or a congested feeling in the throat but on examination the throat is (generally) not swollen or inflamed
- irritability
- fullness or tightness in the chest ('difficulty getting a deep breath')
- women may experience irregular menstruation, premenstrual syndrome or breast tenderness
- in chronic cases there may be signs of heat–flushing, red eyes, tidal fever, dry mouth, short temper

T normal or dark with a thin coat (red edges if there is heat)
P slightly wiry or choppy (rapid with heat)

Treatment principle
Soothe the Liver, move and regulate *qi*
Benefit the throat (clear Heat)

Prescription

XIAO JIANG QI TANG 小降气汤
(*Minor Descending qi Decoction*) modified

This formula is selected for *qi* stagnation without Heat.
- **bai shao** (Radix Paeoniae Lactiflora) 白芍 12g
- **zi su ye** (Fructus Perillae Frutescentis) 紫苏叶 9g
- **mu hu die** (Semen Oroxyli Indici) 木蝴蝶 9g
- **wu yao** (Radix Linderae Strychnifoliae) 乌药 6g
- **chen pi** (Pericarpium Citri Reticulatae) 陈皮 6g
- **jie geng** (Radix Platycodi Grandiflori) 桔梗 6g
- **sheng jiang** (Rhizoma Zingiberis Officinalis Recens) 生姜 3pce
- **da zao** (Fructus Zizyphi Jujubae) 大枣 3pce

Method: Decoction. (Source: *Shi Yong Zhong Yi Nei Ke Xue*)

CHAI HU QING GAN TANG 柴胡清肝汤
(Bupleurum Liver Clearing Decoction) modified

This formula is selected for *qi* stagnation with Heat.

chai hu (Radix Bupleuri) 柴胡	9g
huang qin (Radix Scutellariae Baicalensis) 黄芩	9g
shan zhi zi (Fructus Gardeniae Jasminoidis) 山栀子	9g
lian qiao (Fructus Forsythia Suspensae) 连翘	9g
chuan xiong (Radix Ligustici Chuanxiong) 川芎	6g
ren shen (Panax Ginseng) 人参	9g
jie geng (Radix Platycodi Grandiflori) 桔梗	9g
mu hu die (Semen Oroxyli Indici) 木蝴蝶	9g
gan cao (Radix Glycyrrhizae Uralensis) 甘草	3g

Method: Decoction. (Source: *Shi Yong Zhong Yi Nei Ke Xue*)

Modifications

- To disperse stagnation and nourish the Heart, add **bai he** (Bulbus Lilii) 百合 12g and **dan shen** (Radix Salviae Miltiorrhizae) 丹参 9g.
- To enhance the Liver soothing, *qi* dispersing action, add one or two of the following herbs: **hou po hua** (Flos Magnoliae Officinalis) 厚朴花 9g, **mei gui hua** (Flos Rosae Rugosae) 玫瑰花 6g, **bai ji li** (Fructus Tribuli Terrestris) 白蒺藜 9g or **he huan hua** (Flos Albizziae Julibrissin) 合欢花 9g.
- To redirect *qi* downwards, add **chuan lian zi*** (Fructus Meliae Toosendan) 川楝子 9g.
- If Lung *qi* is stagnant, with Phlegm in the chest, add **su zi** (Fructus Perillae Frutescentis) 苏子 6g and **gua lou pi** (Pericarpium Trichosanthis) 瓜楼皮 12g.
- If worry and anxiety have drained Heart *qi*, causing insomnia with much dreaming, add two or three of the following herbs: **yuan zhi** (Radix Polygalae Tenuifoliae) 远志 6g, **fu shen** (Sclerotium Poriae Cocos Pararadicis) 茯神 12g, **shi chang pu** (Rhizoma Acori Graminei) 石菖蒲 6g, **long chi**ˆ (Dens Draconis) 龙齿 18g or **suan zao ren** (Semen Zizyphi Spinosae) 酸枣仁 12g.

Patent medicines
Xiao Yao Wan 逍遥丸 (Xiao Yao Wan)
Shu Gan Wan 舒肝丸 (Shu Gan Wan)
Chai Hu Shu Gan Wan 柴胡舒肝丸 (Chai Hu Shu Gan Wan)

Acupuncture
Liv.3 (*tai chong*), PC.5 (*jian shi*), PC.6 (*nei guan*), Ht.5 (*tong li*), SJ.6 (*zhi gou*), *yin tang* (M-HN-3)

Clinical notes

- Biomedical conditions that may present as Liver *qi* stagnation type loss of voice or hoarse voice include hysterical aphonia, stage fright, hysteria, stuttering with anger, laryngeal strain, globus hystericus and social awkwardness.
- Episodes respond reasonably well to correct treatment and relaxation. Long term results require an appropriate management plan with relaxation, exercise and stress management.

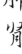

6.6 LUNG AND KIDNEY *YIN* DEFICIENCY

Pathophysiology
- Lung and Kidney *yin* deficiency hoarseness or loss of voice is chronic and develops over a long period of time. It may follow years of other throat or larynx pathology (like recurrent tonsillitis or laryngitis), heavy smoking or years of over use of the voice.

Clinical features
- Chronic or recurrent raspy, hoarse voice with little strength. The voice cannot be used for long before becoming hoarse, and may be lost in some cases. It is worse or recurs in the afternoon or evening and is worse when fatigued. The condition gradually gets worse.
- dry, non-productive cough, dry mouth and throat
- pale red throat and vocal cords; the vocal cord may be thickened
- mild recurrent sore throat that is worse in the afternoon or when fatigued
- malar or facial flushing, night sweats
- a sensation of heat in the palms and soles ('five hearts hot')
- dizziness, tinnitus, insomnia
- lower back ache

T red with little or no coat
P thready and rapid

Treatment principle
Moisten and nourish the Lungs and Kidneys
Clear Heat, benefit the throat

Prescription

BAI HE GU JIN TANG 百合固金汤
(*Lily Combination*) modified

bai he (Bulbus Lilii) 百合	30g
sheng di (Radix Rehmanniae Glutinosae) 生地	15g
shu di (Radix Rehmanniae Glutinosae Conquitae) 熟地	15g
mai dong (Tuber Ophiopogonis Japonici) 麦冬	15g
xuan shen (Radix Scrophulariae Ningpoensis) 玄参	15g
jie geng (Radix Platycodi Grandiflori) 桔梗	10g
bai shao (Radix Paeoniae Lactiflora) 白芍	10g
dang gui (Radix Angelicae Sinensis) 当归	10g
chuan bei mu (Bulbus Fritillariae Cirrhosae) 川贝母	10g
chan tui^ (Periostracum Cicadae) 蝉蜕	10g
he zi (Fructus Terminaliae Chebulae) 诃子	10g
mu hu die (Semen Oroxyli Indici) 木蝴蝶	10g

gan cao (Radix Glycyrrhizae Uralensis) 甘草 6g
Method: Decoction. (Source: *Zhong Yi Nei Ke Lin Chuang Shou Ce*)

MAI WEI DI HUANG WAN 麦味地黄丸
(*Ophiopogon, Schizandra and Rehmannia Formula*), p.148

This formula is selected when Kidney *yin* deficiency is prominent.

Modifications (applied to both prescriptions)
* With severe Heat, add **zhi mu** (Rhizoma Anemarrhenae Asphodeloides) 知母 12g and **huang bai** (Cortex Phellodendri) 黄柏 9g.
* With *qi* deficiency, delete **xuan shen** and **sheng di**, and add **huang qi** (Radix Astragali Membranacei) 黄芪 15g and **tai zi shen** (Radix Pseudostellariae Heterophyllae) 太子参 12g.
* If there are nodules or polyps on the vocal cords, add the herbs suggested in *qi*, Blood and Phlegm stagnation, p.230.

Patent medicines
Ba Xian Chang Shou Wan 八仙长寿丸 (Ba Xian Chang Shou Wan)
Bai He Gu Jin Wan 百合固金丸 (Bai He Gu Jin Wan)
Yang Yin Qing Fei Wan 养阴清肺丸 (Yang Yin Qing Fei Wan)

Gargle
* Decoct equal amounts (9-12 grams is sufficient) of **jie geng** (Radix Platycodi Grandiflori) 桔梗, **gan cao** (Radix Glycyrrhizae Uralensis) 甘草 and **pang da hai** (Semen Sterculiae Scaphigerae) 胖大海, and gargle several times daily.

Acupuncture
Bl.13 (*fei shu* +), Bl.23 (*shen shu* +), K.3 (*tai xi* +), Kid.6 (*zhao hai* +), Lu.7 (*lie que*), Lu.9 (*tai yuan* +)
  • with Heat add Lu.10 (*yu ji* -)

Clinical notes
• Biomedical conditions that may present as *yin* deficiency type loss of voice or hoarse voice include throat cancer, tuberculosis, chronic bronchitis, chronic laryngitis, bronchiectasis, silicosis, polyps, singers throat, post viral syndrome, post glandular fever and post stroke.
• This pattern can be difficult to treat and prolonged therapy is usually necessary for satisfactory results. Often complicated by nodules or polyps on the vocal cords.

肺脾气虚

6.7 LUNG AND SPLEEN *QI* DEFICIENCY

Pathophysiology
- The Lungs have a powerful influence over the throat and the power of expression of the voice. When Lung *qi* is chronically weak there is little force in the voice and what little there is, is easily spent. Weakness of Lung *qi* is compounded if *qi* production is impaired by Spleen weakness.

Clinical features
- chronic hoarse voice which is worse with use, fatigue and in the morning
- weak low voice
- vocal cords appear pale, flaccid and without tone
- shortness of breath on exertion
- spontaneous sweating
- poor appetite
- loose stools
- pale complexion

T pale and swollen with a thin white coat
P deficient and weak

Treatment principle
Tonify Lung and Spleen *qi*
Open and benefit the throat

Prescription

BU ZHONG YI QI TANG 补中益气汤
(*Ginseng and Astragalus Combination*) modified

| zhi huang qi (honey fried Radix Astragali Membranacei) 炙黄芪 15g
| dang shen (Radix Codonopsis Pilosulae) 党参 12g
| chao bai zhu (dry fried Rhizoma Atractylodis Macrocephalae) 炒白术 12g
| zhi gan cao (honey fried Radix Glycyrrhizae Uralensis) 炙甘草 6g
| chen pi (Pericarpium Citri Reticulatae) 陈皮 6g
| dang gui (Radix Angelicae Sinensis) 当归 6g
| sheng ma (Rhizoma Cimicifugae) 升麻 6g
| chai hu (Radix Bupleuri) 柴胡 6g
| he zi (Fructus Terminaliae Chebulae) 诃子 6g
| shi chang pu (Rhizoma Acori Graminei) 石菖蒲 6g

Method: Decoction. (Source: *Zhong Er Bi Hou Ke Xue*)

Modifications
- With Dampness or Phlegm, add **ban xia*** (Rhizoma Pinelliae Ternatae) 半夏 9g, **fu ling** (Sclerotium Poriae Cocos) 茯苓 12g and **bian dou** (Semen Dolichoris Lablab) 扁豆 9g.
- If there are nodules or polyps on the vocal cords, add the herbs suggested in *qi*, Blood and Phlegm stagnation, p.230.

Patent medicines
Bu Zhong Yi Qi Wan 补中益气丸 (Bu Zhong Yi Qi Wan)
Shen Ling Bai Zhu Wan 参苓白术丸 (Shen Ling Bai Zhu Wan)
Shen Qi Da Bu Wan 参芪大补丸 (Shen Qi Da Bu Wan)
Chong Cao Ji Jing 虫草鸡精 (Cordyceps Essence of Chicken)

Gargle
- Decoct equal amounts (9-12 grams is sufficient) of **jie geng** (Radix Platycodi Grandiflori) 桔梗, **gan cao** (Radix Glycyrrhizae Uralensis) 甘草 and **pang da hai** (Semen Sterculiae Scaphigerae) 胖大海, and gargle several times daily.

Acupuncture
LI.4 (*he gu*), St.36 (*zu san li* +▲), Bl.13 (*fei shu* +▲), Lu.9 (*tai yuan* +), Lu.7 (*lie que*), Du.14 (*da zhui* +▲), Sp.6 (*san yin jiao* +)

Clinical notes
- Biomedical conditions that may present as Lung and Spleen *qi* deficiency type loss of voice or hoarse voice include chronic overuse, post viral syndrome, allergic laryngitis (especially in people with food allergies), chronic gastritis, oesophageal reflux, hiatus hernia, chronic asthma and chronic steroid overuse (usually related to chronic rhinitis)
- Generally responds well to correct treatment, more difficult if there are polyps or nodules

6.8 *QI*, BLOOD AND PHLEGM STAGNATION

Pathophysiology
- This pattern represents a complication of chronic throat and vocal cord pathology resulting from *yin* and *qi* deficiency, chronic *qi* stagnation and Phlegm Heat. It involves structural change, that is, thickening and the development of polyps or nodules on the vocal cords.
- In most cases there will be a constitutional pattern in addition to the polyps, typically chronic Phlegm or Phlegm Heat, *yin* deficiency and/or *qi* deficiency. Treatment generally involves adding the herbs listed below to an appropriate constitutional formula.

Clinical features
- relatively severe huskiness and hoarseness of the voice, with a sensation of something in the throat
- frequent clearing of the throat
- polyps on the vocal cords, thickening, lumpiness and darkness of the vocal cords

T according to the accompanying pattern
P according to the accompanying pattern

Treatment principle
Apply the relevant treatment principle for the underlying pattern, with the addition of:
  Invigorate the circulation of *qi* and Blood
  Transform Phlegm

Additional herbs
The herbs below (or appropriate selection thereof) are added to one of the following formulae:

QING YAN NING FEI TANG 清咽宁肺汤
(*Clear the Throat and Calm the Lungs Decoction*, p.221) modified
BAI HE GU JIN TANG 百合固金汤
(*Lily Combination* p.226)
MAI WEI DI HUANG WAN 麦味地黄丸
(*Ophiopogon, Schizandra and Rehmannia Combination* p.148) or
BU ZHONG YI QI TANG 补中益气汤
(*Ginseng and Astragalus Combination* p.228)

    chi shao (Radix Paeoniae Rubrae) 赤芍 6-9g
    mu dan pi (Cortex Moutan Radicis) 牡丹皮 6-12g
    ze lan (Herba Lycopi Lucidi) 泽兰 3-9g
    yu jin (Tuber Curcumae) 郁金 6-9g

chuan bei mu (Bulbus Fritillariae Cirrhosae) 川贝母 3-9g
gua lou ren (Semen Trichosanthis) 瓜楼仁 9-12g
fu hai shi (Pumice) 浮海石 6-15g

Acupuncture
LI.18 (*fu tu* -), SI.17 (*tian rong* -), Lu.7 (*lie que* -), Ren.22 (*tian tu*)

Clinial notes
- This condition is difficult to cure with TCM alone.

SUMMARY OF GUIDING FORMULAE FOR LOSS OF VOICE AND HOARSE VOICE

Acute patterns
Wind Cold - *Liu Wei Tang* 六味汤

Wind Heat - *Shu Feng Qing Re Tang* 疏风清热汤

Lung Dryness - *Sang Xing Tang* 桑杏汤
- with severe dryness or following a febrile upper respiratory tract infection - *Qing Zao Jiu Fei Tang* 清燥救肺汤

Phlegm Heat - *Qing Yan Ning Fei Tang* 清咽宁肺汤

Liver *qi* stagnation - *Xiao Jiang Qi Tang* 小降气汤
- with stagnant Heat - *Chai Hu Qing Gan Tang* 柴胡清肝汤

Chronic patterns
Lung and Kidney *yin* deficiency - *Bai He Gu Jin Wan* 百合固金丸

Lung and Spleen *qi* deficiency - *Bu Zhong Yi Qi Tang* 补中益气汤

Endnote

For more information regarding herbs marked with an asterisk*, an open circle° or a hat^, see the tables on pp.944-952

Disorders of the Lung

7. Sinusitis and Nasal Congestion

Excess conditions
Wind Cold
Wind Heat
Liver *qi* stagnation with stagnant Heat
Liver and Gall Bladder Fire
Phlegm Heat

Deficient conditions
Lung *qi* deficiency
Spleen *qi* deficiency
Kidney deficiency
Blood stagnation

7 SINUSITIS AND NASAL CONGESTION
bi yuan 鼻渊, *bi zhi* 鼻窒

The terms *bi yuan* and *bi zhi* refer to a group of disorders characterised by nasal discharge, nasal congestion, sinus pain and frontal headache. *Bi yuan* is associated with infection and inflammation of the sinuses and nasal cavity, and thus correlates closely with acute sinusitis. *Bi zhi* describes the chronic nasal congestion which can linger with or without infection.

Chronic sinusitis and nasal congestion are common and distressing conditions that are quite often intractable to antibiotic therapy. Similarly, acute sinusitis can be difficult to resolve completely with antibiotic treatment alone. For this reason, these conditions are commonly seen in TCM clinics in the Western world. Allergic and perennial rhinitis (*bi qiu* 鼻鼽) are covered in the next chapter.

DIFFERENTIAL DIAGNOSIS

- **Rhinitis:** rhinitis is a disorder with two components. The first (hayfever) is a seasonal allergy characterised by sneezing, nasal itch, watery nasal discharge, sore, dry throat and red, sore, itchy eyes. It tends to re-occur at much the same time each year in response to seasonal allergens. The second (perennial rhinitis) exhibits the same set of symptoms but may exist all year round. Sinusitis and nasal congestion generally do not have the itchiness or sneezing typical of rhinitis, and do have more supraorbital and maxilliary pain.

AETIOLOGY
External pathogens
Wind Heat (or Wind Cold transforming into Heat) is the most common external cause of sinusitis, while Wind Cold (without Heat) is a common cause of nasal congestion. Invasion of Wind disrupts the functioning of the Lung system, in this case obstructing and preventing drainage of the normal fluids (*ti* 涕) of the sinuses and nasal passages.

If Heat is present, these fluids quickly condense to form the thick, sticky yellow or green mucus (Phlegm Heat) present in *bi yuan*. Recurrent flareups of sinusitis will occur with further attacks of Wind Heat if this accumulated mucus is not cleared from the sinuses.

Liver *qi* stagnation with stagnant Heat
Ongoing stress and repressed emotions disrupt the circulation of Liver *qi*. Prolonged *qi* stagnation generates Heat which can rise to the sinuses, drying fluids and causing congestion of the mucous membranes. This type of

sinusitis is characterised by swelling and congestion (rather than discharge), and is clearly worse for stress. The chronic congestion of this pattern provides the ideal environment for the generation of more intense focal Heat. This development is characterised by sinus pain and purulent discharge, and at this point is redefined as Liver and Gall Bladder Fire.

Phlegm Heat

This pattern is caused or prolonged by overconsumption of Heating and/or Phlegm producing substances, such as rich, greasy foods and alcohol. Phlegm Heat may also occur in an individual who accumulates Dampness due to Spleen deficiency (see below). Dampness that stagnates can generate Heat congealing fluids further into Phlegm Heat. If antibiotics (which clear Heat but do not disperse Damp) are used repeatedly, Phlegm and Damp will be retained in the sinuses creating the perfect conditions for recurrent Phlegm Heat.

Lung and Spleen *qi* deficiency

Overwork, excessive worry or mental activity, irregular eating habits, excessive consumption of cold, raw foods or prolonged illness can weaken Spleen (and Lung) *qi*. Chronic cough or upper respiratory tract infections can damage Lung *qi*. Weakened Lung *qi* may be unable to descend adequately, and fluids (that should go to the Kidney) accumulate in the Lungs and sinuses.

When the Lungs and Spleen are weak, food and fluids are poorly processed, and pathological fluids and Damp may accumulate. This can be exacerbated by certain food groups, the most commonly implicated in the Western world being dairy products. The mucus such foods provoke (in the gut epithelium) brings about a generalised Phlegm Damp condition (whereby the respiratory tract membranes also become congested). Repeated antibiotic use can further complicate the picture by weakening the Spleen and allowing more Phlegm to accumulate.

Kidney deficiency

Kidney deficiency is usually a factor in chronic conditions, and almost always in older people. It can be acquired from chronic illness, ageing or overexertion, or it can be inherited. When inherited, patients sometimes describe a history of some atopic condition during childhood. In these cases, Kidney *yang* is not strong enough to support Lung *qi*, to maintain *wei qi* or to regulate body fluids. Thus, respiration and defenses are weak, and fluids easily accumulate in the upper body. These individuals are particularly vulnerable to Wind and environmental irritants. In some old texts, this chronic sinus congestion and discharge is referred to as 'dripping brain' (*nao luo* 脑漏).

TREATMENT

Acute patterns generally respond well to correct treatment. Chronic patterns are more difficult and require persistent effort to resolve. Patients with chronic Phlegm in the sinuses are very prone to repeated attacks of acute sinusitis, so should be encouraged to seek treatment promptly upon catching cold or producing coloured mucus. The earlier the treatment the better and faster the result.

Sinus wash
Sinus congestion and tendency to infection benefits considerably from daily washing of the sinuses with warm salty water (with good quality sea salt). This dislodges thick or hidden mucus and any focal infection, and tones the mucous membranes. Several months of this practice are usually necessary in most chronic cases. The salt water can be introduced into the nose with a dropper or specialised pot (such as a neti pot, used in certain yoga practices), and should come out through the other nostril or mouth.

Table 7.1 Differentiation between excess and deficient patterns

Symptom	Excess	Deficient
Congestion	continuous, sustained	variable, intermittent
Sense of smell	transient decline or loss	variable transient or permanent loss
Headache	generally severe, frontal, maxilliary or temporal	dull or thick, with dizziness
Discharge	thick yellow or green, copious, purulent and malodorous; may be blood streaked	sticky, yellow or white, generally not malodorous
Mucous membranes	red and swollen	pale and swollen

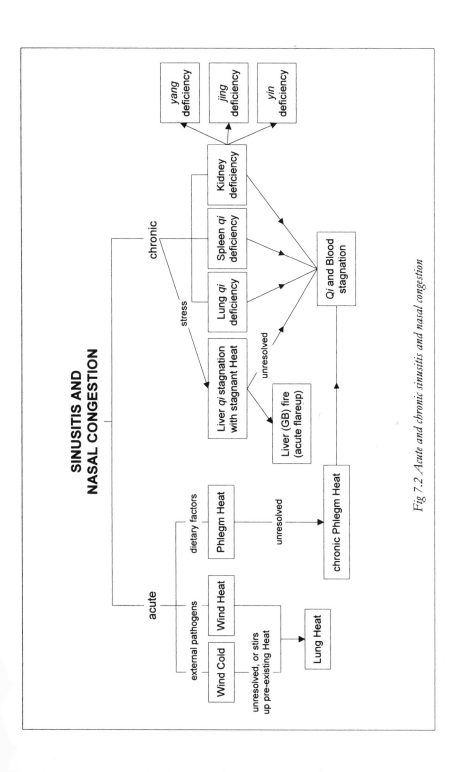

Fig 7.2 Acute and chronic sinusitis and nasal congestion

7.1 WIND COLD

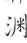

风寒鼻渊

Pathophysiology
- Wind Cold invades the exterior and Lungs, disrupting descent of the normal fluids of the Lung system (*ti* 涕) causing blocked sinuses and nose. This condition often precedes the secondary infection that characterises patterns like Wind Heat or Phlegm Heat.

Clinical features
- nasal congestion, or copious clear or white watery discharge, with discomfort and stuffiness in the nose and sinus region
- reduction or loss of sense of smell
- simultaneous fever and chills
- aversion to cold
- frontal or occipital headache

T normal with a thin white coat
P floating and tight

Treatment principle
Disperse Wind Cold
Redirect Lung *qi* downwards, open the nose

Prescription

XIN YI SAN 辛夷散
(*Magnolia Flower Powder*)

xin yi hua (Flos Magnoliae) 辛夷花	10g
xi xin* (Herba cum Radice Asari) 细辛	10g
gao ben (Rhizoma et Radix Ligustici) 藁本	10g
sheng ma (Rhizoma Cimicifugae) 升麻	10g
chuan xiong (Radix Ligustici Chuanxiong) 川芎	10g
mu tong (Caulis Mutong) 木通	10g
fang feng (Radix Ledebouriellae Divaricatae) 防风	10g
qiang huo (Rhizoma et Radix Notopterygii) 羌活	10g
bai zhi (Radix Angelicae Dahuricae) 白芷	10g
zhi gan cao (honey fried Radix Glycyrrhizae Uralensis) 炙甘草	10g

Method: Grind to a powder and take 6-grams 2-3 times daily with water. May also be decocted. (Source: *Zhong Yi Nei Ke Lin Chuang Shou Ce*)

Patent medicines
Bi Min Gan Wan 鼻敏感丸 (Pe Min Kan Wan)
Gan Mao Ling 感冒灵 (Gan Mao Ling)

Xin Yi San 辛荑散 (Xin Yi San)
Chuan Xiong Cha Tiao Wan 川芎茶调丸 (Chuan Xiong Cha Tiao Wan)
 - with prominent headache

Acupuncture
Lu.7 (*lie que* -), LI.4 (*he gu* -), LI.11 (*qu chi* -), *yin tang* (M-HN-3), LI.20 (*ying xiang*), Du.23 (*shang xing*), Bl.2 (*zan zhu*), *bi tong* (M-HN-14)

Clinical notes
- Biomedical conditions that may present with Wind Cold type sinus congestion include the common cold, influenza and allergic rhinitis.
- This pattern responds very well to correct and timely treatment.

7.2 WIND HEAT

风热鼻渊

Pathophysiology
- Wind Heat (or Wind Cold becoming hot), invades the Lungs, heating and preventing drainage of normal Lung fluids (*ti* 涕) from the sinuses, causing inflammation and congestion. The congestion and nasal discharge is particularly marked when there is pre-existing Phlegm Damp. In contrast to the Phlegm Heat (plus Wind) pattern, the symptoms here tend to be limited to the upper respiratory tract.

Clinical features
- sticky yellow or green purulent and malodorous mucus discharge from the nose, or nasal congestion
- inflamed and swollen nasal mucous membranes
- reduction or loss of sense of smell, nasal voice
- frontal headache and maxillary pain
- cough with yellow sputum
- thirst
- in the early stages there may be fever, or fever and chills

T normal or yellow coat
P floating and/or rapid

Treatment principle
Expel Wind and clear Heat
Open the nose

Prescription

CANG ER ZI SAN 苍耳子散
(*Xanthium Formula*) modified

cang er zi* (Fructus Xanthii Sibirici) 苍耳子	9g
bo he (Herba Mentha Haplocalycis) 薄荷	6g
xin yi hua (Flos Magnoliae) 辛夷花	3g
bai zhi (Radix Angelicae Dahuricae) 白芷	9g
huang qin (Radix Scutellariae Baicalensis) 黄芩	9g
ju hua (Flos Chrysanthemi Morifolii) 菊花	12g
lian qiao (Fructus Forsythia Suspensae) 连翘	15g
ge gen (Radix Puerariae) 葛根	10g

Method: Decoction. (Source: *Zhong Yi Er Bi Hou Ke Xue*)

Modifications
- With severe frontal or maxillary headache, increase the dose of **bai zhi** (Radix Angelicae Dahuricae) 白芷 to 12g and add **man jing zi** (Fructus Viticis) 蔓荆子 9g.

- ♦ With temporal headache, add **chai hu** (Radix Bupleuri) 柴胡 9g.
- ♦ If there is a cough with copious sputum, add **xing ren*** (Semen Pruni Armeniacae) 杏仁 9g, **jie geng** (Radix Platycodi Grandiflori) 桔梗 9g, **gua lou ren** (Semen Trichosanthis) 瓜蒌仁 12g and **dong gua ren** (Semen Benincasae Hispidae) 冬瓜仁 12g.
- ♦ With purulent nasal discharge, add **jin yin hua** (Flos Lonicerae Japonicae) 金银花 15g and **yu xing cao** (Herba Houttuyniae) 鱼腥草 15g.
- ♦ With Lung Heat, add **shi gao** (Gypsum) 石膏 18g and **zhi mu** (Rhizoma Anemarrhenae Asphodeloides) 知母 12g.
- ♦ With pre-existing Phlegm Damp, add **ban xia*** (Rhizoma Pinelliae Ternatae) 半夏 6g, **fu ling** (Sclerotium Poriae Cocos) 茯苓 12g and **chen pi** (Pericarpium Citri Reticulatae) 陈皮 6g.
- ♦ With the remnants of Wind Cold, add **xi xin*** (Herba cum Radice Asari) 细辛 6g, **gao ben** (Rhizoma et Radix Ligustici) 藁本 9g, **fang feng** (Radix Ledebouriellae Divaricatae) 防风 9g and **qiang huo** (Rhizoma et Radix Notopterygii) 羌活 9g.

Patent medicines
Bi Yan Ning 鼻炎宁 (Bi Yen Ning)
Qian Bai Bi Yan Pian 千柏鼻炎片 (Qian Bai Bi Yan Pian)
Niu Huang Jie Du Pian 牛黄解毒片 (Peking Niu Huang Chieh Tu Pien)
  - all the above are good for conditions characterised by congestion or thick yellow mucus and frontal headache

Acupuncture
SJ.5 (*wai guan* -), LI.4 (*he gu* -), GB.20 (*feng chi* -), LI.11 (*qu chi* -), Du.23 (*shang xing*), Bl.2 (*zan zhu*), LI.20 (*ying xiang*), *yin tang* (M-HN-3), *tai yang* (M-HN-9), *bi tong* (M-HN-14)

Snuff
- ♦ **BING LIAN SAN** (*Borneol and Coptis Powder* 冰连散) can be sniffed into each nostril several times daily.
    huang lian (Rhizoma Coptidis) 黄连
    xin yi hua (Flos Magnoliae) 辛夷花
    bing pian (Borneol) 冰片
    Method: Finely powder equal amounts of each herb and store in an airtight container until needed. (Source: *Zhong Yi Er Bi Hou Ke Xue*)

Clinical notes
- • Biomedical conditions that may present with Wind Heat type sinus congestion include acute or chronic sinusitis and acute or chronic rhinitis.
- • This pattern responds well to treatment, but has a tendency to become chronic, particularly with repeated antibiotic treatment.

肝气郁热鼻渊

7.3 LIVER QI STAGNATION WITH STAGNANT HEAT

Pathophysiology
- Chronic stress, emotional turmoil, a high pressure job or lifestyle combined with smoking and sedentary work can contribute to the generation of Liver *qi* stagnation and over time, stagnant Heat. The Heat ascends and lodges in the nasal sinuses, causing inflammation.

Clinical features
- Chronic sinus inflammation and congestion, perhaps with sinus pressure or pain and occasional postnasal discharge. The main feature is the chronic congestion which is worse for stress and emotional upset.
- frontal or temporal headaches, neck and shoulder tension
- red eyes, facial flushing
- irritability, easily angered
- hypochondriac tension or discomfort
- bitter taste in the mouth

T red edges, with red spots and a thin yellow coat
P wiry and possibly rapid

Treatment principle
Soothe Liver *qi*, clear Heat
Open the nose

Prescription

DAN ZHI XIAO YAO SAN 丹栀逍遥散
(*Bupleurum and Paeonia Formula*) modified

chai hu (Radix Bupleuri) 柴胡	12g
cu bai shao (vinegar fried Radix Paeoniae Lactiflora) 醋白芍	12g
fu ling (Sclerotium Poriae Cocos) 茯苓	12g
shan zhi zi (Fructus Gardeniae Jasminoidis) 山栀子	12g
dang gui (Radix Angelicae Sinensis) 当归	10g
bai zhi (Radix Angelicae Dahuricae) 白芷	10g
man jing zi (Fructus Viticis) 蔓荆子	10g
ju hua (Flos Chrysanthemi Morifolii) 菊花	10g
mu dan pi (Cortex Moutan Radicis) 牡丹皮	10g
chuan xiong (Radix Ligustici Chuanxiong) 川芎	6g
bo he (Herba Mentha Haplocalycis) 薄荷	6g

Method: Grind herbs to a fine powder and take in 9-gram doses 2-3 times daily. May also be decocted, in which case **bo he** is added towards the end of cooking (*hou xia* 后下).

Modifications

* With severe congestion, add **cang er zi*** (Fructus Xanthii Sibirici) 苍耳子 6g and **xin yi hua** (Flos Magnoliae) 辛夷花 6g, or combine with **HUO DAN WAN** (*Agastache and Pig Bile Pills* 藿胆丸), a patent pill composed of pigs bile and **huo xiang** (Herba Agastaches seu Pogostemi) 藿香.
* With severe Heat, add **yu jin** (Tuber Curcumae) 郁金 12g and **chuan lian zi*** (Fructus meliae Toosendan) 川楝子 12g. (See also Liver and Gall Bladder Fire, p.244).
* With abdominal distension, poor appetite and/or epigastric discomfort or pain with stress, add **bai zhu** (Rhizoma Atractylodis Macrocephalae) 白术 12g and **mu xiang** 木香 (Radix Aucklandiae Lappae) 12g.
* With constipation, add **da huang** (Radix et Rhizoma Rhei) 大黄 6-9g and **zhi shi** (Fructus Citri Aurantii Immaturus) 枳实 10g.

Patent medicines

Jia Wei Xiao Yao Wan 加味逍遥丸 (Jia Wei Xiao Yao Wan)
Xiao Yao Wan 逍遥丸 (Xiao Yao Wan)
Chai Hu Shu Gan Wan 柴胡舒肝丸 (Chai Hu Shu Gan Wan)
Bi Yan Ning 鼻炎宁 (Bi Yen Ning)
  - usually combined with one of the first three patent formulae
Qian Bai Bi Yan Pian 千柏鼻炎片 (Qian Bai Bi Yan Pian)
  - usually combined with one of the first three patent formulae
Xin Yi San 辛荑散 (Xin Yi San)
  - usually combined with one of the first three patent formulae

Acupuncture

Liv.3 (*tai chong* -), LI.4 (*he gu* -), Liv.2 (*xing jian* -), GB.20 (*feng chi*), SI.3 (*hou xi*), Du.23 (*shang xing*), Bl.2 (*zan zhu*), LI.20 (*ying xiang*), *yin tang* (M-HN-3), *tai yang* (M-HN-9), *bi tong* (M-HN-14)

Clinical notes

* Biomedical conditions that may present with Liver *qi* stagnation type sinus congestion include hypertension, chronic sinusitis, chronic rhinitis and stree induced sinus congestion.
* Daily sinus wash definitely improves results (see p.236).
* This pattern is often difficult and it takes time and effort on the part of the patient to get a good result. Long term results require an appropriate treatment plan which includes lifestyle modification, diet (especially reducing alcohol), relaxation, exercise and stress management.

7.4 LIVER AND GALL BLADDER FIRE

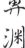

Pathophysiology
- Liver and Gall Bladder Fire is usually an acute aggravation of the previous pattern, Liver *qi* stagnation with stagnant Heat. This pattern usually represents an acute and severe infection of the sinuses.

Clinical features
- thick, sticky, copious yellow or green nasal discharge which is malodorous and maybe purulent
- nasal congestion, reduced sense of smell
- inflamed and swollen nasal mucous membranes
- violent frontal, maxillary or temporal headache or distension
- bitter taste in the mouth
- dry throat
- dizziness, tinnitus
- insomnia, much dreaming
- irritability and restlessness, quick temper
- dry stools or constipation
- feverishness

T red, with a yellow coat
P wiry and rapid

Treatment principle
Clear Fire from the Liver and Gall Bladder
Resolve Dampness, open the nose

Prescription

LONG DAN XIE GAN TANG 龙胆泻肝汤
(*Gentiana Combination*) modified

long dan cao (Radix Gentianae Longdancao) 龙胆草	9g
huang qin (Radix Scutellariae Baicalensis) 黄芩	9g
chai hu (Radix Bupleuri) 柴胡	9g
sheng di (Radix Rehmanniae Glutinosae) 生地	30g
shan zhi zi (Fructus Gardeniae Jasminoidis) 山栀子	9g
che qian zi (Semen Plantaginis) 车前子	9g
jiu dang gui (wine fried Radix Angelicae Sinensis) 酒当归	6g
ze xie (Rhizoma Alismatis Orientalis) 泽泻	6g
mu tong (Caulis Mutong) 木通	3g
ju hua (Flos Chrysanthemi Morifolii) 菊花	12g
bai zhi (Radix Angelicae Dahuricae) 白芷	6g

Method: Decoction. **Che qian zi** is usually cooked in a cloth bag (*bao jian* 包煎)
(Source: *Zhong Yi Nei Ke Lin Chuang Shou Ce*)

Modifications
- With severe headache add **shi jue ming**^ (Concha Haliotidis) 石决明 15g and **gou teng** (Ramulus Uncariae cum Uncis) 钩藤 12g.
- This formula is usually combined with the patent pill **HUO DAN WAN** (*Agastache and Pig Bile Pills* 藿胆丸).

Patent medicines
Long Dan Xie Gan Wan 龙胆泻肝丸 (Long Dan Xie Gan Wan)
Qing Fei Yi Huo Pian 清肺抑火片 (Ching Fei Yi Huo Pien)
Bi Yan Ning 鼻炎宁 (Bi Yen Ning)
   - usually combined with one of the first two patent formulae
Qian Bai Bi Yan Pian 千柏鼻炎片 (Qian Bai Bi Yan Pian)
   - usually combined with one of the first two patent formulae
Huo Dan Wan 藿胆丸 (Agastache and Pig Bile Pills)
   - this patent is combined with the primary prescription
Niu Huang Qing Huo Wan 牛黄清火丸 (Niu Huang Qing Huo Wan)
   - for severe Heat

Acupuncture
SJ.5 (*wai guan* -), LI.4 (*he gu* -), GB.20 (*feng chi* -), Liv.2 (*xing jian* -), GB.39 (*xuan zhong* -), Du.23 (*shang xing*), Bl.2 (*zan zhu*), LI.20 (*ying xiang* -), *yin tang* (M-HN-3), *tai yang* (M-HN-9), *bi tong* (M-HN-14)

Snuff
- **BING LIAN SAN** (see Lung Heat, p.241)

Clinical notes
- Biomedical conditions that may present with Liver Fire type sinus congestion include acute sinusitis, acute rhinitis, stress induced sinus congestion and hypertension.
- Daily sinus wash definitely improves results (see p.236)
- Antibiotics are often prescribed for this type of attack and this type of individual who prefers the quick fix rather than the necessary lifestyle modification. However, prompt treatment with Chinese herbs and acupuncture can certainly be effective in the motivated patient.

7.5 PHLEGM HEAT

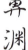

Pathophysiology
- Phlegm Heat type sinusitis can present as an acute attack or a subacute and prolonged congestion.
- It occurs as an acute episode when Phlegm Heat is provoked by extreme overindulgence in rich heating foods and alcohol (sinus following 'the big night out'). In those with specific food intolerances even a small amount (for example one glass of red wine) can set off an attack.
- Acute Phlegm Heat sinusitis also occurs when someone with chronic Phlegm Damp gets a Wind Heat attack. These are the patients who know that as soon as they get a cold, sinusitis will follow.
- Alternatively, this pattern represents chronic nasal congestion with thick sticky yellow mucus. It is usually seen in individuals who eat too much rich and spicy food on a regular basis.
- If this pattern is overenthusiastically treated with antibiotics or bitter cold herbs, the Spleen may be damaged. See also p.252.

Clinical features
- copious sticky, continuous yellow or green nasal discharge, or severe nasal congestion
- inflamed and swollen mucous membranes
- reduction or loss of sense of smell
- vertigo and dizziness
- heavy, woolly-headedness, frontal headache
- heaviness and aches in the body
- lethargy and fatigue
- epigastric and abdominal distension, poor appetite, loose or sluggish stools

T red, with a greasy yellow coat
P soft or slippery and rapid

Treatment principle
Clear and transform Phlegm Heat
Open the nose

Prescription

DAN XI BI YUAN FANG 丹溪鼻渊方
(*Dan Xi's Nasal Congestion Formula*) modified

dan nan xing* (Pulvis Arisaemae cum Felle Bovis) 胆南星	6g
ban xia* (Rhizoma Pinelliae Ternatae) 半夏	9g
cang zhu (Rhizoma Atractylodis) 苍术	9g

bai zhi (Radix Angelicae Dahuricae) 白芷 9g
jiu huang qin (wine fried Radix Scutellariae Baicalensis)
   酒黄芩 9g
shen qu (Massa Fermentata) 神曲 9g
xin yi hua (Flos Magnoliae) 辛夷花 9g
jing jie (Herba seu Flos Schizonepetae Tenuifolia) 荆芥 9g
huo xiang (Herba Agastaches seu Pogostemi) 藿香 12g
bai dou kou (Fructus Amomi Kravanh) 白豆蔻 6g
lian qiao (Fructus Forsythia Suspensae) 连翘 12g
shi chang pu (Rhizoma Acori Graminei) 石菖蒲 6g
Method: Decoction. (Source: *Shi Yong Zhong Yi Nei Ke Xue*)

Modifications

- With severe congestion, add **cang er zi*** (Fructus Xanthii Sibirici) 苍耳子 9g and **bo he** (Herba Mentha Haplocalycis) 薄荷 6g.
- With signs of Wind Heat, add two or three of the following herbs: **jin yin hua** (Flos Lonicerae Japonicae) 金银花 15g, **niu bang zi** (Fructus Arctii Lappae) 牛蒡子 9g, **bo he** (Herba Mentha Haplocalycis) 薄荷 6g or **ju hua** (Flos Chrysanthemi Morifolii) 菊花 12g.
- For cough with copious sputum, add **xing ren*** (Semen Pruni Armeniacae) 杏仁 9g, **jie geng** (Radix Platycodi Grandiflori) 桔梗 6g and **gua lou ren** (Semen Trichosanthis) 瓜蒌仁 9g.
- With a bitter taste in the mouth and dry throat, add **tian hua fen** (Radix Trichosanthes Kirilowii) 天花粉 15g, **zhi mu** (Rhizoma Anemarrhenae Asphodeloides) 知母 9g and **lu gen** (Rhizoma Phragmitis Communis) 芦根 20g.
- With tinnitus and loss of hearing, add **pei lan** (Herba Eupatorii Fortuneii) 佩兰 9g and increase the dose of **shi chang pu** to 9g.
- With insomnia and much dreaming, add **yuan zhi** (Radix Polygalae Tenuifoliae) 远志 6g, **suan zao ren** (Semen Zizyphi Spinosae) 酸枣仁 15g and **ye jiao teng** 夜交藤 15g.

Patent medicines

Bi Yan Ning 鼻炎宁 (Bi Yen Ning)
Qian Bai Bi Yan Pian 千柏鼻炎片 (Qian Bai Bi Yan Pian)
Huang Lian Jie Du Wan 黄连解毒丸 (Huang Lian Jie Du Wan)
Chuan Xin Lian Kang Yan Pian 穿心莲抗炎片
   (Chuan Xin Lian Antiphlogistic Tablets)
Huo Dan Wan 藿胆丸 (Agastache and Pig Bile Pills)
   - this patent is combined with the primary prescription

Acupuncture

LI.4 (*he gu* -), LI.11 (*qu chi* -), GB.20 (*feng chi* -), Sp.9 (*yin ling quan* -), GB.39 (*xuan zhong*), Du.23 (*shang xing*), Bl.2 (*zan zhu*), LI.20 (*ying xiang*), *yin tang* (M-HN-3), *tai yang* (M-HN-9), *bi tong* (M-HN-14)

Snuff

* **BING LIAN SAN** (see Lung Heat, p.241)

Clinical notes

- Biomedical conditions that may present with Phlegm Heat type sinus congestion include acute or chronic sinusitis or rhinitis.
- Daily sinus wash definitely improves results (see p.236)
- Diet is particularly important in this pattern, as many patients will be found to have a Phlegm Damp (Heat) generating diet, frequently dairy products. Avoidance of these items is critical if this is the case.

肺气虚鼻渊

7.6 LUNG *QI* DEFICIENCY

Pathophysiology
- Lung *qi* deficiency follows years of recurrent sinusitis or rhinitis that have weakened Lung *qi*. When Lung *qi* fails to descend, fluids accumulate in the upper respiratory tract and sinuses.

Clinical features
- Chronic nasal and sinus congestion, or discharge of copious thin white or sticky mucus which does not smell (although the patient may perceive it to). The discharge or congestion is variable and aggravated by exposure to wind and cold. When congestion is the main problem, it may be worse at night and when lying down, and better during the day.
- pale, swollen mucous membranes
- diminished sense of smell
- shortness of breath, soft voice or reluctance to speak
- fatigue and spontaneous sweating
- waxy, pale complexion
- weak cough with thin white sputum

T pale with a thin white coat
P weak and forceless

Treatment principle
Tonify and warm Lung *qi*
Disperse Cold, open the nose

Prescription

WEN FEI ZHI LIU DAN 温肺止流丹
(*Warm the Lungs, Stop the Flow Special Pill*) modified

zhi huang qi (honey fried Radix Astragali Membranacei) 炙黄芪	15g
bai zhu (Rhizoma Atractylodis Macrocephalae) 白术	12g
ren shen (Panax Ginseng) 人参	9g
jing jie (Herba seu Flos Schizonepetae Tenuifolia) 荆芥	9g
jie geng (Radix Platycodi Grandiflori) 桔梗	9g
he zi (Fructus Terminaliae Chebulae) 诃子	9g
yu nao shiˆ (Pseudosciaenae Otolithum) 鱼脑石	6g
wu wei zi (Fructus Schizandrae Chinensis) 五味子	6g
xi xin* (Herba cum Radice Asari) 细辛	3g
gan cao (Radix Glycyrrhizae Uralensis) 甘草	3g

Method: Decoction. (Source: *Shi Yong Zhong Yi Nei Ke Xue*)

Modifications

- With frequent colds and spontaneous sweating, double the dose of **zhi huang qi**.
- With headache or dizziness, add **chuan xiong** (Radix Ligustici Chuanxiong) 川芎 6g and **gao ben** (Rhizoma et Radix Ligustici) 藁本 9g.
- If the congestion is very severe, delete **he zi** and **wu wei zi**, and add two or three of the following herbs: **shi chang pu** (Rhizoma Acori Graminei) 石菖蒲 6g, **xin yi hua** (Flos Magnoliae) 辛夷花 9g, **cang er zi** (Fructus Xanthii Sibirici) 苍耳子 9g, **bai zhi** (Radix Angelicae Dahuricae) 白芷 9g, **gui zhi** (Ramulus Cinnamomi Cassiae) 桂枝 9g or **chuan jiao** (Pericarpium Zanthoxyli Bungeani) 川椒 3g.
- With continuous, copious watery nasal discharge, add one or two of the following herbs: **long gu** (Os Draconis) 龙骨 15g, **jin ying zi** (Fructus Rosae Laevigatae) 金樱子 9g, **fu xiao mai** (Semen Tritici Aestivi Levis) 浮小麦 12g or **nuo dao gen** (Radix et Rhizoma Oryzae Glutinosae) 糯稻根 15g.
- With minor signs of Heat or Damp Heat, add **huang lian** (Rhizoma Coptidis) 黄连 3g, **che qian zi** (Semen Plantaginis) 车前子 6g and **mu tong** (Caulis Mutong) 木通 6g.

Variations and additional prescriptions

With a Wind attack

- In a patient with pre-existing Lung *qi* deficiency who catches cold (with mild fever and chills, muscle aches, occipital headache etc.), the correct treatment is to expel Wind Cold and support *qi* with **SHEN SU YIN** (*Ginseng and Perilla Combination* 参苏饮, p.21).

Resistant cases

- If a patient with Lung *qi* deficiency suddenly experiences an aggravation of the congestion, or the primary prescription fails to control the congestion, a more dispersing formula may be used for a short period. **WEN FEI TANG** (*Warm the Lungs Decoction* 温肺汤) may be selected, but because this formula is more dispersing to the *qi*, it is not suitable for prolonged use.

```
huang qi (Radix Astragali Membranacei) 黄芪 .................. 18g
ge gen (Radix Puerariae) 葛根 ................................. 9g
qiang huo (Rhizoma et Radix Notopterygii) 羌活 ............... 9g
fang feng (Radix Ledebouriellae Divaricatae) 防风 ............ 9g
ma huang* (Herba Ephedra) 麻黄 ............................... 6-9g
sheng ma (Rhizoma Cimicifugae) 升麻 .......................... 6g
cong bai (Bulbus Allii Fistulosi) 葱白 ....................... 3pce
ding xiang (Flos Caryophylli) 丁香 ........................... 3g
```

gan cao (Radix Glycyrrhizae Uralensis) 甘草 3g
Method: Decoction. **Cong bai** is added towards the end of cooking (*hou xia* 后下). (Source: *Zhong Yi Er Bi Hou Ke Xue*)

Patent medicines
Yu Ping Feng Wan 玉屏风丸 (Yu Ping Feng Wan)
Xiang Sha Liu Jun Zi Wan 香砂六君子丸 (Xiang Sha Liu Jun Wan))
Bu Zhong Yi Qi Wan 补中益气丸 (Bu Zhong Yi Qi Wan)
Shen Ling Bai Zhu Wan 参苓白术丸 (Shen Ling Bai Zhu Wan)
Shen Qi Da Bu Wan 参芪大补丸 (Shen Qi Da Bu Wan)

Acupuncture
Lu.9 (*tai yuan* ▲ +), St.36 (*zu san li* ▲ +), LI.20 (*ying xiang* +), Du.20 (*bai hui* ▲ +), Du.23 (*shang xing* ▲ +), *yin tang* ▲ (M-HN-3), *bi tong* (M-HN-14), LI.4 (*hegu* +), Bl.2 (*zan zhu* +), GB.20 (*feng chi* +), Bl.13 (*fei shu* ▲).

• Treating *yin tang* with moxa cones over slices of raw ginger is particularly good.

Medicated oil
♦ Particularly good for congestion, these herbs are powdered and steeped in sesame oil for a few days. The oil is filtered and rubbed into the nasal mucosa several times daily.

e bu shi cao (Herba Centipeda) 鹅不食草 30g
hai er cha (Pasta Acaciae seu Uncariae) 孩儿茶 60g
bing pian (Borneol) 冰片 15g
(Source: *Zhong Yi Er Bi Hou Ke Xue*)

Clinical notes
• Biomedical conditions that may present with Lung *qi* deficiency type sinus congestion include chronic sinusitis and allergic rhinitis.
• Sinus wash may be useful, especially if the pattern is aggravated by Wind Cold (see p.236).

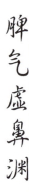

7.7 SPLEEN *QI* DEFICIENCY

Pathophysiology
- Spleen *qi* deficiency is a chronic pattern characterised by congestion and loss of sense of smell. It often follows chronic or recurrent Hot type sinus problems that have been treated with repeated courses of antibiotics. The Phlegm resulting from the weakened Spleen becomes harder and harder to shift and constantly clogs the nasal epithelium, reducing the ability to smell. This pattern often overlaps with Lung *qi* deficiency (p.249). When Spleen deficiency predominates the mucus is thicker and congestion is more severe.

Clinical features
- Chronic, copious and persistent, sticky nasal discharge or nasal congestion. The mucus is sticky and white, not malodorous, and the congestion is relatively severe. The congestion may be worse at night and when lying down, and better during the day and when active.
- pale and swollen mucous membranes
- reduction or loss of sense of smell
- fuzzy-headedness, dizziness
- fatigue, heavy, tired limbs
- poor appetite
- abdominal distension
- pale sallow complexion
- diarrhoea or loose stools

T pale with a thin or thick white coat
P moderate and weak

Treatment principle
Strengthen the Spleen and tonify *qi*
Facilitate the 'raising of clear *yang* and the descent of turbid *yin*'

Prescription

BU ZHONG YI QI TANG 补中益气汤
(*Ginseng and Astragalus Combination*) modified

zhi huang qi (honey fried Radix Astragali Membranacei) 炙黄芪	15g
dang shen (Radix Codonopsis Pilosulae) 党参	12g
chao bai zhu (dry fried Rhizoma Atractylodis Macrocephalae) 炒白术	12g
cang zhu (Rhizoma Atractylodis) 苍术	9g
ze xie (Rhizoma Alismatis Orientalis) 泽泻	9g

zhi gan cao (honey fried Radix Glycyrrhizae Uralensis)
炙甘草 6g
chen pi (Pericarpium Citri Reticulatae) 陈皮 6g
dang gui (Radix Angelicae Sinensis) 当归 6g
sheng ma (Rhizoma Cimicifugae) 升麻 6g
chai hu (Radix Bupleuri) 柴胡 6g
ge gen (Radix Puerariae) 葛根 6g
mu tong (Caulis Mutong) 木通 6g
shi chang pu (Rhizoma Acori Graminei) 石菖蒲 6g
yuan zhi (Radix Polygalae Tenuifoliae) 远志 6g
Method: Decoction. (Source: *Shi Yong Zhong Yi Nei Ke Xue*)

SHEN LING BAI ZHU SAN 参苓白术散
(*Ginseng and Atractylodes Formula*) modified

This formula is selected when gastrointestinal symptoms (particularly diarrhoea or loose stools) are prominent.

dang shen (Radix Codonopsis Pilosulae) 党参 15-30g
bai zhu (Rhizoma Atractylodes Macrocephalae) 白术 10-20g
chao yi ren (dry fried Semen Coicis Lachryma-jobi) 炒苡仁 . 20g
fu ling (Sclerotium Poriae Cocos) 茯苓 15g
chao bian dou (dry fried Semen Dolichos Lablab) 炒扁豆 15g
chao shan yao (dry fried Radix Dioscoreae Oppositae)
炒山药 15g
lian zi (Semen Nelumbinis Nuciferae) 莲子 15g
jie geng (Radix Platycodi Grandiflori) 桔梗 6g
sha ren (Fructus Amomi) 砂仁 6g
shi chang pu (Rhizoma Acori Graminei) 石菖蒲 6g
zhi gan cao (honey fried Radix Glycyrrhizae Uralensis)
炙甘草 3g
Method: Grind the herbs to a powder and take in 9-gram doses 2-3 times daily with warm water. May also be decocted with doses as shown. (Source: *Zhong Yi Er Bi Hou Ke Xue*)

Modifications

- If the Phlegm is sticky white, copious and very persistent, add **ban xia*** (Rhizoma Pinelliae Ternatae) 半夏 9g and **chen pi** (Pericarpium Citri Reticulatae) 陈皮 6g or consider **LIU JUN ZI TANG** (*Six Major Herbs Combination* 六君子汤, p.88).
- If complicated with Phlegm Heat or if the congestion is severe or provoked by trigger foods, add two or three of the following herbs: **huo xiang** (Herba Agastaches seu Pogostemi) 藿香 12g, **xia ku cao** (Spica Prunella Vulgaris) 夏枯草 12g, **cang er zi*** (Fructus Xanthii Sibirici) 苍耳子 6g or **xin yi hua** (Flos Magnoliae) 辛夷花 6g.

Patent medicines
Xiang Sha Liu Jun Zi Wan 香砂六君子丸 (Xiang Sha Liu Jun Wan)
Bu Zhong Yi Qi Wan 补中益气丸 (Bu Zhong Yi Qi Wan)
Shen Ling Bai Zhu Wan 参苓白术丸 (Shen Ling Bai Zhu Wan)
Shen Qi Da Bu Wan 参芪大补丸 (Shen Qi Da Bu Wan)

Acupuncture
LI.20 (*ying xiang* +), Du.20 (*bai hui* +), Du.23 (*shang xing* +), *yin tang* ▲ (M-HN-3), *bi tong* (M-HN-14), LI.4 (*hegu* +), Bl.2 (*zan zhu* +), GB.20 (*feng chi* +), Bl.20 (*pi shu* ▲), St.36 (*zu san li* +), St.40 (*feng long* -), Sp.3 (*tai bai* +)
• *yin tang* (M-HN-3) is treated with moxa cones over slices of raw ginger.

Medicated oil
• see Lung *qi* deficiency, p.251

Clinical notes
• Biomedical conditions that may present with Spleen *qi* deficiency type sinus congestion include chronic sinusitis and chronic rhinitis.
• Dietary modification is very important in this pattern.
• Sinus wash may be useful (see p.236)

7.8 KIDNEY DEFICIENCY

Pathophysiology
- The incessant, chronic mucus typical of Kidney deficiency is part of the systemic failure of fluid movement and metabolism. It can develop from long term sinusitis from any cause, or it may be due to congenital or acquired Kidney weakness, or both.
- This is a very chronic pattern and as such involves the *jing*. Weak *jing* can manifest as either *yin* or *yang* deficiency, depending on the constitution of the patient. With *yin* deficiency there is a tendency to Hot signs and symptoms, with *yang* deficiency a tendency to cold. When both are equally weak, that is *qi* or *jing* deficiency, there may be no obvious tendency to either Heat of Cold.

髓海不充鼻渊

Clinical features
- chronic nasal discharge, worse with exposure to cold
- diminished sense of smell
- dizziness, tinnitus, loss of hearing
- forgetfulness, poor memory
- muddleheaded or slow to learn
- soreness and weakness in the back and spine
- greying lifeless hair
- pale lustreless complexion
- oedema of the lower extremities
- **Kidney *yin* deficiency**: sensation of heat in the palms and soles ('five hearts hot'), insomnia, night sweats, facial or malar flushing, a red, dry tongue with little or no coat and a thready, rapid pulse
- **Kidney *yang* deficiency**: pale complexion, aversion to cold, cold extremities, nocturia, impotence, a pale or blueish and swollen tongue, and a deep, slow pulse

Treatment principle
Tonify the Kidney and supplement *jing*
Benefit the brain and stop discharge

Prescription
7.8.1 Kidney *yin* deficiency

LIU WEI DI HUANG WAN 六味地黄丸
(*Rehmannia Six Formula*) plus
SHENG MAI SAN 生脉散
(*Generate the Pulse Powder*)

This formula is selected when there are obvious Heat signs.

shu di (Radix Rehmanniae Glutinosae Conquitae) 熟地 240g
shan yao (Radix Dioscoreae Oppositae) 山药 120g
shan zhu yu (Fructus Corni Officinalis) 山茱萸 120g
fu ling (Sclerotium Poria Cocos) 茯苓 90g
ze xie (Rhizoma Alismatis Orientalis) 泽泻 90g
mu dan pi (Cortex Moutan Radicis) 牡丹皮 90g
ren shen (Radix Ginseng) 人参 90g
mai dong (Tuber Ophiopogonis Japonici) 麦冬 90g
wu wei zi (Fructus Schizandrae Chinensis) 五味子 60g

Method: Grind the herbs to powder and form into 9-gram pills with honey. The dose is 2-3 pills daily. May also be decocted with a 90% reduction in dosage.
(Source: *Shi Yong Zhong Yi Nei Ke Xue*)

7.8.2 Kidney *yang* deficiency

YOU GUI WAN 右归丸
(*Eucommia and Rehmannia Formula*)

This formula is selected when there are obvious Cold signs.

shu di (Radix Rehmanniae Glutinosae Conquitae) 熟地 250g
shan yao (Radix Dioscoreae Oppositae) 山药 120g
lu jiao jiao^ (Cornu Cervi Gelatinum) 鹿角胶 120g
tu si zi (Semen Cuscutae Chinensis) 菟丝子 120g
gou qi zi (Fructus Lycii) 枸杞子 120g
du zhong (Cortex Eucommiae Ulmoidis) 杜仲 120g
shan zhu yu (Fructus Corni Officinalis) 山茱萸 90g
dang gui (Radix Angelicae Sinensis) 当归 90g
zhi fu zi* (Radix Aconiti Carmichaeli Praeparata)
    制附子 60-180g
rou gui (Cortex Cinnamomi Cassiae) 肉桂 60-120g

Method: Grind herbs to powder and form into 9-gram pills with honey. The dose is one pill 2-3 times daily. May also be decocted with a 90% reduction in dosage, in which case **zhi fu zi** is cooked for 30 minutes before the other herbs are added (*xian jian* 先煎), and **rou gui** is added towards the end of cooking (*hou xia* 后下).

7.8.3 Kidney *qi* or *jing* deficiency

BU NAO WAN 补脑丸
(*Brain Tonic Pills*)

This formula is selected when there are no obvious Heat or Cold signs.

shu di (Radix Rehmanniae Glutinosae Conquitae) 熟地 240g
huang qi (Radix Astragali Membranacei) 黄芪 180g
rou cong rong (Herba Cistanches Deserticolae) 肉苁蓉 180g
fu ling (Sclerotium Poriae Cocos) 茯苓 120g
du zhong (Cortex Eucommiae Ulmoidis) 杜仲 120g

shan yao (Radix Dioscoreae Oppositae) 山药 120g
shan zhu yu (Fructus Corni Officinalis) 山茱萸 120g
gou qi zi (Fructus Lycii) 枸杞子 120g
tu si zi (Semen Cuscutae Chinensis) 菟丝子 120g
lu rong^ (Cornu Cervi Parvum) 鹿茸 120g
ren shen (Radix Ginseng) 人参 90g
mai dong (Tuber Ophiopogonis Japonici) 麦冬 90g
wu wei zi (Fructus Schizandrae Chinensis) 五味子 60g

Method: Grind herbs to powder and form into 9-gram pills with honey. The dose is one pill 2-3 times daily. (Source: *Shi Yong Zhong Yi Nei Ke Xue*)

Patent medicines
Kidney *yang*
Jin Kui Shen Qi Wan 金匮肾气丸 (Sexoton Pills)
You Gui Wan 右归丸 (You Gui Wan)
Ba Ji Yin Yang Wan 巴戟阴阳丸 (Ba Ji Yin Yang Wan)
Ning Xin Bu Shen Wan 宁心补肾丸 (San Yuen Medical Pills)
Zhuang Yao Jian Shen Pian 壮腰健肾片 (Zhuang Yao Jian Shen)

Kidney *yin*
Liu Wei Di Huang Wan 六味地黄丸 (Liu Wei Dihuang Wan)
Zhi Bai Ba Wei Wan 知柏八味丸 (Zhi Bai Ba Wei Wan)

Kidney *jing*
Bu Nao Wan 补脑丸 (Cerebral Tonic Pills)
Chong Cao Ji Jing 虫草鸡精 (Cordyceps Essence of Chicken)

Acupuncture
Bl.23 (*shen shu* +), Du.4 (*ming men* +), Ren.4 (*guan yuan* +), Ren.6 (*qi hai* +), GB.39 (*xuan zhong* +), Du.20 (*bai hui*), Bl.15 (*xin shu*), *yin tang* (M-HN-3), *bi tong* (M-HN-14).

- Use moxa in *jing* and *yang* deficiency. Treating *yin tang* with moxa cones over slices of raw ginger is particularly good.

Clinical notes
- Biomedical conditions that may present with Kidney deficiency type sinus congestion include chronic sinusitis and rhinitis.
- The sinus wash may offer some symptomatic relief (see p.236).

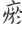

7.9 BLOOD STAGNATION

Pathophysiology
- Blood stagnation sinus congestion is the end result of many years of chronic pathology of the sinus and nasal passages. The mucous membranes develop a distinctive dark and swollen appearance.

Clinical features
- chronic continuous nasal congestion or post nasal drip with sticky yellow or white mucus
- nasal mucous membranes appear swollen, hard and dark or purple (in some cases the same colour as ripe mulberry fruit)
- reduction or loss of sense of smell

T dark red or purple with brown or purple stasis spots
P wiry and thready or choppy

Treatment principle
Harmonise *qi* and Blood
Move stagnation and eliminate Blood stagnation

Prescription

DANG GUI SHAO YAO SAN 当归芍药散
(*Dang Gui and Peonia Formula*) modified

dang gui (Radix Angelicae Sinensis) 当归	12g
fu ling (Sclerotium Poriae Cocos) 茯苓	12g
bai zhu (Rhizoma Atractylodis Macrocephalae) 白术	9g
ze xie (Rhizoma Alismatis Orientalis) 泽泻	9g
xin yi hua (Flos Magnoliae) 辛夷花	9g
ju hua (Flos Chrysanthemi Morifolii) 菊花	9g
di long^ (Lumbricus) 地龙	9g
chuan xiong (Radix Ligustici Chuanxiong) 川芎	6g
bo he (Herba Mentha Haplocalycis) 薄荷	6g
huang qin (Radix Scutellariae Baicalensis) 黄芩	6g
gan cao (Radix Glycyrrhizae Uralensis) 甘草	3g

Method: Decoction. **Bo he** is added towards the end of cooking (*hou xia* 后下).
(Source: *Zhong Yi Er Bi Hou Ke Xue*)

Modifications
- With headache or dizziness, add **bai zhi** (Radix Angelicae Dahuricae) 白芷 10g, **gao ben** (Rhizoma et Radix Ligustici) 藁本 10g, **bai ji li** (Fructus Tribuli Terrestris) 白蒺藜 10g and **man jing zi** (Fructus Viticis) 蔓荆子 10g.

- With cough, add **xing ren*** (Semen Pruni Armeniacae) 杏仁 9g, **jie geng** (Radix Platycodi Grandiflori) 桔梗 9g and **gua lou ren** (Semen Trichosanthis) 瓜蒌仁 12g.

Acupuncture
LI.20 (*ying xiang* +), Du.20 (*bai hui* +), Du.23 (*shang xing* +), *yin tang* ▲ (M-HN-3), *bi tong* (M-HN-14), LI.4 (*hegu* +), Bl.2 (*zan zhu* +), GB.20 (*feng chi* +), Sp.6 (*san yin jiao*), Bl.17 (*ge shu*)
- *yin tang* is treated with direct moxa or moxa cones over slices of raw ginger.

Patent medicines
Xue Fu Zhu Yu Wan 血府逐瘀丸 (Xue Fu Zhu Yu Wan)
Tong Jing Wan 痛经丸 (Tong Jing Wan)
Nei Xiao Luo Li Wan 内消瘰疬丸 (Nei Xiao Luo Li Wan)

Clinical notes
- Biomedical conditions that may present with Blood stagnation type sinus congestion include chronic sinusitis, chronic rhinitis and nasal polyps.
- This is generally a difficult condition to treat successfully, and requires persistence and prolonged treatment for a result.

SUMMARY OF GUIDING FORMULAE FOR SINUSITIS AND NASAL CONGESTION

Wind Cold - *Xin Yi San* 辛荑散

Lung Heat (Wind Heat) - *Cang Er Zi San* 苍耳子散

Liver *qi* stagnation with stagnant Heat - *Dan Zhi Xiao Yao San* 丹栀逍遥散
- Liver Fire - *Long Dan Xie Gan Tang* 龙胆泻肝汤

Damp Heat affecting the Spleen - *Dan Xi Bi Yuan Fang* 丹溪鼻渊方

Lung *qi* deficiency - *Wen Fei Zhi Liu Dan* 温肺止流丹

Spleen *qi* deficiency - *Bu Zhong Yi Qi Tang* 补中益气汤

Kidney deficiency
- *yin* deficiency - *Liu Wei Di Huang Wan* 六味地黄丸 + *Sheng Mai San* 生脉散
- *yang* deficiency - *You Gui Wan* 右归丸
- *jing* deficiency - *Bu Nao Wan* 补脑丸

Qi and Blood stagnation - *Dang Gui Shao Yao San* 当归芍药散

Endnote

For more information regarding herbs marked with an asterisk*, an open circle° or a hatˆ, see the tables on pp.944-952.

Disorders of the Lung

8. Rhinitis

Acute episode
Wind Cold

In between episodes
Lung *qi* deficiency
Lung and Spleen *qi* deficiency (with Phlegm)
Kidney deficiency

8 RHINITIS
bi qiu 鼻鼽

Rhinitis is a seasonal or perennial disorder characterised by episodes of nasal congestion, watery nasal discharge, sneezing and irritation of the conjunctiva throat, and ala nasi. It is due to hypersensitivity of the nasal mucosa to pollen, dust mites, fungal spores, animal dander and saliva, fumes and certain food substances.

When rhinitis occurs in response to allergens like grasses and pollens which have a limited seasonal distribution, it is refered to as seasonal allergic rhinitis, or hayfever. In between episodes of hayfever, patients are usually asymptomatic. The main features are frequent attacks of sneezing with profuse watery nasal discharge and obstruction. The attacks usually last a few hours and can be accompanied by sore watery eyes.

Perennial rhinitis can occur at any time of the year in response to exposure to a variety of mostly non-seasonal allergens, like animal dander, house dust, fungal spores and irritants like cold air, smoke and perfume. Perennial rhinitis may be intermittent or, in some cases, more or less continuous and in general the symptoms are less marked than those in seasonal allergic rhinitis. The main features of perennial rhinitis are low grade itching, irritation and congestion of the nose and eyes, with occasional exacerbations.

Patients with rhinitis usually have swollen nasal mucous membranes, which can prevent sinus drainage, predisposing them to secondary infection and the development of sinusitis (*bi yuan* 鼻淵 p.234). The symptom picture of sinusitis and rhinitis overlap somewhat, but sinusitis usually exhibits maxilliary and supraorbital pain, and less sneezing and itching.

AETIOLOGY

Rhinitis, whether seasonal or perennial, is usually an allergic condition. In TCM terms we relate this concept to deficiency of *wei qi*. The *wei* (or protective) *qi* has its basis in Kidney *yang* and is distributed by the Lungs to all the surfaces of the body. This includes the mucous membranes of the nose and throat. If the functioning of *wei qi* at these surfaces is inadequate, then inappropriate responses to inhaled particles and gases can result, and the area will become irritated and inflamed, provoking mucus production and sneezing.

Allergens

In a TCM context, the allergens which can trigger an episode of rhinitis are a form of external Wind. This Wind is able to invade the nose in the absence of an adequate defense by *wei qi*, and then remain there. The chronic itching and sneezing of rhinitis is due to the persistence of this external Wind in the mucous membranes of the nose. Uncharacteristically for Wind generally, this Wind can remain in the nose for months or years if *wei qi* is too weak to expel it.

Lung *qi* deficiency

Lung *qi* deficiency will be found in individuals who are constitutionally *qi* deficient, have a history of chronic Lung disease or who have damaged Lung *qi* with insufficient or excessive exercise. Lung *qi* is also weakened by excessive or unexpressed sadness and grief.

Those with weak Lung *qi* tend to have weak *wei qi* and will be vulnerable to invasion by, and retention of, external Wind.

Kidney deficiency

Kidney deficiency develops from chronic illness, ageing, overwork or is hereditary. When the Kidney weakness is constitutional, the symptoms of allergic disease often start in childhood. The role the Kidneys play in the aetiology of rhinitis is in the above mentioned role of being the foundation of all the body's *qi* (*zheng qi*) of which *wei qi* is one aspect. Sometimes the *wei qi* deficiency is the only sign of Kidney deficiency.

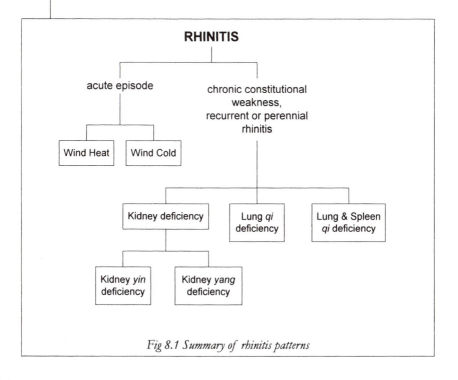

Fig 8.1 Summary of rhinitis patterns

Spleen deficiency

Spleen function is usually damaged by bad eating habits and a diet of cold and Phlegm producing foods. The weakened Spleen function means more Damp and Phlegm accumulation and the rhinitis of this pattern will tend to generate more mucus than the others. Rhinitis that is triggered by fumes and cigarette smoke can fall into this category–it is the nature of strong smells to not only disperse *qi* and irritate mucous membranes, but to also mobilise Phlegm Damp.

TREATMENT

There are two aspects to consider when treating rhinitis–treatment of the acute episodes, in which severe and debilitating symptoms need to be quickly controlled, and treatment between episodes. When symptoms are acute, herbal treatment may need to be administered twice or more per day and acupuncture at least daily. In all except the simple Wind Cold (Heat) category, the treatment should persist between episodes to build the constitution. This is especially important in the months before the hayfever season. Treatment of Lung, Kidney and Spleen type rhinitis can be achieved using the following guiding formula during and after acute episodes (with appropriate modification). Interestingly, in the Kidney deficient types of allergic rhinitis, there may be little in the way of the typical Kidney symptoms. Nevertheless the supposed Kidney *yang* deficiency (manifesting as *wei qi* deficiency) will always be addressed with the addition of a few Kidney *yang* tonic herbs[1]. See also p.151.

---

1. Maciocia G (1994) *The Practice of Chinese Medicine*, Churchill Livingstone, Edinburgh

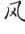

8.1 WIND COLD

Pathophysiology
- A Wind Cold invasion is the most common presentation of an acute episode of rhinitis. Wind Cold invades the nose, obstructs the the passage of normal Lung Fluids (*ti* 涕) and irritates the mucous membranes. The formulae presented here are not suitable for prolonged use as they will eventually aggravate any underlying deficiency, and ultimately make the problem worse. They should be reduced or withdrawn as symptoms improve and appropriate constitutional treatment phased in.

Clinical features
- acute sneezing, nasal itch, runny nose with copious, thin, watery mucus, or nasal obstruction
- reduction or loss of sense of smell
- itchy, irritated, watery eyes
- frontal or maxillary headache

T normal or with a thin white coat
P floating, or floating and tight

Treatment principle
Warm the Lungs and disperse Wind Cold
Warm and transform Phlegm Fluids, redirect Lung *qi* downward

Prescription

XIAO QING LONG TANG 小青龙汤
(*Minor Blue Dragon Combination*)

This prescription is suitable for acute episodes of allergic rhinitis or flareups of perennial rhinitis with copious watery mucus and sneezing.

ma huang* (Herba Ephedra) 麻黄 9g
gui zhi (Ramulus Cinnamomi Cassiae) 桂枝 9g
wu wei zi (Fructus Schizandrae Chinensis) 五味子 9g
bai shao (Radix Paeoniae Lactiflora) 白芍 9g
ban xia* (Rhizoma Pinelliae Ternatae) 半夏 9g
zhi gan cao (honey fried Radix Glycyrrhizae Uralensis)
   炙甘草 6g
gan jiang (Rhizoma Zingiberis Officinalis) 干姜 3g
xi xin* (Herba cum Radice Asari) 细辛 3g
Method: Decoction to be taken hot. (Source: *Shi Yong Zhong Yi Nei Ke Xue*)

Modifications
♦ With severe sneezing and itching nose, add **cang er zi*** (Fructus Xanthii Sibirici) 苍耳子 6g, **bai zhi** (Radix Angelicae Dahuricae) 白芷 9g and

xin yi hua (Flos Magnoliae) 辛夷花 6g.
- With sore, itchy, watery eyes, add **mi meng hua** (Flos Buddleiae Officinalis Immaturus) 蜜蒙花 9g.

Variations and additional prescriptions
- If Wind Cold transforms into Heat, or the initial pathogen is Wind Heat, causing sneezing, sore, itchy or scratchy throat, thirst, thick or coloured nasal discharge and very red, irritated eyes, the correct treatment is to expel Wind Heat with **SANG JU YIN** (*Morus and Chrysanthemum Formula* 桑菊饮) modified. This presentation occurs more in perennial rhinitis.

sang ye (Folium Mori Albae) 桑叶	12g
ju hua (Flos Chrysanthemi Morifolii) 菊花	9g
lu gen (Rhizoma Phragmitis Communis) 芦根	15g
cang er zi* (Fructus Xanthii Sibirici) 苍耳子	9g
bai zhi (Radix Angelicae Dahuricae) 白芷	9g
lian qiao (Fructus Forsythia Suspensae) 连翘	9g
chao xing ren* (dry fried Semen Pruni Armeniacae) 炒杏仁	9g
jie geng (Radix Platycodi Grandiflori) 桔梗	9g
bo he (Herba Mentha Haplocalycis) 薄荷	6g
xin yi hua (Flos Magnoliae) 辛夷花	6g
gan cao (Radix Glycyrrhizae Uralensis) 甘草	3g

    Method: Decoction. Do not cook for more than 20 minutes. **Bo he** is added near the end of cooking (*hou xia* 后下).

Patent medicines
Bi Min Gan Wan 鼻敏感丸 (Pe Min Kan Wan)
Xin Yi San 辛荑散 (Xin Yi San)
Bi Yan Pian 鼻炎片 (Bi Yen Pien)
 - with signs of Heat
Chuan Xiong Cha Tiao Wan 川芎茶调丸 (Chuan Xiong Cha Tiao Wan)
 - with headache

Acupuncture
Lu.7 (*lie que* -), LI.4 (*he gu* -), Bl.12 (*feng men* -Ω), Bl.13 (*fei shu* -Ω), LI.20 (*ying xiang*), Du.23 (*shang xing*), GB.20 (*feng chi* -), *yin tang* ▲ (M-HN-3)
- *yin tang* (M-HN-3) is treated with direct moxa or moxa on ginger (except in cases with Heat)
- with copious mucus, add SP.3 (*tai bai* -) and ST.40 (*feng long* -)
- with Heat, add Lu.10 (*yu ji* -) and LI.11 (*qu chi* -)

Clinical notes
- Biomedical conditions that may present as Wind Cold type rhinitis include acute episodes of hayfever and allergic rhinitis.
- This pattern generally responds well to correct treatment.

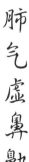

8.2 LUNG *QI* DEFICIENCY

Pathophysiology
- If weak *wei qi*, (which is a subtype of Lung *qi*) does not nourish and protect the lining of the respiratory tract, inhaled particles may cause inappropriate responses causing sneezing and congestion. The deficiency of Lung and *wei qi* predisposes to frequent invasion by Wind.

Clinical features
- transitory, recurrent episodes of paroxysmal sneezing, nasal itch, copious clear watery nasal discharge or congestion
- symptoms initiated or aggravated by exposure to wind and cold air
- reduction or loss of sense of smell
- frequent colds
- soft, low voice
- shortness of breath
- spontaneous sweating
- waxy pale complexion
- in atopic individuals there may be a history of (or concurrent) eczema or asthma

T pale with a thin white coat
P deficient and weak

Treatment principle
Warm and tonify the Lungs
Expel Wind

Prescription

YU PING FENG SAN 玉屏风散
(*Jade Screen Powder*) plus
CANG ER ZI SAN 苍耳子散
(*Xanthium Formula*)

huang qi (Radix Astragali Membranacei) 黄芪 15-30g
bai zhu (Rhizoma Atractylodis Macrocephalae) 白术 9g
fang feng (Radix Ledebouriellae Divaricatae) 防风 9g
cang er zi* (Fructus Xanthii Sibirici) 苍耳子 9g
bai zhi (Radix Angelicae Dahuricae) 白芷 9g
xin yi hua (Flos Magnoliae) 辛夷花 6g
bo he (Herba Mentha Haplocalycis) 薄荷 6g

Method: Decoction or powder. When powdered, the dose is 9-grams 1-2 times daily. When decocted **bo he** is added towards the end of cooking (*hou xia* 后下).
(Source: *Zhong Yi Er Bi Hou Ke Xue*)

Modifications

- Because of the assumed underlying Kidney deficiency (see modifications p.151) in atopic patients, two or three of the following herbs are generally added: **tu si zi** (Semen Cuscutae Chinensis) 菟丝子 12g, **du zhong** (Cortex Eucommiae Ulmoidis) 杜仲 12g, **hu tao ren** (Semen Juglandis Regiae) 胡桃仁 9g, **bu gu zhi** (Fructus Psoraleae Corylifoliae) 补骨脂 12g, **ba ji tian** (Radix Morindae Officinalis) 巴戟天 12g, **xu duan** (Radix Dipsaci Asperi) 续断 12g, **fu pen zi** (Fructus Rubi Chingii) 覆盆子 9g or **wu wei zi** (Fructus Schizandrae Chinensis) 五味子 6g. We also find that powerfully strengthening *wei qi* with large doses of **huang qi** (Radix Astragali Membranacei) 黄芪, is essential, regardless of the prescription. **Huang qi** (and any *yang* tonics) are quite warming, however, and in some cases may need to be balanced with cooling herbs when used for lengthy periods. **Huang qi** is contraindicated in patients with acute exterior patterns, as it can lock the pathogen in, and encourage its internal penetration.
- With severe congestion, add two or three of the following herbs: **xi xin*** (Herba cum Radice Asari) 细辛 3g, **gui zhi** (Ramulus Cinnamomi Cassiae) 桂枝 9g, **chuan jiao** (Pericarpium Zanthoxyli Bungeani) 川椒 3g or **mu xiang** (Radix Aucklandiae Lappae) 木香 6g
- With exhausting paroxysms of sneezing, add one or two of the following herbs: **chan tui^** (Periostracum Cicadae) 蝉蜕 9g, **quan xie*** (Buthus Martensi) 全蝎 1.5g, **she tui^** (Exuviae Serpentis) 蛇蜕 2g or **di long^** (Lumbricus) 地龙 9g
- With continuous, copious, watery nasal discharge, add one or two of the following herbs: **jin ying zi** (Fructus Rosae Laevigatae) 金樱子 9g, **fu xiao mai** (Semen Tritici Aestivi Levis) 浮小麦 12g or **nuo dao gen** (Radix et Rhizoma Oryzae Glutinosae) 糯稻根 15g

Variations and additional prescriptions

- One type of rhinitis is initiated or aggravated by certain foods or wine. This is thought to be due to stagnant Heat affecting the Lung and Large Intestine channels, with a background of Lung deficiency. The formula for this pattern is **XIN YI QING FEI YIN** (*Magnolia Flower Lung Clearing Decoction* 辛夷清肺饮).

    shi gao (Gypsum) 石膏 12-18g
    huang qin (Radix Scutellariae Baicalensis) 黄芩 9g
    shan zhi zi (Fructus Gardeniae Jasminoidis) 山栀子 9g
    zhi mu (Rhizoma Anemarrhenae Asphodeloides) 知母 9g
    sang bai pi (Cortex Mori Albae Radicis) 桑白皮 9g
    xin yi hua (Flos Magnoliae) 辛夷花 9g
    pi pa ye (Folium Eriobotryae Japonicae) 枇杷叶 9g
    bai he (Bulbus Lilii) 百合 9g

mai dong (Tuber Ophiopogonis Japonici) 麦冬 9g
sheng ma (Rhizoma Cimicifugae) 升麻 6g
Method: Decoction. (Source: *Zhong Yi Er Bi Hou Ke Xue*)

Patent medicines
Yu Ping Feng Wan 玉屏风丸 (Yu Ping Feng Wan)
Xiang Sha Liu Jun Zi Wan 香砂六君子丸 (Xiang Sha Liu Jun Wan))
Bu Zhong Yi Qi Wan 补中益气丸 (Bu Zhong Yi Qi Wan)
Shen Ling Bai Zhu Wan 参苓白术丸 (Shen Ling Bai Zhu Wan)
Shen Qi Da Bu Wan 参芪大补丸 (Shen Qi Da Bu Wan)
Bi Min Gan Wan 鼻敏感丸 (Bi Min Gan Wan)
 - combined with one of the five formulae above
Xin Yi San 辛夷散 (Xin Yi San)
 - combined with one of the five formulae above

Acupuncture
GB.20 (*feng chi* -), LI.20 (*ying xiang*), LI.19 (*he liao*), Bl.13 (*fei shu* +), Bl.20 (*pi shu* +), Lu.7 (*lie que*), Lu.9 (*tai yuan* +), St.36 (*zu san li* +), Bl.23 (*shen shu* +), Kid.6 (*zhao hai*), LI.4 (*he gu*)

- Moxibustion on the following points is very useful in chronic cases. Select 3 or 4 per treatment: *yin tang* (M-HN-3), Du.4 (*ming men*), Du.12 (*shen zhu*), Du.23 (*shang xing*), Ren.6 (*qi hai*), Ren.8 (*shen que*), Ren.12 (*zhong wan*), Sp.6 (*san yin jiao*), St.36 (*zu san li*). When treating *yin tang*, moxa cones over slices of ginger is particularly good.

Snuff
- In severe cases **BI YUN SAN** (*Blue Cloud Powder* 碧云散) can be sniffed into each nostril several times daily
    e bu shi cao (Herba Centipeda) 鹅不食草
    chuan xiong (Radix Ligustici Chuanxiong) 川芎
    xi xin* (Herba cum Radice Asari) 细辛
    xin yi hua (Flos Magnoliae) 辛夷花
    qing dai (Indigo Pulverata Levis) 青黛
    Method: Powder equal amounts of each herb and store in an airtight container until needed. (Source: *Zhong Yi Er Bi Hou Ke Xue*)

Paste
- A paste may be made of lanolin and powdered **e bu shi cao** (Herba Centipeda) 鹅不食草 and applied to the nasal mucosa
- powdered **gan jiang** (Rhizoma Zingiberis Officinalis) 干姜 can be mixed with honey and applied to the nasal mucosa

Nasal wash
- In all chronic cases, rinsing the nasal cavity and sinuses with warm salty water to dislodge mucus and tone the mucous membranes is useful (see p.236). Other useful rinses can be made with one of the following herbs: a few shallots (**cong bai** Bulbus Allii Fistulosi 葱白), **e bu shi cao** (Herba Centipeda) 鹅不食草 3g or **xin yi hua** (Flos Magnoliae) 辛夷花 3g

Clinical notes
- Biomedical conditions that may present as Lung *qi* deficiency type rhinitis include acute or chronic rhinitis.
- Can take a while to respond and often needs prolonged treatment for satisfactory results.

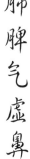

8.3 LUNG AND SPLEEN *QI* DEFICIENCY (WITH PHLEGM)

Pathophysiology
- Lung and Spleen *qi* deficiency with Phlegm is a common pattern occurring frequently in children (although it also occurs in adults) and in Western society is often due to excessive consumption of dairy products and sugar. The main feature here is the quantity and persistence of mucus.

Clinical features
- recurrent episodes of relatively severe nasal congestion or persistent runny nose with thin watery or sticky white mucus
- nasal mucosa swollen and pale or ashen; patients with this pattern often have nasal polyps and children may have upturned noses from frequent wiping upwards with the palm of the hand
- nasal itch, sneezing
- reduction or loss of sense of smell
- fullness and heaviness in the head, woolly headedness
- fatigue, listlessness
- aversion to cold
- tired limbs
- poor appetite, picky eater
- loose stools or diarrhoea

T pale or pale and swollen with tooth marks and a white coat
P soft and weak

Treatment principle
Strengthen the Spleen and tonify *qi*
Tonify the Lungs to consolidate *qi*

Prescription

LIU JUN ZI TANG 六君子汤
(*Six Major Herbs Combination*) modified

This formula can be used for acute exacerbations of a chronic Spleen deficiency (with Phlegm Damp) pattern, and in between episodes. It is suitable for prolonged use.

ren shen (Panax Ginseng) 人参	9g
bai zhu (Rhizoma Atractylodis Macrocephalae) 白术	9g
fu ling (Sclerotium Poria Cocos) 茯苓	9g
gan cao (Radix Glycyrrhizae Uralensis) 甘草	3g
ban xia* (Rhizoma Pinelliae Ternatae) 半夏	9g
chen pi (Pericarpium Citri Reticulatae) 陈皮	6g
huang qi (Radix Astragali Membranacei) 黄芪	15-30g

he zi (Fructus Terminaliae Chebulae) 诃子 9g
xin yi hua (Flos Magnoliae) 辛夷花 9g
wu wei zi (Fructus Schizandrae Chinensis) 五味子 6g
shi chang pu (Rhizoma Acori Graminei) 石菖蒲 6g
Method: Decoction. (Source: *Zhong Yi Er Bi Hou Ke Xue*)

Modifications

- To address the atopy (see modifications p.151), add two or three of the following herbs: **tu si zi** (Semen Cuscutae Chinensis) 菟丝子 12g, **du zhong** (Cortex Eucommiae Ulmoidis) 杜仲 12g, **hu tao ren** (Semen Juglandis Regiae) 胡桃仁 9g, **bu gu zhi** (Fructus Psoraleae Corylifoliae) 补骨脂 12g, **ba ji tian** (Radix Morindae Officinalis) 巴戟天 12g, **xu duan** (Radix Dipsaci Asperi) 续断 12g, **fu pen zi** (Fructus Rubi Chingii) 覆盆子 9g or **wu wei zi** (Fructus Schizandrae Chinensis) 五味子 6g. We also find that powerfully strengthening *wei qi* with large doses of **huang qi** (Radix Astragali Membranacei) 黄芪 is very useful (see modifications p.269)

- With severe congestion, add two or three of the following herbs: **xi xin*** (Herba cum Radice Asari) 细辛 3g, **gui zhi** (Ramulus Cinnamomi Cassiae) 桂枝 9g, **chuan jiao** (Pericarpium Zanthoxyli Bungeani) 川椒 3g, **mu xiang** (Radix Aucklandiae Lappae) 木香 6g or **cang er zi*** (Fructus Xanthii Sibirici) 苍耳子 6g.

- With frontal headache, add **bai zhi** (Radix Angelicae Dahuricae) 白芷 9g.

- With exhausting paroxysms of sneezing, add one or two of the following herbs: **chan tui**^ (Periostracum Cicadae) 蝉蜕 9g, **quan xie*** (Buthus Martensi) 全蝎 1.5g, **she tui**^ (Exuviae Serpentis) 蛇蜕 2g or **di long**^ (Lumbricus) 地龙 9g.

- With continuous, copious, watery nasal discharge, add one or two of the following herbs: **jin ying zi** (Fructus Rosae Laevigatae) 金樱子 9g, **fu xiao mai** (Semen Tritici Aestivi Levis) 浮小麦 12g or **nuo dao gen** (Radix et Rhizoma Oryzae Glutinosae) 糯稻根 15g.

- Once the mucus clears, the principle of treatment should tend more towards tonification. Delete the dispersing, Phlegm cutting herbs (**ban xia, xin yi hua** etc.) as the patient's condition improves, so as not to disperse *qi*.

Variations and additional prescriptions

In children

- In children with perennial rhinitis the formula of choice is **SHEN LING BAI ZHU SAN** (*Ginseng and Atractylodes Formula* 参苓白术散 modified, p.253).

Patent medicines
Xiang Sha Liu Jun Zi Wan 香砂六君子丸 (Xiang Sha Liu Jun Wan)
  - with Phlegm
Bu Zhong Yi Qi Wan 补中益气丸 (Bu Zhong Yi Qi Wan)
Shen Ling Bai Zhu Wan 参苓白术丸 (Shen Ling Bai Zhu Wan)
Shen Qi Da Bu Wan 参芪大补丸 (Shen Qi Da Bu Wan)
Bi Min Gan Wan 鼻敏感丸 (Bi Min Gan Wan)
  - combined with one of the four formulae above
Xin Yi San 辛荑散 (Xin Yi San)
  - combined with one of the four formulae above

Acupuncture
St.40 *(feng long -)*, Sp.3 *(tai bai)*, St.36 *(zu san li +)*, Lu.7 *(lie que)*, Bl.20 *(pi shu +)*, Bl.13 *(fei shu +)*, GB.20 *(feng chi -)*, LI.20 *(ying xiang)*, LI.19 *(he liao)*, Du.23 *(shang xing)*, LI.4 *(he gu)*
- in atopic patients add Bl.23 *(shen shu +)*, Du.4 *(ming men* ▲*)* or Ren.4 *(guan yuan +)*
- Moxibustion on the following points is very useful in chronic cases. Select 3 or 4 per treatment: *yin tang* (M-HN-3), Ren.6 *(qi hai)*, Du.12 *(shen zhu)*, Du.23 *(shang xing)*, Ren.8 *(shen que)*, Ren.12 *(zhong wan)*, Sp.6 *(san yin jiao)*, St.36 *(zu san li)*, Bl.23 *(shen shu)*, Du.4 *(ming men)*, Ren.4 *(guan yuan)*. When treating *yin tang*, moxa cones over slices of ginger are particularly good.

Nasal wash
♦ see p.271

Clinical notes
- Biomedical conditions that may present as Lung and Spleen *qi* deficiency type rhinitis include chronic rhinitis and nasal polyps.
- This is a common pattern in children. It generally responds well to treatment, although dietary change is essential for long term resolution.

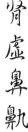

8.4 KIDNEY DEFICIENCY

Pathophysiology
- Kidney deficiency is a very chronic pattern, often present from childhood, and frequently ecountered in atopic patients who may also be subject to asthma and eczema. It may also evolve from one of the previous patterns. Depending on constitutional and environmental factors, it may tend to *yin* or *yang* deficiency, with *yang* deficiency being clinically more common.

Clinical features
- many years of perennial nasal itch, congestion, sneezing, watery nasal discharge, all of which are worse in the morning and evening, after sex or when fatigued
- reduction or loss of sense of smell
- nasal mucosa pale, wet and oedematous
- There may be no accompanying symptoms of Kidney deficiency if deficient *wei qi* is its only manifestation. In other cases Kidney symptoms are obvious and the manifestations will vary depending on the type of deficiency, that is, *yang*, *qi* or *yin* deficiency.

Kidney *yang* deficiency
- cold intolerance, symptoms worse after exposure to cold, weak sore lower back, low libido, impotence, nocturia and frequent urination or oedema and scanty urine, lethargy, pallor, swollen pale tongue and a deep, thready, weak pulse

Kidney *yin* deficiency
- dizziness and tinnitus, forgetfulness, insomnia, heat in the palms and soles ('five hearts hot'), facial flushing, night sweats, a red dry tongue with little or no coat and a thready, rapid pulse

Kidney *qi* or *jing* deficiency
- If tending to neither *yin* or *yang* deficiency, that is, with no obvious Hot or Cold signs, the symptoms reflect general Kidney weakness–sore low back and knees, nocturia, low libido, weak proximal positions on the pulse. If the deficiency is at the level of *jing*, there may be additional symptoms of forgetfulness, poor memory, greying, lifeless or falling hair.

Treatment principle
Tonify and support Kidney *yang* (or *yin*)

Prescriptions
8.3.1 Kidney *yang* deficiency

JIN KUI SHEN QI WAN 金匮肾气丸
(*Rehmannia Eight Formula*) modified

In addition to addressing rhinitis with Kidney *yang* deficiency symptoms, this formula can be used to treat asymptomatic patients prior to the pollen season if they exhibit signs of Cold, or at least no signs of Heat.

shu di (Radix Rehmanniae Glutinosae Conquitae) 熟地	240g
huang qi (Radix Astragali Membranacei) 黄芪	180g
shan yao (Radix Dioscoreae Oppositae) 山药	120g
shan zhu yu (Fructus Corni Officinalis) 山茱萸	120g
fu ling (Sclerotium Poria Cocos) 茯苓	90g
ze xie (Rhizoma Alismatis Orientalis) 泽泻	90g
mu dan pi (Cortex Moutan Radicis) 牡丹皮	90g
wu wei zi (Fructus Schizandrae Chinensis) 五味子	60g
zhi fu zi* (Radix Aconiti Carmichaeli Praeparata) 制附子	60g
rou gui (Cortex Cinnamomi Cassiae) 肉桂	40g

Method: Grind the herbs to powder and form into 9-gram pills with honey. The dose is 2-3 pills daily. May also be decocted with a 90% reduction in dosage. When decocted **zhi fu zi** is cooked for 30 minutes before the other herbs (*xian jian* 先煎). (Source: *Shi Yong Zhong Yi Nei Ke Xue*)

WEN FEI ZHI LIU DAN 温肺止流丹
(*Warm the Lungs, Stop the Flow Special Pill*) modified

This formula is recommended when there is some ongoing congestion, or perennial rhinitis of a *yang* deficiency type. It may also be selected to treat asymptomatic atopic patients prior to the pollen season, provided there are no signs of Heat.

huang qi (Radix Astragali Membranacei) 黄芪	180g
rou cong rong (Herba Cistanches Deserticolae) 肉苁蓉	150g
hu tao ren (Semen Juglandis Regiae) 胡桃仁	120g
jing jie (Herba seu Flos Schizonepetae Tenuifolia) 荆芥	120g
he zi (Fructus Terminaliae Chebulae) 诃子	90g
ren shen (Panax Ginseng) 人参	90g
jie geng (Radix Platycodi Grandiflori) 桔梗	90g
fu pen zi (Fructus Rubi Chingii) 覆盆子	90g
jin ying zi (Fructus Rosae Laevigatae) 金樱子	90g
xi xin* (Herba cum Radice Asari) 细辛	60g
yu nao shi^ (Pseudosciaenae Otolithum) 鱼脑石	60g
wu wei zi (Fructus Schizandrae Chinensis) 五味子	60g
ge jie^ (Gecko) 蛤蚧	60g
gan cao (Radix Glycyrrhizae Uralensis) 甘草	30g

Method: Grind herbs to powder and form into 9-gram pills with honey. The dose is one pill 2-3 times daily. May also be decocted with a 90% reduction in dosage. (Source: *Zhong Yi Er Bi Hou Ke Xue*)

8.3.2 Kidney *yin* deficiency

ZUO GUI WAN 左归丸
(*Achyranthes and Rehmannia Formula*)

This formula is used for chronic rhinitis in a patient with Kidney *yin* deficiency and Heat signs. It may also be selected to treat asymptomatic patients with a tendency to *yin* deficiency prior to the pollen season.

shu di (Radix Rehmanniae Glutinosae Conquitae) 熟地 240g
shan yao (Radix Dioscoreae Oppositae) 山药 120g
shan zhu yu (Fructus Corni Officinalis) 山茱萸 120g
gou qi zi (Fructus Lycii) 枸杞子 120g
tu si zi (Semen Cuscutae Chinensis) 菟丝子 120g
gui ban jiao° (Plastri Testudinis Gelatinum) 龟板胶 120g
lu jiao jiao^ (Cornu Cervi Gelatinum) 鹿角胶 120g
huai niu xi (Radix Achyranthis Bidentatae) 怀牛膝 90g

Method: Grind herbs to powder and form into 9-gram pills with honey. The dose is one pill 2-3 times daily. May also be decocted with a 90% reduction in dosage. In decoction, **lu jiao jiao** and **gui ban jiao** are melted in the strained decoction (*yang hua* 烊化). (Source: *Zhong Yi Er Bi Hou Ke Xue*)

Patent medicines
Kidney *yang* (*qi*) deficiency

Any of these may be selected (in the absence of Heat) for asymptomatic atopic patients

Jin Kui Shen Qi Wan 金匮肾气丸 (Sexoton Pills)
You Gui Wan 右归丸 (You Gui Wan)
Ba Ji Yin Yang Wan 巴戟阴阳丸 (Ba Ji Yin Yang Wan)
Ning Xin Bu Shen Wan 宁心补肾丸 (San Yuen Medical Pills)
Zhuang Yao Jian Shen Pian 壮腰健肾片 (Zhuang Yao Jian Shen)

Kidney *yin* deficiency

Liu Wei Di Huang Wan 六味地黄丸 (Liu Wei Di Huang Wan)
Zhi Bai Ba Wei Wan 知柏八味丸 (Zhi Bai Ba Wei Wan)
Bu Nao Wan 补脑丸 (Cerebral Tonic Pills)
Chong Cao Ji Jing 虫草鸡精 (Cordyceps Essence of Chicken)

Acupuncture

Bl.23 (*shen shu* +), Du.4 (*ming men* +), Ren.4 (*guan yuan* +), Ren.6 (*qi hai* +), GB.39 (*xuan zhong* +), Du.20 (*bai hui*), Bl.15 (*xin shu*), Lu.7 (*lie que*), Kid.6 (*zhao hai*), Lu.9 (*tai yuan*), *yin tang* (M-HN-3), *bi tong* (M-HN-14)

- Use moxa in *jing* and *yang* deficiency.

Clinical notes
- Biomedical conditions that may present as Kidney deficiency type rhinitis include chronic atopic or perennial rhinitis.
- Generally takes prolonged treatment (more than 1 year) to achieve satisfactory results.

SUMMARY OF GUIDING FORMULAE FOR RHINITIS

Acute patterns
Wind Cold - *Xiao Qing Long Tang* 小青龙汤
- with Heat - *Sang Ju Yin* 桑菊饮

Chronic or recurrent patterns
Lung *qi* deficiency
- *Yu Ping Feng San* 玉屏风散 + *Cang Er Zi San* 苍耳子散
- Initiated by food or drink - *Xin Yi Qing Fei Yin* 辛夷清肺饮

Lung and Spleen *qi* deficiency - *Liu Jun Zi Tang* 六君子汤

Kidney deficiency
- *Yang* (*qi*) deficiency (or when asymptomatic but with no Heat signs) - *Jin Kui Shen Qi Wan* 金匮肾气丸 or *Wen Fei Zhi Liu Dan* 温肺止流丹
- *Yin* deficiency - *Zuo Gui Wan* 左归丸

Endnote

For more information regarding herbs marked with an asterisk*, an open circle° or a hatˆ, see the tables on pp.944-952.

Disorders of the Lung

9. Sore Throat

Acute patterns
Wind Heat
Lung and Stomach Heat

Chronic patterns
Lung and Kidney *yin* deficiency
Spleen *qi* deficiency

Appendix – Throat abscess

9 SORE THROAT
hou bi 喉痹

This chapter deals with the analysis and treatment of sore throat, regardless of the disease defined by Western medicine. The sore throats most often seen in the clinic are those associated with colds and flu, tonsillitis or pharyngitis. The term *hou bi* (literally 'throat obstruction') is a general expression for throat disorders characterised by swelling and pain.

In the language of Chinese medicine, acute tonsillitis is described as 'milk moth' (*ru e* 乳蛾), a term which relates to the appearance of the tonsils when inflamed, swollen and suppurative.

AETIOLOGY

In Chinese medicine terms the most important cause of sore throat is Heat. The Heat may be excess, in which case the sore throat is acute and usually intense, or the Heat may be deficient in which case the sore throat is more chronic and recurrent. In severe cases, Toxins can be generated by the focal intensity of the Heat, causing local destruction of tissues and the development of pus. Toxins may also give rise to significant systemic symptoms—fever, anorexia and malaise (see also Throat Abscess, p.301).

Wind Heat (& Damp)

Wind Heat is the most common cause of acute sore throat. Wind Heat invades through the mouth and lodges in the throat inflaming the local tissues. This causes redness, swelling and pain of the throat and/or tonsils. If the Heat is intense enough, Toxins may be generated giving rise to suppuration, which can be observed on the tonsils or the rear of the throat.

Wind Heat can combine with Dampness as well, producing a slightly different picture. Unlike Wind Heat, the presence of the Damp prevents full expression of the Heat, and the disorder may develop slowly. The Dampness complicates and prolongs the Heat elements and tends to linger once the Heat has dissipated. The Damp can also lead to various swellings (glands, liver, spleen etc.). Unlike straight Wind Heat, this pattern may be associated with quite prolonged illness and may become latent, reappearing when the patient is run down or under stress.

Lung and Stomach Heat

Smoking is the most common cause of internal Lung Heat. Similarly, Stomach Heat can be generated by overconsumption of spicy, rich foods or alcohol. Prolonged Liver *qi* stagnation that gives rise to Heat will also have the effect of producing Stomach Heat via the controlling (*ke* 克, p.70) cycle.

Such Heat can smoulder at a low level, damaging the tissues of the upper respiratory and digestive tract, and thus causing low grade inflammation of the throat. Prolonged Heat retained in the throat, can suddenly flare into a particularly severe and suppurative sore throat, if provoked by an invasion of Wind.

Deficient Heat

Sore throat due to *yin* deficient Heat is chronic and recurrent, and usually milder than the acute types. The deficient Heat that causes sore throats is the result of Lung and Kidney *yin* deficiency. Lung *yin* is easily damaged in those who smoke or live in very dry environments, who use bronchodilating medication or in those with recurrent or severe Lung disease of a Hot nature. A hot and spicy diet may also contribute by continually heating the Stomach, damaging the *yin* Fluids of the Stomach and Lung.

Kidney *yin* is consumed by overwork, ageing, excessive sexual activity or drug use, or after febrile diseases. Frequent episodes of acute sore throat from Wind Heat or Lung and Stomach Heat will eventually develop into the chronic type as Lung *yin* is repeatedly damaged.

> **BOX 9.1 SOME BIOMEDICAL CAUSES OF SORE THROAT**
>
> - acute infection (bacterial or viral laryngitis, tonsillitis), quinsy, pharyngeal abscess, diptheria, gonococcus, syphilis, hepatitis, measles, chicken pox, epiglottitis, oral herpes simplex)
> - glandular fever
> - oral thrush
> - HIV
> - foreign body
> - postnasal drip from chronic sinus congestion
> - apthous ulcers
> - leukaemia
> - agranulocytosis
> - angina, myocardial infarction
> - tobacco smoke
> - antiseptic lozenges
> - reflux oesophagitis
> - mouth breathing
> - carcinoma of the oropharynx
> - trauma from overuse or burns from hot food

Spleen deficiency (with lingering pathogens)

This pattern is mostly due to overuse of antibiotic drugs in the treatment of repeated sore throats or other upper respiratory tract infections. The cooling nature of the drugs clears Heat, but not any of the associated pathogens. Antibiotics also damage the Spleen, predisposing to more Damp accumulation, setting the stage for recurrent infections.

> **BOX 9.2 KEY DIAGNOSTIC POINTS**
>
> **Appearance of the throat**
> - red and swollen - Wind Heat
> - red, swollen with pus - Lung and Stomach Heat, Wind Heat with local Toxic Heat
> - not red or pale red - *yin* deficiency or *qi* deficiency
>
> **Aggravation**
> - with fatigue - *yin* deficiency
> - with spicy food - any Heat pattern, particularly *yin* deficiency
>
> **Amelioration**
> - with rest - *yin* deficiency
>
> **Frequency**
> - continuous pain (during an episode) - Wind Heat, Lung and Stomach Heat, Toxic Heat
> - worse in the morning - *qi* deficiency
> - worse in the evening - *yin* deficiency

9. SORE THROAT

风热喉痹

9.1 WIND HEAT

Pathophysiology
- Wind Heat is the most frequent type of acute sore throat, and is the most commonly identified TCM pathogen (especially at an early stage) in viral infections (like colds and flu) and bacterial infections (such as tonsillitis and pharyngitis).

Clinical features
- acute sore throat, worse with swallowing and coughing
- the throat and tonsils are (perhaps only slightly) swollen and red, and there may or may not be a white or yellow exudate on their surfaces
- swollen cervical lymph nodes
- fever and chills, with fever predominant
- headache
- nasal obstruction
- fatigue, poor appetite, malaise
- productive cough

T red tip with a thin white or slightly yellow coat
P floating and rapid

Treatment principle
Expel Wind and Heat
Eliminate Toxins and benefit the throat

Prescription

SHU FENG QING RE TANG 疏风清热汤
(Dispel Wind, Clear Heat Decoction)

jin yin hua (Flos Lonicerae Japonicae) 金银花	30g
lian qiao (Fructus Forsythia Suspensae) 连翘	15g
tian hua fen (Radix Trichosanthes Kirilowii) 天花粉	15g
xuan shen (Radix Scrophulariae Ningpoensis) 玄参	15g
huang qin (Radix Scutellariae Baicalensis) 黄芩	12g
sang bai pi (Cortex Mori Albae Radicis) 桑白皮	12g
jie geng (Radix Platycodi Grandiflori) 桔梗	12g
chi shao (Radix Paeoniae Rubrae) 赤芍	10g
jing jie (Herba seu Flos Schizonepetae Tenuifolia) 荆芥	10g
fang feng (Radix Ledebouriellae Divaricatae) 防风	10g
zhe bei mu (Bulbus Fritillariae Thunbergii) 浙贝母	10g
niu bang zi (Fructus Arctii Lappae) 牛蒡子	10g
gan cao (Radix Glycyrrhizae Uralensis) 甘草	10g

Method: Decoction. (Source: *Zhong Yi Nei Ke Lin Chuang Shou Ce*)

Variations and additional prescriptions

With Damp Heat
* When combined with Dampness, the symptom picture more closely resembles a Warm Disease (*wen bing*). The patient has a sore throat, fever, lethargy and malaise, loss of appetite, generalised lymphadenopathy, nausea, headaches and a red tongue with a thick coat. The treatment is to clear Damp Heat, ease the throat and eliminate Toxin. When the Heat elements are prominent (fever, sore throat), the primary prescription is suitable. When the Damp elements are prominent (nausea, loss of appetite, lassitude and malaise), consider **LIAN PO YIN** (*Coptis and Magnolia Bark Decoction* 连朴饮, p.14) with the addition of Toxic Heat clearing herbs like **bai hua she she cao** (Herbs Oldenlandia Diffusa) 白花蛇舌草 30g, **ban lan gen** (Radix Isatidis seu Baphicacanthi) 板蓝根 15g or **da qing ye** (Folium Daqingye) 大青叶 20g.

With Wind Cold
* Occasionally, sore throat may occur as part of a Wind Cold pattern. Although the pain associated with Wind Cold is generally mild, it may be severe in some cases. The treatment is to disperse Wind Cold with **JING FANG BAI DU SAN** (*Schizonepeta and Ledebouriella Powder to Overcome Pathogenic Influences* 荆防败毒散, p.6).

Patent medicines

Yin Qiao Jie Du Pian 银翘解毒片 (Yin Chiao Chieh Tu Pien)
Niu Huang Jie Du Pian 牛黄解毒片 (Peking Niu Huang Chieh Tu Pien)
    - commonly used for early stage febrile disorder with sore throat, mouth ulcers, conjunctivitis, otitis and suppurative skin infections
Ban Lan Gen Chong Ji 板蓝根冲剂 (Ban Lan Gen Chong Ji)
Chuan Xin Lian Kang Yan Pian 穿心莲抗炎片
    (Chuan Xin Lian Antiphlogistic Tablets)
Shuang Liao Hou Feng San 双料喉风散 (Superior Sore Throat Powder)
    - for topical use
Xi Gua Shuang 西瓜霜 (Watermelon Frost)
    - for topical use

Acupuncture

LI.4 (*he gu* -), St.44 (*nei ting* -), LI.11 (*qu chi* -), Lu.10 (*yu ji* -), Lu.11 (*shao shang* ↓), Ren.22 (*tian tu*), Lu.7 (*lie que*), LI.18 (*fu tu* -)
Ear points: throat, tonsils ↓

Powders

* The powders described here are finely ground herbs that are blown

directly onto the tonsils or throat with a straw or other appropriate implement. They are useful in severe cases that develop swiftly. Both the following powders are available in prepared form. In milder cases **BING PENG SAN** (*Borneol and Borax Powder* 冰硼散) is appropriate.

    bing pian (Borneol) 冰片 1.5g
    zhu sha* (Cinnabaris) 朱砂 1.8g
    xuan ming fen (Mirabilitum Purum) 玄明粉 15g
    peng sha (Borax) 硼砂 15g
    Method: Grind herbs to a powder. Blow a small amount onto affected area 2-3 times daily. Also useful for mouth ulcers. (Source: *Zhong Yi Er Bi Hou Ke Xue*)

- In serious cases with severe pain and ulceration **ZHU HUANG SAN** (*Mother of Pearl and Cow Gallstone Powder* 珠黄散) is selected.
    ma bo (Fructificatio Lasiosphaerae seu Calvatiae) 马勃 15g
    qing dai (Indigo Pulverata Levis) 青黛 3g
    hai er cha (Pasta Acaciae seu Uncariae) 孩儿茶 3g
    peng sha (Borax) 硼砂 3g
    huang lian (Rhizoma Coptidis) 黄连 1.5g
    xuan ming fen (Mirabilitum Purum) 玄明粉 1.5g
    bo he (Herba Mentha Haplocalycis) 薄荷 1.5g
    niu huang^ (Calculus Bovis) 牛黄 1g
    wu mei (Fructus Pruni Mume) 乌梅 1g
    zhen zhu^ (Margarita) 珍珠 1g
    Method: Grind herbs to a powder. Blow a small amount onto affected area 2-3 times daily. Also useful for mouth ulcers. (Source: *Zhong Yi Er Bi Hou Ke Xue*)

Gargles

- Decoct equal portions of **jin yin hua** (Flos Lonicerae Japonicae) 金银花, **jie geng** (Radix Platycodi Grandiflori) 桔梗 and **lian qiao** (Fructus Forsythia Suspensae) 连翘, and gargle several times daily.

Lozenges

- Lozenges are boluses of powdered herbs, which are held in the mouth and sucked slowly, releasing the ingredients over the tonsils. They are useful for patients prone to sore throat to carry while travelling etc. Formulae include **TIE DI WAN** (*Iron Whistle Pill* 铁笛丸).
    jie geng (Radix Platycodi Grandiflori) 桔梗 60g
    zhe bei mu (Bulbus Fritillariae Thunbergii) 浙贝母 60g
    mai dong (Tuber Ophiopogonis Japonici) 麦冬 30g
    xuan shen (Radix Scrophulariae Ningpoensis) 玄参 30g
    gan cao (Radix Glycyrrhizae Uralensis) 甘草 60g
    he zi (Fructus Terminaliae Chebulae) 诃子 30g
    gua lou pi (Pericarpium Trichosanthis) 瓜蒌皮 30g

fu ling (Sclerotium Poria Cocos) 茯苓 30g
qing guo (Fructus Canariae Album) 青果 12g
Method: Grind herbs to a powder and form into 3-gram pills with honey.
(Source: *Zhong Yi Er Bi Hou Ke Xue*)

RUN HOU WAN (*Moisten the Throat Pill* 润喉丸)
gan cao (Radix Glycyrrhizae Uralensis) 甘草 300g
wu mei (Fructus Pruni Mume) 乌梅 750g
peng sha (Borax) 硼砂 15g
shi yan (salt) 食盐 15g
xuan ming fen (Mirabilitum Purum) 玄明粉 30g
Method: Grind herbs to a powder and form into 3-gram pills with water chestnut powder and honey. (Source: *Zhong Yi Er Bi Hou Ke Xue*)

Clinical notes

- Biomedical conditions that may present as Wind Heat type sore throat include tonsillitis, pharyngitis, influenza, common cold, epiglottitis, glandular fever and scarlet fever
- Unresolved or resistant cases may go on to develop abscesses of the throat, thus the timing of treatment is important - the earlier the intervention the better and faster the result.
- This pattern generally responds well to correct and timely treatment.

Table 9.1 Differentiation of Wind Heat and acute Lung and Stomach Heat

	Wind Heat	Acute Lung and Stomach Heat
Throat and tonsils	red and swollen with or without suppuration	very red and swollen with obvious suppuration
General features	sore throat, fever, chills, cough	severe sore throat, high fever, thirst, constipation
Tongue	normal or red tipped, thin white or yellow coat	red with a thick yellow coat
Pulse	floating, rapid	flooding, big, slippery, rapid

肺胃热盛喉痹

9.2 LUNG AND STOMACH HEAT (TOXIC HEAT)

Pathophysiology
- Wind Heat (or Cold that transforms into Heat) is usually the trigger that provokes latent Lung and Stomach Heat to flare in the throat. The main characteristic of this pattern is the severity of the pain and swelling, the clear development of Toxic Heat (in the form of pus) and the systemic symptoms.

Clinical features
- Acute sore throat. The pain is usually severe, and radiates to the lower jaw or ears. On examination the throat or tonsils are swollen and red with a white or yellow exudate on their surfaces. In severe cases, swelling significantly narrows the throat causing difficulty swallowing.
- swollen tender cervical lymph nodes
- high fever
- thirst
- constipation
- scanty concentrated urine
- bad breath
- abdominal distension
- hoarse voice
- cough with thick yellow sputum

T deep red, with a thick greasy yellow coat
P flooding, big and rapid

Treatment principle
Clear and drain Toxic Heat
Reduce swelling and benefit the throat

Prescription

PU JI XIAO DU YIN 普济消毒饮
(*Universal Benefit Decoction to Eliminate the Toxins*) modified

ban lan gen (Radix Isatidis seu Baphicacanthi) 板蓝根	30g
lian qiao (Fructus Forsythia Suspensae) 连翘	20g
xuan shen (Radix Scrophulariae Ningpoensis) 玄参	20g
jiu huang qin (wine fried Radix Scutellariae Baicalensis) 酒黄芩	15g
huang lian (Rhizoma Coptidis) 黄连	15g
jiang can^ (Bombyx Batryticatus) 僵蚕	10g
ma bo (Fructificatio Lasiosphaerae seu Calvatiae) 马勃	10g
niu bang zi (Fructus Arctii Lappae) 牛蒡子	10g

chi shao (Radix Paeoniae Rubrae) 赤芍 10g
chen pi (Pericarpium Citri Reticulatae) 陈皮 6g
jie geng (Radix Platycodi Grandiflori) 桔梗 6g
bo he (Herba Mentha Haplocalycis) 薄荷 6g
gan cao (Radix Glycyrrhizae Uralensis) 甘草 3g

Method: Decoction. **Bo he** is added just before the end of cooking (*hou xia* 后下), **ma bo** is usually cooked in a muslin bag (*bao jian* 包煎). (Source: *Zhong Yi Nei Ke Lin Chuang Shou Ce*)

Modifications

- With very high, persistent fever, add **shi gao** (Gypsum) 石膏 30g, **tian zhu huang** (Concretio Silicea Bambusae Textillis) 天竺黄 10g and **jin yin hua** (Flos Lonicerae Japonicae) 金银花 30g.
- With severe thirst, add **tian hua fen** (Radix Trichosanthes Kirilowii) 天花粉 15g and **mai dong** (Tuber Ophiopogonis Japonici) 麦冬 10g.
- If there is a cough with copious sticky Phlegm, add **quan gua lou** (Fructus Trichosanthis) 全栝楼 15g, **she gan** (Rhizoma Belamacandae) 射干 15g and **zhe bei mu** (Bulbus Fritillariae Thunbergii) 浙贝母 10g.
- With constipation, add **da huang** (Radix et Rhizoma Rhei) 大黄 6-9g and **mang xiao** (Mirabilitum) 芒硝 6g.
- With dizziness, blurred vision and red, sore eyes, add **sang ye** (Folium Mori Albae) 桑叶 10g, **ju hua** (Flos Chrysanthemi Morifolii) 菊花 15g and **xia ku cao** (Spica Prunellae Vulgaris) 夏枯草 15g.
- If the urine is concentrated and scanty, add **zhu ye** (Herba Lophatheri Gracilis) 竹叶 6g and **lu gen** (Rhizoma Phragmitis Communis) 芦根 30g.

Patent medicines

Niu Huang Jie Du Pian 牛黄解毒片 (Peking Niu Huang Chieh Tu Pien)
  - commonly used for early stage febrile disorder with sore throat, mouth ulcers, conjunctivitis, otitis and suppurative skin infections

Chuan Xin Lian Kang Yan Pian 穿心莲抗炎片
  (Chuan Xin Lian Antiphlogistic Tablets)

Niu Huang Qing Huo Wan 牛黄清火丸 (Niu Huang Qing Huo Wan)
  - severe cases

Da Bai Du Jiao Nang 大败毒胶囊 (DBD Capsule)
  - severe cases

Shuang Liao Hou Feng San 双料喉风散 (Superior Sore Throat Powder)
  - for topical use

Xi Gua Shuang 西瓜霜 (Watermelon Frost)
  - for topical use

Acupuncture
L.I.4 (*he gu* -), St.44 (*nei ting* -), L.I.11 (*qu chi* -), S.J.5 (*wai guan* -), Lu.11 (*shao shang* ↓), Ren.22 (*tian tu*), Lu.7 (*lie que*), Lu.10 (*yu ji* -), S.I.17 (*tian rong* -), L.I.18 (*fu tu* -)
Ear points: throat, tonsils ↓
- Treatment needs to be quite frequent in this pattern–1-2 strong treatments daily may be necessary.

Topical treatment
- The same powders, gargles and lozenges that are used for Wind Heat, p.286-288 can be used for Lung and Stomach Heat.

Clinical notes
- Biomedical conditions that may present as Lung and Stomach or Toxic Heat type sore throat include tonsillitis, pharyngitis, epiglottitis, developing peritonsillar abscess and retropharyngeal abscess.
- Unresolved or resistant cases frequently go on to develop abscesses of the throat (see p.301).
- This pattern can respond well to correct, frequent and timely treatment.

9.3 LUNG AND KIDNEY *YIN* DEFICIENCY

Pathophysiology
- The Lung and Kidney *yin* deficiency pattern represents a chronic sore throat which gets worse when the patient is tired. Lung and Kidney *yin* deficiency leads to dryness and Heat in the throat, causing recurrent low grade inflammation of the tonsils and surrounding tissues. Depending on the initial conditions and the patient's constitution, the deficiency may tend towards either the Lung or Kidney, although in practice it is often difficult to differentiate between them, and there are mostly elements of both. In some patients there will be a history of repeated acute throat infections.

Clinical features
General
- chronic sore throat, which gets worse in the afternoon or evening, and with fatigue
- possibly swollen tonsils; if the tonsils are squeezed with a tongue depressor there may be a whitish or yellowish watery exudate
- the throat is dry and feels blocked or hoarse
- itchy irritating sensations in the throat
- afternoon fever or malar flushing
- tiredness and weakness
- sensation of heat in the palms and soles ('five hearts hot')

T red and dry with little or no coat
P thready and rapid

If Lung *yin* deficiency predominates there is:
- mild throat soreness, dry mouth and throat with little or no desire to drink, red lips, dry cough with little or no sputum, shortness of breath, the throat may appear a dull or darkish red

If Kidney *yin* deficiency predominates there is:
- sore, dry throat that tends to be worse than in Lung *yin* deficiency, and with more deficient Heat, low back and knees weak and sore, restlessness, insomnia, dizziness, blurred vision, tinnitus, the throat appears dull or darkish red and dry, or shiny and atrophic with some scab like crusting

9.3.1 Lung *yin* deficiency
Treatment principle
Nourish Lung *yin*, clear Heat
Generate fluids and moisten dryness

Prescription

GAN LU YIN 甘露饮
(Sweet Dew Decoction)

sheng di (Radix Rehmanniae Glutinosae) 生地	15g
shu di (Radix Rehmanniae Glutinosae Conquitae) 熟地	15g
yin chen (Herba Artemisiae Yinchenhao) 茵陈	12g
mai dong (Tuber Ophiopogonis Japonici) 麦冬	10g
tian dong (Tuber Asparagi Cochinchinensis) 天冬	10g
shi hu (Herba Dendrobii) 石斛	10g
zhi ke (Fructus Citri Aurantii) 枳壳	10g
pi pa ye (Folium Eriobotryae) 枇杷叶	10g
huang qin (Radix Scutellariae Baicalensis) 黄芩	10g
gan cao (Radix Glycyrrhizae Uralensis) 甘草	6g

Method: Decocotion. (Source: *Zhong Yi Er Bi Hou Ke Xue*)

9.3.2 Kidney *yin* deficiency
Treatment principle

Nourish Kidney *yin*, redirect Fire downwards
Clear and benefit the throat

Prescription

LIU WEI DI HUANG WAN 六味地黄丸
(Rehmannia Six Formula) modified

shu di (Radix Rehmanniae Glutinosae Conquitae) 熟地	24g
shan yao (Radix Dioscoreae Oppositae) 山药	20g
fu ling (Sclerotium Poriae Cocos) 茯苓	15g
shan zhu yu (Fructus Corni Officinalis) 山茱萸	12g
xuan shen (Radix Scrophulariae Ningpoensis) 玄参	12g
shi hu (Herba Dendrobii) 石斛	12g
mu dan pi (Cortex Moutan Radicis) 牡丹皮	9g
ze xie (Rhizoma Alismatis Orientalis) 泽泻	9g
mai dong (Tuber Ophiopogonis Japonici) 麦冬	9g

Method: Decoction. (Source: *Zhong Yi Er Bi Hou Ke Xue*)

Modifications

- If Fire flares strongly add **zhi mu** (Rhizoma Anemarrhenae Asphodeloides) 知母 9-12g and **huang bai** (Cortex Phellodendri) 黄柏 6-9.

Variations and additional prescriptions

Yin and Blood deficiency
- In cases with both *yin* and Blood deficiency causing chronic sore, dry throat, visual disturbances, numbness in the extremities, pale lips etc. (a

pattern common in post-partum women), the correct treatment is to first nourish Blood and *yin*, and moisten dryness with **SI WU TANG** (*Dang Gui Four Combination* 四物汤) modified.

    shu di (Radix Rehmanniae Glutinosae Conquitae) 熟地 18g
    bai shao (Radix Paeoniae Lactiflora) 白芍 12g
    dang gui (Radix Angelicae Sinensis) 当归 9g
    he shou wu (Radix Polygoni Multiflori) 何首乌 9g
    mai dong (Tuber Ophiopogonis Japonici) 麦冬 9g
    chuan xiong (Radix Ligustici Chuanxiong) 川芎 6g
    e jiao^ (Gelatinum Corii Asini) 阿胶 6g
    Method: Decoction. **E jiao** is melted before being added to the strained decoction (*yang hua* 烊化).

Qi and yin *deficiency*

- When Lung *qi*, fluids and *yin* are damaged, causing a chronic sore, dry throat, poor appetite, shortness of breath, low voice or weak cough, the treatment is to tonify *qi* and generate fluids with **SI JUN ZI TANG** (*Four Major Herbs Combination* 四君子汤) modified.

    ren shen (Radix Ginseng) 人参 9g
    bai zhu (Rhizoma Atractylodes Macrocephalae) 白术 9g
    fu ling (Sclerotium Poria Cocos) 茯苓 9g
    gan cao (Radix Glycyrrhizae Uralensis) 甘草 6g
    huang qi (Radix Astragali Membranacei) 黄芪 18g
    shan yao (Radix Dioscoreae Oppositae) 山药 12g
    huang jing (Rhizoma Polygonati) 黄精 12g
    shi hu (Herba Dendrobii) 石斛 9g
    yu zhu (Rhizoma Polygonati Odorati) 玉竹 9g
    bai he (Bulbus Lilii) 百合 9g
    da zao (Fructus Zizyphi Jujubae) 大枣 3pce
    Method: Decoction. (Source: *Zhong Yi Er Bi Hou Ke Xue*)

Kidney yang *deficiency*

- There is another type of sore throat that is attributed to Kidney *yang* deficiency. This type of sore throat is characterised by a feeling of discomfort and vulnerability in the throat, rather than inflammation. In a *yang* deficient person insufficient *yang* rises to the neck and head, the area of the body that in normal circumstances is 'the meeting point of all the *yang*'. A lack of *yang* reaching the head can also inhibit clarity of thought. This mild sore throat (often worse in the morning) and muddled thinking can be part of a post viral or chronic fatigue syndrome. There may also be accompanying Cold signs and symptoms, such as cold extremities, cold intolerance, loose stools or diarrhoea and a pale swollen tongue. Use the formula **JIN KUI SHEN QI WAN** (*Rehmannia Eight Formula* 金匮肾气丸, p.150) to warm and invigorate Kidney *yang*.

Patent medicines
Ba Xian Chang Shou Wan 八仙长寿丸 (Ba Xian Chang Shou Wan)
Bai He Gu Jin Wan 百合固金丸 (Bai He Gu Jin Wan)
Qing Yin Wan 清音丸 (Qing Yin Wan)
Liu Wei Di Huang Wan 六味地黄丸 (Liu Wei Di Huang Wan)
Zhi Bai Ba Wei Wan 知柏八味丸 (Zhi Bai Ba Wei Wan)
Jin Kui Shen Qi Wan 金匮肾气丸 (Sexoton Pills)
- for Kidney *yang* deficiency

Topical treatments
TIE DI WAN (*Iron Whistle Pill* 铁笛丸)
RUN HOU WAN (*Moisten the Throat Pill* 润喉丸)
- see Wind Heat, p.274-275

Acupuncture
Kidney *yin* deficiency
LI.4 (*he gu*), LI.11 (*qu chi*), St.36 (*zu san li* +), St.6 (*jia che*), Lu.7 (*lie que*), Kid.6 (*zhao hai* +), Kid.3 (*tai xi* +), Lu.10 (*yu ji*), Bl.23 (*shen shu* +), Bl.13 (*fei shu* +), Lu.9 (*tai yuan* +), LI.18 (*fu tu*), bai lao (M-HN-30)

Kidney *yang* deficiency
Du.14 (*da zhui* ▲), Du.20 (*bai hui*), Bl.23 (*shen shu* ▲), Bl.43 (*gao huang shu* ▲), Kid.27 (*shu fu*), Du.4 (*mong men* ▲)

Clinical notes
- Biomedical conditions that may present as Lung and Kidney deficiency type sore throat include chronic laryngitis, pharyngitis, tonsillitis, smokers throat, chronic fatigue syndrome, immune system deficiency and post glandular fever sore throat.
- Can require prolonged treatment for a satisfactory result.
- Sipping pear juice frequently can help to moisten the throat.

9.4 SPLEEN *QI* DEFICIENCY

脾气虚喉痹

Pathophysiology
- Spleen *qi* deficiency sore throat is a chronic pattern and frequently a direct result of overuse of antibiotic drugs. Clinically this is most frequently seen in children who receive repeated courses of medication for tonsillitis. Antibiotics clear the Heat associated with the throat infection, but do not clear Damp or disperse other pathogens, that remain in the throat. These lingering pathogenic factors encourage repeated episodes of infection, which may occur as soon as the course of medication ceases. Repeated courses of antibiotics become less effective at combating the infection, but still damage Spleen *yang qi*. As a result more Damp can accumulate and production of *zheng* and *wei qi* is inhibited. *Wei qi* deficiency allows repeated Wind invasion, which simply aggravates the latent pathogens, until the throat is constantly sore and irritated. Eventually the tonsils may be removed, but the Spleen deficiency remains.

Clinical features
- chronic sore throat, which is worse in the morning and when tired
- the throat appears slightly red or pale and swollen, possibly with a sheen of mucus
- frequent or continual swollen glands in the neck
- frequent colds and upper respiratory tract infections
- poor appetite, picky eating, abdominal distension
- tiredness, lack of vitality
- loose stools or diarrhoea
- nausea or vomiting
- runny nose, puffy eyes, mild oedema
- pale complexion

T pale and possibly swollen and coated
P weak

Treatment principle
Tonify and strengthen Spleen *qi*
Leach out and dry Dampness and benefit the throat

Prescription

SHEN LING BAI ZHU SAN 参苓白术散
(*Ginseng and Atractylodes Formula*) modified

dang shen (Radix Codonopsis Pilosulae) 党参	12g
bai zhu (Rhizoma Atractylodes Macrocephalae) 白术	12g
fu ling (Sclerotium Poriae Cocos) 茯苓	12g

chao bian dou (dry fried Semen Dolichos Lablab)
炒扁豆 12g
chao shan yao (dry fried Radix Dioscoreae Oppositae)
炒山药 15g
chao yi ren (dry fried Semen Coicis Lachryma-jobi)
炒苡仁 15g
lian zi (Semen Nelumbinis Nuciferae) 莲子 9g
jie geng (Radix Platycodi Grandiflori) 桔梗 6g
chen pi (Pericarpium Citri Reticulatae) 陈皮 6g
mu hu die (Semen Oroxyli Indici) 木蝴蝶 6g
sha ren (Fructus Amomi) 砂仁 3g
zhi gan cao (honey fried Radix Glycyrrhizae Uralensis)
炙甘草 3g

Method: Grind the herbs to a powder and take 9 grams (or proportionately less for children) 2-3 times daily with warm water. May also be decocted, in which case **sha ren** is added at the end of cooking (*hou xia* 后下). (Source: *Zhong Yi Nei Ke Lin Chuang Shou Ce*)

Modifications

* With frequent colds, add **huang qi** (Radix Astragali Membranacei) 黄芪 15g and **fang feng** (Radix Ledebouriellae Divaricatae) 防风 9g.
* With copious Phlegm, add **ban xia*** (Rhizoma Pinelliae Ternatae) 半夏 9g.
* With swollen glands, add **zhe bei mu** (Bulbus Fritillariae Thunbergii) 浙贝母 9g, **xuan shen** (Radix Scrophulariae Ningpoensis) 玄参 12g and **cang er zi*** (Fructus Xanthii Sibirici) 苍耳子 9g. See also section on paediatric asthma (p.162) for the swollen gland formula 'Gungy Gland Mix'.

Patent medicines

Shen Ling Bai Zhu Wan 参苓白术丸 (Shen Ling Bai Zhu Wan)
Jian Pi Wan 健脾丸 (Jian Pi Wan)
Bu Zhong Yi Qi Wan 补中益气丸 (Bu Zhong Yi Qi Wan)
Fu Zi Li Zhong Wan 附子理中丸 (Li Chung Yuen Medical Pills)
  - for Spleen *yang* deficiency
Li Zhong Wan 理中丸 (Li Zhong Wan)
  - *yang* deficiency

Acupuncture

St.36 (*zu san li* +▲), LI.11 (*qu chi* +▲), Bl.20 (*pi shu* +▲), Lu.9 (*tai yuan* +), Bl.13 (*fei shu* +▲), Ren.12 (*zhong wan* +▲)
  • with Phlegm add St.40 (*feng long* -)
  • with frequent colds add Du.14 (*da zhui* ▲)

Clinical notes

- Biomedical conditions that may present as Spleen *qi* deficiency type sore throat include chronic tonsillitis, immune dysfunction, chronic fatigue syndrome and post glandular fever sore throat.
- Children with this pattern are often subject to repeated attacks of Wind Heat, so timely treatment with a convenient formula (like Peking Niu Huang Chieh Tu Pien), can help prevent chronic tonsillitis and tonsillectomy.

Table 9.2 *Summary of the main sore throat patterns and treatments*

	Pattern	Main Signs & Symptoms	Appearance of the throat	Guiding Formula
A C U T E	Wind Heat	sore throat, difficulty swallowing, fever & chills, red tipped tongue with thin white or yellow coat	slightly red or red & swollen, maybe with suppuration	SHU FENG QING RE TANG
	Lung & Stomach Heat	severe sore throat, high fever, thirst, constipation, bad breath, concentrated urine, red tongue with a thick yellow coat	very red & swollen with obvious suppuration	PU JI XIAO DU YIN
C H R O N I C	Lung *yin* deficiency	sore, irritated, scratchy throat, worse in the afternoon & evening, dry cough, red lips, facial flushing, thready rapid pulse, red, dry tongue with little or no coat	dull or darkish red	GAN LU YIN
	Kidney *yin* deficiency	sore throat worse in the afternoon & evening, lower back ache, insomnia, tinnitus, dizziness, flushing, night sweats, thready rapid pulse, red dry tongue with little or no coat	dull or darkish red & dry, or shiny & atrophic with a scab-like crusting	LIU WEI DI HUANG WAN
	Kidney *yang* deficiency	sore throat, worse in the morning, pale complexion, oedema, cold intolerance, nocturia, loose stools, pale wet swollen tongue	neither red nor swollen, may be pale & atrophic	JIN KUI SHEN QI WAN
	Spleen *qi* deficiency	sore congested throat, worse in the morning, throat clearing, poor appetite, abdominal distension, pale complexion, frequent colds, pale tongue	possibly pale & swollen, with a coating of mucous	SHEN LING BAI ZHU SAN

SUMMARY OF GUIDING FORMULAE FOR SORE THROAT

Wind Heat - *Shu Feng Qing Re Tang* 疏风清热汤
- Wind Cold - *Jing Fang Bai Du San* 荆防败毒散

Lung and Stomach Heat - *Pu Ji Xiao Du Yin* 普济消毒饮

Lung *yin* deficiency - *Gan Lu Yin* 甘露饮
- with Blood deficiency - *Si Wu Tang* 四物汤
- with *qi* deficiency - *Si Jun Zi Tang* 四君子汤

Kidney *yin* deficiency - *Liu Wei Di Huang Wan* 六味地黄丸
- Kidney *yang* deficiency - *Jin Kui Shen Qi Wan* 金匮肾气丸

Spleen *qi* deficiency - *Shen Ling Bai Zhu San* 参苓白术散

Endnote

For more information regarding herbs marked with an asterisk*, an open circle° or a hat^, see the tables on pp.944-952.

Appendix
THROAT ABSCESS (*hou yong* 喉痈)

A throat abscess is a suppurative, space occupying lesion that usually follows an unresolved bacterial throat infection (primarily tonsillitis). Once an abscess has formed, the main focus of therapy is to eliminate Toxic Heat and expel pus. There are several different prescriptions used depending on the stage and severity of the disorder, and whether the abscess is forming, or has ruptured.

Clinical features
- sore throat with marked one sided swelling and medial displacement of the uvula and (usually) one tonsil, difficulty swallowing, swollen and tender cervical lymph nodes
- in the early stages there will usually be signs of Wind Heat–fever, chills, headache, malaise, floating rapid pulse, yellow tongue coat
- in later stages, as the pathogen moves internally (usually affecting *yang ming* and in serious cases, the Pericardium), the severity of the systemic symptoms increases–high fever, severe headache, constipation, dark urine, bad breath, a flooding, rapid pulse and a red tongue with a thick yellow coat

Treatment principle
Expel Wind, clear Toxic Heat, reduce swelling, stop pain

Prescription

WU WEI XIAO DU YIN 五味消毒饮
(*Five Ingredient Decoction to Eliminate Toxin*) modified

This prescription is used in the early stages of the abscess, when pus is being formed and the abscess is still developing. At this stage, although the throat is very sore, red and swollen, the systemic symptoms are generally relatively mild, reflecting a Wind Heat pattern.

jin yin hua (Flos Lonicerae Japonicae) 金银花 15-30g
zi hua di ding (Herba cum Radice Violae Yedeonsitis)
紫花地丁 15-30g
pu gong ying (Herba Taraxici Mongolici) 蒲公英 15-30g
ye ju hua (Flos Chrysanthemi Indici) 野菊花 12g
jing jie (Herba seu Flos Schizonepetae Tenuifolia) 荆芥 12g
zi bei tian kui (Herba Begoniae Fimbristipulatae) 紫北天葵 . 9g
fang feng (Radix Ledebouriellae Divaricatae) 防风 9g
bai zhi (Radix Angelicae Dahuricae) 白芷 9g
Method: Decoction. (Source: *Zhong Yi Er Bi Hou Ke Xue*)

QING YAN LI GE TANG 清咽利膈汤
(*Clear the Throat, Benefit the Diaphragm Decoction*) modified

This formula is used when the pathogen penetrates deeper into the body and the systemic symptoms are more severe.

lian qiao (Fructus Forsythia Suspensae) 连翘	15g
jin yin hua (Flos Lonicerae Japonicae) 金银花	15g
shan zhi zi (Fructus Gardeniae Jasminoidis) 山栀子	12g
xuan shen (Radix Scrophulariae Ningpoensis) 玄参	12g
jing jie (Herba seu Flos Schizonepetae Tenuifolia) 荆芥	9g
fang feng (Radix Ledebouriellae Divaricatae) 防风	9g
huang qin (Radix Scutellariae Baicalensis) 黄芩	9g
huang lian (Rhizoma Coptidis) 黄连	6g
jie geng (Radix Platycodi Grandiflori) 桔梗	9g
gan cao (Radix Glycyrrhizae Uralensis) 甘草	6g
niu bang zi (Fructus Arctii Lappae) 牛蒡子	9g
da huang (Radix et Rhizoma Rhei) 大黄	6g
mang xiao (Mirabilitum) 芒硝	6g
bo he (Herba Mentha Haplocalycis) 薄荷	6g

Method: Decoction. **Bo he** is added towards the end of cooking (*hou xia* 后下). **Mang xiao** is added to the strained decoction (*chong fu* 冲服). If there is no constipation delete **da huang** and **mang xiao**. (Source: *Zhong Yi Er Bi Hou Ke Xue*)

XIAN FANG HUO MING YIN 仙方活命饮
(*Sublime Formula for Sustaining Life*) modified

The focus of this formula is on clearing Toxic Heat, reducing swelling and invigorating Blood. It is selected when swelling and pain are severe, the abscess has ripened and pus is copious.

jin yin hua (Flos Lonicerae Japonicae) 金银花	15-30g
jing jie (Herba seu Flos Schizonepetae Tenuifolia) 荆芥	12g
dang gui wei (tail of Radix Angelicae Sinensis) 当归尾	9g
chi shao (Radix Paeoniae Rubrae) 赤芍	9g
zhe bei mu (Bulbus Fritillariae Thunbergii) 浙贝母	9g
bai zhi (Radix Angelicae Dahuricae) 白芷	9g
zao jiao ci (Spina Gleditsiae Sinensis) 皂角刺	9g
ru xiang (Gummi Olibanum) 乳香	6g
mo yao (Myrrha) 没药	6g
chuan shan jia° (Squama Manitis Pentadactylae) 穿山甲	6g
fang feng (Radix Ledebouriellae Divaricatae) 防风	6g
chen pi (Pericarpium Citri Reticulatae) 陈皮	6g
gan cao (Radix Glycyrrhizae Uralensis) 甘草	6g

Method: Decoction. (Source: *Zhong Yi Er Bi Hou Ke Xue*)

Variations and additional prescriptions

Heat in the Blood
- If the Toxic Heat progresses further into the body and enters the Blood, affecting the Pericardium and *shen* and causing bleeding or clouded consciousness, the correct treatment is to clear Toxic Heat, cool Blood and clear *ying* with **XI JIAO DI HUANG TANG** (*Rhinoceros Horn and Rehmannia Decoction* 犀角地黄汤, p.41) or **QING YING TANG** (*Clear the Ying Decoction* 清营汤, p.38).

With delirium or disturbances of consciouness
- If there is delirium or loss of consciousness, a resucitation formula like **AN GONG NIU HUANG WAN** (*Calm the Palace Pill with Cattle Gallstone* 安宫牛黄丸, p.914) or **ZI XUE DAN** (*Purple Snow Special Pill* 紫雪丹, p.707) is appropriate.

Slow to heal ulcerations following rupture in the post acute phase
- If, after the throat abscess has ruptured, there is residual ulceration that is slow to heal (usually in run down patients), the treatment is to tonify *qi* and Blood, and expel residual toxin. With non-healing ulceration and residual thin discharge use **DANG GUI BU XUE TANG** (*Dang Gui Decoction to Tonify the Blood* 当归补血汤) modified.
    huang qi (Radix Astragali Membranacei) 黄芪 30g
    dang gui (Radix Angelicae Sinensis) 当归 6g
    jin yin hua (Flos Lonicerae Japonicae) 金银花 15g
    gan cao (Radix Glycyrrhizae Uralensis) 甘草 9g
    Method: Decoction.

Chronic abscess that do not rupture
- For chronic painful, hot abscesses with pus, but which do not readily rupture, the treatment is to tonify *qi* and Blood to expel Toxins and pus. The formula (a variation of the previous formula) is **TOU NONG SAN** (*Discharge Pus Powder* 透脓散).
    huang qi (Radix Astragali Membranacei) 黄芪 15-24g
    dang gui (Radix Angelicae Sinensis) 当归 9g
    chuan shan jia° (Squama Manitis Pentadactylae) 穿山甲 9g
    zao jiao ci (Spina Gleditsiae Sinensis) 皂角刺 9g
    chuan xiong (Radix Ligustici Chuanxiong) 川芎 6g
    Method: Decoction with a 50:50 mixture of water and yellow wine. (Source: *Shi Yong Fang Ji Xue*)

Chronic non healing ulceration
- For prolonged non-healing ulceration in a patient with no residual Toxin and severe deficiency, the treatment is to warm and tonify *qi* and Blood

with **SHI QUAN DA BU TANG** (*Ginseng and Dang Gui Ten Combination* 十全大补汤, p.529).

Clinical notes

- The types of biomedical condition that may present as a TCM defined throat abscess include quinsy, peritonsillar abscess and retropharyngeal abscess.
- In severe cases surgical drainage of the abscess and administration of antibiotics may be indicated, in addition to herbs.
- The same gargles and topical treatments that apply to Wind Heat sore throat (p.286-288) may be used in throat abscess.

Disorders of the Lung

10. Tuberculosis

Yin deficiency with Lung Heat
Lung and Kidney *yin* deficiency
Qi and *yin* deficiency
Yin and *yang* deficiency
Symptomatic treatment

10 TUBERCULOSIS
fei lao 肺癆

The TCM term *fei lao* is usually translated as Lung consumption or Lung asthenia, and corresponds to pulmonary tuberculosis.

Tuberculosis is a chronic disorder of the Lungs characterised by cough, haemoptysis, tidal fever, nightsweats, weakness and emaciation. Such a collection of symptoms was described by Sun Si-miao in the *Qian Jin Fang* 千金方 (Thousand Ducat Prescriptions) in the Tang dynasty, and he perceptively ascribed the condition to Lung 'worms' (*chong* 虫). Today of course, we know that the bacillus *Mycobacterium tuberculosis* is the pathogenic organism responsible for tuberculosis infection.

Until a few years ago tuberculosis was almost eradicated in the developed world. Now we are encountering it more frequently as migration from and travel to developing countries increases. Drug resistant varieties are appearing at various locations around the world.

AETIOLOGY
Pathogens
As noted by Sun Si-miao, it has long been recognised that a special type of pathogen was responsible for *fei lao*. We now know that the early stages of tuberculosis are generally symptomless, although in some cases there may be a vague illness associated with a cough. This most likely corresponds with an invasion of Wind Heat that is never cleared and becomes a latent or hidden (*fu* 伏) pathogen. The usual initial presentation is one of Lung *yin* deficiency (Fig 10.1).

Deficiency
The body's ability to protect itself and contain the pathogen is of primary importance in the development of tuberculosis. If *zheng qi* is intact, the disease may remain silent for years. As *zheng qi* declines, the pathogen opportunistically reactivates, and thus tuberculosis is more common in those too weak to mount a strong defense. Tuberculosis is more common amongst the homeless, the poor, the malnourished and the immuno-compromised. Zhu Dan-xi, writing during the Yuan dynasty, noted that *yin* deficiency was the main predisposing and presenting feature.

TREATMENT
Tuberculosis generally develops gradually and has a long course. Most cases begin with mild, intermittent and often vague symptoms like cough, fevers,

sweats and malaise. As the disease progresses, the pattern becomes more obviously one of *yin* deficiency affecting first the Lungs, then Kidneys. Often the Spleen will also be involved. In advanced disease both *yin* and *yang* are depleted.

The fundamental principle of treatment is to vigorously replenish *yin* (and *qi* or *yang*) while eliminating the pathogen. Today, the principle of eliminating the pathogen is usually acheived with specific antibiotic therapy (usually a combination of rifampicin, isoniazid and pyrazinamide). Because tuberculosis can be so debilitating and in many cases ultimately fatal, the most rational approach is to combine the precision of Western chemotherapy with the constitution strengthening benefits of Chinese medicine.

There are numerous herbs that inhibit the tuberculosis bacillus (Table 10.1). The prescriptions recommended in the source texts, however, concentrate almost entirely on the constitutional patterns evident and not on the pathogen. Presumably, an appropriate selection of known antitubercular herbs can be added to the primary constitutional formula or may be used as a first line treatment in cases of drug resistant tuberculosis. There are, however, certain cautions to be observed in the use of these herbs (see Table 10.1, p.309).

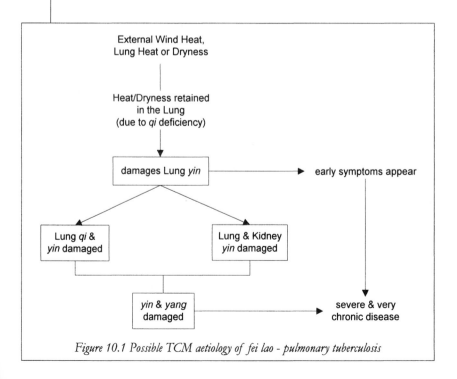

Figure 10.1 Possible TCM aetiology of fei lao - pulmonary tuberculosis

Symptomatic treatment
The symptoms of tuberculosis can be very distressing and may serve to further weaken the patient. When severe they should be controlled with specific herbal combinations added to the main prescription, or treated vigorously first with a specific symptomatic formula (see p.318) before dealing with the constitutional pattern. The treatments outlined in this section are not specific to tuberculosis, and may be adapted to suit any pattern presenting with these symptoms.

Table 10.1 Herbs which inhibit Mycobacterium tuberculosis (from *Shi Yong Zhong Yi Nei Ke Xue*)

Herb	Flavour & Nature, dose	Properties	Adverse effects
Shi Da Gong Lao Ye (Folium Mahoniae Bealei)	bitter, cool 10-15g	Important herb for TB. Nourishes Lung *yin*, alleviates deficient Heat	
Chuan Xin Lian (Herba Andrographitis Paniculatae)	bitter, cold 9-15g	clear Damp Heat	Prolonged use can significantly damage the Spleen. Can be made into a syrup with honey or dates to alleviate this tendency.
Huang Qin (Radix Scutellariae Baicalensis)	bitter, cold 6-15g		
Huang Lian (Rhizoma Coptidis)	bitter, cold 3-9g		
Xia Ku Cao (Spica Prunellae Vulgaris)	bitter, acrid, cold, 9-15g	clears Heat & Toxins, dissipates accumulations	Can weaken the Spleen & Stomach, although not as much as the previous herbs.
Jin Yin Hua (Flos Lonicerae Japonicae)	sweet, cold 9-30g		
Da Suan (Bulbus Alli Sativi)	acrid, warm 3-5 cloves	Kills parasites	Can deplete *yin*. May be taken in rice congee to alleviate this tendency.
Bai Guo (Semen Ginkgo Bilobae)	sweet, bitter, astringent, slightly toxic, 6-9g	Expels Phlegm, Stops wheezing, eliminates Dampness	Caution with hard to expectorate sputum. Long term use can cause toxic side effects.
Di Yu (Radix Sanguisorbae Officinalis)	bitter, sour, cool, 6-15g	Cools the Blood & stops bleeding, Clears Heat	
Shi Liu Pi (Pericarpium Punicae Granati)	sour, astringent, warm, toxic, 3-9g	Kills parasites, astringes the intestines	Can aggravate cases with Heat. Caution with hard to expectorate sputum.
Bai Bu (Radix Stemonae)	sweet, bitter, slightly warm 3-9g	Moistens the Lungs, stops cough, kills parasites	Can aggravate Spleen deficiency.
An Xi Xiang (Benzoinum)	acrid, bitter, neutral, 0.3-1.5g	Opens the orifices, moves *qi* & Blood	Can aggravate *yin* deficiency.

10.1 LUNG *YIN* DEFICIENCY WITH HEAT

Pathophysiology
- In Lung *yin* deficiency with Heat, the Heat is confined to the chest and the *yin* deficiency to the Lungs. This is generally the early stage and initial presentation of infection, before other complications intervene.

Clinical features
- dry cough with little or no mucus or recurrent haemoptysis with frothy fresh red blood
- chest pain with coughing
- afternoon or tidal fever
- night sweats
- sensation of heat in the palms, soles and chest ('five hearts hot')
- malar flush
- warm dry skin
- red lips, dry throat
- emaciation
- insomnia, dream disturbed sleep
- irritability and restlessness, easy anger

T scarlet red or crimson
P thready and rapid

Treatment principle
Nourish *yin*, moisten the Lung, clear Heat
Kill pathogens

Prescription

YUE HUA WAN 月华丸
(*Moonlight Pill*) modified

sha shen (Radix Adenophorae seu Glehniae) 沙参	30g
mai dong (Tuber Ophiopogonis Japonici) 麦冬	30g
tian dong (Tuber Asparagi cochinchinensis) 天冬	30g
sheng di (Radix Rehmanniae Glutinosae) 生地	30g
shu di (Radix Rehmanniae Glutinosae Conquitae) 熟地	30g
bai bu* (Radix Stemonae) 百部	30g
shan yao (Radix Dioscoreae Oppositae) 山药	30g
e jiaoˆ (Gelatinum Corii Asini) 阿胶	30g
chuan bei mu (Bulbus Fritillariae Cirrhosae) 川贝母	30g
fu ling (Sclerotium Poriae Cocos) 茯苓	15g
san qi (Radix Notoginseng) 三七	15g
sang ye (Folium Mori Albae) 桑叶	60g

ju hua (Flos Chrysanthemi Morifolii) 菊花 60g
Method: Grind the herbs to a fine powder and form into 9-gram pills with honey. The dose is five pills daily. May also be decocted with an appropriate reduction in dose. (Source: *Shi Yong Zhong Yi Nei Ke Xue*)

Modifications
- To target the pathogen directly, add two or three herbs from Table 10.1, p.309.
- For a guide to other approaches to symptomatic relief see symptomatic treatment, p.318.

Patent medicines *(as adjunct or symptomatic therapy only)*
Yang Yin Qing Fei Wan 养阴清肺丸 (Yang Yin Qing Fei Wan)
Bai He Gu Jin Wan 百合固金丸 (Bai He Gu Jin Wan)
Chuan Xin Lian Kang Yan Pian 穿心莲抗炎片
(Chuan Xin Lian Antiphlogistic Tablets) - used in addition to one of the patent medicines above

Acupuncture
Lu.5 (*chi ze* -), Bl.13 (*fei shu* -), Bl.43 (*gao huang shu* +▲), St.36 (*zu san li* +)
- with bone steaming fever add Du.14 (*da zhui*), Kid.3 (*tai xi*), PC.8 (*lao gong*), Lu.10 (*yu ji*)
- with night sweats add Ht.6 (*yin xi*), Kid.7 (*fu liu*)
- with haemoptysis add Lu.6 (*kong zui*), Bl.17 (*ge shu*)
- with hoarse voice add Lu.9 (*tai yuan*), LI.18 (*fu tu*)

Clinical notes
- This pattern represents an early stage of pulmonary tuberculosis.
- At this stage, the condition usually responds well to correct treatment.

肺肾阴虚肺痨

10.2 LUNG AND KIDNEY *YIN* DEFICIENCY

Pathophysiology
- Lung and Kidney *yin* deficiency is very similar to the previous Lung *yin* deficiency, the difference being the addition of obvious Kidney deficiency signs. The Heat eventually damages Lung *yin* sufficiently to deplete Kidney *yin* via the generative (*sheng* 生, p.70) cycle. There is a gradual transition between Lung *yin* deficiency and combined Lung and Kidney *yin* deficiency, with more Kidney symptoms progressively appearing.

Clinical features
- irritating cough with scanty, sticky yellow mucus or recurrent haemoptysis with frothy fresh red blood
- bone steaming or tidal fever
- night sweats, malar flush
- lower back soreness and weakness
- dizziness, tinnitus
- restlessness, irritability, easy anger
- insomnia
- sensation of heat in the palms, soles and chest ('five hearts hot')
- in men involuntary seminal emission, in women amenorrhoea
- emaciation
- chest or hypochondriac pain

T red or crimson, with a peeled or cracked surface
P thready, rapid and weak

Treatment principle
Tonify and nourish the Lung and Kidney
Nourish *yin* and purge Fire
Kill pathogens

Prescription

BAI HE GU JIN TANG 百合固金汤
(*Lily Combination*) modified

bai he (Bulbus Lilii) 百合	30g
mai dong (Tuber Ophiopogonis Japonici) 麦冬	30g
xuan shen (Radix Scrophulariae Ningpoensis) 玄参	30g
bai bu* (Radix Stemonae) 百部	30g
shi da gong lao ye (Folium Mahoniae Bealei) 十大功劳叶	18g
sheng di (Radix Rehmanniae Glutinosae) 生地	18g
gui ban° (Plastrum Testudinis) 龟板	15g
shu di (Radix Rehmanniae Glutinosae Conquitae) 熟地	15g

bai shao (Radix Paeoniae Lactiflora) 白芍 15g
chuan bei mu (Bulbus Fritillariae Cirrhosae) 川贝母 12g
dang gui (Radix Angelicae Sinensis) 当归 10g
jie geng (Radix Platycodi Grandiflori) 桔梗 10g
e jiao^ (Gelatinum Corii Asini) 阿胶 10g
dong chong xia cao^ (Cordyceps Sinensis) 冬虫夏草 10g
gan cao (Radix Glycyrrhizae Uralensis) 甘草 6g

Method: Grind the herbs to a fine powder form into 9-gram pills with honey. The dose is 3-5 pills daily. May also be decocted, in which case **e jiao** is melted before being added to the strained decoction (*yang hua* 烊化). (Source: *Zhong Yi Nei Ke Lin Chuang Shou Ce*)

Modifications

- To target the pathogen directly, add two or three herbs from Table 10.1, p.309, taking extra care with the Spleen and Stomach in emaciated patients.
- For a guide to other approaches to symptomatic relief see symptomatic treatment, p.318.

Patent medicines *(as adjunct or symptomatic therapy only)*

Chong Cao Ji Jing 虫草鸡精 (Cordyceps Essence of Chicken)
Liu Wei Di Huang Wan 六味地黄丸 (Liu Wei Di Huang Wan)
Zhi Bai Ba Wei Wan 知柏八味丸 (Zhi Bai Ba Wei Wan)
Chuan Xin Lian Kang Yan Pian 穿心莲抗炎片
  (Chuan Xin Lian Antiphlogistic Tablets) - used in addition to one of the patent medicines above

Acupuncture

Lu.5 (*chi ze* -), Bl.13 (*fei shu* -), Bl.23 (*shen shu* +),
Bl.43 (*gao huang shu* +▲), St.36 (*zu san li* +), Kid.2 (*ran gu* -), Kid.6 (*zhao hai*)

- with bone steaming fever add Du.14 (*da zhui*), Kid.3 (*tai xi*), PC.8 (*lao gong*), Lu.10 (*yu ji*)
- with night sweats add Ht.6 (*yin xi*), Kid.7 (*fu liu*)
- with haemoptysis add Lu.6 (*kong zui*), Bl.17 (*ge shu*)
- with hoarse voice add Lu.9 (*tai yuan*), LI.18 (*fu tu*)

Clinical notes

- This pattern represents a more advanced stage of pulmonary tuberculosis.

10.3 LUNG *QI* AND *YIN* DEFICIENCY

气阴亏耗肺痨

Pathophysiology
- Lung *qi* and *yin* deficiency represents another variation on the possible development of this disease. Because the Lungs have a close relationship with *qi*, deficiency of *qi* is a frequent complication of any Lung pathology.

Clinical features
- weak dry cough with watery or scanty mucus or recurrent haemoptysis with frothy fresh red blood
- aversion to wind and cold
- spontaneous sweating
- night sweats
- poor appetite
- abdominal distension
- loose stools
- shortness of breath
- low voice
- waxy pale complexion
- chest pain
- malar flush, mild afternoon or tidal fevers
- dry mouth and throat

T pale pink or red and swollen with teeth marks, a cracked surface and a thin or peeled coat
P thready, weak and may be rapid

Treatment principle
Tonify *qi* and *yin*
Strengthen the Lung and Spleen
Kill pathogens

Prescription

BAO ZHEN TANG 保真汤
(*Preserve the True Decoction*) modified

huang qi (Radix Astragali Membranacei) 黄芪	30g
bai he (Bulbus Lilii) 百合	30g
ren shen (Radix Ginseng) 人参	18g
fu ling (Sclerotium Poriae Cocos) 茯苓	18g
mai dong (Tuber Ophiopogonis Japonici) 麦冬	15g
tian dong (Tuber Asparagi cochinchinensis) 天冬	15g
sheng di (Radix Rehmanniae Glutinosae) 生地	15g
shu di (Radix Rehmanniae Glutinosae Conquitae) 熟地	15g

dong chong xia cao^ (Cordyceps Sinensis) 冬虫夏草 15g
di gu pi (Cortex Lycii Chinensis) 地骨皮 12g
bai zhu (Rhizoma Atractylodis Macrocephalae) 白术 10g
chen pi (Pericarpium Citri Reticulatae) 陈皮 10g
dang gui (Radix Angelicae Sinensis) 当归 10g
bai shao (Radix Paeoniae Lactiflora) 白芍 10g
bai bu* (Radix Stemonae) 百部 10g
wu wei zi (Fructus Schizandrae Chinensis) 五味子 6g
zi he che^ (Placenta Hominis) 紫河车 6g
zhi gan cao (honey fried Radix Glycyrrhizae Uralensis)
 炙甘草 6g

Method: Grind the herbs to a fine powder and form into 9-gram pills with honey. The dose is 3-5 pills daily. May also be decocted in which case **zi he che** is taken separately in pill or powder form. (Source: *Zhong Yi Nei Ke Lin Chuang Shou Ce*)

Modifications
- To target the pathogen directly, add two or three herbs from Table 10.1, p.309. Extra care must be taken with additions in this pattern to avoid aggravating Spleen damage.
- For a guide to other approaches to symptomatic relief, see p.318.

Patent medicines *(as adjunct or symptomatic therapy only)*
Chong Cao Ji Jing 虫草鸡精 (Cordyceps Essence of Chicken)
Hua Qi Shen Ji Jing 花旗参鸡精 (American Ginseng Essence of Chicken)
Sheng Mai Wan 生脉丸 (Sheng Mai Wan)
Chuan Xin Lian Kang Yan Pian 穿心莲抗炎片
 (Chuan Xin Lian Antiphlogistic Tablets) - used in addition to one of the patent medicines above

Acupuncture
Lu.5 (*chi ze* -), Bl.13 (*fei shu* -), Bl.23 (*shen shu* +), Ren.6 (*qi hai*), Bl.43 (*gao huang shu* +▲), St.36 (*zu san li* +), Lu.9 (*tai yuan*), Ren.12 (*zhong wan*),
- with bone steaming fever add Du.14 (*da zhui*), Kid.3 (*tai xi*), PC.8 (*lao gong*), Lu.10 (*yu ji*)
- with night sweats add Ht.6 (*yin xi*), Kid.7 (*fu liu*)
- with haemoptysis add Lu.6 (*kong zui*), Bl.17 (*ge shu*)
- with hoarse voice add Lu.9 (*tai yuan*), LI.18 (*fu tu*)

Clinical notes
- Another variation of advanced pulmonary tuberculosis.

10.4 YIN AND YANG BOTH DEFICIENT

Pathophysiology
- Yin and yang deficiency is an advanced stage of tuberculosis. The Lung, Spleen and Kidney are significantly weakened.

Clinical features
- cough and wheeze worse with exertion, with expectoration of frothy or dark streaked mucus
- mild tidal fever
- cold body, aversion to cold
- spontaneous sweating, night sweats
- superficial and facial oedema
- mouth and tongue ulcers
- emaciation
- anxiety, nervousness
- dark lips
- poor appetite, loose stools or cockcrow diarrhoea
- amenorrhoea, impotence

T depending on the balance of *yin* and *yang* the tongue will be either red, dry, peeled or cracked, or pale, purplish and swollen with toothmarks
P minute, thready and rapid or deficient and large

Treatment principle
Nourish *yin*, tonify *yang*
Support *yuan qi*, consolidate the root
Kill pathogens

Prescription

BU TIAN DA ZAO WAN 补天大造丸
(*Tonify Heaven Great Creation Pill*)

shu di (Radix Rehmanniae Glutinosae Conquitae) 熟地	100g
huang qi (Radix Astragali Membranacei) 黄芪	50g
bai zhu (Rhizoma Atractylodis Macrocephalae) 白术	40g
suan zao ren (Semen Ziziphi Spinosae) 酸枣仁	40g
bai shao (Radix Paeoniae Lactiflora) 白芍	40g
shan yao (Radix Dioscoreae Oppositae) 山药	40g
fu ling (Sclerotium Poriae Cocos) 茯苓	40g
gui ban° (Plastrum Testudinis) 龟板	40g
lu jiao jiao^ (Cornu Cervi Gelatinum) 鹿角胶	30g
dang gui (Radix Angelicae Sinensis) 当归	30g
ren shen (Radix Ginseng) 人参	30g

gou qi zi (Fructus Lycii) 枸杞子 30g
yuan zhi (Radix Polygalae Tenuifoliae) 远志 20g
zi he che^ (Placenta Hominis) 紫河车 6g
Method: Grind the herbs to a fine powder and form into 9-gram pills with honey. The dose is 3-5 pills daily. May also be decocted in which case **zi he che** is taken separately in pill or powder form and **lu jiao jiao** is melted before being added to the strained decoction (*yang hua* 烊化). (Source: *Shi Yong Zhong Yi Nei Ke Xue*)

Modifications

- To target the pathogen directly, add two or three herbs from Table 10.1, p.309, taking extra care with the Spleen and Stomach.
- With cockcrow diarrhoea, add **wu zhu yu** (Fructus Evodiae Rutaecarpae) 吴茱萸 15g, **rou dou kou** (Semen Myristicae Fragrantis) 肉豆蔻 40g and **bu gu zhi** (Fructus Psoraleae Corylifoliae) 补骨脂 40g
- For a guide to other approaches to symptomatic relief, see p.318.

Patent medicines *(as adjunct or symptomatic therapy only)*

Chong Cao Ji Jing 虫草鸡精 (Cordyceps Essence of Chicken)
Hua Qi Shen Ji Jing 花旗参鸡精 (American Ginseng Essence of Chicken)
Zhuang Yao Jian Shen Pian 壮腰健肾片 (Zhuang Yao Jian Shen)
Wu Ji Bai Feng Wan 乌鸡白凤丸 (Wuchi Paifeng Wan)
Chuan Xin Lian Kang Yan Pian 穿心莲抗炎片
 (Chuan Xin Lian Antiphlogistic Tablets) - used in addition to one of the patent medicines above

Acupuncture

Bl.43 (*gao huang shu* ▲), Bl.13 (*fei shu* ▲), Bl.17 (*ge shu* ▲), Bl.19, Bl.15 (*xin shu* ▲), Ren.6 (*qi hai* ▲)
- with bone steaming fever add Du.14 (*da zhui*), Kid.3 (*tai xi*), PC.8 (*lao gong*), Lu.10 (*yu ji*)
- with night sweats add Ht.6 (*yin xi*), Kid.7 (*fu liu*)
- with haemoptysis add Lu.6 (*kong zui*), Bl.17 (*ge shu*)
- with hoarse voice add Lu.9 (*tai yuan*), LI.18 (*fu tu*)

Clinical notes

- This pattern represents advanced and difficult pulmonary tuberculosis.
- Treatment is difficult at this stage.

10.5 Symptomatic treatment

Treatment may focus specifically on a particularly distressing symptom, especially in cases where palliative treatment is most appropriate. Treatment strategy, thus focuses first on the manifestations and second on the underlying pattern. The following modifications apply to all preceding prescriptions. If any of the following herbs appear in the primary prescription, the dosage may simply be altered depending on the severity of the symptoms.

10.5.1 Night sweats, spontaneous sweating

- In mild cases, add one or two of the following herbs: **fu xiao mai** (Semen Tritici Aestivi Levis) 浮小麦 15g, **ma huang gen** (Radix Ephedrae) 麻黄根 9g, **wu wei zi** (Fructus Schizandrae Chinensis) 五味子 6g, **wu bei zi^** (Galla Rhois Chinensis) 五倍子 6g, **shan zhu yu** (Fructus Corni Officinalis) 山茱萸 12g, **long gu^** (Os Draconis) 龙骨 15g or **mu li^** (Concha Ostreae) 牡蛎 15g.

- When night sweats are severe, combine with **MU LI SAN** (*Oyster Shell Formula* 牡蛎散).
    mu li^ (Concha Ostreae) 牡蛎
    fu xiao mai (Semen Tritici Aestivi Levis) 浮小麦
    ma huang gen (Radix Ephedrae) 麻黄根
    huang qi (Radix Astragali Membranacei) 黄芪
    Method: Grind equal amounts of the herbs to a fine powder and take 9 grams as a draft twice daily. May also be decocted.

- When spontaneous sweating is severe, combine with **MU LI SAN** (above) and **YU PING FENG SAN** (*Jade Screen Powder* 玉屏风散).
    huang qi (Radix Astragali Membranacei) 黄芪 60-90g
    bai zhu (Rhizoma Atractylodis Macrocephalae) 白术 60g
    fang feng (Radix Ledebouriellae Divaricatae) 防风 60g
    Method: Grind the herbs to a fine powder and take 9 grams as a draft twice daily. May be decocted with an appropriate reduction in dosage.

- When choosing to initially treat the nightsweats only, use **DANG GUI LIU HUANG WAN** (*Dang Gui and Six Yellow Pills* 当归六黄丸) modified.
    dang gui (Radix Angelicae Sinensis) 当归 9g
    huang qi (Radix Astragali Membranacei) 黄芪 30g
    sheng di (Radix Rehmanniae Glutinosae) 生地 20g
    shu di (Radix Rehmanniae Glutinosae Conquitae) 熟地 18g
    huang lian (Rhizoma Coptidis) 黄连 6g
    huang qin (Radix Scutellariae Baicalensis) 黄芩 9g
    huang bai (Cortex Phellodendri) 黄柏 6g

fu xiao mai (Semen Tritici Aestivi Levis) 浮小麦 30g
mu li^ (Concha Ostreae) 牡蛎 30g
Method: Grind the herbs to a fine powder and form into 9-gram pills with honey. The dose is 3-5 pills daily. May also be decocted. (Source: *Lin Chuang Shou Ce Zhong Yi Nei Ke*)

10.5.2 Bone steaming fever, tidal fever

♦ In mild cases, add one or two of the following herbs: **qin jiao** (Radix Gentianae Qinjiao) 秦艽 9g, **qing hao** (Herba Artemesiae Annuae) 青蒿 15g, **bie jia**° (Carapax Amydae Sinensis) 鳖甲 15g, **yin chai hu** (Radix Stellariae Dichotomae) 银柴胡 9g, **hu huang lian** (Rhizoma Picrorhizae) 胡黄连 9g or **di gu pi** (Cortex Lycii Chinensis) 地骨皮 12g.

♦ When choosing to initially treat the fever only, use **QIN JIAO BIE JIA SAN** (*Gentiana Qinjiao and Soft-shelled Turtle Powder* 秦艽鳖甲散) modified.
bie jia° (Carapax Amydae Sinensis) 鳖甲 30g
di gu pi (Cortex Lycii Chinensis) 地骨皮 30g
shu di (Radix Rehmanniae Glutinosae Conquistae) 熟地 30g
suan zao ren (Semen Zizyphi Spinosae) 酸枣仁 30g
sheng di (Radix Rehmanniae Glutinosae) 生地 30g
xuan shen (Radix Scrophulariae Ningpoensis) 玄参 30g
fu xiao mai (Semen Tritici Aestivi Levis) 浮小麦 30g
yin chai hu (Radix Stellariae Dichotomae) 银柴胡 12g
qing hao (Herba Artemesiae Annuae) 青蒿 12g
qin jiao (Radix Gentianae Qinjiao) 秦艽 9g
hu huang lian (Rhizoma Picrorhizae) 胡黄连 9g
Method: Grind the herbs to a fine powder and form into 9-gram pills with honey. The dose is 3-5 pills daily. May also be decocted. (Source: *Zhong Yi Nei Ke Lin Chuang Shou Ce*)

10.5.3 Haemoptysis

♦ In mild cases, add one or two of the following herbs: **bai mao gen** (Rhizoma Imperatae Cylindricae) 白茅根 18g, **bai ji** (Rhizoma Bletillae Striatae) 白芨 12g, **ou jie** (Nodus Nelumbinis Nuciferae) 藕节 9g, **xian he cao** (Herba Agrimoniae Pilosae) 仙鹤草 12g, **xiao ji** (Herba Cephalanoplos) 小蓟 9g, **ce bai ye** (Cacumen Biotae Orientalis) 侧柏叶 12g, **xue yu tan**^ (Crinis Carbonisatus Hominis) 血余炭 6g, or **YUN NAN BAI YAO** (*Yun Nan White Powder* 云南白药).

♦ A useful formula that can be taken as a powder in addition to the primary formula in cases of recurrent haemoptysis is **ZHI FEI JIE HE KE TAN XUE FANG** (*Tuberculosis and Haemoptysis Formula* 治肺结核咳痰血方).
bai bu* (Radix Stemonae) 百部 120g
bai ji (Rhizoma Bletillae Striatae) 白芨 120g

chuan bei mu (Bulbus Fritillariae Cirrhosae) 川贝母 60g
zi he che^ (Placenta Hominis) 紫河车 60g
san qi (Radix Notoginseng) 三七 30g
Method: Grind herbs to a powder and take 3 grams three times daily, one hour after eating. (Source: *Shi Yong Zhong Yao Xue*)

10.5.4 Cough

- In mild cases, add two or three of the following herbs: **chuan bei mu** (Bulbus Fritillariae Cirrhosae) 川贝母 9g, **xing ren*** (Semen Pruni Armeniacae) 杏仁 9g, **sang bai pi** (Cortex Mori Albae Radicis) 桑白皮 12g, **ma dou ling*** (Fructus Aristolchiae) 马兜铃 6g, **kuan dong hua** (Flos Tussilagi Farfarae) 款冬花 9g or **bai bu*** (Radix Stemonae) 百部 12g.

- When choosing to initially treat only the cough, use **ZI WAN TANG** (*Aster Decoction* 紫菀汤).
    zi wan (Radix Asteris Tatarici) 紫菀 12g
    zhi mu (Rhizoma Anemarrhenae Asphodeloides) 知母 12g
    fu ling (Sclerotium Poriae Cocos) 茯苓 12g
    chuan bei mu (Bulbus Fritillariae Cirrhosae) 川贝母 9g
    jie geng (Radix Platycodi Grandiflori) 桔梗 9g
    e jiao^ (Gelatinum Corii Asini) 阿胶 9g
    wu wei zi (Fructus Schizandrae Chinensis) 五味子 6g
    gan cao (Radix Glycyrrhizae Uralensis) 甘草 3g
    Method: Decoction. **E jiao** is melted before being added to the strained decoction (*yang hua* 烊化). (Source: *Shi Yong Zhong Yi Nei Ke Xue*)

10.5.5 Chest pain

- This usually occurs with severe coughing. If distressing, add one or two of the following herbs: **si gua luo** (Fasciculus Vascularis Luffae) 丝瓜络 12g, **yu jin** (Tuber Curcumae) 郁金 9g or **yan hu suo** (Rhizoma Corydalis Yanhusuo) 延胡索 9g.

10.5.6 Nocturnal seminal emission

- In mild cases, add two or three of the following herbs: **mu li^** (Concha Ostreae) 牡蛎 15g, **long gu^** (Os Draconis) 龙骨 15g, **jin ying zi** (Fructus Rosae Laevigatae) 金樱子 12g, **lian xu** (Stamen Nelumbinis Nuciferae) 莲须 9g, **wu wei zi** (Fructus Schizandrae Chinensis) 五味子 6g.

- In severe cases, combine with **JIN SUO GU JING WAN** (*Metal Lock Pill to Stabilize the Essence* 金锁固精丸).
    sha yuan ji li (Semen Astragali Complanati) 沙苑蒺藜 90g
    qian shi (Semen Euryales Ferocis) 芡实 90g

lian xu (Stamen Nelumbinis Nucifera) 莲须 90g
duan long gu^ (calcined Os Draconis) 煅龙骨 30g
duan mu li^ (calcined Concha Ostreae) 煅牡蛎 30g

Method: Grind the herbs to a fine powder and form into 9-gram pills with honey. The dose is three pills daily. May also be decocted. (Source: *Shi Yong Zhong Yao Xue*)

Endnote

For more information regarding herbs marked with an asterisk*, an open circle° or a hat^, see the tables on pp.944-952.

Disorders of the Kidney

11. Lower Back Pain

Acute patterns
Wind Cold
Wind Heat
Wind Damp
Damp Heat

Chronic patterns
Kidney deficiency
Liver *qi* stagnation
Spleen deficiency

Acute or Chronic
Cold Damp
Blood stagnation

11 | LOWER BACK PAIN
yao tong 腰痛

The term lower back pain in Chinese medicine encompasses pain, aching, discomfort or weakness in one or both sides of the low thoracic, lumbar and sacral region, and buttocks (Fig. 11.1). The pain may radiate into the posterior or lateral thighs.

Pain originating from the lumbar spine or musculature is one of the commonest complaints in the clinic, affecting an estimated 80% of people at some stage of their lives. Diagnosis is almost entirely subjective for non-pathological lower back pain, that is, lower back pain that has little or no evidence of structural defect or other abnormality. Even in cases with an identifiable pathology, there is generally a poor correlation between x-ray and CT findings, and symptoms. The exception for pain originating from the spine is true disc herniation and sciatica, where neurological signs correlate with radiological findings. In these cases, a firm diagnosis can be made. This is also the case for viscerogenic lower back pain, that is, pain caused from carcinoma, pelvic inflammation or kidney stones.

Even though a large percentage of patients with lower back pain will remain undiagnosed, the types of conditions that may be responsible include rheumatoid and osteo-arthritis, degenerative spinal disorders, facet joint syndrome, soft tissue injury, prolapsed intervertebral discs, kidney diseases like pyelonephritis, kidney stones and polycystic kidneys, tumours, intestinal and gynaecological diseases.

AETIOLOGY

The Chinese noticed that disorders affecting the Kidneys often gave rise to lower back pain and thus called the lower back the 'palace of the Kidney'. In practice, this means that a large proportion of lower back aches have a component of Kidney deficiency, either as a predisposing factor to back injury or as a result of chronic pathogenic influence. In general, there are two broad types of back pain, excess and deficiency. Excess patterns are due to the presence of a pathogenic influence, commonly Cold, Damp, stagnant *qi* or stagnant Blood.

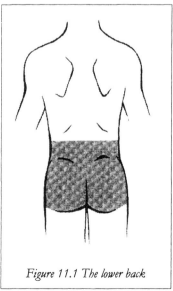

Figure 11.1 The lower back

Deficient patterns are associated with weakness of Kidney *yin*, *yang* or *qi*. Frequently, deficient and excess types will co-exist, as weakness of the Kidney enables pathogens to penetrate through the channels of the back.

External pathogens

The external pathogens, Wind, Cold, Dampness and Damp Heat (see below) may penetrate the channels traversing the lower back, impeding the circulation of *qi* and Blood, causing pain. Cold and Dampness are the most common, and these pathogens can invade the body after exposure to environmental cold damp, for example sitting on cold damp ground, wearing damp clothing, exercising vigorously and sweating in cold damp weather and prolonged immersion in cold water. Once Cold Damp is lodged in the channels of the back, it tends to be persistent. The key feature of the Cold Damp (or external Damp Heat) types is their responsiveness to changes of weather.

Invasion of Cold and Dampness is facilitated where there is pre-existing Kidney weakness. The presence of these pathogens (especially Cold) will in turn drain and weaken Kidney *yang*. In most cases, especially chronic ones, a mixture of excess and deficiency arises. If the circulation of *qi* and Blood is impeded for a long time, Heat may occasionally be generated giving rise to Damp Heat type lower back pain.

Wind Damp, and less commonly Wind Cold and Wind Heat, can also cause pain in the back although in practice the latter two are more likely to affect the upper back and neck. Wind Damp, with the modifying heaviness of the Dampness, tends to sink to the lower back. These patterns are different from the Cold Damp type, in that they are usually associated with colds or flu and are therefore generally self limiting, even without treatment.

Damp Heat

Damp Heat lower back pain corresponds to either inflammation of the spine and/or soft tissues of the lower back, or internal organs that refer pain to the lower back. The source of the Damp Heat may be external or internal. The external Damp Heat pattern may be associated with a direct invasion of Damp Heat into the channels of the lower back, or a transformation of pre-existing Cold Damp. The former is associated with some variety of acute arthritis or myositis; the latter with an inflammatory flareup of a chronic condition. In either case, it is the tissues of the lower back that are affected. External Damp Heat can also cause lower back pain indirectly, by causing inflammation of pelvic organs, like the bladder or kidney. This is more likely to present with symptoms such as painful urination or vaginal discharge, rather than lower back pain.

Internally generated Damp Heat is more likely to cause inflammation of an organ or pelvic structure, which then refers pain to the lower back. Typical examples are the inflammatory stage of kidney stones or infection of the kidneys. Internally generated Damp Heat (compared to external Damp Heat) tends to produce more systemic symptoms, reflecting the original source of the Damp Heat, usually the middle *jiao*.

Blood stagnation

Traumatic injury can lead to acute stagnation of *qi* and Blood in the channels of the lower back. Sudden twisting or bending (such as swinging golf clubs or throwing a ball), lifting or pulling with the spine flexed, exercising vigorously before the body is warmed, or doing heavy work when tired are common causes of acute trauma to the lower back. In practice, however, there may be no discernible trigger, even though the pattern is clearly acute Blood stasis. Often there will be predisposing factors like Kidney or Spleen weakness or Liver *qi* stagnation. Blood stagnation can also be more chronic, manifesting in chronic lower

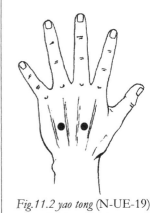

Fig.11.2 yao tong (N-UE-19) Back pain points

BOX 11.1 KEY DIAGNOSTIC POINTS

Duration
- acute pain - invasion of pathogens, Blood stagnation
- chronic pain - Kidney deficiency, or combined Kidney deficiency and pathogenic invasion, Spleen defiency with Damp

Nature of the pain
- sharp, stabbing and fixed - Blood stagnation
- vague, mobile, variable - Liver *qi* stagnation, Wind patterns
- dull ache - Cold Damp, Spleen Damp or Kidney deficiency

Aggravation
- with cold or wet weather - Cold Damp
- not influenced by weather - Liver *qi* stagnation, Blood stagnation, Kidney deficiency
- with activity or movement - Blood stagnation, deficiency patterns
- after sex - Kidney deficiency
- in the morning - Spleen deficiency with Damp
- with stress - Liver *qi* stagnation

Amelioration
- with rest - Kidney deficiency
- with exercise - Liver *qi* stagnation, Spleen deficiency with Damp
- with heat - Cold or Cold Damp, Kidney *yang qi* deficiency

back pain that gradually deteriorates into fixed stabbing pain with systemic signs of stagnant Blood.

Liver *qi* stagnation

Liver *qi* stagnation is caused by repressed emotion, frustration, anger and resentment. Prolonged *qi* stagnation leads to generalised hypertonicity of both skeletal and smooth muscle, which further restricts the circulation of *qi* and Blood to all tissues. This effects the nutrition and elasticity of muscles, particularly those of the lower back. In this case, this chronic muscular tension predisposes the lower back to injury.

Spleen deficiency

This pattern is associated with lack of exercise and poor diet which damage Spleen *qi*, causing a generalised hypotonicity and malnutrition of smooth and skeletal muscle (compare with Liver *qi* stagnation). The loss of muscle tone leads to loss of mechanical support and hypermobility of the lumbar spine. Ligaments, facet joints and other spinal structures may be subject to excessive strain. Patients with this pattern are usually sedentary, with lifestyles involving long periods of sitting or inactivity. They may have a high percentage

---

BOX 11.2 DISTAL POINTS FOR ACUTE PAIN

- **Liv.3 (*tai chong*), LI.4 (*he gu*) and Du.26 (*ren zhong*)** - Calms the *shen*, soothes *qi*, stops pain and relieves muscle tension. These points are treated with the patient lying supine with a pillow under the knees. A particularly good combination for acute back sprain in patients who are very distressed and unable to comfortably lie prone. This is a popular treatment for backs that are so locked up that the patient cannot flex or extend. Usually treated with an even method.
- **Du.26 (*ren zhong*)** - Needled with the patient sitting up or walking while gently flexing and extending as far as they can manage. For pain that is centred on the midline.
- **yao tong xue (N-UE-19, Fig 11.2)** - Found at the proximal junction of the second and third and the fourth and fifth metacarpal bones, needled with the patient sitting or standing while gently flexing and extending as far as they can manage. These points are for pain that is one sided and that restricts mobility markedly. Select the most tender point on the affected side and needle strongly.
- **Bl.40 (*wei zhong*)** - Needled with or without bleeding, when there is localised stabbing pain, particularly along the course of the Bladder channel. This may be done with the patient standing and gently flexing and extending. Bl.40 (*wei zhong*) may be bled with a lancet or three edged needle when there is venous congestion in the popliteal fossa. The latter technique is best performed with the patient lying prone.

> **BOX 11.3 DISTAL POINTS FOR ACUTE OR CHRONIC PAIN**
>
> - **Bl.60 (*kun lun*)** - good for low back and neck pain
> - **Bl.58 (*fei yang*)** - *luo* connecting point, very often tender in chronic pain
> - **Bl.59 (*fu yang*)** - *xi* accumulation point of *yang qiao mai*, very often tender in chronic pain
> - **Bl.36 (*cheng fu*)** and **Bl.37 (*yin men*)** - for pain radiating down the Bladder channel.
> - **GB.30 (*huan tiao*)** - a major point for back pain with a Gall Bladder and Urinary Bladder channel distribution, particularly with buttock pain or pain radiating down the sciatic nerve
> - **GB.31 (*feng shi*)**, **GB.34 (*yang ling quan*)** and **GB.39 (*xuan zhong*)** - for pain radiating down the Gall Bladder channel
> - **Sl.3 (*hou xi*)** and **Bl.62 (*shen mai*)** - needled on the affected side, particularly when there is pain radiating out from the midline

of body fat and are often overweight. Depending on the degree of Spleen weakness, puffiness or fluid retention of the tissues of the waist may be a feature.

Kidney deficiency

Kidney deficiency is a common cause of chronic back ache. Kidney deficiency back aches are often the ones that defy biomedical diagnosis and Western medical treatment. Weak Kidney *qi* makes the back more vulnerable to invasion by pathogenic factors and predisposes it to traumatic injury. There are several specific factors that can contribute to Kidney deficiency lower back pain. These include excessive physical work, particularly that involving overuse of the lumbar muscles, such as heavy lifting and bending and prolonged standing. Prolonged exposure to cold weakens Kidney *yang*. Chronic fear or a sudden severe fright or shock can weaken the Kidneys, predisposing the back to injury or pathogenic invasion.

In addition to the specific factors, the Kidneys are depleted by excessive activity of any kind (the Kidneys are the ultimate store of the body's energy).

> **BOX 11.4 COMMON LOCAL POINTS**
>
> - ***Ah Shi* points** (points of tenderness)
> - **Bl.23 (*shen shu*)** - Kidney *shu* point, used in every chronic case
> - **Bl.25 (*da chang shu*)** - this point is needled deeply to give strong needle sensation in the lumbosacral and buttock area
> - **Bl.54 (*zhi bian*)** - for pain radiating to the upper buttocks
> - **Bl.28 (*pang guang shu*)** - for sacroiliac pain or pain radiating to the sacrum
> - ***shi qi zhui xia* (M-BW-25)** - an extra point between the fifth lumbar and first sacral vertebra. For pain originating at this juncture and for back pain related to menstruation.
> - ***hua tuo jia ji* points, L1-L5** - especially when tender.

This is often seen in sportspeople and professional athletes who often use more *qi* in their activity than they acquire from food and rest. Runners are very prone to back ache as the physical pounding also strains the lower back. The Kidneys are also depleted by pregnancies, either too close together or without adequate recuperation following labour, by miscarriage, termination and sexual activity that is excessive for an individual's constitution.

ACUPUNCTURE TREATMENT

Acupuncture is very effective for lower back pain and is the treatment of choice in acute cases. Point selection depends on the location and radiation of the pain and the channel or channels involved. For a full discussion of the TCM acupuncture approach to lower back pain, see Legge (1997); for the myofacial approach see Baldry (1993) and Travell and Simons (1983).

Principles of point selection

Acute pain
The main principle of treatment in acute pain is to invigorate the circulation of *qi* and Blood, remove obstruction, unblock the channels and stop pain. In general, the main focus of treatment in acute pain is distal points, which should be stimulated strongly with a reducing method. In very acute and painful cases, only distal points are used for the first treatment or two, until the lower back is more relaxed and accessible. Local points can then be chosen on the basis of tenderness and according to channel involvement. As the pain improves, more local points are chosen as appropriate.

Cupping is very useful on *ah shi* points to draw out the stagnation. When cups are used the patient should be informed about the sometimes dramatic purple bruising he or she is likely to have following an effective treatment. The bruising usually subsides after a few days. **Bleeding**, usually applied on Bl.40 (*wei zhong*), may be useful especially when there is venous congestion in the popliteal fossa.

Chronic pain
The main principle in chronic pain is to expel any pathogens, invigorate the circulation of *qi* and Blood, and tonify any underlying deficiency. The point selection is focused on the painful area with one or two distal points in support. Local points are selected according to the degree of tenderness to pressure, the channels involved and the type of deficiency being supplemented. Acupuncture is supplemented in Cold or *yang* deficient patterns by moxa, either on the needle or in a moxa box.

11.1 COLD DAMP

Pathophysiology
- This type of lower back pain may follow exposure to cold and damp environmental conditions, or there may be no obvious cause. The patient is unaware of any mechanical strain. Either way, the key feature is the clear relationship to weather changes. The Cold Damp pathogen invades the channels of the lower back region. The presence of Cold Damp gradually drains Kidney *yang*.
- This pattern may be acute or, more commonly, chronic. In both the acute and chronic patterns there is usually some degree of Kidney deficiency.

Clinical features
- The lower back region feels cold to touch, or the patient may perceive it as feeling cold, aching and heavy. The pain is often described as a 'deep ache', unremitting in nature. The pain is occasionally severe. Twisting and bending are difficult and the symptoms tend to gradually get worse. The pain may radiate down the leg.
- the pain is clearly aggravated by cloudy, wet or cold days and is not improved by rest or lying down

T greasy white coat, particularly on the root
P deep and slow or moderate

Treatment principle
Expel Cold and Damp
Warm and open the channels, support the Kidneys

Prescription

GAN JIANG LING ZHU TANG 甘姜苓术汤
(*Licorice, Ginger, Hoelen and Atractylodes Decoction*) plus
DU HUO JI SHENG TANG 独活寄生汤
(*Du Huo and Vaecium Combination*) modified

This formula is best for chronic patterns with a component of Kidney deficiency. In very acute cases, see also Wind Damp, p.335

sang ji sheng (Ramulus Sangjisheng) 桑寄生	30g
fu ling (Sclerotium Poria Cocos) 茯苓	30g
xu duan (Radix Dipsaci Asperi) 续断	15g
du huo (Radix Angelicae Pubescentis) 独活	15g
bai zhu (Rhizoma Atractylodis Macrocephalae) 白术	15g
niu xi (Radix Achyranthis Bidentatae) 牛膝	15g
chuan xiong (Radix Ligustici Chuanxiong) 川芎	12g
dang gui (Radix Angelicae Sinensis) 当归	12g

du zhong (Cortex Eucommiae Ulmoidis) 杜仲 12g
gan jiang (Rhizoma Zingiberis Officinalis) 干姜 10g
gui zhi (Ramulus Cinnamomi Cassiae) 桂枝 10g
xi xin* (Herba cum Radice Asari) 细辛 3g
Method: Decoction. (Source: *Zhong Yi Nei Ke Lin Chuang Shou Ce*)

Modifications

- With Wind (mobile pain, usually in the early stages of the pattern), add **fang feng** (Radix Ledebouriellae Divaricatae) 防风 9g, **qin jiao** (Radix Gentianae Qinjiao) 秦艽 9g and **qiang huo** (Rhizoma et Radix Notopterygii) 羌活 6g.
- With severe Cold Damp (the area or the patient feels very cold, the pain is severe and significantly relieved with warmth), add **cang zhu** (Rhizoma Atractylodis) 苍术 10g and **zhi fu zi*** (Radix Aconiti Carmichaeli Praeparata) 制附子 6-9g.
- With obvious signs of Kidney deficiency (nocturia, low libido), add **ba ji tian** (Radix Morindae Officinalis) 巴戟天 12g, **xian ling pi** (Herba Epimedii) 仙灵脾 12g and **xian mao** (Rhizoma Curculiginis Orchioidis) 仙茅 9g.

Variations and additional prescriptions

- When the Cold aspect of this pattern has been successfully cleared, patients are occasionally left with residual Dampness, as Damp is sticky and harder to shift. Very persistent Dampness is thought to congeal even further into Phlegm. Extreme overuse of moxa may also congeal Dampness into Phlegm. If the Damp has an internal component there may be digestive symptoms (see also Spleen deficiency, p.343). The treatment is to dry Dampness and transform Phlegm with **SHEN SHI TANG** (*Leach out Dampness Decoction* 渗湿汤)

    cang zhu (Rhizoma Atractylodis) 苍术 10g
    fu ling (Sclerotium Poria Cocos) 茯苓 12g
    bai zhu (Rhizoma Atractylodis Macrocephalae) 白术 12g
    gan jiang (Rhizoma Zingiberis Officinalis) 干姜 10g
    gan cao (Radix Glycyrrhizae Uralensis) 甘草 6g
    chen pi (Pericarpium Citri Reticulatae) 陈皮 6g
    ding xiang (Flos Carophylli) 丁香 3g
    Method: Decoction. (Source: *Shi Yong Zhong Yi Nei Ke Xue*)

Patent medicines

Du Huo Ji Sheng Wan 独活寄生丸 (Du Huo Ji Sheng Wan)
Xiao Huo Luo Dan 小活络丹 (Xiao Huo Luo Dan)
- This formula is very hot and should only be used where Cold is very obvious. Its use should be monitored carefully. Watch for signs of

yin damage.

Zhuang Yao Jian Shen Pian 壮腰健肾片 (Zhuang Yao Jian Shen)
Die Da Zhi Tong Gao 跌打止痛膏 (Plaster for Bruise and Analgesic)
- for local application

Acupuncture

In addition to points selected according to the nature and location of the pain (see Boxes 11.2-4, pp.327-328), use plenty of moxa, either a moxa box or, better, warm needle technique. Up to three 1cm lengths of moxa stick should be used on each of three to four points per treatment.

Clinical notes

- The lower back pain in this pattern may be associated with disorders such as fibrositis, fibromyalgia, osteoarthritis and myositis.
- This is not an uncommon presentation, and the patient will usually not be aware of any particular strain or episode of mechanical stress but will often relate in their history a distinct association between getting wet, or, more usually, hot and sweaty and then getting cold. The back pain generally starts within 24 hours of such an event. Apart from the treatments mentioned in the text, this kind of patient does well with a thermal lumbar support. Gentle mobilisation exercises following a hot shower are also useful.
- Weight loss is important if appropriate.
- When travelling, these patients should be advised to use a hot water bottle on the lower back.

11.2 DAMP HEAT

Pathophysiology
- Damp Heat lower back pain is usually acute, and may be the result of invasion of a Damp Heat pathogen through the *tai yang* channels, chronic Cold Damp stagnation which transforms into Heat or referred pain from an inflamed internal organ.
- When from external Damp Heat, this pattern corresponds to inflammation of the lumbar spine and/or surrounding soft tissues.
- When from internal Damp Heat, the pain may be associated with an inflammatory or infectious process in the structures of the pelvic basin or kidneys, or with kidney stones. There may be symptoms reflecting the source (usually the middle *jiao*) and current location of the Damp Heat.

Clinical features
- the lower back area is sore and feels hot, either to the patient, the practitioner or both and may appear red and swollen
- the pain is clearly aggravated by hot, humid or rainy weather and is not improved by rest
- irritability, feverishness, thirst
- when Damp Heat affects a pelvic organ, there may be symptoms reflecting its location, for example vaginal discharge, dark urine, diarrhoea, etc.

T greasy yellow coating
P soft and rapid

Treatment principle
Clear Heat and dry Dampness
Ease the Tendons, stop pain

Prescription

JIA WEI ER MIAO SAN 加味二妙散
(*Augmented Two Marvel Powder*)

huang bai (Cortex Phellodendri) 黄柏	12g
cang zhu (Rhizoma Atractylodis) 苍术	15g
niu xi (Radix Achyranthis Bidentatae) 牛膝	12g
dang gui wei (tail of Radix Angelicae Sinensis) 当归尾	12g
fang ji (Radix Stephaniae Tetrandrae) 防己	10g
bi xie (Rhizoma Dioscoreae Hypoglaucae) 萆解	12g
yi ren (Semen Coicis Lachryma-jobi) 苡仁	20g
gan cao (Radix Glycyrrhizae Uralensis) 甘草	6g

Method: Decoction. (Source: *Zhong Yi Nei Ke Lin Chuang Shou Ce*)

Modifications
- If the Damp Heat is external, add **chai hu** (Radix Bupleuri) 柴胡 9g, **fang feng** (Radix Ledebouriellae Divaricatae) 防风 12g, **qiang huo** (Rhizoma et Radix Notopterygii) 羌活 9g and **chuan xiong** (Radix Ligustici Chuanxiong) 川芎 6g.
- In severe cases, add **hai tong pi** (Cortex Erythrinae) 海桐皮 12g, **ren dong teng** (Ramus Lonicerae Japonicae) 忍冬藤 15g and **qin jiao** (Radix Gentianae Qinjiao) 秦艽 9g.
- If the back pain is associated with Damp Heat in the Urinary Bladder or kidney stones, see Painful Urination Syndrome, pp.359, 370.

Patent medicines
Qian Jin Zhi Dai Wan 千金止带丸 (Chienchin Chih Tai Wan)
Yu Dai Wan 愈带丸 (Yudai Wan)
    - these formulae are designed to treat Damp Heat leucorrhoea but can be used to treat general Dampness and Heat in the lower *jiao*
Huang Lian Jie Du Wan 黄连解毒丸 (Huang Lian Jie Du Wan)

Acupuncture
In addition to points selected according to the nature and location of the pain (Box 11.2-4, pp.327-328), add Sp.9 (*yin ling quan*), Kid.7 (*fu liu*) and GB.34 (*yang ling quan*).

Clinical notes
- The lower back pain in this pattern may be associated with disorders such as inflammatory arthritis, acute rheumatoid arthritis, inflammatory stage of chronic osteoarthritis, inflammation of soft tissues, kidney stones, pelvic inflammatory disease, urinary tract infection, rheumatic fever, infectious arthritis, gout and osteomyelitis.
- In cases where infectious arthritis is suspected, appropriate investigations and antibiotic therapy should be instituted promptly as destruction of the affected joint may occur quickly.
- Damp Heat is a less common presentation of lower back pain than Cold Damp. In addition to the treatments in the text, the application of ice, massage and stretching may be useful.
- If the aetiology is external Damp Heat and the syndrome is untreated or unresponsive to treatment, it may progress into atrophy syndrome (*wei zheng* 痿证). This appears clinically as a condition like poliomyelitis or the sequelae of other central nervous system infections. If joints other than those of the lower back are involved the condition is reclassified as Hot painful obstruction syndrome (*bi zheng* 痹症).

11.3 WIND (DAMP, COLD OR HEAT)

外风证

Pathophysiology
- These three patterns are acute and due to invasion of Wind with either Damp, Cold or Heat into *tai yang* channels. Most commonly the upper back and neck are affected, however, the Urinary Bladder channel passes through the lower back and may be affected at that level, particularly in the presence of Kidney deficiency. Wind Damp is most likely to cause lower back ache because of the heavy nature and sinking tendency of Damp. Wind Cold lower back pain is less common and Wind Heat lower back pain is rare.
- In contrast to acute Cold Damp (p.330), which frequently becomes chronic, these patterns are self limiting, usually reflecting a viral or influenza like illness.

11.3.1 WIND DAMP

风湿

Clinical features
- acute lower back pain, heaviness or ache and stiffness, unrelieved by changing position or stretching
- generalised sensation of heaviness in the body
- headache or woolly headedness
- mild fever and chills
- maybe mild superficial oedema

T generally normal, or with a thin greasy white coat
P floating

Treatment principle
Expel Wind Damp

Prescription

QIANG HUO SHENG SHI TANG 羌活胜湿汤
(*Notopterygium Decoction to Overcome Dampness*)

qiang huo (Rhizoma et Radix Notopterygii) 羌活	9g
du huo (Radix Angelicae Pubescentis) 独活	9g
gao ben (Rhizoma et Radix Ligustici) 藁本	6g
fang feng (Radix Ledebouriellae Divaricatae) 防风	6g
chuan xiong (Radix Ligustici Chuanxiong) 川芎	6g
man jing zi (Fructus Viticis) 蔓荆子	6g
zhi gan cao (honey fried Radix Glycyrrhizae Uralensis) 炙甘草	3g

Method: Decoction. (Source: *Formulas and Strategies*)

Modifications
- With Cold, add **gui zhi** (Ramulus Cinnamomi Cassiae) 桂枝 6g and **ma huang*** (Herba Ephedrae) 麻黄 6g.
- With severe Damp, add **cang zhu** (Rhizoma Atractylodis) 苍术 9g.
- With severe pain, add **zhi fu zi*** (Radix Aconiti Carmichaeli Praeparata) 制附子 6g.

Patent medicines
Du Huo Ji Sheng Wan 独活寄生丸 (Du Huo Ji Sheng Wan)
Gan Mao Qing Re Chong Ji 感冒清热冲剂 (Gan Mao Qing Re Chong Ji)

Acupuncture
Lu.6 (*kong zui* -), LI.4 (*he gu* -), SJ.6 (*zhi gou* -), Sp.9 (*yin ling quan* -), Ren.12 (*zhong wan* -), St.36 (*zu san li* -)

11.3.2 WIND COLD

Clinical features
- acute lower back ache, unrelieved by changing position or stretching
- high fever and chills or shivering
- generalised myalgia
- stiff neck, occipital headache
- no sweating
- cough
- nasal obstruction, or runny nose with thin watery mucus
- sneezing

T normal or with a thin or greasy white coat
P floating and soggy, or floating and tight

Treatment principle
Disperse Wind Cold

Prescription

JING FANG BAI DU SAN 荆防败毒散
(*Schizonepeta and Ledebouriella Powder to Overcome Pathogenic Influences*)

jing jie (Herba seu Flos Schizonepetae Tenuifolia) 荆芥	10g
fang feng (Radix Ledebouriellae Divaricatae) 防风	10g
qiang huo (Rhizoma et Radix Notopterygii) 羌活	8g
du huo (Radix Angelicae Pubescentis) 独活	6g
chuan xiong (Radix Ligustici Chuanxiong) 川芎	8g
jie geng (Radix Platycodi Grandiflori) 桔梗	10g
qian hu (Radix Peucedani) 前胡	10g

chao xing ren* (dry fried Semen Pruni Armeniacae)
炒杏仁 6g
zhi ke (Fructus Citri Aurantii) 枳壳 9g
sheng jiang (Rhizoma Zingiberis Officinalis Recens)
生姜 3g

Method: Decoction. The herbs should be gently simmered with a lid on for no longer than 20 minutes. Take hot or follow with hot porridge or congee to induce sweating. (Source: *Formulas and Strategies*)

Modifications

♦ With internal Damp (fullness and distension in the chest and epigastrium, poor appetite and nausea), add **zhi xiang fu** (prepared Rhizoma Cyperi Rotundi) 制香附 10g, **zi su ye** (Folium Perillae Frutescentis) 紫苏叶 12g and **chen pi** (Pericarpium Citri Reticulatae) 陈皮 10g.

Patent medicines

Gan Mao Ling 感冒灵 (Gan Mao Ling)
Chuan Xiong Cha Tiao Wan 川芎茶调丸 (Chuan Xiong Cha Tiao Wan)
  - with headache
Gan Mao Qing Re Chong Ji 感冒清热冲剂 (Gan Mao Qing Re Chong Ji)

Acupuncture

LI.4 (*he gu* -), Lu.7 (*lie que* -), GB.20 (*feng chi* -), Bl.12 (*feng men* - Ω), Bl.13 (*fei shu* - Ω). Cups can be applied to *ah shi* points on the lower back.

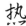

11.3.3 WIND HEAT
Clinical features

• acute lower back pain or heat, unrelieved by changing position or stretching
• fever
• mild sweating
• dry mouth, thirst
• sore throat
T normal or with a red tip
P floating and rapid

Treatment principle

Dispel Wind Heat

Prescription

XIAO CHAI HU TANG 小柴胡汤
(*Minor Bupleurum Combination*) modified

chai hu (Radix Bupleuri) 柴胡	12g
huang qin (Radix Scutellariae Baicalensis) 黄芩	9g
qiang huo (Rhizoma et Radix Notopterygii) 羌活	9g
xu duan (Radix Dipsaci Asperi) 续断	9g
hei dou (Semen Glycines Nigrum) 黑豆	9g
ren shen (Radix Ginseng) 人参	6g
sheng jiang (Rhizoma Zingiberis Officinalis Recens) 生姜	3pce
da zao (Fructus Zizyphi Jujubae) 大枣	3pce

Method: Decoction. (Source: *Shi Yong Zhong Yi Nei Ke Xue*)

Modifications

- With constipation, add **da huang** (Radix et Rhizoma Rhei) 大黄 3-6g.

Patent medicines

Yin Qiao Jie Du Pian 银翘解毒片 (Yin Chiao Chieh Tu Pien)
Gan Mao Zhi Ke Chong Ji 感冒止咳冲剂 (Gan Mao Zhi Ke Chong Ji)
Gan Mao Ling 感冒灵 (Gan Mao Ling)
Xiao Chai Hu Wan 小柴胡丸 (Xiao Chai Hu Wan)

Acupuncture

Du.14 (*da zhui* -Ω), Bl.12 (*feng men* -Ω), LI.11 (*qu chi* -), LI.4 (*he gu* -), SJ.5 (*wai guan* -). Cups can be applied to *ah shi* points on the lower back.
- If the throat is very sore and swollen add Lu.11 (*shao shang* ↓) and SI.17 (*tian rong* -)

Clinical notes

- The lower back pain in this pattern may be associated with disorders such as the common cold, influenza, tonsillitis, upper respiratory tract infection, acute bronchitis, early stage of measles, encephalitis or meningitis.
- Strong cupping is very useful in any early stage Wind disorder.
- The back pain of an external Wind pattern may precede the systemic symptoms by a day or two and persist when other symptoms appear.

瘀血腰痛

11.4 BLOOD STAGNATION

Pathophysiology
- This type of lower back pain is usually acute and follows some trauma or injury, typically lifting a heavy object, or twisting and bending while lifting. The precipitating event may be trivial and pain may occur one or two days after a mild sprain, or even coughing or sneezing. In practice there is often no discernible event.
- Stagnant Blood can also intervene in prolonged lower back pain due to some other pathogenic process, such as chronic Cold Damp.

Clinical features
- Sharp, piercing lower back pain that is fixed in location and aggravated by pressure and palpation. In severe cases movement is difficult or very painful and the range of movement is very restricted. The pain may be worse in the evening and is unaffected by weather or temperature changes.

T in acute cases the tongue may be unremarkable; in chronic cases it may have a purplish tinge, or purplish spots
P choppy or wiry

Treatment principle
Invigorate the circulation of Blood, eliminate stagnant Blood
Regulate *qi* and stop pain

Prescription

HUO LUO XIAO LING DAN 活络校灵丹
(*Fantastically Effective Pill to Invigorate the Collaterals*) modified

dan shen (Radix Salviae Miltiorrhizae) 丹参	25g
dang gui (Radix Angelicae Sinensis) 当归	12g
chuan niu xi (Radix Cyathulae Officinalis) 川牛膝	12g
yan hu suo (Rhizoma Corydalis Yanhusuo) 延胡索	12g
tao ren (Semen Persicae) 桃仁	12g
ru xiang (Gummi Olibanum) 乳香	10g
mo yao (Myrrha) 没药	10g
hong hua (Flos Carthami Tinctorii) 红花	10g
chuan xiong (Rhizoma Ligustici Chuanxiong) 川芎	10g
gan cao (Radix Glycyrrhizae Uralensis) 甘草	10g
di bie chong (Eupolyphaga seu Opisthoplatia) 地鳖虫	6g

Method: Decoction. (Source: *Zhong Yi Nei Ke Lin Chuang Shou Ce*)

Modifications
- With Dampness (thick tongue coat, a sensation of heaviness as well as severe lower back pain), add **du huo** (Radix Angelicae Pubescentis) 独活 9g, **wei ling xian*** (Radix Clematidis) 威灵仙 9g and **qin jiao** (Radix Gentianae Qinjiao) 秦艽 9g.
- With Kidney weakness, add **xu duan** (Radix Dipsaci Asperi) 续断 15g and **du zhong** (Cortex Eucommiae Ulmoidis) 杜仲 9g.

Patent medicines
Jin Gu Die Shang Wan 筋骨跌伤丸 (Chin Koo Tieh Shang Wan)
 - used for acute traumatic injury including fractures, sprains and bruising with pain and swelling

Shu Jin Huo Xue Wan 舒筋活血丸 (Shu Jin Huo Xue Wan)
 - good for chronic Blood stagnation patterns

Zheng Gu Shui liniment 正骨水 (Zheng Gu Shui)
 - excellent for acute sprains. Apply liberally and frequently.

Die Da Zhi Tong Gao 跌打止痛膏 (Plaster for Bruise and Analgesic)
 - excellent for local application

Die Da Tian Qi Yao Jiu 跌打田七药酒 (Die Da Tian Qi Yao Jiu)
 - powerful liniment favoured by martial artists

Acupuncture
In addition to points selected according to the nature and location of the pain (Box 11.2-4, pp.311-12), add LI.4 (*he gu* -), Bl.17 (*ge shu* -), Sp.10 (*xue hai* -) and Sp.6 (*san yin jiao* -).

Clinical notes
- The lower back pain in this pattern may be associated with disorders such as acute back sprain, traumatic back injury, vertebral disc herniation and facet joint syndrome.
- Acupuncture is the treatment of choice in acute cases, and the pattern generally responds well to correct treatment.
- The prone position may exacerbate pain, so in the early stages patients are best treated seated and leaning forward. Lying on the side (lateral recumbent) with hips and knees slightly flexed is also usually comfortable. A pillow between the knees in this position is useful.
- In the early stages (for the first few days, or while pressure on the spine elicits sharp pain) pressure and massage are contraindicated.

11.5 LIVER *QI* STAGNATION

肝气郁滞腰痛

Pathophysiology
- This pattern is characterised by generalised hypertonicity of muscles (compare with Spleen *qi* deficiency) and occurs in tense, emotionally repressed or stressed individuals. The chronic 'holding pattern' of emotion locked away in the muscles causes poor elasticity and nutrition and predisposes the lower back to injury.

Clinical features
- Lower back pain which tends to be aggravated by stress and emotional upset and often radiates from the lower back to the lower abdomen or hypochondriac region. The pain is vague and distending, may move from place to place and come and go. When identifying the painful area, the patient often uses the whole hand and indicates a large area. The range of motion may be normal or only slightly restricted.
- other signs of stagnant Liver *qi*, such as irritability, headaches, digestive upset, fullness in the chest, irregular menstruation or premenstrual syndrome may be present

T darkish (*qing* 青) or with red edges and a thin coat
P wiry and thready, or deep and wiry

Treatment principle
Regulate the Liver, move *qi*

Prescription

TIAN TAI WU YAO SAN 天台乌药散
(*Top Quality Lindera Powder*) modified

wu yao (Radix Linderae Strychnifoliae) 乌药	15g
mu xiang (Radix Aucklandiae Lappae) 木香	15g
chao xiao hui xiang (dry fried Fructus Foeniculi Vulgaris) 炒小茴香	15g
qing pi (Pericarpium Citri Reticulatae Viride) 青皮	15g
gao liang jiang (Rhizoma Alpiniae Officinari) 高良姜	15g
chuan lian zi* (Fructus Meliae Toosendan) 川楝子	9g
bing lang (Semen Arecae Catechu) 槟榔	6g

Method: Grind herbs to a powder and take 3 grams as a draft, 2-3 times daily or as a decoction with 30% reduction in dosage. (Source: *Shi Yong Zhong Yi Nei Ke Xue*)

Modifications
- With Dampness, add **cang zhu** (Rhizoma Atractylodis) 苍术 9g and **yi ren** (Semen Coicis Lachryma-jobi) 苡仁 15g.

- With Damp Heat add, **cang zhu** (Rhizoma Atractylodis) 苍术 9g and **huang bai** (Cortex Phellodendri) 黄柏 9g.
- With Spleen deficiency, add **dang shen** (Radix Codonopsis Pilosulae) 党参 12g, **bai zhu** (Rhizoma Atractylodes Macrocephalae) 白术 12g and **gan cao** (Radix Glycyrrhizae Uralensis) 甘草 6g.
- With *yin* deficiency, add **bai shao** (Radix Paeoniae Lactiflora) 白芍 12g and **gou qi zi** (Fructus Lycii) 枸杞子 12g, or combine with **LIU WEI DI HUANG WAN** (*Rehmania Six Formula* 六味地黄丸, p.391).

Patent medicines
Shu Gan Wan 舒肝丸 (Shu Gan Wan)
Chai Hu Shu Gan Wan 柴胡舒肝丸 (Chai Hu Shu Gan Wan)
Mu Xiang Shun Qi Wan 木香顺气丸 (Aplotaxis Carminative Pills)

Acupuncture
In addition to points selected according to the nature and location of the pain (see Boxes 11.2-4, pp.311-12), use Liv.3 (*tai chong*), LI.4 (*he gu*), GB.34 (*yang ling quan*) and PC.6 (*nei guan*)

Clinical notes
- The pathology underlying this type of back pain can predispose an individual to injury as the soft tissues of the back are in a state of chronic tension. The pattern generally responds well to acupuncture treatment and stress management.
- Other therapies that are useful in long term resolution of this pattern are specific exercises for toning the back (and general exercise to move Liver *qi*), for example stretching, massage, yoga and relaxation.

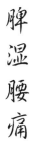

11.6 SPLEEN DEFICIENCY (WITH DAMP)

Pathophysiology
- Spleen deficiency lower back ache is characterised by generalised muscular hypotonicity (compare with Liver *qi* stagnation), loss of mechanical support and hypermobility of the lumbar spine. The weakened Spleen may also fail to produce sufficient *qi* and Blood to nourish the tissues of the lower back, or allow accumulation of Damp.

Clinical features
- aching and heaviness of the lower back region, which may be flabby and with poor muscle tone
- tendency to be overweight, and have poor posture
- depending on the degree of Spleen deficiency, there may be symptoms of digestive weakness or fluid retention

T pale, swollen or with a greasy white coat
P slippery or soft

Treatment principle
Strengthen the Spleen to eliminate Damp

Prescription

BU ZHONG YI QI TANG 补中益气汤
(*Ginseng and Astragalus Combination*) modified

This formula is particularly good for general Spleen deficiency with poor and flabby muscle tone.

huang qi (Radix Astragali Membranacei) 黄芪	15g
bu gu zhi (Fructus Psoraleae Corylifoliae) 补骨脂	12g
xu duan (Radix Dipsaci Asperi) 续断	12g
tu si zi (Semen Cuscutae Chinensis) 菟丝子	12g
dang shen (Radix Codonopsis Pilosulae) 党参	12g
bai zhu (Rhizoma Atractylodes Macrocephalae) 白术	12g
dang gui (Radix Angelicae Sinensis) 当归	9g
chen pi (Pericarpium Citri Reticulatae) 陈皮	6g
zhi gan cao (honey fried Radix Glycyrrhizae Uralensis) 炙甘草	6g
sheng ma (Rhizoma Cimicifugae) 升麻	3g
chai hu (Radix Bupleuri) 柴胡	3g

Method: Decoction. May also be powdered and taken in doses of 9 grams as a draft.

PING WEI SAN 平胃散
(Magnolia and Ginger Formula)

This formula is selected when signs of Spleen Damp (abdominal bloating, diarrhoea, flabby tongue with a greasy tongue coat) are obvious.

    cang zhu (Rhizoma Atractylodis) 苍术 15g
    hou po (Cortex Magnoliae Officinalis) 厚朴 12g
    chen pi (Pericarpium Citri Reticulatae) 陈皮 9g
    gan cao (Radix Glycyrrhizae Uralensis) 甘草 3g
    sheng jiang (Rhizoma Zingiberis Officinalis) 生姜 3pce
    da zao (Fructus Zizyphi Jujubae) 大枣 4pce
    Method: Decoction. (Source: *Shi Yong Zhong Yi Nei Ke Xue*)

FANG JI HUANG QI TANG 防己黄芪汤
(Stephania and Astragalus Combination)

This prescription is selected in cases with mild Damp accumulation (especially when it also affects the knees causing swelling and pain) and easy sweating.

    huang qi (Radix Astragali Membranacei) 黄芪 15g
    fang ji (Radix Stephaniae Tetrandrae) 防己 12g
    bai zhu (Rhizoma Atractylodes Macrocephalae) 白术 12g
    zhi gan cao (honey fried Radix Glycyrrhizae Uralensis)
        炙甘草 3g
    sheng jiang (Rhizoma Zingiberis Officinalis) 生姜 4pce
    da zao (Fructus Zizyphi Jujubae) 大枣 1pce
    Method: Decoction. (Source: *Shi Yong Zhong Yi Nei Ke Xue*)

SHI PI YIN 实脾饮
(Magnolia and Atractylodes Combination) modified

This formula is selected when there are signs of Spleen *yang* deficiency and obvious Damp accumulation (pitting oedema) in the tissues.

    hou po (Cortex Magnoliae Officinalis) 厚朴 30g
    bai zhu (Rhizoma Atractylodes Macrocephalae) 白术 30g
    mu gua (Fructus Chaenomelis) 木瓜 30g
    mu xiang (Radix Aucklandiae Lappae) 木香 30g
    cao guo (Fructus Amomi Tsao-ko) 草果 30g
    bing lang (Semen Arecae Catechu) 槟榔 30g
    zhi fu zi* (Radix Aconiti Carmichaeli Praeparata) 制附子 30g
    fu ling (Sclerotium Poria Cocos) 茯苓 30g
    gan jiang (Rhizoma Zingiberis Officinalis) 干姜 30g
    zhi gan cao (honey fried Radix Glycyrrhizae Uralensis)
        炙甘草 15g

da zao (Fructus Zizyphi Jujubae) 大枣 5pce
Method: Grind herbs to powder and take in 10-12 gram drafts with boiled water. It may also be decocted, with a 60-80% reduction in dosage. When decocted **zhi fu zi** is generally cooked for 30 minutes before adding the other herbs (*xian jian* 先煎). (Source: *Shi Yong Zhong Yi Nei Ke Xue*)

Patent medicines
Bu Zhong Yi Qi Wan 补中益气丸 (Bu Zhong Yi Qi Wan)
 - Spleen *qi* deficiency
Xiang Sha Liu Jun Zi Wan 香砂六君子丸 (Aplotaxis-Ammomum Pills)
 - Spleen *qi* deficiency with Dampness
Fu Zi Li Zhong Wan 附子理中丸 (Li Chung Yuen Medical Pills)
 - with signs of Spleen *yang* deficiency or Cold
Li Zhong Wan 理中丸 (Li Zhong Wan)
 - *yang* deficiency

Acupuncture
In addition to points selected according to the nature and location of the pain (see Box 11.2-4, pp.311-12), add Sp.9 (*yin ling quan*), Sp.3 (*tai bai*), St.40 (*feng long*), St.36 (*zu san li* +) and Bl.20 (*pi shu* +)

Clinical notes
- This type of lower back pain is generally mild and tends to occur in those with an inactive and sedentary lifestyle, or in those who suffer from some immobilising disorder.
- This pattern responds well to correct treatment if the patient also starts exercising and develops correct posture. Excercise is often the key feature of treatment, and results are likely to be poor without it. The patient may also need to change diet and in some cases lose weight. Abdominal exercises are useful, and the patient will be better with a kidney belt or thermal lumbar support.

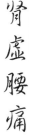

11.7 KIDNEY DEFICIENCY

Pathophysiology
- The Kidneys have a powerful influence over the tissues of the lower back, and (in association with the Spleen's role in general muscle tone) are largely responsible for the strength and integrity of the lower back. Weakness of the Kidneys can lead to inadequate or sluggish circulation of *qi* and Blood through the area, predisposing to injury or allowing invasion by pathogens (especially Cold and Damp).

Clinical features
General features
- chronic dull lower back ache, soreness or weakness, improved by massage and rest
- the pain recurs frequently, and is aggravated by exertion, prolonged standing, sexual activity and fatigue
- weak, sore legs and knees

In addition there may be:

Kidney *qi* deficiency
- clear copious urine, urinary frequency or nocturia, pale lustreless complexion, oedema of the lower extremities, sore knees, a pale or pink tongue with a thin white coat and a deep, thready pulse

Kidney *yang* deficiency
- same as for Kidney *qi* deficiency, with the addition of Cold signs, such as cold extremities, cold intolerance, a wet, swollen tongue with a white coat and slow pulse

Kidney *yin* deficiency
- heat intolerance, occasional urinary irritation or mild discomfort, tinnitus, dizziness, facial flushing, nightsweats, sensation of heat in the palms and soles ('five hearts hot'), a red tongue with little or no coat and a thready, rapid pulse

11.7.1 Kidney *yang* (*qi*) deficiency
Treatment principle
Support and strengthen the lower back
Tonify the Kidneys and support *yang*

Prescription

YOU GUI WAN 右归丸
(*Eucommia and Rehmannia Formula*) modified

shu di (Radix Rehmanniae Glutinosae Conquitae) 熟地	250g
shan yao (Radix Dioscoreae Oppositae) 山药	120g
lu jiao jiao^ (Cornu Cervi Gelatinum) 鹿角胶	120g
tu si zi (Semen Cuscutae Chinensis) 菟丝子	120g
gou qi zi (Fructus Lycii) 枸杞子	120g
du zhong (Cortex Eucommiae Ulmoidis) 杜仲	120g
huai niu xi (Radix Achyranthis Bidentatae) 怀牛膝	120g
xu duan (Radix Dipsaci Asperi) 续断	120g
shan zhu yu (Fructus Corni Officinalis) 山茱萸	90g
dang gui (Radix Angelicae Sinensis) 当归	90g
zhi fu zi* (Radix Aconiti Carmichaeli Praeparata) 制附子	60-180g
rou gui (Cortex Cinnamomi Cassiae) 肉桂	60-120g

Method: Grind herbs to powder and form into 9-gram pills with honey. The dose is one pill 2-3 times daily. May also be decocted with a 90% reduction in dosage, in which case **zhi fu zi** is cooked for 30 minutes before the other herbs are added (*xian jian* 先煎), **rou gui** is added towards the end of cooking (*hou xia* 后下) and **lu jiao jiao** is melted before being added to the strained decoction (*yang hua* 烊化). (Source: *Zhong Yi Nei Ke Lin Chuang Shou Ce*)

Modifications

♦ With few Cold signs (i.e. Kidney *qi* deficiency), delete **zhi fu zi** and **rou gui**, and add **ren shen** (Radix Ginseng) 人参 90g or **dang shen** (Radix Codonopsis Pilosulae) 党参 150g.

11.7.2 Kidney *yin* deficiency

Treatment principle

Tonify the Kidneys and nourish *yin*
Strengthen and support the lower back

Prescription

ZUO GUI WAN 左归丸
(*Achyranthes and Rehmannia Formula*) modified

sheng di (Radix Rehmanniae Glutinosae) 生地	240g
shan yao (Radix Dioscoreae Oppositae) 山药	120g
shan zhu yu (Fructus Corni Officinalis) 山茱萸	120g
gou qi zi (Fructus Lycii) 枸杞子	120g
tu si zi (Semen Cuscutae Chinensis) 菟丝子	120g
gui ban jiao° (Plastri Testudinis Gelatinum) 龟板胶	120g

  lu jiao jiao^ (Cornu Cervi Gelatinum) 鹿角胶 120g
  huai niu xi (Radix Achyranthis Bidentatae) 怀牛膝 90g
  Method: Grind herbs to powder and form into 9-gram pills with honey. The dose is one pill 2-3 times daily. May be decocted with a 90% reduction in dosages. In decoction, **lu jiao jiao** and **gui ban jiao** are melted before being added to the strained decoction (*yang hua* 烊化).

Modifications
- With severe pain, add **sang ji sheng** (Ramulus Sangjisheng) 桑寄生 120g.
- With lots of deficient Heat, add **nu zhen zi** (Fructus Ligustri Lucidi) 女贞子 90g and **han lian cao** (Herba Ecliptae Prostratae) 旱连草 90g, or combine with **DA BU YIN WAN** (*Great Tonify the yin Pill* 大补阴丸, p.407).

Patent medicines
Kidney *yang* (*qi*) deficiency
Jin Kui Shen Qi Wan 金匮肾气丸 (Sexoton Pills)
Zhuang Yao Jian Shen Pian 壮腰健肾片 (Zhuang Yao Jian Shen)
Jian Bu Qiang Shen Wan 健步强身丸 (Jian Bu Qiang Shen Wan)
Xiao Huo Luo Dan 小活络丹 (Xiao Huo Luo Dan)
 - add a small dose when Cold and pain are severe

Kidney *yin* deficiency
Liu Wei Di Huang Wan 六味地黄丸 (Liu Wei Di Huang Wan)
Zhi Bai Ba Wei Wan 知柏八味丸 (Zhi Bai Ba Wei Wan)

Acupuncture
Bl.23 (*shen shu* +), Bl.25 (*da chang shu* +), Du.4 (*ming men* +), Bl.52 (*zhi shi* +), Ren.4 (*qi hai* +), Ren.6 (*guan yuan* +), Kid.3 (*tai xi* +), Bl.60 (*kun lun*), *hua tuo jia ji* (M-BW-35) when tender.
 • add moxa in *yang* deficiency

Clinical notes
- The lower back pain in this pattern may be associated with disorders such as chronic back ache, lumbago, chronic nephritis, osteoporosis, chronic disc disorder, ankylosing spondylitis and osteoarthritis of the spine.
- Satisfactory results in these patterns generally take time to achieve and a combination of acupuncture and herbs achieves the best outcome.

SUMMARY OF GUIDING FORMULAE FOR LOWER BACK PAIN

Acute patterns

Cold Damp - *Gan Jiang Ling Zhu Tang* 干姜苓术汤 plus *Du Huo Ji Sheng Tang* 独活寄生汤

Damp Heat - *Jia Wei Er Miao San* 加味二妙散

Wind Damp - *Qiang Huo Sheng Shi Tang* 羌活胜湿汤

Wind Cold - *Jing Fang Bai Du San* 荆防败毒散

Wind Heat - *Xiao Chai Hu Tang* 小柴胡汤

Blood stagnation - *Huo Luo Xiao Ling Dan* 活络效灵丹

Chronic patterns

Liver *qi* stagnation - *Tian Tai Wu Yao San* 天台乌药散

Spleen deficiency - *Bu Zhong Yi Qi Tang* 补中益气汤
- with Spleen Damp - *Ping Wei San* 平胃散
- with knee pain and sweating - *Fang Ji Huang Qi Tang* 防己黄芪汤
- with Cold, Spleen *yang* deficiency and oedema - *Shi Pi Yin* 实脾饮

Kidney deficiency
- *yang* (*qi*) deficiency - *You Gui Wan* 右归丸
- *yin* deficiency - *Zuo Gui Wan* 左归丸

Endnote

For more information regarding herbs marked with an asterisk*, an open circle° or a hat^, see the tables on pp.944-952.

Disorders of the Kidney

12. Painful Urination Syndrome

Heat painful urination
Damp Heat
Liver Fire
Heart Fire

Stone painful urination
asymptomatic stones
with Damp Heat
with Blood stagnation
with Kidney deficiency

Qi painful urination
Qi stagnation
Qi deficiency

Blood painful urination
Heat, Damp Heat
Blood stagnation
Kidney *yin* deficiency

Cloudy painful urination
Damp Heat
Kidney *qi* deficiency

Exhaustion painful urination
Spleen and Kidney *yang* deficiency
Kidney *yin* deficiency
Heart and Kidney *qi* and *yin* deficiency

12 | PAINFUL URINATION SYNDROME
lin zheng 淋证

Painful urination syndrome includes a variety of disorders characterised by pain associated with urination. The *key feature* in painful urination syndrome is pain, and it is the presence of pain that differentiates this group of disorders from other urinary disorders. Blood in the urine with no pain is classified as haematuria, while blood in the urine with pain is classified as Blood painful urination syndrome.

Painful urination is a very common clinical presentation, and may include a variety of symptoms associated with the passage of urine, including suprapubic discomfort and pain, frequency, tenesmus and urinary difficulty. Painful urination syndrome is most common in women.

> **BOX 12.1 TCM CLASSIFICATION OF PAINFUL URINATION**
>
> - **Heat** painful urination is clinically the most common variety, and is characterised by being acute and by rather intense burning pain upon urination. It is thought that in all acute cases of painful urination syndrome there is some degree of Heat. It is further divided into two types, Damp Heat and Fire. Damp Heat may occur alone or be found as a contributing feature in stone, Blood and cloudy painful urination syndrome.
>
> - **Stone** (or **sand** 砂) painful urination is characterised by the presence of urinary calculi or gravel, and, depending on the location of the stones, intense radiating pain and/or obstructed urination.
>
> - **Qi** painful urination is traditionally divided into two types, deficiency (of *qi*) and excess (*qi* stagnation). The deficiency type is associated with Spleen *qi* deficiency and often follows recurrent Heat types that have not been treated or treated with antibiotics or excessively cold natured herbs. It is characterised by a dragging discomfort which is relieved by pressure, or a feeling of burning that improves with warmth and pressure. It is traditionally placed in this category, although it overlaps with the Exhaustion types. The excess type is characterised by painful urination aggravated or initiated by stress and emotional upset.
>
> - **Blood** painful urination is painful urination with bleeding.
>
> - **Cloudy** painful urination is painful urination with cloudy or milky urine.
>
> - **Exhaustion** painful urination is chronic and recurrent, and is initiated or aggravated by sex, overexertion and when fatigued. It is characterised by incomplete or dribbling urination, lumbar pain and weakness, and mild pain, which is often worse following urination.

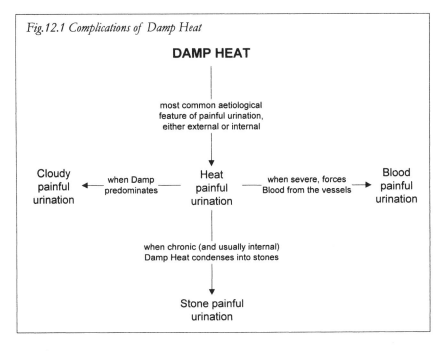

Fig.12.1 Complications of Damp Heat

AETIOLOGY
Heat and Damp Heat in the Bladder

External Heat

Damp Heat causing painful urination syndrome is most commonly due to an external Damp Heat pathogen that invades through the *tai yang* (Urinary Bladder) channel, the leg *yin* channels or the local *luo* channels. The local *luo* channels are small branches of the major channels that spread through the genitourinary system. They can be conduits for infection during sexual intercourse or after bowel movements. In practice, transmission of Damp Heat through the *luo* channels is probably the most common mode of entry, (especially in sexually active individuals).

Internal Heat

Internally generated Heat or Damp Heat can also cause painful urination. Heat affecting the Heart or Liver can be transmitted through their associated channels to the lower *jiao*. Damp Heat generated in the middle *jiao* by overconsumption of rich, greasy or spicy foods and alcohol can simply sink and settle in the lower *jiao*. Damp Heat can also be generated in the lower *jiao* by any prolonged Heat in the system, such as the Heat arising from *yin* deficiency, *qi* stagnation, or by prolonged stagnation of Dampness. Internal Heat can also be caused by stress and emotional turmoil, which disrupt the circulation of Heart and Liver *qi*, giving rise to Heart or Liver Fire. When Heat is generated internally, the symptoms tend to be more systemic, reflecting the original source of the Heat. Heat of external origin, however, tends to produce a more localised pattern, with the focus of symptoms in the bladder and urethra.

Once the Heat/Dampness cycle is established it can give rise to other types of painful urination syndrome (Fig 12.1). For example, long term Damp Heat in the lower *jiao* may congeal into urinary stones. The Heat can injure the Blood vessels of the urinary system causing bleeding. The murky nature of Damp Heat can give rise to opaque or turbid urine–cloudy painful urination syndrome. The Heat types all tend to be more common in women than in men.

> **BOX 12.2 SOME BIOMEDICAL CAUSES OF PAINFUL URINATION**
>
> - urinary infection, cystitis, urethritis
> - severe infections like gonorrhoea, pyelonephritis and herpes
> - urethral syndrome
> - vaginitis
> - neoplasms of the bladder, prostate and urethra
> - Reiter's disease
> - urinary calculi
> - menopausal syndrome
> - prostatitis
> - foreign body in the lower urinary tract
> - acidic urine
> - interstitial cystitis
> - vaginal prolapse
> - urethral stricture
> - chyluria
> - albuminuria

Liver *qi* stagnation, Blood stagnation

Frustration, anger, resentment, sexual tension, repressed emotion and stress can disrupt the circulation of Liver *qi*, and because the Liver channel passes through the lower *jiao*, the movement of lower *jiao qi* is obstructed. When lower *jiao qi* is obstructed, pain and distension may occur and the movement of fluids may be impaired resulting in urinary difficulty.

Liver *qi* stagnation may be complicated by other pathologies. The emotions that give rise to stagnant *qi* (particularly anger and resentment) 'smoulder' in the Liver and create stagnant Heat, which can be transmitted through the Liver channel to the lower *jiao*, or to the Heart and then to the Small Intestine. Obstructed *qi* may fail to lead the Blood, resulting in *qi* and Blood stagnation. Stagnant *qi* can invade the Spleen, causing deficiency and either contributing to exhaustion painful urination or leading to the development of Dampness, which sinks into the lower *jiao*, potentially generating Heat and establishing the Damp Heat cycle.

Pre-existing stagnation (of *qi* and/or Blood) can be transferred from another pelvic organ to the Bladder. This is occasionally observed in women following hysterectomy, myomectomy or removal of ovarian cysts. The organ first affected by the stagnation is removed or repaired, but the *qi* and/or Blood stagnation that gave rise to the initial problem persists. The focus of pelvic symptoms then shifts from the initial site of the stagnation to the Bladder.

Kidney deficiency

Kidney deficiency can be either *yang* or *yin* deficiency. It may be inherited, or it may develop as a result of age, chronic illness or excessive sexual activity. It can also develop in women who have many pregnancies close together, regardless of whether these result in live birth, miscarriage or termination.

Kidney *yang* or *qi* is particularly affected by prolonged exposure to cold conditions or excessive lifting or standing (particularly if this occurs in a cold environment or on cold floors or at night). In some cases, particularly in younger people, Kidney *qi* may be weakened while Kidney *yang* remains intact, in which case the cold symptoms are not seen.

Kidney *yin* is damaged through overwork (especially while under stress), insufficient sleep, febrile diseases, insufficient hydration and the use of some prescription and recreational drugs. The Kidney and Bladder are closely related, so weakness of the Kidney can affect the Bladder. When Kidney *qi* is weak, the Bladder is vulnerable to pathogenic invasion (through the *tai yang*, leg *yin* channels or local *luo* channels), especially by Damp Heat.

BOX 12.3 KEY DIAGNOSTIC POINTS

Colour of urine
- dark, concentrated urine - Heat, Damp Heat or *yin* deficiency
- pale - Kidney *yang* deficiency, Spleen *qi* deficiency or *qi* stagnation
- cloudy and murky - Dampness or Damp Heat
- pale pink to bright red or purple - bleeding due to Fire, Damp Heat, stagnant Blood, Kidney *yin* deficiency or stones

Pain
- burning - Heat or Damp Heat (severe, like 'passing glass'), or *yin* deficiency (mild)
- stabbing and localised, with or without flecks of blood - Blood stagnation or urinary stones
- mild or dragging, or 'empty discomfort' following urination - *qi* deficiency

Frequency
- frequent, urgent and concentrated - Heat or Damp Heat
- frequent and pale - Kidney *yang* or *qi* deficiency
- frequent and pale with a weak or broken stream - Kidney *yang* deficiency

Timing of the pain
- during urination - excess conditions
- before urination - *qi* stagnation
- after urination - deficient conditions

Spleen deficiency

Spleen deficiency patterns may result from frequent use of antibiotics of bitter cold herbs (both of which easily weaken the Spleen) in the treatment of recurrent Damp Heat or Heat types of painful urination. This pattern may also follow lower abdominal surgery or be associated with prolapse of the bladder or uterus. In these latter cases the sensation is generally one of pressure and discomfort in the suprapubic region rather than urethral pain with urination.

TREATMENT

Personal hygiene is very important. In particular, correct wiping after bowel movements (front to back) is important for girls and women to avoid contamination of the urethra and bladder with intestinal bacteria. Synthetic and tight underwear should be avoided. Some women are prone to bladder infection or irritation after sexual intercourse–these women should be advised to empty the bladder immediately after sex and to experiment with different positions. Partners should also be examined so as to eliminate them as a chronic carrier, who may be the source of reinfection. Plenty of fluid is essential, approximately 1.5-2 litres per day and more during an episode of painful urination syndrome.

Acute cases of Damp Heat type painful urination (clinically the most common) are often accompanied by apparent external symptoms, especially fever and chills. It was noted however, as early as the Han Dynasty by *Zhang Zhong-jing*, that diaphoresis is contraindicated. The rationale is that the fever and chills are the result of the 'steam' produced by the struggle between Damp Heat and *zheng qi* in the Bladder, and because of the Heat, *yin* fluids have already been damaged. Causing a sweat will only damage fluids further and aggravate the condition.

All patients with recurrent urinary tract disorder or persistent haematuria should be referred to a urologist for appropriate investigations, for example cystoscopy or intravenous pyelography (IVP) to exclude neoplasm.

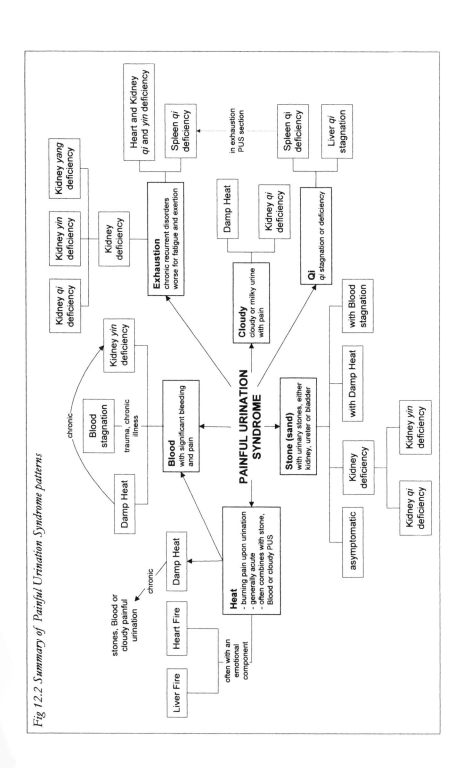

Fig 12.2 Summary of Painful Urination Syndrome patterns

12.1 HEAT PAINFUL URINATION SYNDROME

- Damp Heat
- Heart Fire
- Liver Fire

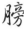

12.1.1 DAMP HEAT IN THE URINARY BLADDER

Pathophysiology
- Damp Heat painful urination is most commonly due to invasion of pathogenic Heat (or Cold, which turns to Heat once inside) through the *tai yang* channels (Bladder and Small Intestine), leg *yin* channels or the local *luo* channels into the urethra and Bladder. Invasion by external pathogens may be facilitated by a pre-existing Kidney deficiency.
- When transmission of Damp Heat is direct (i.e. external Damp Heat that enters through the local *luo* channels, *tai yang* or leg *yin* channels), quite often the systemic symptoms listed below (nausea, fever, epigastric fullness etc.) are not experienced. Systemic symptoms may be more numerous in cases of painful urination due to internally generated Damp Heat.

Clinical features
- Painful, frequent and urgent urination; the pain is often described as burning or like 'passing glass', and may radiate to the umbilical area, and is generally worse when pressure is applied. The urine is dark, concentrated and strong smelling and may be accompanied by a feeling of incomplete emptying or dripping.
- suprapubic fullness and discomfort
- lower back pain
- fullness or discomfort in the chest and epigastrium
- nausea, loss of appetite
- bitter taste in the mouth
- thirst with little desire to drink
- a tendency to constipation or alternating loose and sluggish stools
- maybe fever (especially afternoon fever), or alternating fever and chills

T greasy yellow coat, especially on the root
P slippery and rapid or soft and rapid

Treatment principle
Ease painful urination, eliminate Dampness
Clear Heat and promote urination

Prescription

BA ZHENG SAN 八正散
(Dianthus Formula)

che qian zi (Semen Plantaginis) 车前子	12g
hua shi (Talcum) 滑石	12g
bian xu (Herba Polygoni Avicularis) 篇蓄	9g
qu mai (Herba Dianthi) 瞿麦	9g
shan zhi zi (Fructus Gardeniae Jasminoidis) 山栀子	6g
mu tong (Caulis Mutong) 木通	6g
zhi da huang (Radix et Rhizoma Rhei) 制大黄	6g
gan cao shao (tips of Radix Glycyrrhizae Uralensis) 甘草梢	3g
deng xin cao (Medulla Junci Effusi) 灯心草	2g

Method: Decoction. **Che qian zi** is usually cooked in a muslin bag (*bao jian* 包煎). This is a useful prescription to also have handy in powder form for those prone to recurrent Hot painful urination syndrome. (Source: *Shi Yong Zhong Yi Nei Ke Xue*)

Modifications

- With severe abdominal distension and constipation, increase the dose of **zhi da huang** (Radix et Rhizoma Rhei) 制大黄 to 9g and add **zhi shi** (Fructus Immaturus Citri Aurantii) 枳实 9g.
- With abdominal fullness and loose stools, delete **zhi da huang**.
- With lower abdominal pain, add **chuan lian zi*** (Fructus Meliae Toosendan) 川楝子 3-9g and **wu yao** (Radix Linderae Strychnifoliae) 乌药 3-9g.
- With mild bleeding, add **xiao ji** (Herba Cephalanoplos) 小蓟 9g and **bai mao gen** (Rhizoma Imperatae Cylindricae) 白茅根 12g.

Variations and additional prescriptions

With shaoyang *involvement*

- Alternating fever and chills, nausea and dizziness indicate that Damp Heat is obstructing the *shao yang* level. Add **chai hu** (Radix Bupleuri) 柴胡 9g, **huang qin** (Radix Scutellariae Baicalensis) 黄芩 9g and **ban xia*** (Rhizoma Pinelliae Ternatae) 半夏 6g to harmonise *shao yang*, or use **CHAI LING TANG** (*Bupleurum and Hoelen Combination* 柴苓汤) modified.

chai hu (Radix Bupleuri) 柴胡	12g
ban xia* (Rhizoma Pinelliae Ternatae) 半夏	12g
huang qin (Radix Scutellariae Baicalensis) 黄芩	9g
ren shen (Radix Ginseng) 人参	9g
ze xie (Rhizoma Alismatis Orientalis) 泽泻	15g
fu ling (Sclerotium Poriae Cocos) 茯苓	12g
zhu ling (Sclerotium Polypori Umbellati) 猪苓	12g
bai zhu (Rhizoma Atractylodes Macrocephalae) 白术	12g

    gui zhi (Ramulus Cinnamomi Cassiae) 桂枝 6g
    zhi gan cao (honey fried Radix Glycyrrhizae Uralensis)
        炙甘草 6g
    lian qiao (Fructus Forsythiae Suspensae) 连翘 12g
    pu gong ying (Herba Taraxaci Mongolici) 蒲公英 12g
    ye ju hua (Flos Chrysanthemi Indici) 野菊花 9g
    Method: Decoction. (Source: *Shi Yong Zhong Yi Nei Ke Xue*)

With yin *deficiency*

- With mild *yin* deficiency, either from the Heat damaging *yin* or a Damp Heat episode on a background of *yin* deficiency, the correct treatment is to promote urination, clear Heat and nourish *yin* with **ZHU LING TANG** (*Polyporus Combination* 猪苓汤). See also Kidney *yin* deficiency, p.390.
    zhu ling (Sclerotium Polypori Umbellati) 猪苓 9g
    fu ling (Sclerotium Poria Cocos) 茯苓 9g
    ze xie (Rhizoma Alismatis Orientalis) 泽泻 9g
    hua shi (Talcum) 滑石 9g
    e jiao^ (Gelatinum Corii Asini) 阿胶 9g
    Method: Decoction. E jiao is melted before being added to the strained decoction (*yang hua* 烊化). (Source: *Shi Yong Zhong Yi Nei Ke Xue*)

During pregnancy

- During pregnancy, the use of **qu mai, da huang, che qian zi** and **hua shi** is contraindicated. **WU LIN SAN** (*Gardenia and Hoelen Formula* 五淋散) modified, may be used instead instead of **BA ZHENG SAN**. **WU LIN SAN** is also suitable for Damp Heat painful urination in patients with Blood deficiency.
    chi fu ling (Sclerotium Poriae Cocos Rubrae) 赤茯苓 12g
    jiao shan zhi zi (blackened Fructus Gardeniae Jasminoidis)
      焦山栀子 9g
    dang gui (Radix Angelicae Sinensis) 当归 9g
    huang qin (Radix Scutellariae Baicalensis) 黄芩 9g
    chao bai shao (dry fried Radix Paeoniae Lactiflorae)
      炒白芍 9g
    sheng di (Radix Rehmanniae Glutinosae) 生地 9g
    ze xie (Rhizoma Alismatis Orientalis) 泽泻 9g
    gan cao shao (tips of Radix Glycyrrhizae Uralensis)
      甘草梢 6g
    Method: Decoction. (Source: *Shi Yong Zhong Yi Fu Ke Xue*)

Heat in the Blood

- With severe systemic Heat, from Heat penetrating into the Blood, with skin rashes, bleeding, manic behaviour, a red tongue and a rapid slippery pulse, the correct treatment is to clear Toxic Heat and Fire with a combination of **HUANG LIAN JIE DU TANG** (*Coptis and Scute Combination* 黄连解毒汤, p.838) and **WU WEI XIAO DU YIN** (*Five Ingredient Decoction to Eliminate Toxin* 五味消毒饮, p.710).

Patent medicines

Ming Mu Shang Qing Pian 明目上清片 (Ming Mu Shang Ching Pien)
Long Dan Xie Gan Wan 龙胆泻肝丸 (Long Dan Xie Gan Wan)
Dao Chi Pian 导赤片 (Tao Chih Pien)
Chuan Xin Lian Kang Yan Pian 穿心连抗炎片
　　(Chuan Xin Lian Antiphlogistic Tablets)

Table 12.1 Comparison of Heat Painful Urination patterns

Pattern	Aetiology	Features	Guiding Prescription
Damp Heat	external invasion of Damp Heat, or less commonly internally generated Damp Heat	suprapubic fullness, loss of appetite, nausea, constipation or alternating loose and sluggish stools, thirst with little desire to drink, greasy yellow tongue coat, slippery rapid pulse	**Main Rx: BA ZHENG SAN** · with mild *yin* deficiency **ZHU LING TANG** · during pregnancy or with Blood deficiency **WU LIN SAN** · with *shao yang* symptoms **CHAI LING TANG** · with Toxic Heat **HUANG LIAN JIE DU TANG** **plus WU WEI XIAO DU YIN**
Heart Fire	emotional turmoil, particularly prolonged anxiety and worry	red complexion, palpitations, insomnia, dream disturbed sleep, anxiety, irritability, thirst, mouth ulcers, red tongue with a redder tip, rapid big pulse, especially in the distal position	**DAO CHI SAN**
Liver Fire	emotional turmoil, particularly severe or repressed frustration, resentment and anger	extreme irritability or temper, dizziness, sore bloodshot eyes, temporal headache, hypochondriac discomfort, red tongue with redder edges and a dry yellow coat, wiry, rapid pulse	**LONG DAN XIE GAN TANG**

Acupuncture

Ren.3 (*zhong ji* -), Liv.5 (*li gou* -), Ht.8 (*shao fu* -), Sp.9 (*yin ling quan* -), Sp.6 (*san yin jiao* -), Bl.28 (*pang guang shu* -), Liv.2 (*xing jian* -)
- for alternating fever and chills add SJ.5 (*wai guan*) and GB.39 (*xuan zhong*)

Clinical notes

- Biomedical conditions that may present as Damp Heat type Painful Urination include urethritis, cystitis, pyelonephritis, gonorrhoeal urethritis, prostatitis, non-specific urethritis, Reiter's syndrome, and glomerulonephritis.
- Generally responds well to correct treatment. Simple measures, such as increasing fluid intake and drinking a decoction of **chi xiao dou** (adzuki beans, boiled for 30 minutes) may be useful in the early stages of this pattern.

心火淋证

12.1.2 HEART FIRE

Pathophysiology
- Heart Fire is usually the result of a significant emotional shock, trauma or persistent anxiety and worry. These emotions can impede the circulation of Heart *qi* and over time generate Heat, which can be transmitted to the Small Intestine (the *yang* partner organ of the Heart) and then to the Bladder, resulting in painful urination.

Clinical features
- urination that is burning, painful, concentrated, urgent and frequent
- red complexion
- mouth and tongue ulcers, particularly on the tip of the tongue
- thirst with a desire for cold drinks
- sensation of heat in the chest
- irritablity, restlessness, agitation, anxiety
- palpitations
- insomnia, dream disturbed sleep

T red with a redder tip. The tongue may be ulcerated, especially on the tip. The coat is dry and yellow.
P rapid and big, especially in the distal position

Treatment principle
Clear Heat from the Heart and promote urination

Prescription

DAO CHI SAN 导赤散
(*Rehmannia and Akebia Formula*) modified

sheng di (Radix Rehmanniae Glutinosae) 生地	15g
dan zhu ye (Herba Lophatheri Gracilis) 淡竹叶	9g
mu tong (Caulis Mutong) 木通	6g
huang lian (Rhizoma Coptidis) 黄连	6g
gan cao shao (tips of Radix Glycyrrhizae Uralensis) 甘草梢	3g
deng xin cao (Medulla Junci Effusi) 灯心草	2g

Method: Decoction.

Modifications
- With *yin* deficiency, add **shi hu** (Herba Dendrobii) 石斛 6-12g and **zhi mu** (Rhizoma Anemarrhenae Asphodeloidis) 知母 6-12g.
- With traces of blood in the urine, add **bai mao gen** (Rhizoma Imperatae Cylindricae) 白茅根 9-15g and **han lian cao** (Herba Ecliptae

Prostratae) 旱连草 9-15g.
- With painful mouth ulcers combine with **XIE HUANG SAN** (*Drain the Yellow Powder* 泻黄散).
   shi gao (Gypsum) 石膏 15g
   fang feng (Radix Ledebouriellae Divaricatae) 防风 9g
   huo xiang (Herba Agastaches seu Pogostemi) 藿香 9g
   shan zhi zi (Fructus Gardeniae Jasminoidis) 山栀子 6g
   gan cao (Radix Glycyrrhizae Uralensis) 甘草 3g
   Method: Decoction.

Patent medicines
Ming Mu Shang Qing Pian 明目上清片 (Ming Mu Shang Ching Pien)
Long Dan Xie Gan Wan 龙胆泻肝丸 (Long Dan Xie Gan Wan)
Dao Chi Pian 导赤片 (Tao Chih Pien)
Chuan Xin Lian Kang Yan Pian 穿心连抗炎片
    (Chuan Xin Lian Antiphlogistic Tablets)
Da Bai Du Jiao Nang 大败毒胶囊 (DBD Capsule)
 - severe cases

Acupuncture
Ren.3 (*zhong ji* -), St.28 (*shui dao* -), Sp.6 (*san yin jiao* -), Ht.8 (*shao fu* -), Sp.9 (*yin ling quan* -), PC.8 (*lao gong* -), Kid.6 (*zhao hai*), PC.6 (*nei guan*), *yin tang* (M-HN-3)

Clinical notes
- Biomedical conditions that may present as Damp Heat type Painful Urination include urethritis, cystitis, pyelonephritis, prostatitis and Behçet's syndrome.
- This pattern frequently overlaps with Liver Fire types and is often associated with emotional or psychological factors. In these cases counselling may be necessary for long term resolution.
- Acupuncture is very effective for clearing Heat from the Heart and calming restlessness.

肝胆火旺

12.1.3 LIVER FIRE
Pathophysiology
- The Liver channel passes through the lower *jiao*. Heat in the Liver is mostly produced by chronic Liver *qi* stagnation, and, like the Heart Fire pattern, is frequently emotional in origin. In addition to the emotional aspect, development of Liver Fire is promoted by excessive consumption of hot foods and alcohol. In contrast to the Heart Fire pattern, the emotions most likely to give rise to Liver *qi* stagnation and Fire are repressed or severe anger, frustration and resentment. Liver Fire can be transmitted in either direction–to the lower *jiao* or head (or both).

Clinical features
- burning, painful, concentrated, urgent and/or frequent urination
- extreme irritablity, anger outbursts
- dizziness
- tinnitus
- bloodshot, painful eyes
- temporal headaches
- thirst, dry throat
- constipation
- hypochondriac tension, discomfort or pain
- in some patients ulcerations, a tendency to herpes genitalia or eczema in the groin and on the genitals

T red or with red edges and a thick, dry, yellow coat
P wiry, rapid and strong

Treatment principle
Drain Fire from the Liver and promote urination

Prescription

LONG DAN XIE GAN TANG 龙胆泻肝汤
(*Gentiana Combination*)

jiu long dan cao (wine fried Radix Gentianae Longdancao) 酒龙胆草	6g
che qian zi (Semen Plantaginis) 车前子	9g
huang qin (Radix Scutellariae Baicalensis) 黄芩	9g
shan zhi zi (Fructus Gardeniae Jasminoides) 山栀子	9g
sheng di (Radix Rehmanniae Glutinosae) 生地	9g
ze xie (Rhizoma Alismatis Orientalis) 泽泻	9g
dang gui (Radix Angelicae Sinensis) 当归	6g
mu tong (Caulis Mutong) 木通	6g

chai hu (Radix Bupleuri) 柴胡 6g
gan cao (Radix Glycyrrhizae Uralensis) 甘草 6g
Method: Decoction. **Che qian zi** is usually cooked in a muslin bag (*bao jian* 包煎).
(Source: *Shi Yong Fang Ji Xue*)

Patent medicines
Ming Mu Shang Qing Pian 明目上清片 (Ming Mu Shang Ching Pien)
Long Dan Xie Gan Wan 龙胆泻肝丸 (Long Dan Xie Gan Wan)
Dao Chi Pian 导赤片 (Tao Chih Pien)
Chuan Xin Lian Kang Yan Pian 穿心连抗炎片
    (Chuan Xin Lian Antiphlogistic Tablets)
Da Bai Du Jiao Nang 大败毒胶囊 (DBD Capsule)
- severe cases

Acupuncture
Bl.28 (*pang guang shu* -), Ren.3 (*zhong ji* -), SJ.6 (*zhi gou* -), Liv.5 (*li gou* -), Liv.2 (*xing jian* -), Liv.3 (*tai chong* -)

Clinical notes
- Biomedical conditions that may present as Damp Heat type Painful Urination include urethritis, cystitis, pyelonephritis, systemic lupus erythematosus, Reiter's syndrome, prostatitis, orchitis and genital herpes.
- This pattern frequently overlaps with Heart Fire. Treatment is directed to the system most affected, or a combination of prescriptions is given when the distinction is unclear. When (perhaps traumatic) emotional aspects are involved, counselling may be necessary for long term resolution.
- Acupuncture is very effective in treating the emotional aspects of this pattern (although needling very angry people requires a great degree of sensitivity). Acupuncture or appropriate herbal treatment should be continued (for at least one course or several months) after resolution of the acute symproms in those prone to this pattern so as to prevent reoccurence.

石
淋

12.2 STONE PAINFUL URINATION SYNDROME

- urinary tract stones in asymptomatic patients
- with Damp Heat
- with Blood stagnation
- with Kidney deficiency

Formation of urinary tract stones

- Calculi or gravel may form in the urinary system due to a variety of factors, including excess dietary calcium (dairy foods) or oxalates (some fruit and vegetables), urates (organ meat) or the overuse of vitamin D preparations. Medical conditions, such as hyperparathyroidism, gout or Cushing's syndrome, can predispose to stone formation, as does prolonged immobilisation. Insufficient consumption of water or excessive loss through sweat (causing increased concentration of salts in the blood and their precipitation out of solution) may also contribute.
- Western medical diagnosis of stones is usually made according to their appearance in the urine, or the nature, location and radiation of the pain. Kidney stones however, may be present for years without giving rise to symptoms, and are sometimes discovered during radiological examination for another disorder. Knowing that stones are present (even in asymptomatic patients) enables the addition of a number of very specific stone dissolving herbs to any suitable prescription. X-rays and ultrasound diagnosis will reveal the size and extent of the stones. Large staghorn or renal medulla stones are not readily amenable to TCM treatment and require lithotripsy or surgery. Small stones (<5mm) and gravel are amenable to treatment.
- Stones may appear as fine sandy sediment in the urine, or as larger particles that lodge in the ureter during their passage from the kidney, causing broken urine stream or urinary retention, and acute pain.
- Once stones are dislodged and begin to move, the pain is often severe, and may radiate down to the inner thighs, genitals, lower back or lower abdomen. If a calculus damages the urinary tract endothelium, there may be blood in the urine.

12.2.1 ASYMPTOMATIC STONES

Treatment principle

The basic treatment for urinary gravel and sand in otherwise asymptomatic patients (usually those with accidentally discovered stones) is to dissolve stones and gravel and promote urination. Symptomatic patients with small stones are differentiated and treated according to the three categories on the following pages.

Prescription

SHI WEI SAN 石苇散
(*Pyrrosia Powder*) modified

shi wei (Folium Pyrrosiae) 石苇	6g
che qian zi (Semen Plantaginis) 车前子	9g
qu mai (Herba Dianthi) 瞿麦	6g
hua shi (Talcum) 滑石	9g
dong kui zi (Semen Abutili seu Malvae) 冬葵子	6g
jin qian cao (Herba Lysimachiae) 金钱草	30-120g
hai jin sha (Spora Lygodii Japonici) 海金砂	30g
ji nei jin^ (Endothelium Corneum Gigeriae Galli) 鸡内金	15g

Method: Decoction. **Ji nei jin** is powdered and added to the strained decoction (*chong fu* 冲服). **Hai jin sha** and **che qian zi** are usually decocted in a cloth bag (*bao jian* 包煎). This prescription should be taken for a minimum of one month and is often required for several months to be effective. (Source: *Shi Yong Zhong Yi Nei Ke Xue*)

Alternative formula
Although probably less effective than the main prescription, a popular approach (more convenient and cost effective given the length of time required for success) is to simply brew **jin qian cao** (Herba Lysimachiae) 金钱草 60-120g as tea several times daily.

Patent medicines
Te Xiao Pai Shi Wan 特效排石丸 (Specific Drug Passwan)
Shi Lin Tong Pian 石淋通片 (Shi Lin Tong Pian)

Acupuncture
Asymptomatic patients
In asymptomatic patients, acupuncture may be applied to strengthen the Kidneys, improve urinary function and promote urination, in conjuction with herbs (noted above) to dissolve the stones. Points may be selected primarily from the Kidney, Spleen, Liver and Urinary Bladder channels. The electro-acupuncture protocol outlined below is reserved for cases of acute pain, i.e. when urinary tract stones are moving.

Electro-acupuncture for patients with acute pain
The following electro-acupuncture point prescriptions are suitable for all types of small urinary stones with pain. Electro-acupuncture is generally applied only when the patient is experiencing pain as the stones move in the urinary tract. In asymptomatic patients, the use of electro-acupuncture may dislodge a large stone causing obstruction and pain. Use a high frequency (reducing) current on the main points

connected (~). The negative electrode (-ve) is usually attached to the proximal point. Auxilliary points should be needled with a strong reducing method. Treatment may be given once or twice daily in severe cases.

Kidney stones
- Bl.23 (*shen shu* -ve) ~ Sp.9 (*yin ling quan* +ve) on the same side of the body.
- Auxiliary points: Bl.28 (*pang guang shu* -), Kid.6 (*zhao hai* -), St.25 (*tian shu* -), GB.25 (*jing men* -)

Ureter stones
1. **Upper ureter:** Bl.23 (*shen shu* -ve) ~ Bl.28 (*pang guang shu* +ve) on the same side of the body.
- Auxiliary points: Ren.6 (*qi hai* -), Bl.22 (*san jiao shu* -)
2. **Lower ureter:** Bl.23 (*shen shu* -ve) ~ St.28 (*shui dao* +ve) on the same side of the body.
- Auxiliary points: Ren.3 (*zhong ji* -), Bl.32 (*ci liao* -)

Bladder or urethra stones
- Ren.4 (*guan yuan* -ve) or Ren.3 (*zhong ji* -ve) ~ St.28 (*shui dao* +ve) or Sp.6 (*san yin jiao* +ve).
- Auxiliary points: Kid.8 (*jiao xin* -), Sp.14 (*fu jie* -), PC.6 (*nei guan* -)
Ear points (suitable for all locations): kidney, urinary bladder, *shen men*, subcortex. Strong manual or electro-stimulation.

Clinical notes
- Success in getting rid of urinary tract stones depends on several factors. The higher in the urinary tract the stones are, the more difficult they are to shift. Staghorn stones in the renal pelvis are generally not amenable to TCM treatment. The size and shape of the stone are also important. Rounded stones are easier to move than irregular or angular stones. Stones larger than 5mm are difficult. The prognosis is good for small rounded stones with persistent treatment. A course of at least several months is generally recommended before judgement is made on the success (or otherwise) of the treatment.
- Maintaining adequate (or increasing) fluid intake is useful with small stones.
- Depending on the type of stone, certain food groups should be avoided and others are beneficial. In the case of oxalate stones foods to avoid or restrict are those with oxalic acid–rhubarb, spinach, swiss chard, beet greens, potatoes, plums, cranberries and chocolate.

Beneficial foods include parsley and radishes. For uric acid stones patients should restrict alcohol and protein (excess meat, particularly organ meats and tinned fish).

12.2.2 STONES WITH DAMP HEAT

Pathophysiology
- Persistent Damp Heat in the lower *jiao* is the most common aetiological factor for stones in the urinary tract. The drying and congealing nature of Heat can condense the Dampness into stones.
- A rich diet and excess alcohol consumption is usually the source of the Damp Heat in this pattern.

Clinical features
- acute, chronic or recurrent lower back or loin pain, or pain that radiates to the inner thigh, lower abdomen or genitals
- difficult urination
- concentrated, burning urine
- thirst with no desire to drink
- alternating constipation and diarrhoea

T red body with a thick, greasy, yellow coat, especially on the root
P rapid, slippery or wiry

Treatment principle
Clear Heat and alleviate Dampness
Ease painful urination and expel stones

Prescription

NIAO LU PAI SHI TANG #2 尿路排石汤二号
(*Expel Urinary Stones #2 Decoction*)

This is a strong cooling formula for Damp Heat with urinary tract stones. Once Damp Heat has subsided, the previous prescription (for asymptomatic stones) may be more appropriate.

jin qian cao (Herba Lysimachiae) 金钱草	30-120g
hua shi (Talcum) 滑石	12g
che qian zi (Semen Plantaginis) 车前子	12g
shi wei (Folium Pyrrosiae) 石苇	9g
bian xu (Herba Polygoni Avicularis) 篇蓄	9g
shan zhi zi (Fructus Gardeniae Jasminoidis) 山栀子	9g
niu xi (Radix Achyranthis Bidentatae) 牛膝	9g
zhi shi (Fructus Immaturus Citri Aurantii) 枳实	9g
mu tong (Caulis Mutong) 木通	6g

12. PAINFUL URINATION SYNDROME - Stone

zhi da huang (Radix et Rhizoma Rhei) 制大黄 6g
gan cao shao (tips of Radix Glycyrrhizae Uralensis)
甘草梢 6g

Method: Decoction. **Che qian zi** is usually cooked in a muslin bag (*bao jian* 包煎). (Source: *Shi Yong Zhong Yi Nei Ke Xue*)

SAN JIN TANG 三金汤
(*Three Golden Herbs Decoction*) modified

This formula is milder than the primary prescription and most suited to urinary tract stones with mild Damp Heat.

guang jin qian cao (Herba Desmodii Styracifolii)
广金钱草 60g
jin sha teng (Herba Lygondii Japonici) 金沙藤 30g
dong kui zi (Semen Abutili seu Malvae) 冬葵子 12g
qu mai (Herba Dianthi) 瞿麦 12g
ji nei jin^ (Endothelium Corneum Gigeriae Galli)
鸡内金 9g
shi wei (Folium Pyrrosiae) 石苇 9g

Method: Decoction. **Ji nei jin** is powdered and added to the strained decoction (*chong fu* 冲服). (Source: *Formulas and Strategies*)

Patent medicines

Te Xiao Pai Shi Wan 特效排石丸 (Specific Drug Passwan)
Shi Lin Tong Pian 石淋通片 (Shi Lin Tong Pian)

Acupuncture

During episodes of pain use the electro-acupuncture treatment outlined on p.352. Points to clear Damp Heat from the Bladder can also be selected: Liv.5 (*li gou* -), Ht.8 (*shao fu* -), Liv.2 (*xing jian* -), SJ.5 (*wai guan*), GB.39 (*xuan zhong*)

Clinical notes

- The Damp Heat pattern often occurs as an acute inflammatory exacerbation of asymptomatic urinary tract stones, often provoked by excess consumption of alcohol and rich food.
- In general, herbs are used to dissolve urinary stones and acupuncture used to manage pain. Both are useful for clearing Damp Heat. Reduction or avoidance of alcohol and Damp Heat generating foods is essential for long term results.

血瘀石淋

12.2.3 STONES WITH BLOOD STAGNATION

Pathophysiology
- Blood stagnation in the urinary tract can be the result of the long term presence of urinary tract stones, trauma (including surgery) or the result of long term Damp Heat, *qi* stagnation or deficiency.

Clinical features
- acute or chronic lower back or loin pain which is fixed and stabbing
- flecks of purplish blood, or copious dark blood in the urine

T purplish body with stasis spots
P wiry and tight or moderate and choppy

Treatment principle
Dissolve stones and promote urination
Move *qi* and eliminate stagnant Blood

Prescription

NIAO LU PAI SHI TANG #1 尿路排石汤一号
(*Expel Urinary Stones #1 Decoction*)

jin qian cao (Herba Lysimachiae) 金钱草	30-120g
hai jin sha (Spora Lygodii Japonici) 海金砂	15g
che qian zi (Semen Plantaginis) 车前子	12g
chi shao (Radix Paeoniae Rubrae) 赤芍	12g
hua shi (Talcum) 滑石	12g
wu yao (Radix Linderae Strychnifoliae) 乌药	9g
chuan lian zi* (Fructus Meliae Toosendan) 川楝子	9g
niu xi (Radix Achyranthis Bidentatae) 牛膝	9g
mu tong (Caulis Mutong) 木通	6g
gan cao shao (tips of Radix Glycyrrhizae Uralensis) 甘草梢	6g

Method: Decoction. **Hai jin sha** and **che qian zi** are usually decocted in a muslin bag (*bao jian* 包煎). (Source: *Shi Yong Zhong Yi Nei Ke Xue*)

Patent medicines
Te Xiao Pai Shi Wan 特效排石丸 (Specific Drug Passwan)
Shi Lin Tong Pian 石淋通片 (Shi Lin Tong Pian)
Yun Nan Bai Yao 云南白药 (Yunnan Paiyao)
　　- this medicine is specific for stopping bleeding and can be taken in addition to the main formula. The red pill is reserved for severe cases.

Acupuncture

During episodes of pain use the electro-acupuncture treatment outlined on p.368-369. Points to move stagnant Blood from the urinary tract are also selected: Sp.10 (*xue hai* -), St.29 (*gui lai* -), Bl.32 (*ci liao* -)
- In general, herbs are used to dissolve urinary stones and acupuncture used to manage pain.

Clinical notes

- This pattern corresponds to conditions such as damage to urinary tract endothelium by stones, obstruction of urinary tract, history of renal tuberculosis or congenital malformation of urinary tract.
- If there is severe damage caused to the urinary tract by the stones manifesting as persisent bleeding, then surgery and antibiotic therapy should be considered.

12.2.4 STONES WITH KIDNEY DEFICIENCY

12.2.4.1 Kidney *qi* deficiency
Pathophysiology
- Kidney *qi* is weakened by prolonged disease, the long term presence of stones or by inappropriate or excessive use of bitter cold herbs in the treatment of Damp Heat stone disorders.

Clinical features
- long history of recurrent colicky low back or loin pain, with aching lower back in between episodes
- aching, empty feeling in the lower abdomen
- waxy pale complexion
- shortness of breath
- weakness and fatigue

T pale and swollen, with toothmarks
P thready, small and forceless

Treatment principle
Dissolve stones and tonify Kidney *qi*

Prescription

NIAO LU PAI SHI TANG #3 尿路排石汤三号
(*Expel Urinary Stones #3 Decoction*)

jin qian cao (Herba Lysimachiae) 金钱草	30-120g
hai jin sha (Spora Lygodii Japonici) 海金砂	15g
huang qi (Radix Astragali Membranacei) 黄芪	15g

hua shi (Talcum) 滑石 12g
shu di (Radix Rehmanniae Glutinosae Conquitae) 熟地 12g
che qian zi (Semen Plantaginis) 车前子 12g
bai shao (Radix Paeoniae Lactiflorae) 白芍 12g
dang shen (Radix Codonopsis Pilosulae) 党参 12g
tu si zi (Semen Cuscutae Chinensis) 菟丝子 12g
wu yao (Radix Linderae Strychnifoliae) 乌药 9g
chuan lian zi* (Fructus Meliae Toosendan) 川楝子 9g
niu xi (Radix Achyranthis Bidentatae) 牛膝 9g
han lian cao (Herba Ecliptae Prostratae) 旱莲草 9g
bu gu zhi (Fructus Psoraleae Corylifoliae) 补骨脂 9g
mu tong (Caulis Mutong) 木通 6g
gan cao shao (tips of Radix Glycyrrhizae Uralensis) 甘草稍 6g
Method: Decoction, powder or pills. **Che qian zi** and **hai jin sha** are cooked in a muslin bag (*bao jian* 包煎). (Source: *Shi Yong Zhong Yi Nei Ke Xue*)

Patent medicines
Jin Kui Shen Qi Wan 金匮肾气丸 (Sexoton Pills) plus either
Te Xiao Pai Shi Wan 特效排石丸 (Specific Drug Passwan) or
Shi Lin Tong Pian 石淋通片 (Shi Lin Tong Pian)

Acupuncture
During episodes of pain use the electro-acupuncture treatment outlined on p.368-369. Points to tonify Kidney *qi* are also selected:
St.36 (*zu san li* +▲) and Ren.4 (*guan yuan* +▲)

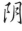

12.2.4.2 Kidney *yin* deficiency
Pathophysiology
- Kidney *yin* deficiency may follow long term Damp Heat that has gradually consumed *yin*, or may be a result of overwork, excessive sex, prolonged or severe illness or constitutional factors. When Kidney *yin* is deficient, body fluids may be concentrated to such a point that crystals and salts precipitate out of solution.

Clinical features
- long history of colicky low back or loin pain
- aching, empty feeling in the lower abdomen
- dull low back ache
- dark concentrated urine
- sensation of heat in the palms and soles ('five hearts hot')
- night sweats
- insomnia
- dry mouth and throat

T red, dry, with little or no coat
P thready and rapid

Treatment principle
Dissolve stones and tonify Kidney *yin*

Prescription

ZHI BAI BA WEI WAN 知柏八味丸
(*Anemarrhena, Phellodendron and Rehmannia Formula*) modified

> **shu di** (Radix Rehmanniae Glutinosae Conquitae) 熟地 24g
> **shan yao** (Radix Dioscoreae Oppositae) 山药 12g
> **shan zhu yu** (Fructus Corni Officinalis) 山茱萸 12g
> **fu ling** (Sclerotium Poria Cocos) 茯苓 9g
> **mu dan pi** (Cortex Moutan Radicis) 牡丹皮 9g
> **ze xie** (Rhizoma Alismatis Orientalis) 泽泻 9g
> **zhi mu** (Rhizoma Anemarrhenae Asphodeloidis) 知母 9g
> **yan huang bai** (salt fried Cortex Phellodendri) 盐黄柏 9g
> **che qian zi** (Semen Plantaginis) 车前子 15g
> **yi ren** (Semen Coicis Lachryma-jobi) 苡仁 12g
> **mai dong** (Tuber Ophiopogonis Japonici) 麦冬 9g
> Method: Decoction or pills. **Che qian zi** is cooked in a muslin bag (*bao jian* 包煎).

Patent medicines
Zhi Bai Ba Wei Wan 知柏八味丸 (Zhi Bai Ba Wei Wan) plus either
Te Xiao Pai Shi Wan 特效排石丸 (Specific Drug Passwan) or
Shi Lin Tong Pian 石淋通片 (Shi Lin Tong Pian)

Acupuncture
During episodes of pain use the electro-acupuncture treatment outlined on p.369-369. Points to strengthen Kidney *yin* are also selected: Kid.6 (*zhao hai*) and Kid.3 (*tai xi*)

- Care must be taken with very deficient patients as strong electro-acupuncture may disperse *qi*. Gentle treatment may be better tolerated.

Clinical notes
- In cases of stones with significant underlying deficiency, there are usually elements of both Kidney *qi* and *yin* deficiency.
- Long term therapy will usually be required.

12.3 *QI* PAINFUL URINATION SYNDROME

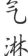

- Liver *qi* stagnation
- Spleen *qi* deficiency, which is traditionally included in this category, overlaps with the Spleen pattern of exhaustion painful urination syndrome and is described there (p.394).

12.3.1 LIVER *QI* STAGNATION
Pathophysiology
- Liver *qi* stagnation painful urination is usually due to emotional factors like repressed emotion, anger, resentment and frustration that disrupt the smooth circulation of Liver *qi* generally, and as the Liver channel passes through the lower *jiao*, in this case the Bladder.

Clinical features
- lower abdominal fullness and pain that may radiate to the tops of the thighs, is initiated or aggravated by emotions, and which eases with relaxation and urination
- urination may feel uncomfortable, the stream may be weak or broken and may be hard to get started or feel incomplete
- tightness or fullness in the chest, often described as difficulty in drawing a satisfying breath, temporarily relieved by frequent sighing
- hypochondriac discomfort or tightness
- dizziness
- occasional fatigue (although the patient feels better for exercise)
- irritability or depression
- abdominal distension, flatulence, alternating constipation and diarrhoea
- women may experience irregular menstruation, premenstrual syndrome and breast tenderness
- all symptoms tend to be aggravated by stress

T normal or darkish
P deep and wiry

Treatment principle
Soothe and regulate Liver *qi*
Ease painful urination and disperse stagnant *qi*

Prescription

CHEN XIANG SAN 沉香散
(*Aquillaria Powder*) modified

chen xiang (Lignum Aquilariae) 沉香	1.5g
shi wei (Folium Pyrrosiae) 石苇	20g

12. PAINFUL URINATION SYNDROME - Qi

chao bai shao (dry fried Radix Paeoniae Lactiflorae)
炒白芍 20g
hua shi (Talcum) 滑石 20g
dong kui zi (Semen Abutili seu Malvae) 冬葵子 15g
wang bu liu xing (Semen Vaccariae Segetalis) 王不留行 15g
dang gui (Radix Angelicae Sinensis) 当归 12g
chen pi (Pericarpium Citri Reticulatae) 陈皮 10g
sheng gan cao (Radix Glycyrrhizae Uralensis) 生甘草 6g
Method: Powder or decoction. If powdered, the dose is 6 grams as a draft twice daily. (Source: *Zhong Yi Nei Ke Lin Chuang Shou Ce*)

Modifications
- With severe lower abdominal distension and fullness, add **mu xiang** (Radix Aucklandiae Lappae) 木香 6g, **qing pi** (Pericarpium Citri Reticulatae Viride) 青皮 6g and **wu yao** (Radix Linderae Strychnifoliae) 乌药 6g.
- With stagnant Blood (very chronic cases, occasional stabbing pain, purplish spots on the tongue, venous congestion around the inner ankles and Sp.9 *yin ling quan*), add **hong hua** (Flos Carthami Tinctorii) 红花 6g, **chi shao** (Radix Paeoniae Rubrae) 赤芍 9g and **chuan niu xi** (Radix Cyathulae Officinalis) 川牛膝 9g.
- With Damp Heat, add **shan zhi zi** (Fructus Gardeniae Jasminoidis) 山栀子 9g.
- With Spleen deficiency, add **bai zhu** (Rhizoma Atractylodes Macrocephalae) 白术 12g, **huang qi** (Radix Astragali Membranacei) 黄芪 15g and **dang shen** (Radix Codonopsis Pilosulae) 党参 12g.
- If there is *yin* deficiency, add **zhi mu** (Rhizoma Anemarrhenae Asphodeloidis) 知母 9g and **huang bai** (Cortex Phellodendri) 黄柏 9g.

Patent medicines
Chai Hu Shu Gan Wan 柴胡舒肝丸 (Chai Hu Shu Gan Wan)
Shu Gan Wan 舒肝丸 (Shu Gan Wan)
Xiao Yao Wan 逍遥丸 (Xiao Yao Wan)
Jia Wei Xiao Yao Wan 加味逍遥丸 (Jia Wei Xiao Yao Wan)
Qian Lie Xian Wan 前列腺丸 (Prostate Gland Pills)
   - very useful added to one of the above formulae in men with prostate swelling

Acupuncture
PC.6 (*nei guan*), Bl.18 (*gan shu* -), Bl.22 (*san jiao shu* -), Liv.5 (*li gou* -), Bl.28 (*pang guang shu* -), Ren.5 (*shi men*), Liv.3 (*tai chong* -), St.30 (*qi chong* -).

Clinical notes
- Biomedical conditions that may present as Liver *qi* stagnation type

Painful Urination include stress related dysuria.
- Liver *qi* stagnation can appear alone or complicate other pathogenic entities like Dampness, Damp Heat, Spleen deficiency or *yin* deficiency.
- Acupuncture is especially effective in *qi* stagnation patterns.
- Stress management and relaxation techniques (or psychotherapy in severe cases) may be very useful.

12.4. BLOOD PAINFUL URINATION SYNDROME

- Blood painful urination syndrome is defined by the quantity of blood expelled in the urine, that is, the urine should look pink or red. In cases where a patient complains of painful urination and a urine test reveals small traces of blood (although the urine colour is normal), then another category of painful urination (Heat, *qi*, stone painful urination etc.), should be selected according to the prominent symptoms present. The appropriate formula could then be modified by the addition of styptic herbs. Substantial urinary bleeding with minimal or no pain is diagnosed as haematuria (p.458).
- Heavy exercise (especially the repetitive pounding of long distance running) and drug induced (warfarin, cyclophosphamide) Blood painful urination should be excluded. Urinary tract stones can cause Blood painful urination.
- There are three general patterns of Blood painful urination:
  - Heat or Damp Heat
  - Blood stagnation
  - Kidney *yin* deficiency

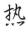

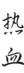

12.4.1 HEAT, DAMP HEAT
Pathophysiology
- Heat or Damp Heat causing Blood painful urination is basically the same as the Damp Heat (p.358) or Fire varieties of Heat painful urination (pp.363, 365), but accompanied by significant bleeding. Once Damp Heat, Heat (or Fire) are present, Blood is quickened and it may be forced from the *luo* channels of the Bladder.

Clinical features
- Painful, frequent, urgent urination (like 'passing glass') with urine that is fresh red or purplish red with blood. The intensity of the colour will depend on the degree of bleeding, which, if copious, makes it seem as if pure blood is being passed. In some cases there may be clotted threads, or small blood clots.
- fever, or alternating fever and chills
- lower back pain
- nausea, vomiting
- bitter taste in the mouth
- constipation
- thirst

T yellow greasy coat and a red tip
P slippery or soft, rapid and strong

Treatment principle
Stop bleeding
Clear Heat and Dampness

Prescription

XIAO JI YIN ZI 小蓟饮子
(*Cephalanoplos Decoction*) modified

This prescription is suitable for all excess Heat types of Blood painful urination. After bleeding stops, the underlying pattern should be identified and treated.

xiao ji (Herba Cephalanoplos) 小蓟	30g
sheng di (Radix Rehmanniae Glutinosae) 生地	30g
hua shi (Talcum) 滑石	30g
bai mao gen (Rhizoma Imperatae Cylindricae) 白茅根	30g
xian he cao (Herba Agrimoniae Pilosae) 仙鹤草	25g
ou jie (Nodus Nelumbinis Nuciferae Rhizomatis) 藕节	15g
dan zhu ye (Herba Lophatheri Gracilis) 竹叶	12g
chao pu huang (dry fried Pollen Typhae) 炒蒲黄	10g
shan zhi zi (Fructus Gardeniae Jasminoidis) 山栀子	10g
mu tong (Caulis Mutong) 木通	6g
gan cao shao (tips of Radix Glycyrrhizae Uralensis) 甘草梢	6g

Method: Decoction. (Source: *Zhong Yi Nei Ke Lin Chuang Shou Ce*)

Modifications

- With mild Blood stasis, add **san qi fen** (powdered Radix Notoginseng) 三七粉 6g, **hu po fen** (powdered Succinum) 琥珀粉 1g and **chuan niu xi** (Radix Cyathulae Officinalis) 川牛膝 6g.
- With severe Heat, add **pu gong ying** (Herba Taraxaci Mongolici) 蒲公英 15g, **huang bai** (Cortex Phellodendri) 黄柏 9g and **jin yin hua** (Flos Lonicerae Japonicae) 金银花 15g.

Patent medicines

Ming Mu Shang Qing Pian 明目上清片 (Ming Mu Shang Ching Pien)
Long Dan Xie Gan Wan 龙胆泻肝丸 (Long Dan Xie Gan Wan)
Chuan Xin Lian Kang Yan Pian 穿心连抗炎片
   (Chuan Xin Lian Antiphlogistic Pills)
Yun Nan Bai Yao 云南白药 (Yunnan Paiyao)
  - this medicine is specific for stopping bleeding and can be taken in addition to the main formula selected. The red pill is reserved for severe cases.

Acupuncture

Ren.3 (*zhong ji* -), Sp.6 (*san yin jiao* -), Bl.17 (*ge shu* -),
BL.28 (*pang guang shu* -), Ht.8 (*shao fu* -), Sp.10 (*xue hai* -)

Clinical notes

- Biomedical conditions that may present as Heat type Blood Painful Urination include urinary tract infection, renal calculi, bladder tumours, renal tuberculosis, Goodpasture's syndrome, glomerulonephritis, Henoch Schönlein purpura, prostatitis and interstitial cystitis.

- Once treatment has stopped the bleeding, a clearer picture should emerge and other underlying patterns may need to be addressed.

12.4.2 BLOOD STAGNATION

Pathophysiology
- Blood stagnation type Blood painful urination may follow an acute trauma to the groin, lower back or pelvis. Other long term genitourinary pathology, such as *qi* deficiency or *qi* stagnation, recurrent Damp Heat or *yin* deficiency can also lead to stagnant Blood.
- Stagnant Blood is a physical obstruction that blocks Blood circulation. Blood behind the obstruction is forced from the vessels and causes bleeding.

Clinical features
- sharp, stabbing, rough pain during urination, without burning
- urine that is purple or may have purplish clots
- fixed, stabbing lower abdominal pain
- there may be palpable masses, which may or may not be painful
- dark or purplish spider naevi or broken vessels on the trunk and around the inner ankle and knee
- dark, ashen, sallow or purplish complexion, dark or purplish lips and conjunctiva, dark ring under the eyes

T purple or with brown or purple stasis spots, sublingual veins dark and distended

P thready and choppy

Treatment principle
Invigorate Blood circulation, eliminate stagnant Blood
Warm *yang* and break through painful obstruction

Prescription

SHAO FU ZHU YU TANG 少腹逐瘀汤
(*Drive Out Blood Stasis in the Lower Abdomen Decoction*)

This formula is designed for Blood stagnation with Cold.

dang gui (Radix Angelicae Sinensis) 当归	9g
chi shao (Radix Paeoniae Rubrae) 赤芍	9g
sheng pu huang (Pollen Typhae) 生蒲黄	9g
chao wu ling zhi^ (dry fried Excrementum Trogopteri seu Pteromi) 炒五灵脂	9g
yan hu suo (Rhizoma Corydalis Yanhusuo) 延胡索	9g
chuan xiong (Radix Ligustici Chuanxiong) 川芎	6g
xiao hui xiang (Fructus Foeniculi Vulgaris) 小茴香	6g
mo yao (Myrrha) 没药	4.5g
rou gui (Cortex Cinnamomi Cassiae) 肉桂	3g

12. PAINFUL URINATION SYNDROME - Blood

pao jiang (quick fried Rhizoma Zingiberis Officinalis) 炮姜 .. 3g
Method: Decoction. (Source: *Fluid Physiology and Pathology in Traditional Chinese Medicine*)

Modifications

- If there are post surgical adhesions with pain, add **san qi fen** (powdered Radix Notoginseng) 三七粉 3g, **hong hua** (Flos Carthami Tinctorii) 红花 9g and **ze lan** (Herba Lycopi Lucidi) 泽兰 9g.
- If the pain follows a traumatic injury, add **san qi fen** (powdered Radix Notoginseng) 三七粉 3g and **wang bu liu xing** (Semen Vaccariae Segetalis) 王不留行 9g.

Patent medicines

Sheng Tian Qi Pian 生田七片 (Raw Tian Qi Ginseng Pills)
Xue Fu Zhu Yu Wan 血府逐瘀丸 (Xue Fu Zhu Yu Wan)
Fu Ke Wu Jin Wan 妇科乌金丸 (Woo Garm Yuen Medical Pills)
Yun Nan Bai Yao 云南白药 (Yunnan Paiyao)
 - this medicine is specific for stopping bleeding and can be taken in addition to the main formula selected. The red pill is reserved for severe cases.

Acupuncture

Bl.28 (*pang guang shu* -), Ren.3 (*zhong ji* -), Sp.10 (*xue hai* -), Sp.1 (*yin bai* -), St.29 (*gui lai* -), Ren.4 (*guan yuan* -), Sp.6 (*san yin jiao*), Bl.17 (*ge shu* -)

Clinical notes

- Biomedical conditions that may present as Blood stagnation type Blood Painful Urination include urethral stricture, bladder or prostatic cancer, bladder polyps, nephrotic syndrome and bladder stones.
- Patients presenting with this pattern should be assumed to have a potentially dangerous condition and referred accordingly for appropriate investigations.
- This pattern is generally difficult to treat, especially when chronic bladder disease has caused Blood stasis. Blood stagnation from trauma responds better, and the prognosis is usually good (depending on the extent of the trauma). Tumours of the genitourinary tract should be treated with a combination of Western medicine and TCM. If bladder stones are present refer to Stone painful urination with Blood stagnation, p.372.

12.4.3 KIDNEY *YIN* DEFICIENCY

Pathophysiology
- Kidney *yin* deficiency type Blood painful urination is a chronic condition that occurs when damaged Kidney *yin* fails to maintain the integrity of the *luo* channels of the lower *jiao*. Heat generated by the deficiency can force Blood from the vessels. The disease course is prolonged and usually recurrent.

Clinical features
- pale or occasionally bright red blood in the urine with mild urinary pain
- bleeding is mild and recurrent
- weakness or soreness of the lower back; weak, sore knees and heel pain
- sensation of heat in the palms and soles ('five hearts hot')
- facial flushing, malar flush
- night sweats
- insomnia
- dry mouth and throat
- all symptoms tend to be worse in the afternoon and evening

T pale red, or red and dry with little coat
P thready and rapid

Treatment principle
Nourish *yin*, clear Heat, stop bleeding

Prescription

ZHI BAI BA WEI WAN 知柏八味丸
(*Anemarrhena, Phellodendron and Rehmannia Formula*) modified

zhi mu (Rhizoma Anemarrhenae Asphodeloidis) 知母	10g
huang bai (Cortex Phellodendri) 黄柏	10g
sheng di (Radix Rehmanniae Glutinosae) 生地	20g
shu di (Radix Rehmanniae Glutinosae Conquitae) 熟地	20g
fu ling (Sclerotium Poria Cocos) 茯苓	20g
shan yao (Radix Dioscoreae Oppositae) 山药	30g
shan zhu yu (Fructus Corni Officinalis) 山茱萸	15g
han lian cao (Herba Ecliptae Prostratae) 旱连草	20g
xiao ji (Herba Cephalanoplos) 小蓟	20g
ze xie (Rhizoma Alismatis Orientalis) 泽泻	12g
mu dan pi (Cortex Moutan Radicis) 牡丹皮	12g
e jiao^ (Gelatinum Corii Asini) 阿胶	12g
gan cao (Radix Glycyrrhizae Uralensis) 甘草	6g

Method: Decoction, powder or pills. Usually a decoction will be used until the bleeding has stopped and then pills or powder will be administered. In decoction,

e jiao is melted before being added to the strained decoction (*yang hua* 烊化). (Source: *Zhong Yi Nei Ke Lin Chuang Shou Ce*)

Modifications

- If there is Liver *qi* stagnation with hypochondriac tightness, tenderness or fullness and abdominal distension, add **bai shao** (Radix Paeoniae Lactiflorae) 白芍 12g and **chai hu** (Radix Bupleuri) 柴胡 9g.

Patent medicines

Zhi Bai Ba Wei Wan 知柏八味丸 (Zhi Bai Ba Wei Wan)

Yun Nan Bai Yao 云南白药 (Yunnan Paiyao)
- this medicine is specific for stopping bleeding and can be taken in addition to the main formula selected. The red pill is reserved for severe cases.

Acupuncture

Bl.23 (*shen shu* +), Ren.3 (*zhong ji* +), Ren.4 (*guan yuan* +), Kid.6 (*zhao hai* +), Kid.10 (*yin gu* +), Sp.6 (*san yin jiao*), Liv.1 (*da dun* ▲), Sp.1 (*yin bai* ▲)

Clinical notes

- Biomedical conditions that may present as Kidney *yin* deficiency type Blood Painful Urination include urinary tract infection, menopausal vaginitis and bladder or prostatic cancer
- This pattern can be difficult to treat successfully and prolonged therapy is needed for satisfactory results. Resistant or recurrent cases should be referred for investigation to exclude neoplasm.
- Urinary alkalysing agents like barley water or alfalfa tea are useful for reducing the discomfort.

12.5 CLOUDY PAINFUL URINATION SYNDROME

- Damp Heat
- Kidney *qi* deficiency

12.5.1 DAMP HEAT
Pathophysiology
- Damp Heat cloudy painful urination occurs when Damp Heat disrupts the transformation of Bladder *qi* and the separation of clear and turbid fluids.
- In contrast to other Damp Heat conditions where Heat may predominate, in this case the relative preponderance of Dampness causes cloudiness of the urine.

Clinical features
- urine that is either scanty and cloudy (like rice water or diluted milk) or cloudy and yellow, and that may contain globules of fatty material
- burning and painful urination
- fullness and discomfort in the chest and epigastrium
- bitter taste in the mouth, thirst or dry mouth with no desire to drink
- tendency to constipation or alternating loose and sluggish stools

T red body with greasy yellow coat
P rapid and slippery or soft

Treatment principle
Clear Heat and Dampness
Alleviate cloudiness and turbidity

Prescription

BEI XIE FEN QING YIN 萆解分清饮
(*Tokoro Combination*) modified

bei xie (Rhizoma Dioscoreae Hypoglaucae) 萆解	15g
che qian zi (Semen Plantaginis) 车前子	30g
fu ling (Sclerotium Poria Cocos) 茯苓	30g
shi wei (Folium Pyrrosiae) 石苇	20g
shi chang pu (Rhizoma Acori Graminei) 石菖蒲	6g
huang bai (Cortex Phellodendri) 黄柏	6g
gan cao (Radix Glycyrrhizae Uralensis) 甘草	6g
lian zi xin (Plumula Nelumbinis Nuciferae) 莲子心	3g
deng xin cao (Medulla Junci Effusi) 灯心草	3g

Method: Decoction. **Che qian zi** is cooked in a muslin bag (*bao jian* 包煎).
(Source: *Zhong Yi Nei Ke Lin Chuang Shou Ce*)

Modifications

- With significant Heat and pain, add **long dan cao** (Radix Gentianae Longdancao) 龙胆草 6g, **mu tong** (Caulis Mutong) 木通 6g and **shan zhi zi** (Fructus Gardeniae Jasminoidis) 山栀子 9g.
- With lower abdominal fullness and pain, add **wu yao** (Radix Linderae Strychnifoliae) 乌药 9g and **yi zhi ren** (Fructus Alpiniae Oxyphyllae) 益智仁 6g.
- With mild bleeding, add **xiao ji** (Herba Cephalanoplos) 小蓟 9g, **bai mao gen** (Rhizoma Imperatae Cylindricae) 白茅根 9g and **ou jie** (Nodus Nelumbinis Nuciferae Rhizomatis) 藕节 9g.

Patent medicines

Ming Mu Shang Qing Pian 明目上清片 (Ming Mu Shang Ching Pien)
Long Dan Xie Gan Wan 龙胆泻肝丸 (Long Dan Xie Gan Wan)
Dao Chi Pian 导赤片 (Tao Chih Pien)
Chuan Xin Lian Kang Yan Pian 穿心连抗炎片
   (Chuan Xin Lian Antiphlogistic Tablets)
Qian Jin Zhi Dai Wan 千金止带丸 (Chien Chin Chih Tai Wan)
   - recurrent or chronic cases
Bi Xie Fen Qing Wan 萆解分清丸 (Bi Xie Fen Qing Wan)
   - mild recurrent or chronic cases

Acupuncture

Bl.28 (*pang guang shu* -), Bl.22 (*san jiao shu* -), Ren.3 (*zhong ji* -), Sp.9 (*yin ling quan* -), Sp.6 (*san yin jiao* -), St.28 (*shui dao* -), GB.34 (*yang ling quan* -), St.40 (*feng long* -), Kid.7 (*fu liu*)

Clinical notes

- Biomedical conditions that may present as Damp Heat type cloudy Painful Urination include urethritis, cystitis, pyelonephritis, chyluria, prostatitis, gonorrhoea, nephrotic syndrome, myeloma and amyloidosis.
- Herbs are often best at leaching out Dampness. Depending on the associated biomedical disease, this pattern can respond well to TCM treatment. Amyloidosis and myeloma are difficult to treat with TCM alone and TCM treatment is probably best as a supportive treatment with Western medicine.

12.5.2 KIDNEY *QI* DEFICIENCY

肾气不足

Pathophysiology
- Kidney *qi* deficiency cloudy painful urination may occur when recurrent or chronic Damp Heat cloudy painful urination gradually weakens Kidney energy. Kidney *qi* is drained and so fails to separate the clear and turbid fluids, which then appear as cloudiness associated with uncomfortable urination.

Clinical features
- the urine is cloudy or oily; the cloudiness may be intermittent
- urination may be difficult, painful or uncomfortable as well as frequent, perhaps to the point of incontinence
- lower back pain, weak sore knees
- dizziness
- weakness and fatigue
- emaciation and pallor

T pale with a greasy coat
P thready and weak

Treatment principle
Tonify and consolidate Kidney *qi*
Leach out residual Dampness

Prescription

LIU WEI DI HUANG WAN 六味地黄丸
(*Rehmannia Six Formula*) plus
JIN SUO GU JING WAN 金锁固精丸
(*Metal Lock Pill to Stabilize the Essence*) modified

shu di (Radix Rehmanniae Glutinosae Conquitae) 熟地	240g
shan zhu yu (Fructus Corni Officinalis) 山茱萸	120g
shan yao (Radix Dioscoreae Oppositae) 山药	120g
fu ling (Sclerotium Poria Cocos) 茯苓	90g
ze xie (Rhizoma Alismatis Orientalis) 泽泻	90g
duan long gu^ (calcined Os Draconis) 煅龙骨	90g
duan mu li^ (calcined Concha Ostreae) 煅牡蛎	90g
sha yuan ji li (Semen Astragali Complanati) 沙苑蒺藜	60g
qian shi (Semen Euryales Ferocis) 芡实	60g
lian xu (Stamen Nelumbinis Nucifera) 莲须	60g

Method: Grind herbs into powder and form into 9-gram pills with honey. The dose is one pill 2-3 times daily. May also be decocted with a 90% reduction in dosage. (Source: *Shi Yong Zhong Yi Nei Ke Xue*)

Patent medicines
Jin Kui Shen Qi Wan 金匱肾气丸 (Sexoton Pills) plus
Jin Suo Gu Jing Wan 金锁固精丸 (Chin So Ku Ching Wan)

Acupuncture
Bl.28 (*pang guang shu*), Ren.3 (*zhong ji*), Ren.4 (*guan yuan* +),
Sp.9 (*yin ling quan*), Kid.3 (*tai xi* +), Ren.6 (*qi hai* ▲), Du.20 (*bai hui* ▲),
si feng (M-UE-9), St.40 (*feng long*)

Clinical notes
- Biomedical conditions that may present as Kidney *qi* deficiency type cloudy Painful Urination include albuminuria, chyluria, chronic nephritis, incontinence and weakness of bladder musculature.
- While acupuncture is useful to ease the discomfort associated with urination and to strengthen Kidney function, prolonged treatment with herbs may be necessary to fully address the Kidney deficiency.

12.6 EXHAUSTION PAINFUL URINATION SYNDROME

Pathophysiology

This group of patterns develops when a urinary disorder of any origin persists for long enough to cause damage to other organ systems. As well as the general features of a deficient type urinary disorder, there will be symptoms reflecting damage to the Kidney, Spleen or Heart. Patients with one (or more) of these patterns will generally be found to have presented repeatedly to their physician with 'cystitis', and probably have had numerous courses of antibiotics. The three main patterns are:

- Kidney *yin*, *qi* or *yang* deficiency
- Spleen *qi* deficiency (traditionally grouped in the *qi* painful urination category, this pattern is more consistent with this group)
- Heart and Kidney *qi* and *yin* deficiency

General clinical features

- chronic and recurrent, mild urinary discomfort that is aggravated or initiated by exertion, fatigue and sexual activity
- the urine is generally pale
- there may be urinary difficulty, dripping or mild incontinence

12.6.1 KIDNEY DEFICIENCY

Kidney *yin* deficiency

- mild lower back ache, frequent urination that feels hot but may or may not be concentrated, occasional urinary irritation or mild discomfort, sensation of heat in the palms and soles ('five hearts hot')

T red with little or no coat
P thready and rapid

Kidney *qi* deficiency

- lower abdominal discomfort that may be relieved by warmth, lower back soreness and weakness, clear urine, pale lustreless complexion, oedema of the lower extremities

T pale with a thin white coat
P deep and thready

Kidney *yang* deficiency

- same as for Kidney *qi* deficiency, with the addition of Cold signs, such as lower abdominal discomfort that is relieved by warmth, cold extremities, cold intolerance

T pale and swollen with toothmarks
P slow

Treatment principle
Tonify the Kidney and ease painful urination

Prescription
12.6.1.1 Kidney *yin* deficiency

LIU WEI DI HUANG WAN 六味地黄丸
(*Rehmannia Six Formula*)

> **shu di** (Radix Rehmanniae Glutinosae Conquitae) 熟地 240g
> **shan yao** (Radix Dioscoreae Oppositae) 山药 120g
> **shan zhu yu** (Fructus Corni Officinalis) 山茱萸 120g
> **fu ling** (Sclerotium Poria Cocos) 茯苓 90g
> **ze xie** (Rhizoma Alismatis Orientalis) 泽泻 90g
> **mu dan pi** (Cortex Moutan Radicis) 牡丹皮 90g
> Method: Grind the herbs to powder and form into 9-gram pills with honey. The dose is 2-3 pills daily. May also be decocted with a 90% reduction in dosage.
> (Source: *Shi Yong Zhong Yi Nei Ke Xue*)

Modifications
- With significant Heat, add **zhi mu** (Rhizoma Anemarrhenae Asphodeloidis) 知母 90g and **huang bai** (Cortex Phellodendri) 黄柏 90g.
- With lower back pain, add **xu duan** (Radix Dipsaci Asperi) 续断 90g, **gou ji** (Rhizoma Cibotii Barometz) 狗脊 90g and **sang ji sheng** (Ramulus Sangjisheng) 桑寄生 120g.
- With some Damp Heat, causing relatively more pain or burning upon urination, add **che qian zi** (Semen Plantaginis) 车前子 90g and **ren dong teng** (Ramus Lonicerae Japonicae) 忍冬藤 120g.

Patent medicines
Liu Wei Di Huang Wan 六味地黄丸 (Liu Wei Di Huang Wan)
Zhi Bai Ba Wei Wan 知柏八味丸 (Zhi Bai Ba Wei Wan)

Acupuncture
BL.23 (*shen shu* +), Bl.28 (*pang guang shu* +), Ren.2 (*qu gu* +), Kid.3 (*tai xi* +), Kid.2 (*ran gu* -), Kid.6 (*zhao hai* +).

Prescription
12.6.1.2 Kidney *qi* deficiency

WU BI SHAN YAO WAN 无比山药丸
(*Incomparable Dioscorea Pill*) modified

> **shan yao** (Radix Dioscoreae Oppositae) 山药 30g
> **fu ling** (Sclerotium Poria Cocos) 茯苓 20g
> **shu di** (Radix Rehmanniae Glutinosae Conquitae) 熟地 20g

shan zhu yu (Fructus Corni Officinalis) 山茱萸 20g
tu si zi (Semen Cuscutae Chinensis) 菟丝子 20g
ze xie (Rhizoma Alismatis Orientalis) 泽泻 15g
rou cong rong (Herba Cistanches Deserticolae) 肉苁蓉 15g
ba ji tian (Radix Morindae Officinalis) 巴戟天 15g
du zhong (Cortex Eucommiae Ulmoidis) 杜仲 15g
wu wei zi (Fructus Schizandrae Chinensis) 五味子 10g
gan cao (Radix Glycyrrhizae Uralensis) 甘草 6g

Method: Grind herbs into powder and form into 9-gram pills with honey. The dose is one pill 2-3 times daily. May also be decocted with the doses as given.
(Source: *Zhong Yi Nei Ke Lin Chuang Shou Ce*)

Patent medicines
Jin Kui Shen Qi Wan 金匮肾气丸 (Sexoton Pills)

Acupuncture
Du.4 (*ming men* +▲), Bl.23 (*shen shu* +▲), Bl.28 (*pang guang shu* +), Kid.3 (*tai xi* +▲), Kid.7 (*fu liu* +▲), Ren.4 (*guan yuan* +▲), Sp.6 (*san yin jiao* +), Lu.7 (*lie que*), Kid.6 (*zhao hai*)

Prescription
12.6.1.3 Kidney *yang* deficiency

JIN KUI SHEN QI WAN 金匮肾气丸
(*Rehmannia Eight Formula*)

shu di (Radix Rehmanniae Glutinosae Conquitae) 熟地 240g
shan yao (Radix Dioscoreae Oppositae) 山药 120g
shan zhu yu (Fructus Corni Officinalis) 山茱萸 120g
fu ling (Sclerotium Poria Cocos) 茯苓 90g
ze xie (Rhizoma Alismatis Orientalis) 泽泻 90g
mu dan pi (Cortex Moutan Radicis) 牡丹皮 90g
zhi fu zi* (Radix Aconiti Carmichaeli Praeparata) 制附子 60g
rou gui (Cortex Cinnamomi Cassiae) 肉桂 40g

Method: Grind the herbs to powder and form into 9-gram pills with honey. The dose is 2-3 pills daily. May also be decocted with a 90% reduction in dosage. When decocted, **zhi fu zi** is cooked for 30 minutes before the other herbs are added (*xian jian* 先煎), **rou gui** is added towards the end of cooking (*hou xia* 后下).
(Source: *Shi Yong Zhong Yi Nei Ke Xue*)

Patent medicines
Jin Kui Shen Qi Wan 金匮肾气丸 (Sexoton Pills)

Acupuncture
Du.4 (*ming men* +▲), Bl.23 (*shen shu* +▲), Bl.28 (*pang guang shu* +),

Kid.3 (*tai xi* +▲), Kid.7 (*fu liu* +▲), Ren.4 (*guan yuan* +▲), Sp.6 (*san yin jiao* +), Lu.7 (*lie que*), Kid.6 (*zhao hai*)

Clinical notes

- Biomedical conditions that may present as Damp Heat type cloudy Painful Urination include chronic glomerular disease, end stage kidney disease, diabetic nephropathy and uraemic syndrome.
- In all the exhaustion patterns, treatment needs to be long term to achieve a satisfactory result. Depending on the severity of the deficiency, one or two years may not be excessive.
- Rest is essential for success, and bladder training programs may be useful in some patients. Stress management and reduction of irritants or diuretic drinks like tea and coffee will also help. Urinary alkalysing agents like barley water or alfalfa tea are useful.
- Urine cultures will usually fail to find any pathogen.

12.6.2 SPLEEN *QI* DEFICIENCY

Pathophysiology
- Spleen *qi* deficiency type chronic dysuria is usually found in the elderly, post menopausal women and in patients who have had recurrent urinary tract disorders that have been treated with many courses of antibiotics or bitter cold herbs. This pattern is sometimes associated with prolapse of pelvic organs and poor muscle tone generally.
- This pattern is traditionally placed with *qi* stagnation pattern in the *qi* painful urination section.

Clinical features
- suprapubic pain, fullness or discomfort–the pain is vague or dull and dragging and is relieved by pressure and warmth over the bladder area
- frequent clear urine with a dull or 'empty' pain following voiding
- urinary dribbling or mild incontinence
- all symptoms are worse for overexertion and when fatigued
- there may be a history of prolapses or lower abdominal surgery
- pale complexion
- puffy eyelids and oedema of the extremities, particularly the fingers
- abdominal distension
- poor appetite
- loose stools
- fatigue
- shortness of breath

T pale
P deficient, thready and weak

Treatment principle
Tonify Spleen and Stomach
Benefit and raise *qi*

Prescription

BU ZHONG YI QI TANG 补中益气汤
(*Ginseng and Astragalus Combination*)

This formula is particularly good when prolapses are part of the pattern.
- **huang qi** (Radix Astragali Membranacei) 黄芪 15g
- **dang shen** (Radix Codonopsis Pilosulae) 党参 12g
- **bai zhu** (Rhizoma Atractylodes Macrocephalae) 白术 12g
- **dang gui** (Radix Angelicae Sinensis) 当归 9g
- **chen pi** (Pericarpium Citri Reticulatae) 陈皮 6g

zhi gan cao (honey fried Radix Glycyrrhizae Uralensis)
炙甘草 6g
sheng ma (Rhizoma Cimicifugae) 升麻 3g
chai hu (Radix Bupleuri) 柴胡 3g
Method: Decoction or powdered and taken in doses of 9-grams as a draft.
(Source: *Shi Yong Zhong Yi Nei Ke Xue*)

Modifications

- This pattern is frequently associated with Kidney *qi* deficiency; if so, combine with **WU BI SHAN YAO WAN** (*Incomparable Dioscorea Pill* 无比山药丸, p.391).
- If Lung *qi* is weak, add **mai dong** (Tuber Ophiopogonis Japonici) 麦冬 9g and **wu wei zi** (Fructus Schizandrae Chinensis) 五味子 6g.
- If Heart *qi* is weak and there are no signs of Damp Heat, **GUI PI TANG** (*Ginseng and Longan Combination* 归脾汤, p.554) may be used.
- If the dripping and incontinence are severe, add **sang piao xiao˘** (Ootheca Mantidis) 桑螵蛸 9g and **sha yuan ji li** (Semen Astragali Complani) 沙苑蒺藜 12g.

Patent medicines

Bu Zhong Yi Qi Wan 补中益气丸 (Bu Zhong Yi Qi Wan)
Bi Xie Fen Qing Wan 萆解分清丸 (Bi Xie Fen Qing Wan)

Acupuncture

Ren.4 (*guan yuan* ▲), St.36 (*zu san li* +), LI.4 (*he gu* +),
Sp.6 (*san yin jiao* +), Ren.6 (*qi hai* +), Bl.32 (*ci liao* +), Du.20 (*bai hui* ▲),
Lu.7 (*lie que*), Kid.6 (*zhao hai*)

Clinical notes

- Biomedical conditions that may present as Spleen *qi* deficiency type cloudy Painful Urination include interstitial cystitis, chronic nephritis, and bladder, vaginal or uterine prolapse
- In all the exhaustion patterns, treatment needs to be long term to achieve a satisfactory result. Depending on the severity of the deficiency, one or two years may not be excessive.
- Rest is essential for success, and bladder training programs may be useful in some patients. Stress management and reduction of irritants or diuretic drinks like tea and coffee will also help. Urinary alkalysing agents like barley water or alfalfa tea are useful.
- In some patients, the dysuria will not improve until prolapses are surgically repaired.

12.6.3 HEART AND KIDNEY *QI* AND *YIN* DEFICIENCY

Pathophysiology
- Heart and Kidney *qi* and *yin* deficiency is a variation of the Kidney deficiency type. This type is characterised by being worse for anxiety, overexcitement and excessive stimulation.

Clinical features
- chronic intermittent urinary discomfort or pain with a feeling of incomplete voiding, aggravated or initiated by overexertion, anxiety or overexcitement
- mild lower abdominal fullness
- palpitations, shortness of breath
- insomnia with much dreaming
- dry mouth and tongue
- fatigue and tiredness

T pink or only slightly red and swollen with numerous surface cracks, or the tip of the tongue is red; the coating is absent or thin and white
P thready and weak and possibly slightly rapid

Treatment principle
Nourish and strengthen *qi* and *yin*
Re-establish communication between the Heart and Kidney

Prescription

QING XIN LIAN ZI YIN 清心莲子饮
(*Lotus Seed Combination*)

huang qi (Radix Astragali Membranacei) 黄芪	15g
fu ling (Sclerotium Poria Cocos) 茯苓	12g
dang shen (Radix Codonopsis Pilosulae) 党参	12g
huang qin (Radix Scutellariae Baicalensis) 黄芩	9g
mai dong (Tuber Ophiopogonis Japonici) 麦冬	9g
di gu pi (Cortex Lycii Radicis) 地骨皮	9g
che qian zi (Semen Plantaginis) 车前子	9g
lian zi xin (Plumula Nelumbinis Nuciferae) 莲子心	6g
zhi gan cao (honey fried Radix Glycyrrhizae Uralensis) 炙甘草	3g

Method: Decoction or powdered and taken as a draft. **Che qian zi** is cooked in a muslin bag (*bao jian* 包煎). (Source: *Shi Yong Zhong Yi Nei Ke Xue*)

Modifications
- If there is significant intermittent pain upon urination combine (during painful episodes) with **DAO CHI SAN** (*Rehmannia and Akebia Formula*

导赤散 p.363).

Patent medicines
Tian Wang Bu Xin Dan 天王补心丹 (Tian Wang Bu Xin Dan)
Zhi Bai Ba Wei Wan 知柏八味丸 (Zhi Bai Ba Wei Wan)
Zuo Gui Wan 左归丸 (Zuo Gui Wan)

Acupuncture
BL.23 (*shen shu* +), Bl.28 (*pang guang shu* +), Ren.2 (*qu gu* +), Kid.3 (*tai xi* +), Kid.2 (*ran gu* -), Ren.4 (*guan yuan* +), Ren.6 (*qi hai* +), Ht.7 (*shen men*), Kid.9 (*zhu bin*)

Clinical notes
- In all the exhaustion patterns treatment needs to be long term to achieve a satisfactory result. Depending on the severity of the deficiency, one or two years may not be excessive
- Rest is essential for success, and bladder training programs may be useful in some patients. Stress management and reduction of irritants or diuretic drinks like tea and coffee will also help. Urinary alkalysing agents like barley water or alfalfa tea are useful.

SUMMARY OF GUIDING FORMULAE FOR PAINFUL URINATION

Heat painful urination
- Damp Heat - *Ba Zheng San* 八正散
- Heart Fire - *Dao Chi San* 导赤散
- Liver Fire - *Long Dan Xie Gan Tang* 龙胆泻肝汤

Stone painful urination
- In otherwise asymptomatic patients - *Shi Wei San* 石苇散
- with Damp Heat - *Niao Lu Pai Shi Tang* #2 尿路排石汤二号 or *San Jin Tang* 三金汤
- with Blood stagnation - *Niao Lu Pai Shi Tang* #1 尿路排石汤一号
- with Kidney deficiency
    - *qi* deficiency - *Niao Lu Pai Shi Tang* #3 尿路排石汤三号
    - *yin* deficiency - *Zhi Bai Ba Wei Wan* 知柏八味丸

Liver *qi* stagnation painful urination
- *Chen Xiang San* 沉香散

Blood painful urination
- Heat - *Xiao Ji Yin Zi* 小蓟饮子
- Kidney *yin* deficiency - *Zhi Bai Ba Wei Wan* 知柏八味丸

Cloudy painful urination
- Damp Heat - *Bei Xie Fen Qing Yin* 萆解分清饮
- Kidney *qi* deficiency - *Liu Wei Di Huang Wan* 六味地黄丸 plus *Jin Suo Gu Jin Wan* 金锁固精丸

Exhaustion painful urination
- Kidney *yin* deficiency - *Liu Wei Di Huang Wan* 六味地黄丸
- Kidney *qi* deficiency - *Wu Bi Shan Yao Wan* 无比山药丸
- Kidney *yang* deficiency - *Jin Kui Shen Qi Wan* 金匮肾气丸
- Spleen *qi* deficiency - *Bu Zhong Yi Qi Tang* 补中益气汤
- Heart and Kidney *qi* and *yin* deficiency - *Qing Xin Lian Zi Yin* 清心莲子饮

Endnote

For more information regarding herbs marked with an asterisk*, an open circle° or a hatˆ, see the tables on pp.944-952.

Disorders of the Kidney

13. Cloudy Urination

Excess patterns
Damp Heat

Deficient patterns
Spleen deficiency with sinking *qi*
Kidney *yang* deficiency
Kidney *yin* deficiency

13 CLOUDY URINATION
niao zhuo 尿浊

Cloudy urination refers to urine that appears milky or cloudy like rice water, or urine that may appear clear but precipitates sediment if allowed to stand. There is no, or only very mild pain associated with urination. If pain is predominant, see cloudy painful urination syndrome p.386.

AETIOLOGY

Damp Heat
This type of cloudy urine is most often a manifestation of lower *jiao* Damp Heat of internal origin. That is, the Damp Heat has been produced in the middle *jiao* by excessive consumption of rich food and alcohol and has then sunk into the lower *jiao*. The Damp Heat can also arise directly in the lower *jiao* by the condensing action of internal Heat on Fluids. Such internal Heat is produced by *yin* deficiency or long term *qi* or Damp stagnation.

Less often, Damp Heat type cloudy urine may be the result of external Damp Heat pathogen that invades through the *tai yang* (Bladder) channel, the leg *yin* channels or the local *luo* channels. External Damp Heat typically causes acute painful urination. However, if the Damp Heat is unresolved or lingering, the urine may become cloudy.

Spleen deficiency
Overwork, excessive worry or mental activity, irregular dietary habits or prolonged illness can weaken Spleen *qi*; Spleen *qi* naturally ascends creating the appropriate equilibrium for the descent of turbid waste materials, so it is said the Spleen governs 'the raising of the clear and descent of the turbid'. If this activity fails, the 'clear and turbid' intermingle and sink, settling in the lower *jiao* and Bladder. Also, when the Spleen is weak, food and fluids are poorly processed and Dampness may accumulate.

Kidney deficiency
Kidney deficiency manifests as either *yang* or *yin* deficiency. A tendency to Kidney weakness can be inherited and it certainly increases with age. Chronic illness, excessive sexual activity and many pregnancies also weaken the

---

BOX 13.1 KEY DIAGNOSTIC POINTS

Colour
- cloudy, concentrated, scanty - Damp Heat or *yin* deficiency
- milky, opaque, copious - Spleen or Kidney *qi* or *yang* deficiency

Kidneys.

Kidney *yang* or *qi* is particularly affected by prolonged exposure to cold conditions or excessive lifting or standing. In some cases, particularly in younger people, Kidney *qi* may be weakened while Kidney *yang* remains intact, in which case the cold symptoms are not seen.

Kidney *yin* is damaged through overwork (especially while under stress), insufficient sleep, febrile diseases, insufficient hydration and the use of some prescription and recreational drugs.

> **BOX 13.2 SOME BIOMEDICAL CAUSES OF CLOUDY URINE**
>
> - chyluria
> - nephrotic syndrome
> - urinary tract infection
> - inflammation of the genitourinary system
> - filariasis
> - tuberculosis of the kidneys
> - toxaemia of pregnancy
> - sarcoidosis
> - amyloidosis
> - tumours
> - albuminuria

The Kidney and Bladder are closely related, so weakness of the Kidney can affect the Bladder. When Kidney *qi* is weak, the Bladder is vulnerable to pathogenic invasion (through the *tai yang*, leg *yin* channels or local *luo* channels), especially Damp Heat.

13.1 DAMP HEAT

Pathophysiology

- Damp Heat cloudy urination is most commonly due to overconsumption of rich and greasy foods and alcohol, which generate Dampness and Heat in the middle *jiao*. The Damp Heat sinks and settles in the lower *jiao* disrupting Bladder *qi* and the separation of clear and turbid fluids. Cloudiness also occurs in acute attacks of external Damp Heat. However, in these cases painful urination is usually the main symptom and the clinical analysis proceeds from painful urination syndrome (p.386). Cloudy urine is more likely to follow an unresolved or subacute case of external Damp Heat.
- Depending on whether Dampness or Heat predominates, the pattern will vary. If Dampness predominates the urine will be white and cloudy. If Heat predominates the urine will still be cloudy, but more scanty and concentrated and there is more likely to be mild pain.

Clinical features

- cloudy, whitish urine, like the water after washing rice, or cloudy, yellow and scanty urine; in some cases there may be mild bleeding, in which case the urine is pink and opaque
- suprapubic fullness and discomfort
- lower back pain
- fullness in the chest and epigastrium
- poor appetite, nausea
- bitter taste in the mouth
- thirst with little desire to drink
- a tendency to constipation or alternating loose and sluggish stools
- some cases may have afternoon fever or alternating fever and chills

T greasy yellow coat
P soft and rapid

Treatment principle

Clear and transform Dampness and Heat

Prescription

CHENG SHI BEI XIE FEN QING YIN 程氏萆解分清饮
(*Tokoro Formula from the Cheng Clan*)

    bei xie (Rhizoma Dioscoreae Hypoglaucae) 萆解 12g
    fu ling (Sclerotium Poria Cocos) 茯苓 12g
    che qian zi (Semen Plantaginis) 车前子 12g
    bai zhu (Rhizoma Atractylodes Macrocephalae) 白术 9g

dan shen (Radix Salviae Miltiorrhizae) 丹参 9g
huang bai (Cortex Phellodendri) 黄柏 6g
shi chang pu (Rhizoma Acori Graminei) 石菖蒲 6g
lian zi xin (Plumula Nelumbinis Nuciferae) 莲子心 3g

Method: Decoction. **Che qian zi** is cooked in a muslin bag (*bao jian* 包煎).
(Source: *Shi Yong Zhong Yi Nei Ke Xue*)

Modifications

- If Heat predominates, add **mu tong** (Caulis Mutong) 木通 6g, **shan zhi zi** (Fructus Gardeniae Jasminoidis) 山栀子 9g and **hua shi** (Talcum) 滑石 12-18g.
- If Dampness predominates, add **cang zhu** (Rhizoma Atractylodis) 苍术 9g, **hou po** (Cortex Magnoliae Officinalis) 厚朴 9g, **ban xia*** (Rhizoma Pinelliae Ternatae) 半夏 9g and **chen pi** (Pericarpium Citri Reticulatae) 陈皮 6g.

Patent medicines

Ming Mu Shang Qing Pian 明目上清片 (Ming Mu Shang Ching Pien)
Long Dan Xie Gan Wan 龙胆泻肝丸 (Long Dan Xie Gan Wan)
Dao Chi Pian 导赤片 (Tao Chih Pien)
Chuan Xin Lian Kang Yan Pian 穿心连抗炎片
    (Chuan Xin Lian Antiphlogistic Tablets)

Acupuncture

Sp.6 (*san yin jiao* -), Sp.9 (*yin ling quan* -), Sp.4 (*gong sun* -),
BL.22 (*san jiao shu* -), Ren.3 (*zhong ji* -), Bl.28 (*pang guang shu* -),
Liv.5 (*li gou* -), Kid.7 (*fu liu*), GB.41 (*zu lin qi* -), SJ.5 (*wai guan* -)

Clinical notes

- Biomedical conditions that may present as Damp Heat type cloudy urination include urinary tract infection, acute or chronic prostatitis, cystitis, urethritis, orchitis, nephrotic syndrome, chyluria and amyloidosis.
- This pattern can respond well to TCM treatment, although conditions like amyloidosis are best treated with combined Western and Chinese medicine.
- While acupuncture can be useful, herbs are particularly effective for leaching Damp from the body.

脾虛氣陷尿濁

13.2 SPLEEN *QI* DEFICIENCY WITH SINKING *QI*

Pathophysiology
- When the Spleen is weak, inefficient digestion can lead to an accumulation of Dampness or a failure to properly separate the 'pure and turbid', which may then sink and settle in the lower *jiao* and appear as cloudy urine.

Clinical features
- chronic and recurrent cloudy urine that is like rice water, or urine that precipitates a sediment; the condition is aggravated or initiated by fatigue and consumption of oily or rich foods
- dragging or sinking feeling in the lower abdomen
- oedema of the eyelids or upper extremities (especially the fingers) that is worse in the morning
- sallow or pale complexion
- lethargy
- shortness of breath
- poor appetite
- loose stools
- possibly prolapses of various structures, such as the uterus, bladder and rectum

T pale and swollen, with tooth marks
P deficient and soft

Treatment principle
Raise and strengthen Spleen *qi*

Prescription

BU ZHONG YI QI TANG 补中益气汤
(*Ginseng and Astragalus Combination*) modified

huang qi (Radix Astragali Membranacei) 黄芪	18g
fu ling (Sclerotium Poria Cocos) 茯苓	15g
long gu^ (Os Draconis) 龙骨	15g
dang shen (Radix Codonopsis Pilosulae) 党参	12g
bai zhu (Rhizoma Atractylodes Macrocephalae) 白术	9g
cang zhu (Rhizoma Atractylodis) 苍术	9g
xiao hui xiang (Fructus Foeniculi Vulgaris) 小茴香	9g
chen pi (Pericarpium Citri Reticulatae) 陈皮	6g
dang gui (Radix Angelicae Sinensis) 当归	6g
chuan lian zi* (Fructus Meliae Toosendan) 川楝子	6g
chai hu (Radix Bupleuri) 柴胡	3g
sheng ma (Rhizoma Cimicifugae) 升麻	3g

zhi gan cao (honey fried Radix Glycyrrhizae Uralensis)
炙甘草 3g
Method: Decoction. (Source: *Shi Yong Zhong Yi Nei Ke Xue*)

Modifications
- If there is some residual or co-existing Damp Heat, add **huang bai** (Cortex Phellodendri) 黄柏 9g and **bei xie** (Rhizoma Dioscoreae Hypoglaucae) 萆解 9g.

Patent medicines
Bu Zhong Yi Qi Wan 补中益气丸 (Bu Zhong Yi Qi Wan)
Shen Ling Bai Zhu Wan 参苓白术丸 (Shen Ling Bai Zhu Wan)
Bi Xie Fen Qing Wan 萆解分清丸 (Bi Xie Fen Qing Wan)

Acupuncture
Ren.6 (*qi hai* +), Liv.13 (*zhang men* +), Bl.23 (*shen shu* +), Kid.3 (*tai xi* +), Du.20 (*bai hui* ▲), Sp.6 (*san yin jiao* +), Bl.20 (*pi shu*), Du.4 (*ming men* ▲), Lu.7 (*lie que*)

Clinical notes
- Biomedical conditions that may present as Spleen *qi* deficiency type cloudy urination include chyluria, albuminuria, nephrotic syndrome, amyloidosis, sarcoidosis, prolonged bed rest, chronic nephritis and chronic renal failure.
- Conditions like amyloidosis and sarcoidosis are difficult to treat with TCM alone.

13.3 KIDNEY *YIN* DEFICIENCY

Pathophysiology
- Kidney *yin* deficiency cloudy urine is due to the Heat generated by *yin* deficiency, which concentrates fluids and causes precipitation of solids from solution causing the urine to appear cloudy.

Clinical features
- chronic cloudy, scanty, yellow urine or recurrent milky, opaque urine like rice water
- sensations of heat in the palms and soles ('five hearts hot')
- facial flushing, malar flush
- nightsweats
- dry mouth and throat
- restlessness
- insomnia
- dizziness
- tinnitus
- soreness or weakness of the lower back and knees, heel pain
- tendency to dry stools or constipation

T red and dry with little or no coat
P thready and rapid

Treatment principle
Nourish Kidney *yin*, clear Heat

Prescription

ZHI BAI BA WEI WAN 知柏八味丸
(*Anemarrhena, Phellodendron and Rehmannia Formula*) modified

shu di (Radix Rehmanniae Glutinosae Conquitae) 熟地	24g
shan yao (Radix Dioscoreae Oppositae) 山药	12g
shan zhu yu (Fructus Corni Officinalis) 山茱萸	12g
bei xie (Rhizoma Dioscoreae Hypoglaucae) 萆解	12g
fu ling (Sclerotium Poria Cocos) 茯苓	9g
mu dan pi (Cortex Moutan Radicis) 牡丹皮	9g
ze xie (Rhizoma Alismatis Orientalis) 泽泻	9g
lian zi xin (Plumula Nelumbinis Nuciferae) 莲子心	9g
zhi mu (Rhizoma Anemarrhenae Asphodeloidis) 知母	9g
yan huang bai (salt fried Cortex Phellodendri) 盐黄柏	9g
gan cao (Radix Glycyrrhizae Uralensis) 甘草	3g

Method: Decoction, powder or pills. (Source: *Shi Yong Zhong Yi Nei Ke Xue*)

DA BU YIN WAN 大补阴丸
(*Great Tonify the yin Pill*)

This formula is particularly good when the deficient Heat aspects, particularly bone steaming fever and nightsweats, are severe.

shu di (Radix Rehmanniae Glutinosae Conquitae) 熟地 180g
zhi gui ban° (honey fried Plastrum Testudinis) 炙龟板 180g
yan huang bai (salt fried Cortex Phellodendri) 盐黄柏 120g
yan zhi mu (salt fried Rhizoma Anemarrhenae Asphodeloidis)
盐知母 120g

Method: Grind herbs to a fine powder and form into 9-gram pills with honey. The dose is one pill 2-3 times daily.

Patent medicines
Zhi Bai Ba Wei Wan 知柏八味丸 (Zhi Bai Ba Wei Wan)
Liu Wei Di Huang Wan 六味地黄丸 (Liu Wei Di Huang Wan)
Zuo Gui Wan 左归丸 (Zuo Gui Wan)

Acupuncture
Bl.23 (*shen shu* +), Ren.4 (*guan yuan* +), St.28 (*shui dao* +),
Kid.6 (*zhao hai* +), Kid.2 (*ran gu* -)

Clinical notes
- Biomedical conditions that may present as Kidney *yin* deficiency type cloudy urination include chronic nephritis, nephrotic syndrome, chronic glomerulonephritis, renal tuberculosis, toxaemia of pregnancy, hypertension, myeloma, amyloidosis and sarcoidosis.
- Symptoms of Kidney *yin* deficiency often respond well to lengthy treatment. Conditions like amyloidosis, myeloma and sarcoidosis are difficult to treat with TCM alone.

13.4 KIDNEY *YANG* DEFICIENCY

肾阳虚衰尿浊

Pathophysiology
- When Kidney *yang* is weak, there is a general failure of fluid transformation and metabolism–in essence, the 'distillation' Fire (*ming men huo* 命门火) required for processing fluids for excretion and redistribution is inadequate. Excess of untransformed fluids gives rise to Damp in the Bladder, which appears as cloudiness.

Clinical features
- chronic and recurrent cloudy or opaque urine that is frequent and copious
- waxy pale complexion with dark rings under the eyes
- oedema, particularly below the waist and in the ankles
- listlessness, lethargy
- increased desire to sleep
- coldness and aching in the lower back and knees
- cold extremities
- low libido, impotence
- nocturia

T pale and swollen with a white coat
P deep, weak and thready

Treatment principle
Warm and consolidate the Kidneys
Tonify Kidney *yang*

Prescription

LU RONG BU SE WAN 鹿角补涩丸
(*Deer Horn Pills to Tonify and Astringe*)

lu jiao jiao^ (Cornu Cervi Gelatinum) 鹿角胶	120g
fu ling (Sclerotium Poria Cocos) 茯苓	120g
huang qi (Radix Astragali Membranacei) 黄芪	120g
long gu^ (Os Draconis) 龙骨	120g
bu gu zhi (Fructus Psoraleae Corylifoliae) 补骨脂	120g
tu si zi (Semen Cuscutae Chinensis) 菟丝子	120g
ren shen (Radix Ginseng) 人参	100g
zhi fu zi* (Radix Aconiti Carmichaeli Praeparata) 制附子	60g
sang bai pi (Cortex Mori Albae Radicis) 桑白皮	60g
rou gui (Cortex Cinnamomi Cassiae) 肉桂	60g
lian zi (Semen Nelumbinis Nuciferae) 莲子	60g
sang piao xiao^ (Ootheca Mantidis) 桑螵蛸	40g

wu wei zi (Fructus Schizandrae Chinensis) 五味子 40g

Method: Powder the herbs and form into 9-gram pills with honey. The dose 2-3 pills daily. May also be decocted with a 90% reduction in dosage. When decocted **zhi fu zi** is cooked for 30 minutes prior to the other herbs (*xian jian* 先煎) and **lu jiao jiao** is melted before being added to the strained decoction (*yang hua* 烊化). (Source: *Shi Yong Zhong Yi Nei Ke Xue*)

JIN KUI SHEN QI WAN 金匮肾气丸
(Rehmannia Eight Formula)

This is the basic Kidney *yang* strengthening formula, and is excellent as a general *yang* tonic. While not as specific as the principal formula, it is cheaper and widely available in patent medicine form.

shu di (Radix Rehmanniae Glutinosae Conquitae) 熟地 240g
shan yao (Radix Dioscoreae Oppositae) 山药 120g
shan zhu yu (Fructus Corni Officinalis) 山茱萸 120g
fu ling (Sclerotium Poria Cocos) 茯苓 90g
ze xie (Rhizoma Alismatis Orientalis) 泽泻 90g
mu dan pi (Cortex Moutan Radicis) 牡丹皮 90g
zhi fu zi* (Radix Aconiti Carmichaeli Praeparata) 制附子 60g
rou gui (Cortex Cinnamomi Cassiae) 肉桂 40g

Method: Grind the herbs to powder and form into 9-gram pills with honey. The dose is 2-3 pills daily. May also be decocted with a 90% reduction in dosage. When decocted **zhi fu zi** is cooked for 30 minutes before the other herbs (*xian jian* 先煎), **rou gui** is added towards the end of cooking (*hou xia* 后下). (Source: *Shi Yong Zhong Yi Nei Ke Xue*)

Modifications

- If there is some blood in the urine, add **pao jiang tan** (roasted Rhizoma Zingiberis Officinalis) 炮姜炭 60g and **ce bai ye** (Cacumen Biotae Orientalis) 侧柏叶 90g.

Variations and additional prescriptions

- With less (or no) Cold and evidence of Heart involvement (frequent and cloudy urination, forgetfulness, disorientation, a pale tongue with a thin white coat and a thready weak pulse), the correct treatment is to regulate and tonify the Heart and Kidneys, stabilise *jing* and clear turbidity with **SANG PIAO XIAO SAN** (*Mantis Egg Case Powder* 桑螵蛸散)

    sang piao xiao^ (Ootheca Mantidis) 桑螵蛸 9g
    fu ling (Sclerotium Poria Cocos) 茯苓 9g
    dang gui (Radix Angelicae Sinensis) 当归 9g
    yuan zhi (Radix Polygalae Tenuifoliae) 远志 6g
    shi chang pu (Rhizoma Acori Graminei) 石菖蒲 6g
    duan long gu^ (Calcined Os Draconis) 煅龙骨 12g
    dang shen (Radix Codonopsis Pilosulae) 党参 12g

zhi gui ban° (honey fried Plastrum Testudinis) 炙龟板 15g
Method: Decoction. (Source: *Shi Yong Zhong Yao Xue*)

Patent medicines
Jin Kui Shen Qi Wan 金匮肾气丸 (Sexoton Pills)
You Gui Wan 右归丸 (You Gui Wan)
Ba Ji Yin Yang Wan 巴戟阴阳丸 (Ba Ji Yin Yang Wan)
Jin Suo Gu Jing Wan 金锁固精丸 (Chin So Ku Ching Wan)
 - added to one of the three patents above

Acupuncture
Ren.6 (*qi hai* +▲), Ren.4 (*guan yuan* +▲), Kid.3 (*tai xi* +▲), Bl.23 (*shen shu* +▲), Du.4 (*ming men* +▲), Kid.7 (*fu liu*), Sp.4 (*gong sun*)

Clinical notes
- Biomedical conditions that may present as Kidney *yin* deficiency type cloudy urination include chronic nephritis, nephrotic syndrome, amyloidosis and sarcoidosis.
- *Yang* deficiency patterns often respond well to treatment with moxa and warming herbs and cloudiness of the urine should resolve with treatment. However, if the kidney is severely structurally damaged or the disorder is very advanced the prognosis is poor. Conditions like amyloidosis and sarcoidosis are difficult to treat with TCM alone.

SUMMARY OF GUIDING FORMULAE FOR CLOUDY URINATION

Damp Heat - *Cheng Shi Bei Xie Fen Qing Yin* 程氏萆解分清饮

Spleen *qi* deficiency - *Bu Zhong Yi Qi Tang* 补中益气汤

Kidney *yin* deficiency - *Zhi Bai Ba Wei Wan* 知柏八味丸
- with deficient Heat - *Da Bu Yin Wan* 大补阴丸

Kidney *yang* deficiency
 - *Lu Rong Bu Se Wan* 鹿茸补涩丸 or *Jin Kui Shen Qi Wan* 金匮肾气丸
- with Heart and Kidney *qi* deficiency - *Sang Piao Xiao San* 桑螵蛸散

Endnote

For more information regarding herbs marked with an asterisk*, an open circle° or a hat^, see the tables on pp.944-952.

Disorders of the Kidney

14. Difficult Urination and Urinary Retention

Excess patterns
Damp Heat
Lung *qi* obstruction
Liver *qi* stagnation
Blood stagnation

Deficient patterns
Spleen *yang* deficiency
Kidney *yang* deficiency
Kidney *yin* deficiency

14 DIFFICULT URINATION, URINARY RETENTION
long bi 癃闭

Difficult urination (*long* 癃) refers to reduced volume of urine with difficulty in voiding the bladder. The patient may experience difficulty in starting urination or have a weak or broken stream and a feeling of incomplete voiding.

Urinary retention (*bi* 闭) is severe difficulty urinating even though the bladder is full. Generally no urine at all or only a few drops are passed.

The term *long bi*, therefore, refers to a continuum of states from difficult urination to complete retention. Because *bi* can lead to serious kidney damage, it is a medical emergency and should be treated in a hospital.

In ancient times multiple treatment methods were recognised and used accordingly - Sun Si-miao of the Tang Dynasty (618-907AD) applied a catheter composed of the tubal leaf of a spring onion in addition to herbal decoction.

AETIOLOGY
Damp Heat
External Heat
Damp Heat causing urinary difficulty or retention can result from an external Damp Heat pathogen that invades through the *tai yang* (Urinary Bladder) channel, the leg *yin* channels or the local *luo* channels. In practice, transmission of Damp Heat through the *luo* channels is probably the most common mode of entry (especially in sexually active individuals). The presence of Damp Heat blocks *qi* transformation in the bladder and obstructs the free passage of urine. When external Damp Heat is the cause of the urinary difficulty, the symptoms are frequently localised in the bladder and the systemic symptoms of Damp Heat diminished or absent.

Internal Heat
Internally generated Heat or Damp Heat can also cause urinary difficulty or retention. Heat affecting the Heart or Liver can be transmitted through their associated channels to the lower *jiao*. Damp Heat generated in the middle *jiao* by overconsumption of rich, greasy or spicy foods and alcohol can simply sink and settle in the lower *jiao*. Damp Heat can also be generated in the lower *jiao* by any prolonged Heat in the system, such as the Heat arising from *yin* deficiency, *qi* stagnation, or by prolonged stagnation of Dampness. When the Heat is generated internally, the symptoms tend to be more systemic, reflecting the original source of the Heat. Heat of external origin,

however, tends to produce a more localised pattern, with the focus of symptoms in the bladder and urethra. An important cause of urinary difficulty in chronic Damp Heat patterns is the development of urinary tract stones which easily obstruct the passage of urine.

Spleen deficiency

Overwork, excessive worry or mental activity, irregular dietary habits or prolonged illness can weaken Spleen *qi*. Spleen *qi* naturally ascends, creating the appropriate equilibrium for the descent of turbid waste materials, so it is said the Spleen governs 'the raising of the clear and descent of the turbid'. If this activity fails, the 'clear and turbid' intermingle, and in this case neither descend or ascend (or if they do descend into the bladder they appear as cloudy urine). If Spleen *qi* deficiency persists, or there is overconsumption of cold raw foods, Spleen *yang* deficiency may develop. When Spleen *yang* is weak, fluid metabolism and movement is impaired and instead of going to the Bladder for processing, fluids congeal into Dampness or accumulate in the limbs and tissues as oedema. Weak *yang* is also responsible for general weakness of *qi* movement, and thus forceless expulsion of urine.

> **BOX 14.1 SOME BIOMEDICAL CAUSES OF DIFFICULT URINATION OR URINARY RETENTION**
>
> - urinary tract infection
> - tumours of the bladder, prostate or kidney
> - urethral scarring
> - prostatic hypertrophy
> - pressure from gynaecological tumours like fibroids
> - obstruction by urinary calculi
> - transverse myelitis
> - multiple sclerosis
> - extreme cold
> - alcohol
> - faecal impaction
> - foreign body
> - anticholinergic drugs

Kidney deficiency

Weak Kidney *yang* or *qi* may be an inherited condition, or may develop as a result of age, chronic illness, too much exposure to cold conditions or excessive lifting or standing (particularly if this occurs in a cold environment or on cold floors or at night). Kidney *yang* or *qi* may also be damaged by excessive sexual activity, or in women who have many pregnancies. In some cases, particularly in younger people, Kidney *qi* may be weakened while Kidney *yang* remains intact, in which case the cold symptoms are not seen.

Kidney *yin* becomes damaged through febrile disease, overwork (especially while under stress), insufficient sleep, and the use of recreational drugs. Kidney *yin* may also be weakened by ageing and excessive sexual activity, or in women who have many pregnancies.

Obstruction of Lung *qi*

The Lungs, as one of the organs involved in the fluid cycle, play a role in the smooth excretion of urine. The Lungs send a portion of the fluids (sent upwards by the Spleen) to the skin and a portion to the Kidneys for reprocessing. If the natural descent of Lung *qi* is obstructed by some pathogenic factor (usually Wind or Heat), fluids can fail to reach the lower *jiao* and will accumulate in the upper *jiao*.

Liver *qi* stagnation, Blood stagnation

Frustration, anger, resentment, prolonged emotional turmoil, repressed emotions and stress can disrupt the circulation of Liver *qi*, and because the Liver channel passes through the lower *jiao*, Bladder *qi* can also be disrupted. Once Bladder *qi* is blocked, urine will not pass smoothly and the Blood stagnation that can eventuate may reflect serious disorders like stones or malignancy.

Liver *qi* stagnation can give rise to other complications. Prolonged Liver *qi* stagnation creates Heat which can travel through the Liver channel to the lower *jiao* condensing Bladder Fluids into Dampness or Damp Heat. Liver *qi* may also damage the Spleen, predisposing to Dampness which sinks to the lower *jiao*. This Damp can obstruct the Bladder or predispose to Damp Heat.

Pre-existing stagnation (of *qi* and Blood) can be transferred from another pelvic organ to the Bladder. This is most commonly observed in women following hysterectomy, myomectomy or removal of ovarian cysts. The organ primarily affected by the stagnation is removed or repaired, but the underlying *qi* and Blood stagnation that gave rise to the initial problem persists. The focus of pelvic symptoms then shifts from, for example the uterus, causing heavy periods and pain, to the Bladder.

DIFFERENTIAL DIAGNOSIS

Painful urination syndrome (*lin zheng* 淋证): Difficult urination frequently accompanies painful urination, the difference being the prominence and degree of dysuria. Difficult urination and retention are not painful or only minimally painful.

Guan Ge syndrome (*guan ge* 关格): A group of patterns characterised by simultaneous anuria, constipation and vomiting. *Guan ge* may include (with appropriate presentation) kidney disorders like uraemia, chronic renal failure, chronic pyelonephritis, glomerularsclerosis, renal tuberculosis and diabetic nephropathy, as well as conditions like shock, crush injuries, severe burns and severe infections.

Oedema (*shui zhong* 水肿): Oedema is fluid accumulation in subcutaneous tissues. When oedema is significant, there is a decrease in fluids being processed by the Kidney and smaller volumes excreted. However, there is usually no difficulty in urinating.

Ascites/Drum-like Abdominal distension (*gu zhang* 臌胀): *Gu zhang* is fluid accumulation in the abdominal cavity, with a decrease in urinary output. *Gu zhang* occurs in such conditions as hepatic cirrhosis, schistosomiasis, abdominal and liver cancer, chronic malaria and tuberculous peritonitis.

In addition, excessive fluid loss through diarrhoea, sweating and inadequate fluid replacement can cause reduced urination, though again, generally without difficulty.

TREATMENT

The two general approaches to treatment in urinary difficulty reflect the underlying pathology. In the excess patterns, Damp Heat and Liver *qi* stagnation, removal of the pathogen or moving *qi* will usually quickly alleviate the condition. In the deficient patterns, gradual strengthening of the organs involved in fluid metabolism and propulsion is the therapeutic aim. In this case persisent treatment must be given, often for a number of months, to produce a lasting result.

In cases of acute retention, *tui na* or electro-acupuncture therapy may be applied. If this fails, hospitalisation and catheterisation will be required as kidney damage can occur quite quickly. In mild cases (especially in children) sitting in a warm bath or listening to a running tap can induce urination.

Tui na
Ren.6 (*qi hai*), Ren.5 (*shi men*), Ren.4 (*guan yuan*)
Press from above towards the pubic bone. Be sure to have some implement to contain the urine, as this technique may cause immediate release.

Electro-acupuncture
St.28 (*shui dao*) ~ Sp.6 (*san yin jiao*) or Sp.9 (*yin ling quan*) with high frequency stimulation. St.28 (*shui dao*) should be needled cautiously and superficially in those with very distended bladders. This technique may cause immediate release of urine.

14.1 DAMP HEAT

Pathophysiology
- Damp Heat in the Bladder causes difficult urination in two ways. First, Damp, being a *yin* pathogen, obstructs the movement of fluid, and second, Heat burns the delicate tissues of the urethra causing pain. If pain is the prominent feature, see Painful Urination Syndrome, p.358.
- Chronic or unresolved Damp Heat can lurk in the Bladder and eventually congeal into urinary stones (see Stone Painful Urination Syndrome p.370) which will obstruct the passage of urine.

Clinical features
- acute, scanty, concentrated urine that is difficult to pass and comes in drips; urination may be hot or burning and in severe cases almost no urine is passed
- suprapubic fullness and discomfort
- lower back pain
- fullness in the chest and epigastrium
- poor appetite, nausea
- bitter taste in the mouth
- thirst with little desire to drink
- tendency to constipation or alternating loose and sluggish stools
- in some cases there may be fever (especially in the afternoon), or alternating fever and chills

T red with a greasy yellow coat
P slippery and rapid or soft and rapid

Treatment principle
Clear Damp Heat
Promote urination

Prescription

BA ZHENG SAN 八正散
(*Dianthus Formula*) modified

qu mai (Herba Dianthi) 瞿麦	20g
hua shi (Talcum) 滑石	15g
che qian zi (Semen Plantaginis) 车前子	15g
bian xu (Herba Polygoni Avicularis) 萹蓄	15g
shan zhi zi (Fructus Gardeniae Jasminoidis) 山栀子	9g
gan cao (Radix Glycyrrhizae Uralensis) 甘草	6g
mu tong (Caulis Mutong) 木通	6g
zhi da huang (Radix et Rhizoma Rhei) 制大黄	6g

Method: Decoction. **Che qian zi** is cooked in a muslin bag (*bao jian* 包煎).
(Source: *Zhong Yi Nei Ke Lin Chuang Shou Ce*)

Modifications

- With severe difficulty urinating, or urinary retention, increase the dosage of **mu tong** (Caulis Mutong) 木通, **hua shi** (Talcum) 滑石 and **bian xu** (Herba Polygoni Avicularis) 篇蓄 by 30% and add **huang bai** (Cortex Phellodendri) 黄柏 9g and **rou gui** (Cortex Cinnamomi Cassiae) 肉桂 3g.
- If the bowels are loose, delete **da huang** (Radix et Rhizoma Rhei).
- If the tongue coat is very thick, yellow and greasy, add **huang bai** (Cortex Phellodendri) 黄柏 12g and **cang zhu** (Rhizoma Atractylodis) 苍术 12g.
- Irritability, restlessness, insomnia, mouth and tongue ulcers and erosions indicate that Heat is affecting the Heart–add **sheng di** (Radix Rehmanniae Glutinosae) 生地 15g and **huang lian** (Rhizoma Coptidis) 黄连 6g.
- Alternating fever and chills, nausea and dizziness indicate that Damp Heat is obstructing the *shao yang* level. Add **chai hu** (Radix Bupleuri) 柴胡 9g, **huang qin** (Radix Scutellariae Baicalensis) 黄芩 9g and **ban xia*** (Rhizoma Pinelliae Ternatae) 半夏 6g to harmonise *shao yang*.
- With mild bleeding, add **xiao ji** (Herba Cephalanoplos) 小蓟 9g and **bai mao gen** (Rhizoma Imperatae Cylindricae) 白茅根 12g.
- In prolonged cases, Damp Heat can damage *yin*. If there are signs of Kidney *yin* deficiency in addition to Damp Heat (peeled tongue or peeled tongue root, nightsweats, afternoon fever and heat in the palms and soles), add **sheng di** (Radix Rehmanniae Glutinosae) 生地 20g, **huai niu xi** (Radix Achyranthis Bidentatae) 怀牛膝 12g and **nu zhen zi** (Fructus Ligustri Lucidi) 女贞子 12g, or nourish *yin* and clear Damp Heat with **ZI SHEN TONG GUAN WAN** (*Nourish Kidney, Open the Gate Pill* 滋肾通关丸) modified.

    sheng di (Radix Rehmanniae Glutinosae) 生地 15g
    che qian zi (Semen Plantaginis) 车前子 12g
    niu xi (Radix Achyranthis Bidentatae) 牛膝 12g
    zhi mu (Rhizoma Anemarrhenae Asphodeloidis) 知母 12g
    huang bai (Cortex Phellodendri) 黄柏 9g
    rou gui (Cortex Cinnamomi Cassiae) 肉桂 3g
    Method: Decoction. **Che qian zi** is cooked in a muslin bag (*bao jian* 包煎)
    (Source: *Shi Yong Zhong Yi Nei Ke Xue*)

Variations and additional prescriptions

Toxic Damp

- If the Damp Heat obstructs and impedes the transformation of *san jiao qi*, leading to accumulation of Toxic Dampness, there will be symptoms of difficult urination or anuria, darkish complexion, no appetite, lethargy, listlessness, fullness in the chest, irritability, nausea, vomiting, bad breath that smells of urine, and in severe cases delerium and confusion. In such cases, the correct treatment is to clear turbidity and harmonise the Stomach, clear Damp Heat, and open the bowels to drain Toxins with **HUANG LIAN WEN DAN TANG** (*Coptis Decoction to Warm the Gall Bladder* 黄连温胆汤) modified.

> **huang lian** (Rhizoma Coptidis) 黄连 6g
> **zhu ru** (Caulis Bambusae in Taeniis) 竹茹 9g
> **zhi shi** (Fructus Immaturus Citri Aurantii) 枳实 9g
> **ban xia*** (Rhizoma Pinelliae Ternatae) 半夏 9g
> **chen pi** (Pericarpium Citri Reticulatae) 陈皮 9g
> **fu ling** (Sclerotium Poriae Cocos) 茯苓 12g
> **che qian zi** (Semen Plantaginis) 车前子 12g
> **bai mao gen** (Rhizoma Imperatae Cylindricae) 白茅根 30g
> **mu tong** (Caulis Mutong) 木通 6g
> **da huang** (Radix et Rhizoma Rhei) 大黄 6g
> **gan cao** (Radix Glycyrrhizae Uralensis) 甘草 3g
>
> Method: Decoction. **Che qian zi** is cooked in a muslin bag (*bao jian* 包煎).
> (Source: *Shi Yong Zhong Yi Nei Ke Xue*)

Patent medicines

Ming Mu Shang Qing Pian 明目上清片 (Ming Mu Shang Ching Pien)
Long Dan Xie Gan Wan 龙胆泻肝丸 (Long Dan Xie Gan Wan)
Dao Chi Pian 导赤片 (Tao Chih Pien)
Chuan Xin Lian Kang Yan Pian 穿心连抗炎片
    (Chuan Xin Lian Antiphlogistic Tablets)
Qian Lie Xian Wan 前列腺丸 (Prostate Gland Pills)
    - combined with one of the above formulae for prostate swelling

Acupuncture

GB.41 (*zu lin qi*), SJ.5 (*wai guan*), Ren.3 (*zhong ji* -), Sp.6 (*san yin jiao* -), Sp.9 (*yin ling quan* -), Kid.6 (*zhao hai*), BL.28 (*pang guang shu* -), Bl.22 (*san jiao shu* -), Kid.7 (*fu liu* -), St.28 (*shui dao* -)

Clinical notes

- Biomedical conditions that may present as Damp Heat type difficult urination include urethritis, cystitis, the inflammatory stage of urinary calculi, pyelonephritis and prostatitis.
- Because this is an acute condition treatment needs to be prompt and frequent. Acupuncture can be applied twice a day or more if necessary and herbs the same. With acute retention, strong stimulation should be applied to acupuncture points on the abdomen so that *de qi* travels to the bladder. A useful way to approach treatment is to use acupuncture to move Bladder *qi* and relieve the retention, followed by herbs to

clear Damp Heat.
- Sometimes this treatment can induce sudden emptying of the bladder. It should be remembered that complete retention of urine constitutes a medical emergency and catheterisation is necessary if other therapies fail.
- In cases with severe infection, especially that involving the kidneys, antibiotics may be necessary to quickly cool Heat. Once the infection is controlled, treatment may be given to clear Damp.

14.2 OBSTRUCTION OF LUNG *QI*

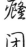

Pathophysiology
- This condition often (but not always) follows an acute febrile disease, usually a sore throat or upper respiratory tract infection. The pathogenic factor (generally Heat) obstructs the Lungs and prevents the normal descent of Lung *qi*. The fluids the Lungs should send to the Kidneys accumulate in the upper *jiao*. This pattern is also known as Wind oedema.

Clinical features
- difficult or scanty urination initially accompanied by orbital and facial oedema; this may be followed by oedema of the limbs or whole body; any urine that is passed tends to be pale
- fever and chills
- dry sore throat
- cough
- dyspnoea
- aching joints and muscles, heaviness in the limbs

T thin white coat
P floating and tight, or floating, slippery and rapid

Treatment principle
Restore the descent of Lung *qi*
Open the water passages

Prescription

YUE BI JIA ZHU TANG 越婢加术汤
(*Atractylodes Combination*)

This formula is selected when the exterior symptoms are obvious.
- **shi gao** (Gypsum) 石膏 30g
- **ma huang*** (Herba Ephedrae) 麻黄 12g
- **bai zhu** (Rhizoma Atractylodes Macrocephalae) 白术 12g
- **sheng jiang** (Rhizoma Zingiberis Officinalis) 生姜 9g
- **gan cao** (Radix Glycyrrhizae Uralensis) 甘草 6g
- **da zao** (Fructus Zizyphi Jujubae) 大枣 5pce

Method: Decoction. (Source: *Fluid Physiology and Pathology in Traditional Chinese Medicine*)

Modifications
- Without obvious Heat, or with obvious Cold (i.e. chilliness, muscle aches, no sweating and a floating, tight pulse), delete **shi gao**.

QING FEI YIN 清肺饮
(Clear the Lungs Decoction)

This formula is selected if internal Heat affects the Lungs. The pattern is characterised by difficult urination or anuria, fullness or tightness in the chest, shortness of breath, rapid rough breathing, thirst, dry mouth and throat, cough, possible constipation, a yellow tongue coat and a slippery or soft and rapid pulse. The correct treatment is to clear Heat from the Lungs and aid the descent of Lung *qi*.

sang bai pi (Cortex Mori Albae Radicis) 桑白皮	20g
fu ling (Sclerotium Poria Cocos) 茯苓	20g
huang qin (Radix Scutellariae Baicalensis) 黄芩	15g
mai dong (Tuber Ophiopogonis Japonici) 麦冬	15g
che qian zi (Semen Plantaginis) 车前子	15g
shan zhi zi (Fructus Gardeniae Jasminoidis) 山栀子	9g
mu tong (Caulis Mutong) 木通	6g
dan zhu ye (Herba Lophatheri Gracilis) 淡竹叶	3g

Method: Decoction. **Che qian zi** is cooked in a muslin bag (*bao jian* 包煎).
(Source: *Zhong Yi Nei Ke Lin Chuang Shou Ce*)

Modifications

- With irritability, restlessness and a red tongue tip (indicating some Heat affecting the Heart), add **lian zi xin** (Plumula Nelumbinis Nuciferae) 莲子心 2g and **huang lian** (Rhizoma Coptidis) 黄连 6g.
- If Lung *yin* has been damaged (red dry tongue with little or no coat), add **sha shen** (Radix Adenophorae seu Glehniae) 沙参 12g and **bai he** (Bulbus Lilii) 百合 12g.
- With constipation, add **da huang** (Radix et Rhizoma Rhei) 大黄 9g and **xing ren*** (Semen Pruni Armeniacae) 杏仁 9g.
- With nasal obstruction and headache, add **bo he** (Herba Mentha Haplocalycis) 薄荷 6g and **jie geng** (Radix Platycodi Grandiflori) 桔梗 6g.

Variations and additional prescriptions

With qi *deficiency*

- If neither of the above treatments begin to increase urinary output and decrease the oedema within a few days, or if the patient is lethargic, feels heavy and is sweating freely, indications are that *qi* is too weak to move fluids correctly. The correct treatment is to bolster *wei qi* and promote urination with **FANG JI HUANG QI TANG** (*Stephania and Astragalus Combination* 防己黄芪汤) modified.

huang qi (Radix Astragali Membranacei) 黄芪	30g
bai zhu (Rhizoma Atractylodes Macrocephalae) 白术	12g

fu ling (Sclerotium Poriae Cocos) 茯苓	12g
fang ji (Radix Stephaniae Tetrandrae) 防己	9g
gui zhi (Ramulus Cinnamomi Cassiae) 桂枝	9g
zhi gan cao (honey fried Radix Glycyrrhizae Uralensis) 炙甘草	3g
sheng jiang (Rhizoma Zingiberis Officinalis) 生姜	4pce
da zao (Fructus Zizyphi Jujubae) 大枣	1pce

Method: Decoction. (Source: *Fluid Physiology and Pathology in Traditional Chinese Medicine*)

Patent medicines
Fang Feng Tong Sheng Wan 防风通圣丸 (Fang Feng Tong Sheng Wan)
Ma Xing Zhi Ke Pian 麻杏止咳片 (Ma Hsing Chih Ke Pien)
Zhi Sou Ding Chuan Wan 止嗽定喘丸 (Zhi Sou Ding Chuan Wan)

Acupuncture
Lu.7 (*lie que* -), Sp.9 (*yin ling quan* -), Ren.3 (*zhong ji* -), BL.13 (*fei shu* -), Bl.24 (*qi hai shu* -), Bl.32 (*ci liao* -), Sp.6 (*san yin jiao* -), Ren.9 (*shui fen* ▲)
- for Wind Cold add LI.4 (*he gu* -)
- for Wind Heat add Lu.5 (*chi ze* -) and Lu.10 (*yu ji* -)

Clinical notes
- Biomedical conditions that may present as Lung *qi* obstruction type difficult urination include acute (post streptococcal) glomerulonephritis.
- Treatment needs to be prompt and frequent. In some patients with mild obstruction, a sneeze may be enough to get the urine flowing.

14.3 LIVER *QI* STAGNATION

Pathophysiology
- Difficulty with urination can be caused by disruptions to the circulation of Liver *qi* because the Liver channel passes through the genitals and Bladder area. Sudden rage (expressed or more likely unexpressed) may provoke an acute episode of urinary difficulty or retention. It may also occur as repeated difficulty in someone who is stressed or frustrated.

Clinical features
- urinary difficulty or retention that is initiated or aggravated by anger or stress
- sensation of tightness or fullness in the chest (often described as difficulty in drawing a satisfying breath)
- hypochondriac discomfort or tightness
- frequent sighing
- dizziness
- occasional fatigue (although the patient may feel better for exercise)
- irritability or depression
- abdominal distension, flatulence
- alternating constipation and diarrhoea
- women may experience irregular menstruation, premenstrual syndrome and breast tenderness
- all symptoms are aggravated by stress

T normal or dark (*qing* 青)
P wiry

Treatment principle
Regulate and invigorate Liver *qi*
Promote urination

Prescription

CHAI HU SHU GAN SAN 柴胡舒肝散
(*Bupleurum and Cyperus Formula*) plus
WEI LING TANG 胃苓汤
(*Magnolia and Hoelen Combination*)

This prescription is suitable for mild cases or recurrent urinary difficulty with stress.

chai hu (Radix Bupleuri) 柴胡	9g
bai shao (Radix Paeoniae Lactiflorae) 白芍	12g
zhi ke (Fructus Citri Aurantii) 枳壳	9g
xiang fu (Rhizoma Cyperi Rotundi) 香附	9g

fu ling (Sclerotium Poria Cocos) 茯苓 9g
ze xie (Rhizoma Alismatis Orientalis) 泽泻 9g
zhu ling (Sclerotium Polypori Umbellati) 猪苓 9g
bai zhu (Rhizoma Atractylodes Macrocephalae) 白术 9g
cang zhu (Rhizoma Atractylodis) 苍术 9g
chuan xiong (Radix Ligustici Chuanxiong) 川芎 6g
chen pi (Pericarpium Citri Reticulatae) 陈皮 6g
gui zhi (Ramulus Cinnamomi Cassiae) 桂枝 6g
hou po (Cortex Magnoliae Officinalis) 厚朴 6g
zhi gan cao (honey fried Radix Glycyrrhizae Uralensis)
  炙甘草 3g

Method: Decoction. (Source: *Fluid Physiology and Pathology in Traditional Chinese Medicine*)

CHAI HU SHU GAN SAN 柴胡舒肝散
(*Bupleurum and Cyperus Formula*) plus
CHEN XIANG SAN 沉香散
(*Aquillaria Powder*)

This prescription is selected for more severe or acute cases with significant urinary difficulty or retention.

shi wei (Folium Pyrrosiae) 石苇 30g
wang bu liu xing (Semen Vaccariae Segetalis) 王不留行 15g
dong kui zi (Semen Abutili seu Malvae) 冬葵子 15g
hua shi (Talcum) 滑石 15g
bai shao (Radix Paeoniae Lactiflorae) 白芍 9g
chai hu (Radix Bupleuri) 柴胡 9g
dang gui (Radix Angelicae Sinensis) 当归 9g
zhi ke (Fructus Citri Aurantii) 枳壳 9g
xiang fu (Rhizoma Cyperi Rotundi) 香附 9g
chuan xiong (Radix Ligustici Chuanxiong) 川芎 6g
chen pi (Pericarpium Citri Reticulatae) 陈皮 6g
chen xiang (Lignum Aquilariae) 沉香 3g
zhi gan cao (honey fried Radix Glycyrrhizae Uralensis)
  炙甘草 3g

Method: Decoction. (Source: *Fluid Physiology and Pathology in Traditional Chinese Medicine*)

Modifications (apply to both prescriptions)

- If the patient is robust, add **yu jin** (Tuber Curcuma) 郁金 9g and **wu yao** (Radix Linderae Strychnifoliae) 乌药 9g.
- If stagnant *qi* transforms into Heat, with facial flushing, temper outbursts, red edges on the tongue and a rapid wiry pulse, add **long dan cao** (Radix Gentianae Longdancao) 龙胆草 6g, **mu dan pi** (Cortex

Moutan Radicis) 牡丹皮 9g and **shan zhi zi** (Fructus Gardeniae Jasminoidis) 山栀子 9g.

Patent medicines
Chai Hu Shu Gan Wan 柴胡舒肝丸 (Chai Hu Shu Gan Wan)
Shu Gan Wan 舒肝丸 (Shu Gan Wan)
Mu Xiang Shun Qi Wan 木香顺气丸 (Aplotaxis Carminative Pills)
Xiao Yao Wan 逍遥丸 (Xiao Yao Wan)
Qian Lie Xian Wan 前列腺丸 (Prostate Gland Pills)
  - combined with one of the above formulae for prostate swelling

Acupuncture
Ren.12 (*zhong wan* -), PC.6 (*nei guan* -), Ren.3 (*zhong ji* -), Liv.2 (*xing jian* -), St.30 (*qi chong*), Liv.14 (*qi men*), SJ.6 (*zhi gou* -), GB.34 (*yang ling quan* -), Liv.3 (*tai chong* -)

Clinical notes
- Biomedical conditions that may present as Liver *qi* stagnation type difficult urination include stress related dysuria and hysterical anuria.
- Acupuncture can be very effective at relieving urinary difficulty caused by Liver *qi* stagnation. For recurrent cases herbs may be added. The origin of any emotional imbalance or stress must be addressed to prevent recurrence.

14.4 BLOOD STAGNATION

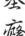

Pathophysiology
- This pattern follows damage to the urinary tract by trauma, surgery, infection or urinary tract stones. Blood stagnation can also follow prolonged *qi* stagnation, Heat or Damp Heat. If there are urinary tract stones, see also Stone Painful Urination Syndrome, p.372.

Clinical features
- difficult urination or periodic obstruction to the passage of urine
- the urinary stream is thin and there may be fixed stabbing pain upon voiding; the urine may be occasionally dark or purplish or contain blood clots
- suprapubic fullness, distension and pain, the pain is localised and stabbing
- there may be lower abdominal masses, and women may experience dysmenorrhoea
- pain in the iliac fossae with palpation
- thin purple vessels (spider naevi) on the abdomen, inner ankle and knee

T darkish, purplish or with purplish or brown spots and a thin coat, sublingual vessels are distended and dark

P choppy or wiry

Treatment principle
Expel Blood stagnation and obstruction
Promote urination

Prescription

DAI DI DANG WAN 代抵当丸
(*Substituted Resistance Pill*) modified

dang gui wei (tail of Radix Angelicae Sinensis) 当归尾	15g
chuan shan jia° (Squama Manitis Pentadactylae) 穿山甲	15g
niu xi (Radix Achyranthis Bidentatae) 牛膝	15g
tao ren (Semen Persicae) 桃仁	10g
da huang (Radix et Rhizoma Rhei) 大黄	10g
mang xiao (Mirabilitum) 芒硝	10g
hong hua (Flos Carthami Tinctorii) 红花	10g

Method: Grind herbs to a powder and form into 6-gram pills with honey. The dose is one pill 2-3 times daily. May also be decocted, in which case **mang xiao** is dissolved in the strained decoction (*chong fu* 冲服). (Source: *Zhong Yi Nei Ke Lin Chuang Shou Ce*)

Modifications
- If the condition is very prolonged and accompanied by *qi* and Blood

deficiency, use **dang gui shen** (main part of the root of Radix Angelicae Sinensis) 当归身 15g, and add **dan shen** (Radix Salviae Miltiorrhizae) 丹参 12g and **huang qi** (Radix Astragali Membranacei) 黄芪 15g.
- With mild haematuria, add **san qi fen** (powdered Radix Notoginseng) 三七粉 6g and **hu po** (Succinum) 琥珀 3g (add both to strained decoction).
- If there are small stones or gravel in the urine, add **jin qian cao** (Herba Lysimachiae) 金钱草 30-60g, **hai jin sha** (Spora Lygodii Japonici) 海金砂 30g, **dong kui zi** (Semen Abutili seu Malvae) 冬葵子 9g, **qu mai** (Herba Dianthi) 瞿麦 9g and **bian xu** (Herba Polygoni Avicularis) 篇蓄 9g. See also Stone Painful Urination Syndrome, pp.367-375.

Patent medicines
Nei Xiao Luo Li Wan 内消瘰疬丸 (Nei Xiao Luo Li Wan)
Tao He Cheng Qi San 桃核承气散 (Persica and Rhubarb Combination)
Sheng Tian Qi Pian 生田七片 (Raw Tian Qi Ginseng Pills)
Dan Shen Pian 丹参片 (Dan Shen Pills)
Fu Ke Wu Jin Wan 妇科乌金丸 (Woo Garm Yuen Medical Pills)
Qian Lie Xian Wan 前列腺丸 (Prostate Gland Pills)
   - combined with one of the above formulae for prostate swelling

Acupuncture
Ren.3 (*zhong ji* -), St.29 (*gui lai* -), St.30 (*qi chong* -), Sp.10 (*xue hai* -), Bl.17 (*ge shu* -), Bl.30 (*bai huan shu* -), Bl.47 (*zhi shi* -), Liv.3 (*tai chong* -), GB.25 (*jing men* -), LI.4 (*he gu* -)

Clinical notes
- This pattern is the result of obstruction to the urinary tract. The cause may be structural (from stones, blood clots, tumours, post traumatic or infectious urethral stricture or stenosis, prostatic hypertrophy) or functional (congenital neuromuscular defects). It can also occur due to endometriosis (endometrial tissue affecting the ureter or bladder) or polyps in the bladder. Referral for full investigation is necessary to assess for malignancy.
- The prognosis in this pattern is variable depending on the underlying cause. Strictures and tumours of the prostate or bladder should be treated with a combination of Western medicine and TCM.

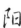

14.5 SPLEEN *YANG* DEFICIENCY

Pathophysiology
- In this pattern, there are several possible mechanisms that can give rise to difficult urination, each with its own distinctive features.
- First, fluid movement and metabolism in general are disturbed, and instead of going to the Bladder for processing, fluids congeal into Dampness or accumulate in the limbs and tissues. In this case there will be oedema and scanty urine. This is the most common mechanism by which Spleen deficiency causes difficult urination.
- Second, weak Spleen *yang* can fail to support the Lungs and *wei qi*. Fluids may be lost through the surface as sweat and not reach the Urinary Bladder at all. In this case there will be excessive sweating in addition to the Spleen *yang* deficiency signs.
- Third, when *yang* is weak the general movement of *qi* will be weak. In this case, the urine will not necessarily be scanty, but will be hard to push out, that is, there is not enough power behind the expulsion of urine. This pattern often occurs post surgically or postpartum and may be associated with bladder prolapse.

Clinical features
- scanty difficult urination, the patient feels the need to urinate but is unable to, or can only urinate a very small amount
- generalised oedema which is more noticeable in the limbs and below the waist, the oedema is usually pitting; in milder cases the patient may only notice puffiness of the hands and may complain that rings feel tight on the fingers
- waxy pale complexion
- fatigue and lethargy
- poor appetite
- abdominal distension
- loose stools with undigested food
- cold extremities
- dragging or sinking sensation in the lower abdomen
- bladder prolapse in some cases

T pale and swollen with a thin or thick white coat
P weak and thready

Treatment principle
Warm the Spleen to promote transformation and distribution of fluids

Prescription

SHI PI YIN 实脾饮
(Magnolia and Atractylodes Combination)

fu ling (Sclerotium Poria Cocos) 茯苓	9g
bai zhu (Rhizoma Atractylodes Macrocephalae) 白术	9g
zhi fu zi* (Radix Aconiti Carmichaeli Praeparata) 制附子	6g
gan jiang (Rhizoma Zingiberis Officinalis) 干姜	6g
mu gua (Fructus Chaenomelis) 木瓜	6g
hou po (Cortex Magnoliae Officinalis) 厚朴	6g
mu xiang (Radix Aucklandiae Lappae) 木香	6g
da fu pi (Pericarpium Arecae Catechu) 大腹皮	6g
cao guo (Fructus Amomi Tsao-ko) 草果	6g
zhi gan cao (honey fried Radix Glycyrrhizae Uralensis) 炙甘草	3g
sheng jiang (Rhizoma Zingiberis Officinalis) 生姜	6g
da zao (Fructus Zizyphi Jujubae) 大枣	3pce

Method: Decoction. Zhi fu zi is cooked for 30 minutes prior to the other herbs (*xian jian* 先煎). (Source: *Fluid Physiology and Pathology in Traditional Chinese Medicine*)

Variations and additional prescriptions

Spleen qi *deficiency*

- With little or no oedema and no obvious Cold symptoms, Spleen *qi* deficiency is the main problem. The severity of the urinary difficulty varies with energy levels. When the patient is rested and relatively more energetic, the urine will be expelled more effectively, when tired the urine will slow or cease. The correct treatment is to 'raise the clear to aid descent of the turbid' by invigorating Spleen *qi* and assisting urination with **BU ZHONG YI QI TANG** (*Ginseng and Astragalus Combination* 补中益气汤) modified.

huang qi (Radix Astragali Membranacei) 黄芪	15g
bai zhu (Rhizoma Atractylodes Macrocephalae) 白术	12g
che qian zi (Semen Plantaginis) 车前子	9g
ren shen (Radix Ginseng) 人参	6g
dang gui (Radix Angelicae Sinensis) 当归	6g
chen pi (Pericarpium Citri Reticulatae) 陈皮	6g
chai hu (Radix Bupleuri) 柴胡	6g
sheng ma (Rhizoma Cimicifugae) 升麻	6g
rou gui (Cortex Cinnamomi Cassiae) 肉桂	6g
tong cao (Medulla Tetrapanacis Papyriferi) 通草	6g
zhi gan cao (honey fried Radix Glycyrrhizae Uralensis) 炙甘草	3g

Method: Decoction. Che qian zi is cooked in a muslin bag (*bao jian* 包煎). (Source: *Zhong Yi Nei Ke Lin Chuang Shou Ce*)

Patent medicines
Fu Zi Li Zhong Wan 附子理中丸 (Li Chung Yuen Medical Pills)
- for Spleen *yang* deficiency

Li Zhong Wan 理中丸 (Li Zhong Wan)
- Spleen *yang* deficiency

Bu Zhong Yi Qi Wan 补中益气丸 (Bu Zhong Yi Qi Wan)
- for *qi* deficiency

Jin Kui Shen Qi Wan 金匮肾气丸 (Sexoton Pills)
- with Kidney *yang* deficiency

Qian Lie Xian Wan 前列腺丸 (Prostate Gland Pills)
- combined with one of the above formulae for prostate swelling

Acupuncture
Ren.6 (*qi hai* +▲), LI.4 (*he gu* +), Sp.6 (*san yin jiao* -), Lu.7 (*lie que*), St.29 (*shui dao* -), Ren.9 (*shui fen* ▲), Du.26 (*ren zhong*), Kid.7 (*fu liu*), Du.20 (*bai hui* ▲), Ren.3 (*zhong ji*), Bl.20 (*pi shu* +▲), Bl.22 (*san jiao shu*), Bl.23 (*shen shu* +▲)

- a useful technique for lower abdominal prolapses in general is to thread a 3-inch needle from Ren.6 (*qi hai*) to Ren.3 (*zhong ji*). The needle is twirled to anchor it, then raised towards the sternum creating a lifting sensation in the lower abdomen. It can be taped (in its lifted position) in place for the duration of the treatment.

Clinical notes
- Biomedical conditions that may present as Spleen *yang* deficiency type difficult urination include chronic glomerular, interstitial or diffuse nephritis, nephrotic syndrome, prolapse of the bladder or uterus, fluid retention associated with hormonal imbalance and premenstrual fluid retention.
- This pattern will often overlap to some degree with Kidney *yang* deficiency.
- Urinary difficulty due to Spleen *qi* and *yang* deficiency can be quite responsive to treatment with both acupuncture and herbs. If prolapses are pronounced, however, surgery may be required.

14.6 KIDNEY *YANG* DEFICIENCY

Pathophysiology
- When weak Kidney *yang* fails to support the metabolism and transformation of fluids, these accumulate in the tissues (particularly of the lower body) as oedema and the volume of urine will be accordingly reduced.
- When *yang* is weak the general movement of *qi* will be weak. In this case, the urine will not necessarily be scanty, but will be hard to push out, that is, there is not enough power behind the expulsion of urine. The same mechanism occurs in Spleen *yang* deficiency, and these patterns often co-exist, especially in chronic cases.

Clinical features
- difficult or forceless expulsion of urine, to the point of retention in severe cases; the urge to void may be frequent, but urination is unable to get started, or once started the stream is weak and broken; urination feels incomplete
- pitting oedema, which is worse below the waist
- waxy pale complexion
- listlessness and fatigue
- aversion to cold, cold extremities
- lower abdominal distension
- constipation or loose stools
- weak, cold and sore lower back and knees

T pale, wet and swollen
P deep and thready or slow and weak, particularly in the proximal positions

Treatment principle
Warm *yang*, benefit *qi*
Tonify the Kidney and promote urination

Prescription

JI SHENG SHEN QI WAN 济生肾气丸
(Kidney Qi Pill from Formulas to Aid the Living)

shan zhu yu (Fructus Corni Officinalis) 山茱萸	30g
shan yao (Radix Dioscoreae Oppositae) 山药	30g
ze xie (Rhizoma Alismatis Orientalis) 泽泻	30g
fu ling (Sclerotium Poria Cocos) 茯苓	30g
mu dan pi (Cortex Moutan Radicis) 牡丹皮	30g
che qian zi (Semen Plantaginis) 车前子	30g
shu di (Radix Rehmanniae Glutinosae Conquitae) 熟地	15g
rou gui (Cortex Cinnamomi Cassiae) 肉桂	15g

zhi fu zi* (Radix Aconiti Carmichaeli Praeparata) 制附子 15g
chuan niu xi (Radix Cyathulae Officinalis) 川牛膝 15g
Method: Grind herbs to a fine powder and form into 9-gram pills with honey. The dose is one pill 2-3 times daily. May also be decocted with a 50% reduction in dosage. When decocted **zhi fu zi** is cooked for 30 minutes before the other herbs (*xian jian* 先煎) and **che qian zi** is decocted in a muslin bag (*bao jian* 包煎). (Source: *Shi Yong Zhong Yi Nei Ke Xue*)

Modifications

- If *yuan qi* is greatly depleted, add **hong shen** (steamed Radix Ginseng) 红参 15g, **lu jiao pian**^ (Cornu Cervi) 鹿角片 12g, **xian mao** (Rhizoma Curculiginis Orchioidis) 仙茅 20g and **xian ling pi** (Herba Epimedii) 仙灵脾 20g.

Variations and additional prescriptions

Acute, following a Wind attack

- Relatively acute urinary difficulty can follow an attack of pathogenic Wind Cold or Wind Heat in a patient with pre-existing Kidney *yang* deficiency. The features are sudden urinary difficulty, aversion to cold (especially on the back), generalised body aches, no sweating, a pale tongue with little coat and a deep, tight, or floating and tight pulse. The correct treatment is to support *yang*, clear the exterior and promote urination with **MA HUANG FU ZI XI XIN TANG** (*Ma Huang, Asarum and Prepared Aconite Decoction* 麻黄附子细辛汤, p.24) plus **niu xi** (Radix Achyranthis Bidentatae) 牛膝 12g and **che qian zi** (Semen Plantaginis) 车前子 12g.

Water Toxin

- If Kidney *yang* is very weak, and the '*qi* transformation' function of the *san jiao* and Bladder is failing, this may lead to accumulation of 'Water Toxin'. The features are very scanty urine or anuria, dizziness, vomiting of clear fluids, loss of appetite, restlessness, and in severe cases, confusion. There may slso be constipation. The correct treatment is to warm and tonify Kidney and Spleen *yang* and stop vomiting (and purge accumulation) with a mixture of **FU ZI LI ZHONG WAN** (*Aconite, Ginseng and Ginger Formula* 附子理中丸, p.56) and **WU ZHU YU TANG** (*Evodia Combination* 吴茱萸汤, p.63). Herbs that promote urination and descend turbidity may also be added, for example **che qian zi** (Semen Plantaginis) 车前子 15g and **mu tong** (Caulis Mutong) 木通 6g. With constipation **da huang** (Radix et Rhizoma Rhei) 大黄 6-9 g may be added.

Patent medicines

Jin Kui Shen Qi Wan 金匱肾气丸 (Sexoton Pills)
Qian Lie Xian Wan 前列腺丸 (Prostate Gland Pills)
  - combined with the above formula for prostate swelling

Acupuncture

Du.26 (*ren zhong*), Du.4 (*ming men* ▲), Bl.23 (*shen shu* +▲),
Ren.3 (*zhong ji*), Kid.7 (*fu liu* -), Sp.6 (*san yin jiao*), Ren.6 (*qi hai* +▲),
Bl.53 (*wei yang* +▲), Ren.9 (*shui fen* ▲)
  • A moxa-box over the lower abdomen may be useful.

Clinical notes

• Biomedical conditions that may present as Kidney *yang* deficiency type difficult urination include chronic glomerular, interstitial or diffuse nephritis, nephrotic syndrome, benign prostatic hypertrophy, hypothyroidism and chronic prostatitis.
• This pattern can respond well to correct treatment, which will usually need to continue for some months. Conditions like hypothyroidism can be difficult and may require a combination of Western and Chinese medicine.

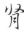
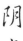

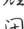

14.7 KIDNEY *YIN* DEFICIENCY

Pathophysiology
- In this pattern, lack of *yin* and fluids and the resulting deficient Heat applied to the remaining fluids in the Bladder, gives rise to scantiness and concentration of urine, and difficult urination.
- This pattern frequently co-exists with Liver *qi* stagnation, Damp Heat or stagnant Blood. Liver *qi* stasis can easily generate Heat which injures *yin*. Damp Heat may smoulder in the lower *jiao* and gradually damage *yin*.

Clinical features
- Scanty, concentrated urine with difficulty initiating a flow, or a frequent desire to urinate with only small amounts of urine expelled. There may also be with mild oedema.
- dry mouth and throat
- restlessness and irritability
- insomnia
- facial flushing, malar flush
- nightsweats
- sensations of heat in the palms and soles ('five hearts hot')
- dizziness and tinnitus
- soreness or weakness of the lower back and knees, heel pain
- tendency to dry stools or constipation

T red and dry with little or no coat
P thready and rapid

Treatment principle
Nourish and tonify Kidney *yin*
Promote urination

Prescription

LIU WEI DI HUANG WAN 六味地黄丸
(*Rehmannia Six Formula*) plus
ZHU LING TANG 猪苓汤
(*Polyporus Combination*)

shu di (Radix Rehmanniae Glutinosae Conquitae) 熟地	24g
shan yao (Radix Dioscoreae Oppositae) 山药	12g
shan zhu yu (Fructus Corni Officinalis) 山茱萸	12g
fu ling (Sclerotium Poria Cocos) 茯苓	9g
mu dan pi (Cortex Moutan Radicis) 牡丹皮	9g
ze xie (Rhizoma Alismatis Orientalis) 泽泻	9g
zhu ling (Sclerotium Polypori Umbellati) 猪苓	9g

hua shi (Talcum) 滑石 9g
e jiao^ (Gelatinum Corii Asini) 阿胶 9g
Method: Decoction. **E jiao** is melted before being added to the strained decoction (*yang hua* 烊化). (Source: *Shi Yong Zhong Yi Nei Ke Xue*)

Modifications
- With Damp Heat, add **zhi mu** (Rhizoma Anemarrhenae Asphodeloidis) 知母 9g and **huang bai** (Cortex Phellodendri) 黄柏 9g.
- With *qi* stagnation, add **wu yao** (Radix Linderae Strychnifoliae) 乌药 6g, **chuan lian zi*** (Fructus Meliae Toosendan) 川楝子 6g and **xiang fu** (Rhizoma Cyperi Rotundi) 香附 9g.

Patent medicines
Liu Wei Di Huang Wan 六味地黄丸 (Liu Wei Di Huang Wan)
Zhi Bai Ba Wei Wan 知柏八味丸 (Zhi Bai Ba Wei Wan)
Qian Lie Xian Wan 前列腺丸 (Prostate Gland Pills)
 - combined with one of the above formulae for prostate swelling

Acupuncture
Bl.23 (*shen shu* +), Ren.3 (*zhong ji* +), Ren.6 (*qi hai* +), Ren.4 (*guan yuan* +), Ht.5 (*tong li*), Kid.3 (*tai xi* +), Kid.6 (*zhao hai*), Lu.7 (*lie que*), Sp.6 (*san yin jiao* +)

Clinical notes
- Biomedical conditions that may present as Kidney *yang* deficiency type difficult urination include menopausal syndrome, chronic interstitial cystitis and post febrile disease retention.
- Kidney *yin* deficiency patterns can respond well to correct treatment, although in most cases treatment needs to continue for prolonged periods. Interstitial cystitis is very difficult to treat successfully.

SUMMARY OF GUIDING FORMULAE FOR DIFFICULT URINATION AND URINARY RETENTION

Damp Heat - *Ba Zheng San* 八正散
- with Toxic Damp - *Huang Lian Wen Dan Tang* 黄连温胆汤

Obstruction of Lung *qi* (by Heat) - *Yue Bi Jia Zhu Tang* 越婢加术汤
- with severe Heat - *Qing Fei Yin* 清肺饮
- in stubborn cases - *Fang Ji Huang Qi Tang* 防己黄芪汤

Liver *qi* stagnation - *Chai Hu Shu Gan San* 柴胡疏肝散
- plus, in mild cases - *Wei Ling Tang* 胃苓汤
- plus, in severe cases - *Chen Xiang San* 沉香散

Blood stagnation - *Dai Di Dang Tang* 代抵当汤

Spleen *yang* deficiency - *Shi Pi Yin* 实脾饮
- Spleen *qi* deficiency - *Bu Zhong Yi Qi Tang* 补中益气汤

Kidney *yang* deficiency - *Ji Sheng Shen Qi Wan* 济生肾气丸
- acute following a Wind attack - *Ma Huang Fu Zi Xi Xin Tang* 麻黄附子细辛汤

Kidney *yin* deficiency
- *Liu Wei Di Huang Wan* 六味地黄丸 plus *Zhu Ling Tang* 猪苓汤

Endnote

For more information regarding herbs marked with an asterisk*, an open circle° or a hatˆ, see the tables on pp.944-952.

Disorders of the Kidney

15. Frequent Urination and Incontinence

Excess patterns
Damp Heat
Liver *qi* stagnation

Deficient patterns
Lung and Spleen *qi* deficiency
Kidney (*qi*) *yang* deficiency
Kidney *yin* deficiency

15 | FREQUENT URINATION, INCONTINENCE
yi niao 遗尿

Frequent urination refers to an obvious increase, over a period of time in the urge to void urine. On average, most people with normal urinary function urinate several times daily, the frequency depending on the volume and (diuretic) nature of fluids consumed, and the weather. In general, however, an increase in frequency is judged subjectively by the patient, rather than by being compared with an objective average rate. Depending on the underlying cause, frequency may develop slowly, or become a problem quite suddenly. In severe cases the urge to void may occur four or five times per hour. The volume of urine may be profuse, normal or scanty.

Incontinence refers to lack of control over urination. Leakage of varying amounts of urine may occur without warning or immediately on perceiving the urge to urinate. The latter is called **urge incontinence**. Leakage which occurs as a result of the increased intra-abdominal pressure caused by sneezing, coughing or jumping is called **stress incontinence**. Incontinence is often a complication of long term frequency.

The mechanisms behind **nocturia** and **nocturnal enuresis** are the same as for frequency and incontinence. Nocturia refers to increased frequency and volume of urine at night. In general, needing to urinate more than once per night is deemed pathological. Nocturia should be carefully distinguished from situations where the patient sleeps poorly and gets up to urinate simply because they are awake. Nocturnal enuresis is urinary incontinence during sleep and is mostly seen in children.

In TCM terms, urinary frequency can be due to the irritating effects of Heat or Liver *qi* stagnation on the Bladder, or from failure of *yang* to fully process and metabolise Fluids. Similarly, nocturia represents a failure of '*yang* within *yin*', that is, the essential *yang* urine concentrating function that continues at night (*yin*) to allow unbroken sleep. Nocturia is mostly associated with weak Kidney *yang*.

Urinary incontinence and nocturnal enuresis have similar mechanisms. As with frequency and nocturia, they may be associated with weakness of the *yang* in transforming fluids, but with the additional feature of weakness of the lower *yin* (in this cases the urethra), which simply cannot hold urine in. Weakness of either the Kidney or Spleen may contribute to this secondary mechanism as the Kidney controls the lower *yin* orifices and the Spleen both quality of muscle tone and the lifting of organs against gravity.

AETIOLOGY

Kidney deficiency

Weak Kidney *yang* or *qi* may be an inherited condition or may develop as a result of age, chronic illness, too much exposure to cold conditions or excessive lifting or standing (particularly if this occurs in a cold environment or on cold floors or at night). Kidney *yang* or *qi* may also be damaged by excessive sexual activity or in women who have many pregnancies. In some cases, particularly in younger people, Kidney *qi* may be weakened while Kidney *yang* remains intact, in which case the Cold symptoms are not seen.

Kidney *yin* becomes damaged through febrile disease, overwork (especially while under stress), insufficient sleep and use of recreational drugs. Kidney *yin* may also be weakened by ageing and excessive sexual activity, or pregnancies. Kidney deficiency can lead to nocturia, frequency, enuresis (especially congenital Kidney deficiency) and incontinence.

> **BOX 15.1 SOME BIOMEDICAL CAUSES OF FREQUENT URINATION/INCONTINENCE**
>
> - cystitis/UTI
> - prostatitis
> - pregnancy
> - diabetes mellitus/insipidus
> - benign prostatic hypertrophy
> - diuretics (including nightcap alcohol or caffeine)
> - essential enuresis
> - hypothyroidism
> - stress
> - trauma
> - multiple sclerosis
> - irritable bladder
> - bladder stones/tumours
> - neurogenic bladder
> - Parkinson's disease
> - post surgery
> - interstitial cystitis
> - post menopausal atrophic changes in the bladder and urethral wall

Damp Heat

Frequency of the Damp Heat type is usually acute, and is due to an external Damp Heat pathogen that invades through the *tai yang* (Bladder) channel, the leg *yin* channels or the local *luo* channels. Clinically, this may be associated with poor genital hygiene or transmission from a sexual partner. The Damp Heat can also be chronic, generated in the middle *jiao* by excessive, irregular or poor diet. Damp Heat in the lower *jiao* can also come from any prolonged Heat in the system, such as the Heat generated by *yin* deficiency, *qi* stagnation, or prolonged stagnation of Dampness. The Damp Heat irritates the Bladder, leading to frequency or in severe cases, incontinence.

Liver *qi* stagnation

Frustration, anger, resentment, prolonged emotional turmoil, repressed emotions and stress disrupt both the circulation of Liver *qi*, and, because the Liver channel passes through the lower *jiao*, Bladder *qi* is affected. Liver *qi* stagnation tends to cause irritation of the Bladder leading to frequency without copious or otherwise unusual urine.

Pre-existing stagnation (of *qi* and Blood) can be transferred from another pelvic organ to the Bladder. This is most commonly observed in women following hysterectomy, myomectomy or removal of ovarian cysts. The organ primarily affected by the stagnation is removed or repaired, but the condition that gave rise to the initial problem (that is *qi* and/or Blood stagnation) persists. The focus of pelvic symptoms then shifts from, for example the uterus with heavy periods and pain, to the Bladder.

Spleen (and Lung) *qi* deficiency

If Spleen *qi* is weak, it will fail to distribute fluids to the extremities and Lungs. These fluids sink to the lower *jiao*, accumulate in the Bladder and cause frequent urination or incontinence. If Lung *qi* is weak (as a direct result of Spleen *qi* deficiency or otherwise), there may be a chronic cough. The repeated coughing increases the downward pressure on the already sinking fluids leading to stress incontinence. In elderly patients there will usually be Kidney deficiency as well.

The Lungs, one of the organs involved in fluid metabolism, also have an energetic connection to the Bladder. Lung *qi* descends and takes a portion of the fluid (sent up by the Spleen) to the Kidneys for reprocessing, and sends a portion to the skin as sweat. If one pathway is unavailable (for example, when the pores are shut during cold weather), fluids will increase along the other. This can be seen in the simple observation that most people tend to urinate more frequently in cold weather. Similarly, when Lung *qi* is weak, allowing excessive sweating, urinary output often decreases.

BOX 15.2 KEY DIAGNOSTIC POINTS

Colour of urine
- concentrated and dark - Damp Heat or *yin* deficiency
- pale or normal - Liver *qi* stagnation, Spleen (and Lung) or Kidney deficiency

Aggravation
- with stress - Liver *qi* stagnation
- with cold - Kidney deficiency
- with cough - Spleen and Lung deficiency
- when fatigued - deficiency patterns

Common patterns
- frequent urination - Kidney deficiency, Lung and Spleen deficiency, Liver *qi* stagnation, Damp Heat
- incontinence - Kidney deficiency, Lung and Spleen deficiency, Damp Heat
- nocturia - Kidney deficiency
- nocturnal enuresis - Kidney deficiency, Liver *qi* stagnation with Heat or Fire

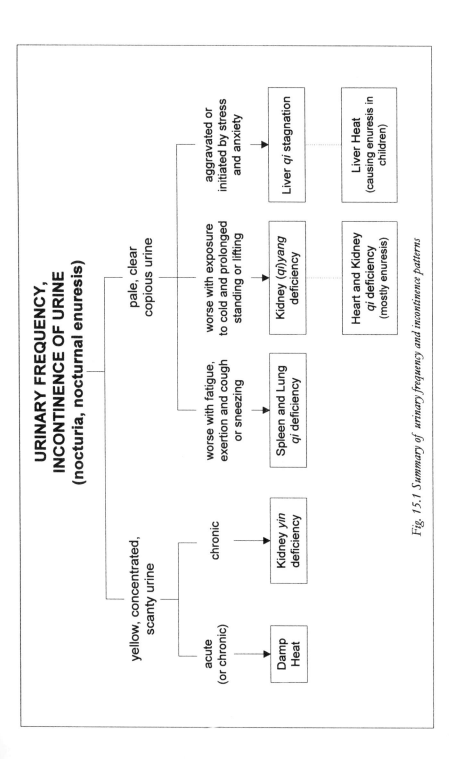

Fig. 15.1 *Summary of urinary frequency and incontinence patterns*

15.1 DAMP HEAT

Pathophysiology

- Damp Heat in the Bladder can be acute or chronic. The chronic variety is more likely due to internally generated Damp Heat (particularly from a rich diet and alcohol), or unresolved, lingering external Damp Heat. Chronic Damp Heat in the Bladder produces milder symptoms than acute Damp Heat. In acute cases the symptoms may be localised in the Bladder and there may be few of the systemic symptoms listed below.
- In either case, the mechanisms are the same. Damp obstructs the normal process of *qi* transformation in the Bladder, while the Heat irritates the Bladder and its expanding nature forces Fluids outward, causing a sense of urgency and frequency.
- Depending on the balance of Dampness and Heat, the features will differ. When Heat predominates, urgency and dark scanty urine result. When Damp predominates, suprapubic fullness, a feeling of incomplete voiding and gastrointestinal symptoms result.

Clinical features

- in acute cases frequent, urgent, burning, scanty urination, which feels incomplete or dripping ; in chronic cases burning and urgency may be mild or absent, or there may be a sense of urethral irritation or a feeling of constantly needing to urinate
- if there is incontinence, the urine is scanty, strong smelling and dark or cloudy
- suprapubic fullness and discomfort, lower back pain
- fullness or discomfort in the chest and epigastrium
- poor appetite, nausea, bitter taste in the mouth
- thirst with little desire to drink
- a tendency to constipation or alternating loose and sluggish stools
- acute cases may have fever (especially in the afternoon), or alternating fever and chills.

T greasy yellow coat
P slippery and rapid or soft and rapid

Treatment principle

Clear and drain Dampness and Heat

Prescription

BA ZHENG SAN 八正散
(*Dianthus Formula*)

che qian zi (Semen Plantaginis) 车前子	12g

hua shi (Talcum) 滑石 12g
bian xu (Herba Polygoni Avicularis) 篇蓄 9g
qu mai (Herba Dianthi) 瞿麦 9g
shan zhi zi (Fructus Gardeniae Jasminoidis) 山栀子 6g
mu tong (Caulis Mutong) 木通 6g
zhi da huang (Radix et Rhizoma Rhei) 制大黄 6g
gan cao shao (tips of Radix Glycyrrhizae Uralensis)
甘草梢 3g
deng xin cao (Medulla Junci Effusi) 灯心草 2g

Method: Decoction. **Che qian zi** is cooked in a muslin bag (*bao jian* 包煎).
(Source: *Shi Yong Zhong Yi Nei Ke Xue*)

Modifications

- Alternating fever and chills, nausea, fatigue and dizziness indicate that Damp Heat is obstructing the *shao yang* level. Add **chai hu** (Radix Bupleuri) 柴胡 9g, **huang qin** (Radix Scutellariae Baicalensis) 黄芩 9g and **ban xia*** (Rhizoma Pinelliae Ternatae) 半夏 6g to harmonise *shao yang*.
- With slight (or occult) haematuria add **xiao ji** (Herba Cephalanoplos) 小蓟 9g and **bai mao gen** (Rhizoma Imperatae Cylindricae) 白茅根 12g.

Patent medicines

Ming Mu Shang Qing Pian 明目上清片 (Ming Mu Shang Ching Pien)
Long Dan Xie Gan Wan 龙胆泻肝丸 (Long Dan Xie Gan Wan)
Dao Chi Pian 导赤片 (Tao Chih Pien)
Chuan Xin Lian Kang Yan Pian 穿心连抗炎片
    (Chuan Xin Lian Antiphlogistic Tablets)

Acupuncture

Ren.3 (*zhong ji* -), Liv.5 (*li gou* -), Ht.8 (*shao fu* -), Sp.6 (*san yin jiao* -), Bl.28 (*pang guang shu* -), Sp.9 (*yin ling quan* -), Liv.2 (*xing jian* -)
- for alternating fever and chills add SJ.5 (*wai guan*) and GB.39 (*xuan zhong*) or GB.41 (*zu lin qi*)

Clinical notes

- Biomedical conditions that may present as Damp Heat type frequent urination include urinary tract infection, urethritis, cystitis, pyelonephritis, gonorrhoeal urethritis and prostatitis.
- Generally responds well. Following resolution of chronic cases, Kidney tonification is useful to prevent recurrence.

肝气郁滞遗尿

15.2 LIVER *QI* STAGNATION

Pathophysiology
- This pattern is usually due to emotional factors, such as repressed anger, resentment and frustration, which disrupt the smooth circulation of Liver *qi* in general, and in particular in the lower *jiao*. As the Liver channel passes through the lower *jiao*, constraint of Liver *qi* can disrupt the smooth flow of Bladder *qi*. The main feature of this pattern is the clear influence of emotions.
- Liver *qi* stagnation often complicates other pathogenic entities, such as Dampness, Damp Heat, Spleen deficiency or *yin* deficiency, in which case a combined approach to treatment is necessary. The relative degree of *qi* stagnation should be assessed from the degree of influence that emotion and stress has on the frequency.

Clinical features
- urinary frequency that is initiated or aggravated by stress or emotional upset, urination feels incomplete or is hesitant
- fullness in the lower abdomen
- tightness or fullness in the chest, difficulty getting a satisfying breath
- hypochondriac discomfort or tightness, frequent sighing
- dizziness
- occasional fatigue (although patients often feel better with exercise)
- irritability or depression
- abdominal distension
- flatulence and alternating constipation and diarrhoea
- women may experience irregular menstruation, premenstrual syndrome and breast tenderness
- all symptoms tend to be aggravated by stress

T normal or dark (*qing* 青)
P wiry

Treatment principle
Move and spread Liver *qi*

Prescription

XIAO YAO SAN 逍遥散
(*Bupleurum and Dang Gui Formula*) modified

chai hu (Radix Bupleuri) 柴胡	9g
dang gui (Radix Angelicae Sinensis) 当归	9g
bai shao (Radix Paeoniae Lactiflorae) 白芍	9g
bai zhu (Rhizoma Atractylodes Macrocephalae) 白术	9g

fu ling (Sclerotium Poria Cocos) 茯苓 9g
pao jiang (roasted Rhizoma Zingiberis Offinalis) 炮姜 6g
zhi gan cao (honey fried Radix Glycyrrhizae Uralensis)
炙甘草 6g
wu yao (Radix Linderae Strychnifoliae) 乌药 6g
bo he (Herba Mentha Haplocalycis) 薄荷 3g

Method: Decoction or powder. When decocted **bo he** is added just before the end of cooking (*hou xia* 后下). (Source: *Fluid Physiology and Pathology in Traditional Chinese Medicine*)

Modifications

- With severe lower abdominal distension and fullness add, **mu xiang** (Radix Aucklandiae Lappae) 木香 6g and **qing pi** (Pericarpium Citri Reticulatae Viride) 青皮 6g.
- With stagnant Blood (purplish spots on the tongue, venous congestion around the inner ankles and Sp.9 *yin ling quan*), add **hong hua** (Flos Carthami Tinctorii) 红花 9g, **chi shao** (Radix Paeoniae Rubrae) 赤芍 12g and **chuan niu xi** (Radix Cyathulae Officinalis) 川牛膝 9g.
- In men with prostatic hypertrophy, add two or three herbs to 'soften hardness and disperse swelling' from the following list: **mu li**^ (Concha Ostreae) 牡蛎 12g, **zhe bei mu** (Bulbus Fritillariae Thunbergii) 浙贝母 9g, **xuan shen** (Radix Scrophulariae) 玄参 12g, **chuan shan jia**° (Squama Manitis) 穿山甲 9g, **wa leng zi**^ (Concha Arcae) 瓦楞子 12g, **wang bu liu xing** (semen Vaccariae Segetalis) 王不留行 9g.

Variations and additional prescriptions

- Enuresis in nervous, anxious, hyperactive or exciteable children may be due to Liver *qi* stagnation with Heat or Fire. The features are frequent enuresis in an energetic child with a ruddy complexion, yellow urine, restlessness at night, insomnia, nightmares, irritability, tendency to constipation, may be a sore or inflamed urinary tract and a red tongue. The treatment is to clear Heat from the Liver with a formula like **LONG DAN XIE GAN TANG** (*Gentiana Combination* 龙胆泻肝汤, p.500) or **CHAI HU JIA LONG GU MU LI TANG** (*Bupleurum and Dragon Bone Combination* 柴胡加龙骨牡蛎汤, p.816) and dietary regulation. Add astringents like **jin ying zi** (Fructus Rosae Laevigatae) 金樱子 and **sang piao xiao**^ (Ootheca Mantidis) 桑螵蛸.

Patent medicines

Chai Hu Shu Gan Wan 柴胡舒肝丸 (Chai Hu Shu Gan Wan)
Shu Gan Wan 舒肝丸 (Shu Gan Wan)
Xiao Yao Wan 逍遥丸 (Xiao Yao Wan)
Jia Wei Xiao Yao Wan 加味逍遥丸 (Jia Wei Xiao Yao Wan)

Long Dan Xie Gan Wan 龙胆泻肝丸 (Long Dan Xie Gan Wan)
- Liver Fire

Qian Lie Xian Wan 前列腺丸 (Prostate Gland Pills)
- very useful added to one of the above formulae in men with prostate swelling

Acupuncture

PC.6 (*nei guan*), Bl.18 (*gan shu*), Bl.22 (*san jiao shu*), Liv.8 (*qu quan*), Bl.28 (*pang guang shu* -), Ren.5 (*shi men*), Liv.5 (*li gou* -), Liv.3 (*tai chong* -)

Clinical notes

- Biomedical conditions that may present as Liver *qi* stagnation type frequent urination include anxiety neurosis, 'nervous bladder' and nocturnal enuresis in children (with Heat)
- Acupuncture can be very effective at relieving urinary frequency caused by Liver *qi* stagnation. For recurrent cases herbs may be added. The origin of any emotional imbalance or stress must be addressed to prevent recurrence.

15.3 KIDNEY (QI) YANG DEFICIENCY

Pathophysiology
- If the *qi* or *yang* of the Kidney is weak, the control of the lower *yin* orifices may be compromised leading to leakage of urine or incontinence. Kidney *yang* plays a very important role in fluid metabolism and transformation, thus weakness of *yang* will result in excess fluid accumulation in the Bladder necessitating frequent voiding of large quantities of urine.
- Kidney deficiency patterns are frequently complicated by Spleen deficiency. When the Spleen is also weak, the muscle tone of the urethral sphincter may be compromised, and urine cannot be held up against gravity. This dual deficiency often leads to incontinence of urine.
- Depending on the degree of deficiency, either *qi* or *yang* may be weak. In younger individuals, *qi* deficiency is more common and there are fewer (or none) cold symptoms.

Clinical features
- frequent, copious or scanty, clear urine, incontinence or nocturia with profuse clear urine
- the urge to urinate may increase with exposure to cold and is worse with prolonged standing and lifting
- when urine is scanty there will be oedema
- waxy pale complexion
- listlessness and fatigue
- aversion to cold, cold extremities
- lower abdominal distension
- constipation or loose stools
- weak, cold and sore lower back and knees

T pale, wet and swollen
P deep and thready or slow and weak, particularly in the proximal positions

Treatment principle
Warm, strengthen and consolidate Kidney *yang*
Astringe fluids as necessary

Prescription

YOU GUI WAN 右归丸
(*Eucommia and Rehmannia Formula*) modified

shu di (Radix Rehmanniae Glutinosae Conquitae) 熟地	240g
lu jiao jiao^ (Cornu Cervi Gelatinum) 鹿角胶	120g
shan yao (Radix Dioscoreae Oppositae) 山药	120g
gou qi zi (Fructus Lycii) 枸杞子	120g

tu si zi (Semen Cuscutae Chinensis) 菟丝子 120g
du zhong (Cortex Eucommiae Ulmoidis) 杜仲 120g
shan zhu yu (Fructus Corni Officinalis) 山茱萸 90g
dang gui (Radix Angelicae Sinensis) 当归 90g
sha yuan ji li (Semen Astragali Complanati) 沙苑蒺藜 90g
fu pen zi (Fructus Rubi Chingii) 复盆子 90g
chao sang piao xiao^ (dry fried Ootheca Mantidis)
    炒桑螵蛸 60g
zhi fu zi* (Radix Aconiti Carmichaeli Praeparata)
    制附子 60-180g
rou gui (Cortex Cinnamomi Cassiae) 肉桂 60-120g

Method: Grind herbs to a fine powder and form into 9-gram pills with honey. The dose is one pill 2-3 times daily. May also be decocted with an 90% reduction in dosage. When decocted **zhi fu zi** is cooked for 30 minutes before the other herbs (*xian jian* 先煎).

SANG PIAO XIAO SAN 桑螵蛸散
(*Mantis Egg Case Powder*)

This formula is selected when Kidney and Heart *qi* deficiency is the main problem. This pattern is common in children or young people (often a congenital weakness). The features are frequent urination or nocturnal enuresis with dream-disturbed sleep, occasional cloudy urine, forgetfulness, disorientation, a pink or pale tongue with a thin white coat and a thready weak pulse.

sang piao xiao^ (Ootheca Mantidis) 桑螵蛸 9g
fu ling (Sclerotium Poria Cocos) 茯苓 9g
dang gui (Radix Angelicae Sinensis) 当归 9g
yuan zhi (Radix Polygalae Tenuifoliae) 远志 6g
shi chang pu (Rhizoma Acori Graminei) 石菖蒲 6g
duan long gu^ (Calcined Os Draconis) 煅龙骨 12g
dang shen (Radix Codonopsis Pilosulae) 党参 12g
zhi gui ban° (honey fried Plastrum Testudinis) 炙龟板 15g

Method: Decoction. (Source: *Shi Yong Zhong Yi Nei Ke Xue*)

Modifications (apply to both formulae, where not already included)
- In stubborn cases, add **yi zhi ren** (Fructus Alpiniae Oxyphyllae) 益智仁 90(9)g and **bu gu zhi** (Fructus Psoraleae Corylifoliae) 补骨脂 90(9)g.
- With Spleen deficiency (diarrhoea with undigested food, abdominal distension, poor appetite, indigestion, daytime frequency and nocturia or incontinence), add two or three of the following herbs: **huang qi** (Radix Astragali Membranacei) 黄芪 180(18)g, **sha yuan ji li** (Semen Astragali Complanati) 沙苑蒺藜 90(9)g, **sheng ma** (Rhizoma Cimicifugae) 升麻 60(6)g, **dang shen** (Radix Codonopsis Pilosulae)

党参 120(12)g, **bai zhu** (Rhizoma Atractylodes Macrocephalae) 白术 90 (9)g and **gan jiang** (Rhizoma Zingiberis Officinalis) 干姜 60(6)g, or combine with **BU ZHONG YI QI TANG** (*Ginseng and Astragalus Combination* 补中益气汤 modified, p.454).

- In men with prostatic hypertrophy, add two or three herbs to 'soften hardness and disperse swelling' from the following: **mu li**^ (Concha Ostreae) 牡蛎 120(12)g, **zhe bei mu** (Bulbus Fritillariae Thunbergii) 浙贝母 90(9)g, **xuan shen** (Radix Scrophulariae) 玄参 120(12)g, **chuan shan jia**° (Squama Manitis) 穿山甲 90(9)g, **wa leng zi**^ (Concha Arcae) 瓦楞子 120(12)g, **wang bu liu xing** (semen Vaccariae Segetalis) 王不留行 90(9)g.

Patent medicines

Jin Kui Shen Qi Wan 金匮肾气丸 (Sexoton Pills)
Ba Ji Yin Yang Wan 巴戟阴阳丸 (Ba Ji Yin Yang Wan)
Ning Xin Bu Shen Wan 宁心补肾丸 (Bo San Yuen Medical Pills)
Jin Suo Gu Jing Wan 金锁固精丸 (Chin So Ku Ching Wan)
 - this last formula (which is primarily astringent) and one
  of the above patent formulae are generally taken together
Qian Lie Xian Wan 前列腺丸 (Prostate Gland Pills)
 - combined with one of the above formulae for prostate swelling

Acupuncture

Bl.23 (*shen shu* +▲), Du.4 (*ming men* +▲), Ren.4 (*guan yuan* +▲), Kid.3 (*tai xi* +), Sp.6 (*san yin jiao* +), SI.3 (*hou xi*), Du.26 (*ren zhong*), Kid.11 (*heng gu*)
 • for enuresis of a Kidney deficiency type in children, SI.3 (*hou xi*) is often enough to strengthen the *du mai* and stop the leakage

Clinical notes

- Biomedical conditions that may present as Kidney *yang* deficiency type frequent urination include chronic glomerular, interstitial or diffuse nephritis, nephrotic syndrome, benign prostatic hypertrophy, hypothyroidism, diabetes insipidis and nocturnal enuresis.
- Kidney *yang* deficiency frequent urination often responds well to correct TCM treatment. Conditions like hypothyroidism can be difficult and may require a combination of Western and Chinese medicine.
- Bladder training programs have a high degree of success in improving incontinence, and are appropriate for chronic syndromes. This approach involves strengthening the muscles of the pelvic floor and desensitising the detrusor muscle. In addition, abstaining from diuretic substances and irritants, like coffee and tea, is important.

15.4 KIDNEY *YIN* DEFICIENCY

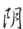
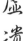

Pathophysiology
- Heat (from Kidney *yin* deficiency) concentrates Fluids in the Bladder, and at the same time, the expanding nature of Heat forces urine out. The weakness of Kidney *yin* also means the 'lower *yin*' orifices are not consolidated, allowing leakage of urine. This pattern is most common in middle aged and elderly women.

Clinical features
- frequent, scanty yellow urine, possibly with a sensation of heat or irritation, incontinence may occur as the deficiency progresses
- dry mouth and throat
- restlessness
- insomnia
- sensations of heat in the palms and soles ('five hearts hot')
- facial flushing, malar flush, nightsweats
- dizziness
- tinnitus
- soreness or weakness of the lower back and knees, heel pain
- tendency to dry stools or constipation

T red and dry with little or no coat
P thready and rapid

Treatment principle
Nourish and tonify Kidney *yin*
Clear deficient Heat

Prescription

ZHI BAI BA WEI WAN 知柏八味丸
(*Anemarrhena, Phellodendron and Rehmannia Formula*)

shu di (Radix Rehmanniae Glutinosae Conquitae) 熟地	240g
shan yao (Radix Dioscoreae Oppositae) 山药	120g
shan zhu yu (Fructus Corni Officinalis) 山茱萸	120g
fu ling (Sclerotium Poria Cocos) 茯苓	90g
ze xie (Rhizoma Alismatis Orientalis) 泽泻	90g
mu dan pi (Cortex Moutan Radicis) 牡丹皮	90g
zhi mu (Radix Anemarrhenae Asphodeloidis) 知母	90g
huang bai (Cortex Phellodendri) 黄柏	90g

Method: Grind the herbs to powder and form into 9-gram pills with honey. The dose is 2-3 pills daily. May also be decocted with a 90% reduction in dosage.
(Source: *Shi Yong Zhong Yi Nei Ke Xue*)

Modifications
- If the urine is very frequent, add two or three of the following astringent herbs: **mu li^** (Concha Ostreae) 牡蛎 90g, **wu wei zi** (Fructus Schizandrae Chinensis) 五味子 60g, **jin ying zi** (Fructus Rosae Laevigatae) 金樱子 90g or **qian shi** (Semen Euryales Ferocis) 芡实 90g.
- In men with prostatic hypertrophy, add two or three herbs to 'soften hardness and disperse swelling' from the following list: **mu li^** (Concha Ostreae) 牡蛎 120g, **zhe bei mu** (Bulbus Fritillariae Thunbergii) 浙贝母 90g, **xuan shen** (Radix Scrophulariae) 玄参 120g, **chuan shan jia°** (Squama Manitis) 穿山甲 90g, **wa leng zi^** (Concha Arcae) 瓦楞子 120g, **wang bu liu xing** (semen Vaccariae Segetalis) 王不留行 90g.

Patent medicines
Liu Wei Di Huang Wan 六味地黄丸 (Liu Wei Di Huang Wan)
Zhi Bai Ba Wei Wan 知柏八味丸 (Zhi Bai Ba Wei Wan)
Qian Lie Xian Wan 前列腺丸 (Prostate Gland Pills)
  - combined with one of the above formulae for prostate swelling

Acupuncture
BL.23 (*shen shu* +), Ren.4 (*guan yuan* +), Sp.6 (*san yin jiao*),
Kid.2 (*ran gu* -), BL.53 (*wei yang*), Kid.3 (*tai xi* +), Kid.6 (*zhao hai*)

Clinical notes
- Biomedical conditions that may present as Kidney *yin* deficiency type frequent urination include chronic nephritis, atrophic vaginitis, diabetes mellitus, chronic urinary tract infection, interstitial cystitis and benign prostatic hypertrophy.
- Kidney *yin* deficiency is a common pattern of urinary frequency or incontinence in menopausal women. The urethra suffers from the decline of oestrogen in much the same way as the vagina does, that is, it becomes thinner and drier and more prone to irritation. This can cause frequent urges to urinate even when the bladder is not full. If the tissue thins and loses elasticity too much, incontinence of urine can result. Herbs that clear Heat and tonify *yin* improve this condition over time. In severe or distressing cases a small amount of oestrogen cream can be applied (usually vaginally) for a short time while the herbs take effect.
- Bladder training programs have a high degree of success, and are very useful in chronic patterns. This approach involves strengthening the muscles of the pelvic floor and desensitising the detrusor muscle. In addition abstaining from diuretic substances and irritants, like coffee and tea, is important.

15.5 SPLEEN (AND LUNG) *QI* DEFICIENCY

脾肺气虚遗尿

Pathophysiology
- This pattern can be due to failure of Spleen and Lung *qi* to metabolise and distribute fluids properly so that they accumulate in the Bladder (and Lung). The Lung involvement is usually secondary to the Spleen weakness.
- It can also be associated with loss of the Spleen's ascending action, that is, the aspect of Spleen function that holds structures in place against the force of gravity. When combined with the hypotonicity of muscles (in this case the urethral sphincter or bladder) so characteristic of a weak Spleen, urine can not be held in properly and frequency or incontinence results.

Clinical features
- frequent, copious, clear urine or incontinence, which is worse with exertion and when fatigued, or with sneezing or coughing
- shortness of breath
- cough with thin watery sputum
- soft, low voice, or reluctance to speak
- fatigue
- poor appetite, abdominal distension with eating, loose stools
- pale complexion and lips
- mild oedema of the eyelids or fingers, worse in the morning

T pale with a white coat
P weak

Treatment principle
Warm and tonify Spleen and Lung *qi*
Aid the ascent of *yang*

Prescription

BU ZHONG YI QI TANG 补中益气汤
(*Ginseng and Astragalus Combination*) modified

huang qi (Radix Astragali Membranacei) 黄芪	15g
mu li^ (Concha Ostreae) 牡蛎	15g
bai zhu (Rhizoma Atractylodes Macrocephalae) 白术	12g
ren shen (Radix Ginseng) 人参	9g
dang gui (Radix Angelicae Sinensis) 当归	6g
chen pi (Pericarpium Citri Reticulatae) 陈皮	6g
sheng ma (Rhizoma Cimicifugae) 升麻	6g
chai hu (Radix Bupleuri) 柴胡	6g
gan jiang (Rhizoma Zingiberis Officinalis) 干姜	6g
yi zhi ren (Fructus Alpiniae Oxyphyllae) 益智仁	6g
wu wei zi (Fructus Schizandrae Chinensis) 五味子	6g

zhi gan cao (honey fried Radix Glycyrrhizae Uralensis)
炙甘草 3g
Method: Decoction. (Source: *Shi Yong Zhong Yi Nei Ke Xue*)

Modifications
- Incontinence following a difficult childbirth usually indicates that the Spleen has been weakened, the Bladder damaged and there is residual stagnation of Blood. Add **tao ren** (Semen Persicae) 桃仁 9g and **hong hua** (Flos Carthami Tinctorii) 红花 9g.

Variations and additional prescriptions
- Sudden increase in urine output in an individual with a pre-existing Spleen and Lung deficiency may indicate that the patient has been influenced by an external pathogen (like Wind Cold). The Cold shuts the pores, causing an increase in the descent of fluids. The correct treatment is to use a diaphoretic formula to expel Wind Cold. The appropriate formula is **SHEN SU YIN** (*Ginseng and Perilla Combination* 参苏饮, p.21).

Patent medicines
Bu Zhong Yi Qi Wan 补中益气丸 (Bu Zhong Yi Qi Wan)
Yu Ping Feng Wan 玉屏风丸 (Yu Ping Feng Wan)
Jin Suo Gu Jing Wan 金锁固精丸 (Chin So Ku Ching Wan)
  - added to one of the above patent formulae

Acupuncture
Du.20 (*bai hui* ▲), Ren.6 (*qi hai* +▲), Ren.4 (*guan yuan* +▲),
Lu.7 (*lie que*), Bl.24 (*qi hai shu* +), St.36 (*zu san li* +p), Sp.6 (*san yin jiao* +),
Ren.12 (*zhong wan* +▲), Bl.20 (*pi shu*)
- a useful technique for lower abdominal prolapses in general is to thread a 3-inch needle from Ren.6 (*qi hai*) to Ren.3 (*zhong ji*). The needle is twirled to anchor it, then raised towards the sternum creating a lifting sensation in the lower abdomen. It can be taped (in its lifted position) in place for the duration of the treatment.

Clinical notes
- Biomedical conditions that may present as Spleen *qi* deficiency type frequent urination include prolapsed uterus exerting pressure on the bladder, prolapsed bladder and stress incontinence.
- Prolapses sometimes occur following lower abdominal surgery, like hysterectomy, if the ligaments supporting the bladder are damaged.
- Bladder training programs have a high degree of success in controlling incontinence, and are particularly useful in patterns characterised by muscular hypotonicity. In addition, abstaining from diuretic substances and irritants, like coffee and tea, is important.

SUMMARY OF GUIDING FORMULAE FOR FREQUENT URINATION AND INCONTINENCE OF URINE

Damp Heat - *Ba Zheng San* 八正散

Liver *qi* stagnation - *Xiao Yao San* 逍遥散
- nocturnal enuresis due to Liver Heat - *Long Dan Xie Gan Tang* 龙胆泻肝汤

Kidney *yang* (*qi*) deficiency - *You Gui Wan* 右归丸
- with Heart and Kidney *qi* deficiency - *Sang Piao Xiao San* 桑螵蛸散

Kidney *yin* deficiency - *Zhi Bai Ba Wei Wan* 知柏八味丸

Spleen (and Lung) *qi* deficiency - *Bu Zhong Yi Qi Tang* 补中益气汤

Endnote

For more information regarding herbs marked with an asterisk*, an open circle° or a hat^, see the tables on pp.944-952.

Disorders of the Kidney

16. Haematuria

Excess patterns
Damp Heat
Heart Fire
Liver Fire
Blood stagnation

Deficient patterns
Spleen and Kidney *qi* deficiency
Kidney *yin* deficiency with deficient Fire

16 HAEMATURIA
niao xue 尿血

Haematuria is the presence of blood or blood clots in the urine without any pain. The appearance of the urine varies with the amount of blood and can be pale pink, smoky, fresh red or dark red. In severe cases there may be blood clots. For haematuria with pain, see Blood Painful Urination Syndrome, p.379.

Traditionally, haematuria implied visible blood in the urine. With more sensitive testing methods, however, non visible traces of blood ('occult blood') can be detected. As these traces are often picked up on a routine urine test in otherwise healthy individuals, it is questionable whether treatment for haematuria is indicated. If blood traces are detected in a patient with some other problem, styptic herbs may be added to whatever prescription is appropriate.

AETIOLOGY

There are three general mechanisms underlying haematuria, and indeed all forms of bleeding.

The first and most common is Heat, which quickens the Blood causing it to spill from the vessels, and which can scorch and damage the delicate *luo* vessels of urinary system. Heat may be associated with external invasion, Toxins, Dampness, *qi* stagnation or *yin* deficiency.

The second is failure of the Spleen *qi* to hold Blood in the vessels. One of Spleen *qi's* primary functions is to exert an external 'pressure' on the walls of blood vessels, holding the Blood in. When this function is weakened or fails, Blood seeps out of the vessels and the bleeding that results is usually mild and recurrent. When weakness of Spleen *qi* is responsible for bleeding, there will often be multiple sites of bleeding, typically easy bruising, uterine bleeding and so on.

The third is stagnant Blood. If stagnant Blood obstructs the circulation of *qi* and Blood, pressure will build up behind the obstruction, and eventually Blood overflows and spills from the vessels.

Heat (Damp Heat) in the Urinary Bladder
External Heat

External pathogenic Heat or Damp Heat (or other external pathogens, like Dampness or Cold, that generate Heat once trapped internally) can invade through the *tai yang* (Urinary Bladder) channel, the leg *yin* channels or the local *luo* channels. The local *luo* channels are small branches of the major channels that spread through the genitourinary system. They can be conduits for infection during sexual intercourse or after bowel movements. Heat of external origin, however, tends to produce a more localised pattern, with the focus of symptoms in the bladder and urethra. Clinically, patients with an external Heat or Damp Heat pattern are in fact more likely to complain of bleeding *and* pain, in which case Blood Painful Urination Syndrome (p.379) should be the starting point for diagnosis. Invasion by external pathogens occurs more easily in someone who has a pre-existing Kidney deficiency.

Internal Heat
When the cause is internal, haematuria can be due to Damp Heat, Heart or Liver Fire or Heat arising from *yin* deficiency. Damp Heat can arise in the middle *jiao* from overconsumption of rich, greasy or spicy foods and alcohol. Because Damp is heavy, it sinks and settles in the lower *jiao*. It may also be generated in the lower *jiao* directly if any Heat arising from *yin* deficiency or *qi* stagnation combines with Dampness already present. Damp Heat, when prolonged, can congeal into stones, which can damage the urinary tract and cause bleeding.

> **BOX 16.1 SOME BIOMEDICAL CAUSES OF HAEMATURIA**
>
> **Common**
> - local infection (cystitis, urethritis, prostatitis)
> - urinary calculi
> - trauma
> - tumours (renal, prostate, bladder)
>
> **Pre-renal**
> - epidemic haemorrhagic diseases
> - blackwater fever
> - thrombocytopoenia
> - sickle cell anaemia
> - systemic lupus erythematosus
> - blood dyscrasia
>
> **Renal**
> - renal infarction
> - polycystic kidneys
> - renal calculi
> - tumours
> - Goodpasture's syndrome
> - glomerulonephritis
> - renal papillary necrosis
> - tuberculosis of the kidneys
>
> **Post-renal**
> - foreign body
> - prostatic varices
> - prostatic hypertrophy
> - following vigorous exercise
> - radiation cystitis
> - endometriosis
> - anticoagulants
> - haemophilia

Stress and emotional turmoil, which cause stagnation of Heart and Liver *qi*, can cause Heart or Liver Fire. It generally requires extreme stress or emotional trauma to create sufficient internal Heat to cause bleeding. If the Heat is internal in origin, the symptoms tend to be more systemic, reflecting the original source of the Heat.

Kidney *yin* deficiency (with deficient Heat)
Kidney *yin* becomes damaged through overwork (especially while under stress), late nights, shift work, insufficient sleep and use of recreational drugs.

Kidney *yin* may also be damaged by febrile disease, ageing and, in men by excessive ejaculation, and in women by having many pregnancies close together. Deficient Kidney *yin* generates Heat, which forces Blood to behave recklessly, causing it to spill from the vessels. Fire can also scorch and damage the delicate *luo* vessels of the urinary system.

Spleen and Kidney *yang* (*qi*) deficiency

Spleen *qi* exerts a consolidating pressure on the walls of blood vessels This pressure is responsible for preventing blood from leaking out. Although in this pattern there are usually signs of both Spleen and Kidney weakness, it is the Spleen's loss of control over Blood vessels that is the primary cause of bleeding.

The Spleen is weakened by overwork, excessive worry or mental activity, irregular dietary habits, excessive consumption of cold, raw foods, prolonged illness or lack of support from the Kidneys.

The Kidney *yang* or *qi* weakness which may accompany this pattern, can be an inherited condition or may develop as a result of age, chronic illness, overexposure to cold conditions, or excessive lifting or standing (particularly if this occurs in a cold environment, on cold floors or at night). Kidney *yang* or *qi* can also be damaged in men by excessive ejaculation, or in women by having many pregnancies close together. In some cases, in particular younger people, Kidney *qi* may be weakened while Kidney *yang* remains intact, in which case the cold symptoms are not seen.

Qi and Blood stagnation

Frustration, anger, resentment, prolonged emotional turmoil, repressed emotions and stress can disrupt the circulation of Liver *qi,* and, because the Liver channel passes through the lower *jiao*, Bladder *qi* can also be disrupted. Once *qi* is obstructed, it fails to lead the Blood resulting in *qi* and Blood stagnation.

In addition, *qi* stagnation can give rise to Heat—the emotions that give rise to stagnant *qi* (particularly anger and resentment) 'smoulder' in the Liver and create Heat (or Fire), which can be transmitted to the Heart or can travel through the Liver channel to the lower *jiao*. Stagnant Liver *qi* can disrupt the function of the Spleen, weakening it and leading to the development of Dampness. This Dampness can sink into the lower *jiao*, potentially generating Heat and establishing the Damp Heat cycle.

Pre-existing stagnation (of *qi* and Blood), can be transferred from another pelvic organ to the Bladder. This may be observed in women following hysterectomy, myomectomy or removal of ovarian cysts. The organ primarily affected by the stagnation is removed or repaired, but the condition that gave rise to the initial problem (that is, *qi* and/or Blood stagnation) persists.

16.2 KEY DIAGNOSTIC POINTS

Colour of the urine
- The colour of the urine is largely due to the quanity of blood present. In excess cases, bleeding is usually significant and the urine can appear quite red, to the point where it seems pure blood.
- pale or pink urine signifies mild bleeding, usually from deficiency
- bright red and copious - Heat, usually excess, less frequently from deficiency
- dark or purplish and clotty - stagnant blood

Location of bleeding
- bleeding at the beginning of urination - from the urethra or prostate
- at the end of urination - from the bladder
- if the bleeding is evenly distributed in the urine stream - possibly from the kidney
- bleeding from other sites as well (bruising etc.) - mostly Spleen deficiency

Caution
- Note that red coloured urine can be due to pigments from red food colourings, beetroot or berries. Vitamin B12 injections and some drugs can colour the urine, and, in some rare cases, so can some metabolic disorders which allow excessive excretion of porphyrins.
- Certain medications, such as anticoagulants, may cause occult haematuria.
- Occult haematuria often occurs in joggers and athletes who exercise vigorously.

The focus of pelvic symptoms then shifts, for example, from the uterus (which was removed because of heavy periods and pain) to the Bladder.

TREATMENT

In general there are several steps to consider when treating a bleeding disorder. The first, and most important step, is to stop the bleeding. When the bleeding is severe, the initial focus of treatment is to use first aid or herbs to quickly staunch the bleeding. This can usually be acheived with the patent medicine *Yun Nan Bai Yao* 云南白药 (Yunnan Paiyao) or a suitable styptic formulae. In practice an appropriate root treatment formula may be combined with *Yun Nan Bai Yao* for severe bleeding.

Once bleeding is under control, the underlying pattern can be dealt with more fully. There are two additional aspects to consider. First, any residual Blood outside the vessels is stagnant Blood and must be moved as it may become pathological if allowed to remain. Herbs to gently invigorate or regulate Blood should be incorporated into the appropriate formula. This is especially important in Heat types of bleeding, as the herbs used to stop bleeding will likely be cold natured and astringent. These herbs congeal Blood. Second, any *qi* or Blood deficiency that exists as a direct result of Blood loss should be supplemented with *qi* and Blood tonic herbs.

16.1 DAMP HEAT

Pathophysiology
- Damp Heat causes haematuria in two ways: first by quickening the Blood and second, by damaging the delicate *luo* vessels of the Bladder.
- This syndrome is differentiated from 'Damp Heat Painful Urination Syndrome', p.358, by the predominance of the bleeding relative to the pain (if there is any).

Clinical features
- scanty, concentrated, strong smelling urine with fresh red or darkish blood
- possible very mild burning with urination and a feeling of incomplete bladder emptying
- suprapubic fullness and discomfort, lower back pain
- fullness or discomfort in the chest and epigastrium
- poor appetite, nausea
- bitter taste in the mouth, thirst with little desire to drink
- a tendency to constipation or alternating loose and sluggish stools
- some cases may have afternoon fever, or alternating fever and chills

T greasy yellow coat
P slippery and rapid or soft and rapid

Treatment principle
Clear Dampness and Heat, promote urination
Cool the Blood and stop bleeding

Prescription

XIAO JI YIN ZI 小蓟饮子
(*Cephalanoplos Decoction*)

sheng di (Radix Rehmanniae Glutinosae) 生地	24g
hua shi (Talcum) 滑石	20g
xiao ji (Herba Cephalanoplos) 小蓟	15g
ou jie (Nodus Nelumbinis Nuciferae Rhizomatis) 藕节	10g
chao pu huang (dry fried Pollen Typhae) 炒蒲黄	10g
dan zhu ye (Herba Lophatheri Gracilis) 淡竹叶	10g
shan zhi zi (Fructus Gardeniae Jasminoidis) 山栀子	10g
dang gui (Radix Angelicae Sinensis) 当归	10g
gan cao shao (tips of Radix Glycyrrhizae Uralensis) 甘草稍	6g
mu tong (Caulis Mutong) 木通	6g

Method: Decoction. (Source: *Fluid Physiology and Pathology in Traditional Chinese Medicine*)

Modifications

- With severe bleeding, add **ce bai ye** (Cacumen Biotae Orientalis) 侧柏叶 9g, **xue yu tan^** (Crinus Carbonisatus Hominis Hominis) 血余炭 6g and **xian he cao** (Herba Agrimoniae Pilosae) 仙鹤草 12g, or combine with **YUN NAN BAI YAO** (*Yun Nan White Powder* 云南白药).
- With exterior signs (chills and fever), add **lian qiao** (Fructus Forsythiae Suspensae) 连翘 9g and **jin yin hua** (Flos Lonicerae Japonicae) 金银花 12g.
- Alternating fever and chills, nausea and dizziness indicate that Damp Heat is obstructing the *shao yang* level. Add **chai hu** (Radix Bupleuri) 柴胡 9g, **huang qin** (Radix Scutellariae Baicalensis) 黄芩 9g and **ban xia*** (Rhizoma Pinelliae Ternatae) 半夏 6g.
- With constipation, add **da huang** (Radix et Rhizoma Rhei) 大黄 6g and **quan gua lou** (Fructus Trichosanthis) 全栝楼 12g.
- With thirst and a bitter taste, add **shi hu** (Herba Dendrobii) 石斛 9g and **lu gen** (Rhizoma Phragmitis Communis) 芦根 15g.

Variations and additional prescriptions

- If the Heat is severe and produces significant systemic symptoms, high fever and chills, arthralgia, severe thirst, irritability, purpura or other sites of bleeding, a thick yellow tongue coat and rapid full pulse, it is redefined as Toxic Heat. The correct treatment is to clear Toxic Heat, cool the Blood and stop bleeding with **HUANG LIAN JIE DU TANG** (*Coptis and Scute Combination* 黄连解毒汤) modified.

　　huang lian (Rhizoma Coptidis) 黄连 3g
　　huang qin (Radix Scutellariae Baicalensis) 黄芩 9g
　　huang bai (Cortex Phellodendri) 黄柏 6g
　　shan zhi zi (Fructus Gardeniae Jasminoidis) 山栀子 9g
　　sheng di (Radix Rehmanniae Glutinosae) 生地 12g
　　jin yin hua (Flos Lonicerae Japonicae) 金银花 12g
　　mu dan pi (Cortex Moutan Radicis) 牡丹皮 9g
　　xiao ji (Herba Cephalanoplos) 小蓟 12g
　　ou jie (Nodus Nelumbinis Nuciferae Rhizomatis) 藕节 12g
　　qing dai (Indigo Pulverata Levis) 青黛 3g

　　Method: Decoction. **Qing dai** is added to the strained decoction (*chong fu* 冲服). (Source: *Shi Yong Zhong Yi Nei Ke Xue*)

Patent medicines

Ming Mu Shang Qing Pian 明目上清片 (Ming Mu Shang Ching Pien)
Long Dan Xie Gan Wan 龙胆泻肝丸 (Long Dan Xie Gan Wan)
Dao Chi Pian 导赤片 (Tao Chih Pien)
Chuan Xin Lian Kang Yan Pian 穿心莲抗炎片
　　(Chuan Xin Lian Antiphlogistic Tablets)

Yun Nan Bai Yao 云南白药 (Yunnan Paiyao)
- this medicine can be taken in addition to the main formula selected. The red pill that accompanies the powder is only used in severe cases.

Acupuncture
GB.41 (*zu lin qi* -), SJ.5 (*wai guan* -), GB.26 (*dai mai*), GB.28 (*wei dao*), Ren.3 (*zhong ji*), Liv.5 (*li gou* -), Sp.6 (*san yin jiao* -), LI.11 (*qu chi* -), Sp.9 (*yin ling quan* -), Ren.5 (*shi men*)

Clinical notes
- Biomedical conditions that may present as Damp Heat type haematuria include urinary tract infection, urethritis, cystitis, pyelonephritis, gonorrhoeal urethritis and prostatitis.
- Generally responds well to correct treatment.

Table 16.1 Comparison of excess patterns of haematuria

Pattern	Aetiology	Features		Guiding formula
Damp Heat	external invasion of Damp Heat, or less commonly internally generated Heat		suprapubic fullness, loss of appetite, nausea, constipation or alternating loose and sluggish stools, thirst with little desire to drink, greasy yellow tongue coat, slippery rapid pulse	XIAO JI YIN ZI with Toxic Heat HUANG LIAN JIE DU TANG
Heart Fire	emotional turmoil, particularly prolonged anxiety and worry	copious bright or dark red blood in the urine	red complexion, palpitations, insomnia, dream disturbed sleep, anxiety, irritability, thirst, mouth ulcers, red tongue with a redder tip, big rapid pulse especially in the distal position	DAO CHI SAN + XIAO JI YIN ZI with yin deficiency TIAN WANG BU XIN DAN
Liver Fire	emotional turmoil, particularly severe or repressed frustration, resentment and anger		extreme irritability, temper, dizziness, sore bloodshot eyes, temporal headache, hypochondriac discomfort, red tongue with redder edges and a dry yellow coat, wiry rapid pulse	LONG DAN XIE GAN WAN

16.2 HEART FIRE

Pathophysiology
- Heart Fire is usually the result of a significant emotional shock or prolonged and severe anxiety, which impedes the circulation of Heart *qi*. This stagnation can generate Heat, which can be transmitted to the Small Intestine (the *yang* partner organ of the Heart), and then to the Bladder.
- Fire quickens the Blood and damages the delicate *luo* vessels of the Bladder.

Clinical features
- hot, concentrated, urgent and frequent urine with fresh red blood
- red complexion
- ulceration of the mouth and tongue, particularly the tongue tip
- thirst with a desire for cold drinks
- sensation of heat in the chest
- irritability, restlessness, anxiety, agitation
- palpitations
- insomnia, dream disturbed sleep

T red with a redder tip and a dry, yellow coat; the tongue may be ulcerated
P rapid and big

Treatment principle
Clear Heart Fire, cool the Blood to stop bleeding

Prescription

DAO CHI SAN 导赤散
(*Rehmannia and Akebia Formula*) plus
XIAO JI YIN ZI 小蓟饮子
(*Cephalanoplos Decoction*) modified

sheng di (Radix Rehmanniae Glutinosae) 生地	30g
xiao ji (Herba Cephalanoplos) 小蓟	20g
ou jie (Nodus Nelumbinis Nuciferae Rhizomatis) 藕节	20g
hua shi (Talcum) 滑石	20g
qu mai (Herba Dianthi) 瞿麦	12g
mu tong (Caulis Mutong) 木通	10g
dan zhu ye (Herba Lophatheri Gracilis) 淡竹叶	10g
shan zhi zi (Fructus Gardeniae Jasminoidis) 山栀子	10g
chao pu huang (dry fried Pollen Typhae) 炒蒲黄	6g
gan cao shao (tips of Radix Glycyrrhizae Uralensis) 甘草梢	6g
hu po fen (powdered Succinum) 琥珀粉	3g

Method: Decoction. **Hu po** powder is added to the strained decoction (*chong fu* 冲服). (Source: *Zhong Yi Nei Ke Lin Chuang Shou Ce*)

Modifications
- With insomnia and irritability, add **huang lian** (Rhizoma Coptidis) 黄连 6g, **mai dong** (Tuber Ophiopogonis Japonici) 麦冬 10g and **ye jiao teng** (Caulis Polygoni Multiflori) 夜胶藤 15g to clear Heart Fire and calm the *shen*.
- With severe bleeding, combine with **YUN NAN BAI YAO** (*Yun Nan White Powder* 云南白药).

Variations and additional prescriptions
With yin *damage*
- In recurrent cases of Heart Fire, *yin* is often damaged and the condition becomes a mixture of deficiency and excess, leading to a loss of communication between the Heart and Kidney. The features are recurrent mouth ulcers and occasional mild or occult haematuria, insomnia, palpitations, anxiety, heat in the palms and soles, flushing, a dry red tongue or red tipped tongue with little or no coat and a thready rapid pulse. The correct treatment is to restore communication between the Heart and Kidneys (and nourish Heart and Kidney *yin*) using **TIAN WANG BU XIN DAN** (*Ginseng and Zizyphus Formula* 天王补心丹, p.852).

Patent medicines
Dao Chi Pian 导赤片 (Tao Chih Pien)
Ming Mu Shang Qing Pian 明目上清片 (Ming Mu Shang Ching Pien)
Long Dan Xie Gan Wan 龙胆泻肝丸 (Long Dan Xie Gan Wan)
Chuan Xin Lian Kang Yan Pian 穿心连抗炎片
   (Chuan Xin Lian Antiphlogistic Pills)
Yun Nan Bai Yao 云南白药 (Yunnan Paiyao)
   - this medicine can be taken in addition to the main formula selected. The red pill that accompanies the powder is only used in severe cases.

Acupuncture
Ren.3 (*zhong ji* -), PC.8 (*lao gong* -), Liv.2 (*xing jian* -), Bl.15 (*xin shu* -), Sp.10 (*xue hai* -), Ht.6 (*yin xi* -), Kid.6 (*zhao hai* +), SI.3 (*hou xi* -)

Clinical notes
- Biomedical conditions that may present as Heart Fire type haematuria include urinary tract infection, pyelonephritis, gonorrhoeal urethritis, prostatitis, Behçet's syndrome and Reiter's syndrome.
- The acute phase generally responds well to treatment to clear Heart Fire. Long term success of treatment, however, depends also on resolution or avoidance of external stressors.
- Heart and Liver Fire often overlap.

16.3 LIVER FIRE

Pathophysiology
- Ongoing obstruction of Liver *qi* by stress and emotional upsets will eventually give rise to Liver Fire. Since the Liver channel passes through the genitourinary area, Liver Fire can damage the delicate *luo* vessels in the urinary tract and quicken the Blood, forcing it from the vessels.

Clinical features
- scanty, dark, burning, urgent urination with fresh blood
- extreme irritability and a tendency to temper outbursts
- temporal headaches
- hypochondriac tightness or pain
- sore, bloodshot eyes
- bitter taste in the mouth
- dizziness
- tinnitus
- thirst
- constipation
- in some patients there may be ulcerations on the genitals, a tendency to herpes genitalia or eczema or rashes in the groin

T red body, with redder edges and a thick dry yellow coat
P wiry, rapid and strong

Treatment principle
Drain Liver Fire, clear Dampness and Heat

Prescription

LONG DAN XIE GAN TANG 龙胆泻肝汤
(*Gentiana Combination*) modified

jiu long dan cao (wine fried Radix Gentianae Longdancao) 酒龙胆草	6g
sheng di (Radix Rehmanniae Glutinosae) 生地	15g
che qian zi (Semen Plantaginis) 车前子	12g
shan zhi zi (Fructus Gardeniae Jasminoides) 山栀子	12g
huang qin (Radix Scutellariae Baicalensis) 黄芩	9g
ze xie (Rhizoma Alismatis Orientalis) 泽泻	9g
dang gui (Radix Angelicae Sinensis) 当归	6g
mu tong (Caulis Mutong) 木通	6g
chai hu (Radix Bupleuri) 柴胡	6g
gan cao (Radix Glycyrrhizae Uralensis) 甘草	6g
chao pu huang (dry fried Pollen Typhae) 炒蒲黄	9g

xiao ji (Herba Cephalanoplos) 小蓟 9g
Method: Decoction. **Che qian zi** is usually cooked in a muslin bag (*bao jian* 包煎).
(Source: *Shi Yong Fang Ji Xue*)

Modifications

- With severe bleeding, add **qian cao gen** (Radix Rubiae Cordifoliae) 茜草根 9g and **ce bai ye** (Cacumen Biotae Orientalis) 侧柏叶 12g, or combine with **YUN NAN BAI YAO** (*Yun Nan White Powder* 云南白药).
- With severe Heat, add **huang lian** (Rhizoma Coptidis) 黄连 6g, **ling yang jiao fen**° (powdered Cornu Antelopis) 羚羊角粉 3g.
- With dryness, add **mai dong** (Tuber Ophiopogonis Japonici) 麦冬 12g, **xuan shen** (Radix Scrophulariae Ningpoensis) 18g and **zhi mu** (Rhizoma Anemarrhenae Asphodeloides) 知母 12g.

Patent medicines

Long Dan Xie Gan Wan 龙胆泻肝丸 (Long Dan Xie Gan Wan)
Ming Mu Shang Qing Pian 明目上清片 (Ming Mu Shang Ching Pien)
Chuan Xin Lian Kang Yan Pian 穿心连抗炎片
   (Chuan Xin Lian Antiphlogistic Pills)
Yun Nan Bai Yao 云南白药 (Yunnan Paiyao)
   - this medicine can be taken in addition to the main formula selected. The red pill that accompanies the powder is only used in severe cases.

Acupuncture

Liv.2 (*xing jian* -), Sp.6 (*san yin jiao* -), Sp.10 (*xue hai* -), Ren.3 (*zhong ji* -), Bl.28 (*pang guang shu* -), GB.34 (*yang ling quan* -), Liv.8 (*qu quan* -), SJ.6 (*zhi gou* -), Liv.1 (*da dun* ↓)

Clinical notes

- Biomedical conditions that may present as Liver Fire type haematuria include urinary tract infection, pyelonephritis, gonorrhoeal urethritis, prostatitis, Reiter's syndrom and Behçet's syndrome.
- Treatment with acupuncture and herbs is usually effective at clearing Liver Heat or Fire, however stress resolution or behavioural modification will be necessary for enduring results.
- Heart and Liver Fire often overlap.

16.4 BLOOD STAGNATION

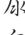

Pathophysiology
- Blood stagnation type haematuria may follow a trauma to the groin, lower back or pelvis, and warrants thorough investigation. Chronic *qi* deficiency, *qi* stagnation, Damp Heat, Cold accumulation or *yin* deficiency can all lead to stagnant Blood.
- Stagnant Blood is a physical obstruction that blocks Blood circulation. Blood behind the obstruction is forced from the vessels and causes bleeding into the Bladder.

Clinical features
- intermittent haematuria with dark or browny red blood and clots; there may be difficult urination or periodic obstruction to the passage of urine
- lower back pain and suprapubic distension and pain, which tends to be worse at night; if there is pain, it is stabbing and fixed
- dark complexion
- dark rings under the eyes
- there may be lower abdominal masses
- thin purple vessels (spider naevi) on the inner ankle and knee

T darkish, purplish or with purplish or brown spots and a thin coat; sublingual vessels are distended and dark

P choppy or wiry

Treatment principle
Transform and expel stagnant Blood
Stop bleeding

Prescription

SHAO FU ZHU YU TANG 少腹逐瘀汤
(*Drive Out Blood Stasis in the Lower Abdomen Decoction*) modified

chi shao (Radix Paeoniae Rubrae) 赤芍	25g
yan hu suo (Rhizoma Corydalis Yanhusuo) 延胡索	12g
tao ren (Semen Persicae) 桃仁	10g
hong hua (Flos Carthami Tinctorii) 红花	10g
pu huang (Pollen Typhae) 蒲黄	10g
wu ling zhi^ (Excrementum Trogopteri seu Pteromi) 五灵脂	10g
xiao hui xiang (Fructus Foeniculi Vulgaris) 小茴香	10g
hu po fen (powdered Succinum) 琥珀粉	3g
san qi fen (powdered Radix Notoginseng) 三七粉	3g

Method: Decoction. **Hu po fen** and **san qi fen** are added to the strained decoction (*chong fu* 冲服). (Source: *Zhong Yi Nei Ke Lin Chuang Shou Ce*)

Modifications

- With Cold (cold sensations or the abdomen feels cold to the touch), add **gui zhi** (Ramulus Cinnamomi Cassiae) 桂枝 6g, **pao jiang** (roasted Rhizoma Zingiberis Offinalis) 炮姜 6g and **ai ye tan*** (charred Folium Artemisiae Argyi) 艾叶炭 3g.
- With Heat (yellow tongue coat, warm feelings in the lower abdomen, strong smelling urine and thirst), add **sheng di** (Radix Rehmanniae Glutinosae) 生地 30g and **mu dan pi** (Cortex Moutan Radicis) 牡丹皮 9g.
- With lower abdominal masses, add **mu li**^ (Concha Ostreae) 牡蛎 15g, **xia ku cao** (Spica Prunellae Vulgaris) 夏枯草 15g, **dan shen** (Radix Salviae Miltiorrhizae) 丹参 15g and **e zhu** (Rhizoma Curcumae Ezhu) 莪术 9g.

QIAN GEN SAN 茜根散
(*Rubia Decoction*) modified

This formula is suitable for milder cases of Blood stagnation complicated by Heat, *yin* deficiency and Phlegm.

gua lou (Fructus Trichosanthis) 栝楼	15g
sheng di (Radix Rehmanniae Glutinosae) 生地	15g
qian cao gen (Radix Rubiae Cordifoliae) 茜草根	9g
e jiao^ (Gelatinum Corii Asini) 阿胶	9g
dang gui (Radix Angelicae Sinensis) 当归	9g
zhe bei mu (Bulbus Fritillariae Thunbergii) 浙贝母	9g
hong hua (Flos Carthami Tinctorii) 红花	9g
pu huang (Pollen Typhae) 蒲黄	9g
yu jin (Tuber Curcumae) 郁金	9g
ce bai ye (Cacumen Biotae Orientalis) 侧柏叶	6g
hu po fen (powdered Succinum) 琥珀粉	3g
san qi fen (powdered Radix Notoginseng) 三七粉	3g
gan cao (Radix Glycyrrhizae Uralensis) 甘草	3g

Method: Decoction. **Hu po fen** and **san qi fen** are added to the strained decoction (*chong fu* 冲服). (Source: *Shi Yong Zhong Yi Nei Ke Xue*)

Variations and additional prescriptions

With qi *deficiency*

- In the elderly or those with very weak *qi*, stagnant Blood may arise because there is insufficient motive force for good circulation–Blood slows and pools. The correct treatment in this case is not simply to disperse Blood stasis–this approach would likely aggravate the condition. Intead, tonifying *qi* to move and hold Blood is appropriate. This can be achieved using **BU ZHONG YI QI TANG** (*Ginseng and Astragalus Combination* 补中益气汤, p.394) plus **san qi** (Radix Notoginseng) 三七.

Patent medicines

Yun Nan Bai Yao 云南白药 (Yunnan Paiyao)
 - this medicine can be taken in addition to the main formula selected. The red pill that accompanies the powder is only used in severe cases.

Sheng Tian Qi Pian 生田七片 (Raw Tian Qi Ginseng Tablets)

Xue Fu Zhu Yu Wan 血府逐瘀丸 (Xue Fu Zhu Yu Wan)

Tong Jing Wan 痛经丸 (Tong Jing Wan)

Tao He Cheng Qi San 桃核承气散 (Persica and Rhubarb Formula)
 - severe Blood stagnation

Jin Gu Die Shang Wan 筋骨跌伤丸 (Chin Koo Tieh Shang Wan)
 - Blood stasis from trauma

Acupuncture

Bl.28 (*pang guang shu* -), St.30 (*qi chong* -), St.29 (*gui lai* -), Bl.34 (*xia liao* -), Bl.32 (*ci liao* -), Sp.10 (*xue hai* -), SJ.6 (*zhi gou* -), St.40 (*feng long* -), Liv.3 (*tai chong* -), SI.4 (*wan gu* -)

Clinical notes

- Biomedical conditions that may present as Blood stagnation type haematuria include bladder cancer, prostate cancer and trauma.
- Other than in the cases of minor trauma with shortlived haematuria, patients presenting with this pattern should be assumed to have a potentially dangerous condition and referred accordingly for appropriate investigations.
- Probably difficult to treat, depending on the underlying cause. Tumours of the genitourinary tract should be treated with a combination of Western medicine and TCM. Bleeding as a result of trauma usually responds quickly to treatment.

16.5 KIDNEY *YIN* DEFICIENCY WITH HEAT (FIRE)

肾阴虚火旺尿血

Pathophysiology
- Like the other Heat patterns, the Heat generated by deficiency quickens the Blood and damages the *luo* vessels. However, the Heat here is the product of a deficient pattern and consequently is less intense and more prolonged.

Clinical features
- episodic haematuria with fresh red blood. The urine may be concentrated
- soreness or weakness of the lower back and knees, heel pain
- sensations of heat in the palms and soles ('five hearts hot')
- dry mouth and throat
- irritability and restlessness
- insomnia
- facial flushing, malar flush
- afternoon fever, bone steaming fever, nightsweats
- dizziness
- tinnitus
- tendency to dry stools or constipation

T red and dry with little or no coat
P thready and rapid

Treatment principle
Nourish Kidney *yin* and clear Fire
Cool the Blood and stop bleeding

Prescription

ZHI BAI BA WEI WAN 知柏八味丸
(*Anemarrhena, Phellodendron and Rehmannia Formula*) modified

zhi mu (Rhizoma Anemarrhenae Asphodeloidis) 知母	10g
huang bai (Cortex Phellodendri) 黄柏	10g
sheng di (Radix Rehmanniae Glutinosae) 生地	30g
shan yao (Radix Dioscoreae Oppositae) 山药	25g
shan zhu yu (Fructus Corni Officinalis) 山茱萸	15g
mu dan pi (Cortex Moutan Radicis) 牡丹皮	10g
xiao ji (Herba Cephalanoplos) 小蓟	20g
da ji (Herba seu Radix Cirsii Japonici) 大蓟	20g
ou jie (Nodus Nelumbinis Nuciferae Rhizomatis) 藕节	15g
han lian cao (Herba Ecliptae Prostratae) 旱莲草	20g
bai mao gen (Rhizoma Imperatae Cylindricae) 白茅根	30g
xian he cao (Herba Agrimoniae Pilosae) 仙鹤草	20g
gan cao (Radix Glycyrrhizae Uralensis) 甘草	6g

Method: Decoction. (Source: *Zhong Yi Nei Ke Lin Chuang Shou Ce*)

Modifications
- With low grade fever, afternoon fever or bone steaming fever, add **bie jia°** (Carapax Amydae Sinensis) 鳖甲 12g, **yin chai hu** (Radix Stellariae Dichotomae) 银柴胡 9g and **di gu pi** (Cortex Lycii Chinensis) 地骨皮 12g.
- With irritability and insomnia, add **suan zao ren** (Semen Zizyphi Spinosae) 酸枣仁 12g, **yuan zhi** (Radix Polygalae Tenuifoliae) 远志 9g and **ye jiao teng** (Caulis Polygoni Multiflori) 夜胶藤 12g.

Patent medicines
Zhi Bai Ba Wei Wan 知柏八味丸 (Zhi Bai Ba Wei Wan)
Liu Wei Di Huang Wan 六味地黄丸 (Liu Wei Di Huang Wan)
Yun Nan Bai Yao 云南白药 (Yunnan Paiyao)
  - this medicine can be taken in addition to the main formula selected. The red pill that accompanies the powder is only used in severe cases.

Acupuncture
Bl.23 (*shen shu* +), Kid.3 (*tai xi* +), Kid.2 (*ran gu* -), Kid.6 (*zhao hai* +), Lu.7 (*lie que* +), Ren.4 (*guan yuan* +), Bl.28 (*pang guang shu* +)

Clinical notes
- Biomedical conditions that may present as Blood stagnation type haematuria include bladder cancer, prostatic cancer and post menopausal urethral atrophy.
- Tumours of the genitourinary tract should be treated with a combination of Western medicine and TCM.
- Recurrent urinary tract infections and pelvic inflammatory disease can predispose individuals to this pattern.

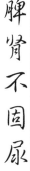

16.6 SPLEEN AND KIDNEY *YANG* (*QI*) DEFICIENCY

Pathophysiology
- When the Spleen is weak, it can fail in its function of holding Blood inside the vessels, thus allowing leakage of Blood into the Bladder. In addition, the Kidney deficiency, by providing insufficient physiological Heat to transform fluids, gives rise to the frequency and increased volume of urine.
- The urine is pale red or pink due to mixing of Blood with Dampness derived from the Spleen deficiency and from the dilution due to the volume of urine.

Clinical features
- frequent, copious pale red or pink urine
- poor appetite
- loose stools or diarrhoea with undigested food
- abdominal distension
- waxy pale or sallow complexion
- fatigue, lethargy, tiredness
- lower back and knee soreness and weakness
- cold intolerance and cold extremities
- dizziness and tinnitus
- easy bruising, bleeding haemorrhoids, melaena, uterine bleeding

T pale with a thin white coat
P deficient and weak

Treatment principle
Strengthen the Spleen, benefit *qi* to hold Blood
Tonify and consolidate Kidney *yang qi*

Prescription

BU ZHONG YI QI TANG 补中益气汤
(*Ginseng and Astragalus Combination*) plus
WU BI SHAN YAO WAN 无比山药丸
(*Incomparable Dioscorea Pill*) modified

huang qi (Radix Astragali Membranacei) 黄芪	30g
shan yao (Radix Dioscoreae Oppositae) 山药	30g
shu di (Radix Rehmanniae Glutinosae Conquitae) 熟地	20g
tu si zi (Semen Cuscutae Chinensis) 菟丝子	20g
dang shen (Radix Codonopsis Pilosulae) 党参	15g
shan zhu yu (Fructus Corni Officinalis) 山茱萸	15g
rou cong rong (Herba Cistanches Deserticolae) 肉苁蓉	15g

chao du zhong (dry fried Cortex Eucommiae Ulmoidis)
炒杜仲 15g
bai zhu (Rhizoma Atractylodes Macrocephalae) 白术 12g
ba ji tian (Radix Morindae Officinalis) 巴戟天 10g
ou jie (Nodus Nelumbinis Nuciferae Rhizomatis) 藕节 10g
sheng ma (Rhizoma Cimicifugae) 升麻 6g
pao jiang (roasted Rhizoma Zingiberis Offinalis) 炮姜 6g
zhi gan cao (honey fried Radix Glycyrrhizae Uralensis)
炙甘草 6g

Method: Decoction. (Source: *Zhong Yi Nei Ke Lin Chuang Shou Ce*)

Modifications
- If the bleeding is persistent, add some astringent herbs, such as **mu li^** (Concha Ostreae) 牡蛎 15g, **long gu^** (Os Draconis) 龙骨 10g and **jin ying zi** (Fructus Rosae Laevigatae) 金樱子 10g.
- With *yang* deficiency and Cold, add **zhi fu zi*** (Radix Aconiti Carmichaeli Praeparata) 制附子 6g and **rou gui** (Cortex Cinnamomi Cassiae) 肉桂 3g.

Follow up treatment
- Once the bleeding has stopped, a suitable formula to tonify Spleen and/or Kidney *yang* should be selected. For Kidney *yang* or *qi* deficiency, **JIN KUI SHEN QI WAN** (*Rehmannia Eight Formula* 金匮肾气丸, p.150) is suitable; for Spleen *yang* deficiency **FU ZI LI ZHONG WAN** (*Aconite, Ginseng and Ginger Formula* 附子理中丸, p.56). Combine the two formulae for mixtures of Spleen and Kidney deficiency.

Patent medicines
Jin Kui Shen Qi Wan 金匮肾气丸 (Sexoton Pills)
Ba Ji Yin Yang Wan 巴戟阴阳丸 (Ba Ji Yin Yang Wan)
Bu Zhong Yi Qi Wan 补中益气丸 (Bu Zhong Yi Qi Wan)
   - Spleen *qi* deficiency
Fu Zi Li Zhong Wan 附子理中丸 (Li Chung Yuen Medical Pills)
   - Spleen *yang* deficiency
Yun Nan Bai Yao 云南白药 (Yunnan Paiyao)
   - this medicine can be taken in addition to the main formula. The red pill that accompanies the powder is only used in severe cases.

Acupuncture
Bl.23 (*shen shu* +▲), Bl.20 (*pi shu* +▲), Bl.17 (*ge shu*), Ren.4 (*guan yuan* ▲), St.36 (*zu san li* +), Sp.6 (*san yin jiao* +), Du.4 (*ming men* ▲), Sp.10 (*xue hai*), Sp.1 (*yin bai* ▲)

Clinical notes

- Biomedical conditions that may present as Spleen and Kidney *yang* deficiency type haematuria include thrombocytopoenia and haemophilia.
- While treatment with herbs and acupuncture may not cure the disease with which the haematuria is associated (for example haemophillia), the bleeding can be effecively controlled.

SUMMARY OF GUIDING FORMULAE FOR HAEMATURIA

Damp Heat - *Xiao Ji Yin Zi* 小蓟饮子
- with Toxic Heat - *Huang Lian Jie Du Tang* 黄连解毒汤

Heart Fire - *Dao Chi San* 导赤散 plus *Xiao Ji Yin Zi* 小蓟饮子

Liver Fire - *Long Dan Xie Gan Tang* 龙胆泻肝汤

Blood stagnation - *Shao Fu Zhu Yu Tang* 少腹逐瘀汤
- with *yin* deficiency - *Qian Gen San* 茜根散
- from *qi* deficiency - *Bu Zhong Yi Qi Tang* 补中益气汤

Kidney *yin* deficiency - *Zhi Bai Ba Wei Wan* 知柏八味丸

Spleen and Kidney *yang qi* deficiency
- *Bu Zhong Yi Qi Tang* 补中益气汤 plus *Wu Bi Shan Yao Wan* 无比山药丸

Endnote

For more information regarding herbs marked with an asterisk*, an open circle° or a hatˆ, see the tables on pp.944-952.

Disorders of the Kidney

17. Impotence

Excess patterns
Liver *qi* stagnation
Damp Heat

Deficient patterns
Kidney *yang* deficiency
Kidney *yin* deficiency
Heart Blood and Spleen *qi* deficiency
Heart and Gall Bladder *qi* deficiency

Appendix – Nocturnal Seminal Emission

17 | IMPOTENCE (Low Libido, Male Infertility)
yang wei 阳痿

Impotence is the inability to achieve erection, ejaculation or both. Men presenting with impotence may have any of a number of complaints; loss of libido, inability to initiate or sustain an erection, ejaculatory failure, inability to achieve orgasm or infertility.

Impotence is often associated with vascular disease and may be complicated by social and emotional factors, like overwork and consequent fatigue, anxiety and depression, disinterest in the sexual partner, fear of sexual incompetence, marital discord or guilt about unconventional sexual impulses.

This chapter can be used to analyse low libido or male infertility even where impotence is not a feature. Low libido and infertility in women are covered elsewhere in the handbook series.

AETIOLOGY

In TCM terms, the ability to get and sustain an erection (and reproduce) is primarily the responsibility of the Kidney and the Liver. Kidney *yang* controls the functional aspect of an erection and Kidney *jing* the ability to reproduce, while the Liver channel passes through the external genitals. Weakness of the Kidney reduces the physiological 'Fire of desire', while stagnation of Liver *qi* reduces the physical ability.

Male sexual function depends not only on sound physiological health but also on the psychological state. Thus, the emotional aspects of the Heart, Liver and Kidney systems can all influence sexual ability. Specifically, mental stress can obstruct the flow of Liver *qi*, which as noted above, can have a very direct and dismal affect on the functioning of the 'ancestral Tendon of the Liver' (as the penis is sometimes known). Anxiety and extremes of emotion, which destabilise the Heart and the *shen*, can also play havoc with the ability to achieve and maintain an erection.

Another TCM category of impotence is related to Kidney dysfunction from fear or shock. In this case, severe fright damages the *zhi* 志 (the aspect of consciousness associated with the Kidney) and the *shen* profoundly, such that timidity and nervousness become constant personality traits. Such traits do not lend themselves to confident and effective sexual encounters.

Damp Heat

The Damp Heat that causes impotence or male infertility is most commonly generated internally. In the Western world, Damp Heat type impotence is primarily a disorder of overconsumption of alcohol and rich foods. It may also be generated in the lower *jiao* by any long term Heat in the system, such as Heat generated by *yin* deficiency, *qi* stagnation or by prolonged stagnation of Dampness. In some cases it may be due to an unresolved or poorly treated external Damp Heat pathogen. In this case, the Damp Heat often lingers in the lower *jiao* as a low grade infection. Whether internal or external, impotence due to Damp Heat is a chronic disorder.

Liver *qi* stagnation

Frustration, anger, resentment, prolonged emotional turmoil and stress disrupt the circulation of Liver *qi*, and, because the Liver channel passes through the penis, insufficient *qi* arrives to enable an erection.

Kidney deficiency

Kidney deficiency is an important cause of impotence, loss of libido and male infertility and can involve either *jing*, *yang*, *yin* or a combination. It can be inherited or may develop as a result of overwork, age, chronic illness or excessive ejaculation.

> **BOX 17.1 SOME BIOMEDICAL CAUSES OF IMPOTENCE & LOSS OF LIBIDO**
>
> - loss of interest, boredom
> - elderly
> - excessive fatigue or stress
> - anxiety (fear of disease, performance)
> - vascular occlusion of the penis
> - diabetes
> - multiple sclerosis
> - debilitating disease
> - hyperprolactinaemia
> - hypogonadism
> - hypothyroidism
> - hypopituitarism
> - orchitis
> - prostatitis
> - spinal cord trauma/disease
>
> **Drugs**
> - anti-hypertensives
> - antipsychotics
> - antidepressants
> - sedatives
> - diuretics
> - steroids
> - alcohol
> - methadone
> - heroin
> - cannabis
> - tobacco

Kidney *yang* or *qi* is particularly affected by prolonged exposure to cold conditions, or excessive lifting or standing. In some cases, particularly in younger men, Kidney *qi* may be weakened while Kidney *yang* remains intact, in which case the cold symptoms are not seen.

Kidney *yin* is damaged through overwork (especially while under stress), late nights, shift work, insufficient sleep, febrile diseases, insufficient hydration and the use of some prescription, recreational and in this case, tonic drugs. Kidney *yin* deficiency type impotence is fairly common in young (in their 30s and 40s) men, who consume large quantities of hot natured *yang* tonic herbs like red ginseng and deer horn in order to increase sexual potency.

Spleen *qi* and Heart Blood deficiency

Overwork, physical and mental exhaustion, worry, irregular diet and too much raw or sweet food can damage the Spleen, which then fails to generate sufficient *qi* and Blood. Similarly, any situation that overwhelms the Spleen's ability to replace *qi* and Blood, like a prolonged or severe illness, can lead to *qi* and Blood deficiency. The primary weakness in this pattern is in the Spleen, which is unable to generate enough Blood to nourish the Heart and stabilise the *shen*. Instability of the *shen* can then be the basis of impotence with psychological components.

Heart and Gall Bladder *qi* deficiency

This pattern describes an anxious or timid personality type, traits that may be congenital or acquired. When congenital, it can be the result of a significant shock or prolonged fearful situation experienced by the mother during pregnancy, or weakness of the parental Kidney *jing*. When acquired, it is the result of some sudden and violent or extreme shock or fright. Other, more insidious events, like emotional or physical abuse or trauma during childhood, may contribute. It may also sometimes follow other debilitating illnesses that plunder *qi*. This pattern, too, underlies impotence of psychogenic origin.

17.1 LIVER *QI* STAGNATION

肝气郁滞阳痿

Pathophysiology
- This type of impotence or loss of libido is typically found in men stressed by overwork or facing the emotional conflicts of a midlife crisis. It is also seen in younger men or adolescents overwrought with sexual anxiety or frustration.

Clinical features
- inability to get or sustain an erection, loss of libido
- sensation of tightness or fullness in the chest (often described as difficulty in drawing a satisfying breath)
- hypochondriac discomfort or tightness
- vague aches and pains
- frequent sighing
- dizziness
- occasional fatigue (although patients often feel better for exercise)
- irritability or depression
- abdominal distension, flatulence
- alternating constipation and diarrhoea

T normal or dark (*qing* 青), maybe with red edges and yellow coat if there is Heat
P wiry

Treatment principle
Regulate and soothe Liver *qi*
Support *yang*

Prescription

XIAO YAO SAN 逍遥散
(*Bupleurum and Dang Gui Formula*) modified

chai hu (Radix Bupleuri) 柴胡	9g
dang gui (Radix Angelicae Sinensis) 当归	9g
bai shao (Radix Paeoniae Lactiflorae) 白芍	12g
bai zhu (Rhizoma Atractylodes Macrocephalae) 白术	9g
fu ling (Sclerotium Poria Cocos) 茯苓	12g
sheng jiang (Rhizoma Zingiberis Officinalis) 生姜	3pce
da zao (Fructus Zizyphi Jujubae) 大枣	3pce
du zhong (Cortex Eucommiae Ulmoidis) 杜仲	12g
tu si zi (Semen Cuscutae Chinensis) 菟丝子	12g

Method: Decoction. (Source: *Shi Yong Zhong Yi Nei Ke Xue*)

Modifications

- With Heat (red face, flushing, red eyes, a tongue with red edges and a yellow coat), add **mu dan pi** (Cortex Moutan Radicis) 牡丹皮 9g and **shan zhi zi** (Fructus Gardeniae Jasminoidis) 山栀子 9g.
- With depression or anxiety, add **he huan pi** (Cortex Albizziae Julibrissin) 合欢皮 9g and **suan zao ren** (Semen Zizyphi Spinosae) 酸枣仁 12g.
- With constipation and abdominal bloating, add **zhi shi** (Fructus Immaturus Citri Aurantii) 枳实 10g and **hou po** (Cortex Magnoliae Officinalis) 厚朴 10g.
- If the patient is robust, with severe irritability, restlessness or insomnia and palpitations, use **CHAI HU JIA LONG GU MU LI TANG** (*Bupleurum and Dragon Bone Combination* 柴胡加龙骨牡蛎汤 p.816).

Patent medicines

Chai Hu Shu Gan Wan 柴胡舒肝丸 (Chai Hu Shu Gan Wan)
Shu Gan Wan 舒肝丸 (Shu Gan Wan)
Mu Xiang Shun Qi Wan 木香顺气丸 (Aplotaxis Carminative Pills)
Xiao Yao Wan 逍遥丸 (Xiao Yao Wan)
  - the above formulae are all suitable for general Liver *qi* stasis
Kang Wei Ling 抗痿灵 (Kang Wei Ling)
  - powerfully invigorates *qi* and Blood. Usually given in short courses of several weeks at a time as an adjunct to other systemic treatment. This pill is suitable for excess types of impotence and works by opening up blood circulation to the penis.

Acupuncture

Ren.6 (*qi hai*), LI.4 (*he gu*), Liv.3 (*tai chong*), Liv.5 (*li gou*), Liv.14 (*qi men*), PC.6 (*nei guan*), Sp.6 (*san yin jiao*), Liv. 8 (*qu quan*)

Clinical notes

- Acupuncture is usually very effective at regulating Liver *qi* and calming the *shen*.
- Much of the impotence experienced in middle age and later is due to vascular disease. The most recent generation of impotence drugs work by preventing the breakdown of chemicals that dilate penile arteries, thus enhancing the strength and longevity of erections. They are effective in helping two out of three men achieve erections but do not improve libido or address the root of the problem. For men who do not wish to use the drugs, encouraging circulation of Liver *qi* (and hence blood) with acupuncture and herbs provides a good alternative.

17.2 DAMP HEAT

Pathophysiology
- Prolonged stagnation of Damp Heat in the lower *jiao* weakens and softens the Tendons (which include the penis as the 'ancestral Tendon of the Liver'), leading to impotence.
- This is most likely due to excessive consumption of alcohol or to a chronic infection like prostatitis. Chronic Damp Heat in the male reproductive tract can predispose to the formation of antisperm antibodies and impaired fertility.

Clinical features
- inability to get or maintain a full erection
- possibly excessive sweating around the scrotum and groin, and itching or pain in the genitals
- there may also be occasional mucopurulent discharge from the urethra, or a history of genital herpes
- loose stools or alternating constipation and diarrhoea
- concentrated urine
- heaviness and aching in the lower limbs
- lethargy, afternoon fatigue
- there may be a poor sperm count or low motility and antisperm antibodies; thick or congealed ejaculate with retarded liquification

T greasy yellow coat, especially over the root
P deep and slippery or soft and slippery, possibly rapid

Treatment principle
Clear Dampness and Heat

Prescription

ER MIAO SAN 二妙散
(*Two Marvel Powder*) modified

che qian zi (Semen Plantaginis) 车前子	30g
shi wei (Folium Pyrrosiae) 石苇	30g
fu ling (Sclerotium Poria Cocos) 茯苓	30g
shan yao (Radix Dioscoreae Oppositae) 山药	30g
gou qi zi (Fructus Lycii) 枸杞子	20g
ze xie (Rhizoma Alismatis Orientalis) 泽泻	15g
bi xie (Rhizoma Dioscoreae Hypoglaucae) 萆解	15g
cang zhu (Rhizoma Atractylodis) 苍术	12g
zhu ling (Sclerotium Polypori Umbellati) 猪苓	12g
yan huang bai (salt fried Cortex Phellodendri) 盐黄柏	10g

yan zhi mu (salt fried Rhizoma Anemarrhenae Asphodeloidis)
盐知母 10g
gan cao (Radix Glycyrrhizae Uralensis) 甘草 6g
Method: Decoction. **Che qian zi** is decocoted in a muslin bag (*bao jian* 包煎).
(Source: *Zhong Yi Nei Ke Lin Chuang Shou Ce*)

Modifications
- If Liver Heat or Fire complicates the Damp Heat, with hypochondriac fullness and discomfort, headaches, red sore eyes, irritability and a wiry pulse, add **long dan cao** (Radix Gentianae Longdancao) 龙胆草 9g and **chai hu** (Radix Bupleuri) 柴胡 9g, or use **LONG DAN XIE GAN TANG** (*Gentiana Combination* 龙胆泻肝汤, p.500).
- With antisperm antibodies, add Blood regulating herbs, such as **dan shen** (Radix Salviae Miltiorrhizae) 丹参 15g, **tao ren** (Semen Persicae) 桃仁 9g or **hong hua** (Flos Carthami Tinctorii) 红花 6g.
- In men with prostatic swelling, add two or three herbs to 'soften hardness and disperse swelling' from the following list: **xia ku cao** (Spica Prunellae Vulgaris) 夏枯草 15g, **mu li**ˆ (Concha Ostreae) 牡蛎 15g, **zhe bei mu** (Bulbus Fritillariae Thunbergii) 浙贝母 9g, **xuan shen** (Radix Scrophulariae) 玄参 15g, **chuan shan jia**° (Squama Manitis) 穿山甲 12g, **wa leng zi**ˆ (Concha Arcae) 瓦楞子 12g, **wang bu liu xing** (semen Vaccariae Segetalis) 王不留行 9g.

Variations and additional prescriptions
- For patients with low fertility, once the Damp Heat is cleared herbs are often prescribed to increase sperm count and motility (see Kidney patterns following).

Patent medicines
Long Dan Xie Gan Wan 龙胆泻肝丸 (Long Dan Xie Gan Wan)
Qian Lie Xian Wan 前列腺丸 (Prostate Gland Pills)
Chuan Xin Lian Kang Yan Pian 穿心连抗炎片
   (Chuan Xin Lian Antiphlogistic Tablets)
Kang Wei Ling 抗痿灵 (Kang Wei Ling)
- see p.484

Acupuncture
Ren.3 (*zhong ji*), Sp.9 (*yin ling quan* -), Liv.5 (*li gou* -), St.30 (*qi chong*), GB.26 (*dai mai* -), GB.41 (*zu lin qi* -), Kid.10 (*yin gu*), SJ.6 (*zhi gou* -), Bl.32 (*ci liao* -)

Clinical notes

- Biomedical conditions that may present as Damp Heat type impotence include acute and chronic prostatitis, excessive alcohol consumption and other genital infections.
- While modern drug therapy claims good success in increasing the ability to achieve erections it does nothing to address underlying causes. Damp Heat, causing inflammation or infection in the prostate, urethra or testicles, can be effectively treated with herbs. Treatment should persist until all signs of Damp Heat have cleared (especially the tongue coat).
- Infertility in this category is amenable to treatment, although successful results are often achieved more readily where antisperm antibodies are not present
- Dietary changes and limiting alcohol intake are strongly advised.
- In some cases antibiotic or antifungal drug therapy may be needed in addition to Damp Heat dispersing TCM treatment.

17.3 KIDNEY *YANG* DEFICIENCY

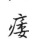

Pathophysiology
- According to TCM, Kidney *yang* is the basis of sexual desire. Kidney *yang* also plays a pivotal role in the mechanics of getting and sustaining an erection. Male infertility frequently falls into this category, sometimes with few of the below mentioned accompanying symptoms.

Clinical features
- low libido, an inability to get an erection or sustain an erection, infertility
- low sperm motility and sperm count, thin watery ejaculate
- waxy pale complexion
- listlessness and fatigue
- cold intolerance, aversion to cold, cold extremities
- urinary frequency, nocturia or oedema of the lower limbs with scanty urine
- lower abdominal distension
- constipation or loose stools
- weak, cold and sore lower back and knees

T pale, wet and swollen
P deep and thready or slow and weak, particularly in the proximal positions

Treatment principle
Tonify the Kidneys, warm and support *yang*

Prescription

WU ZI YAN ZONG WAN 五子衍宗丸
(*Five Seed Ancestral Qi Amplifying Pill*) plus
ZAN YU DAN 赞育丹
(*Special Pill to Aid Fertility*) modified

shu di (Radix Rehmanniae Glutinosae Conquitae) 熟地	240g
gou qi zi (Fructus Lycii) 枸杞子	240g
tu si zi (Semen Cuscutae Chinensis) 菟丝子	240g
chao du zhong (dry fried Cortex Eucommiae Ulmoidis) 炒杜仲	120g
fu pen zi (Fructus Rubi Chingii) 覆盆子	120g
ba ji tian (Radix Morindae Officinalis) 巴戟天	120g
xian ling pi (Herba Epimedii) 仙灵脾	120g
xian mao (Rhizoma Curculiginis Orchioidis) 仙茅	120g
rou gui (Cortex Cinnamomi Cassiae) 肉桂	60g
zhi fu zi* (Radix Aconiti Carmichaeli Praeparata) 制附子	60g
wu wei zi (Fructus Schizandrae Chinensis) 五味子	30g

lu rong^ (Cornu Cervi Parvum) 鹿茸 30g
zhi gan cao (honey fried Radix Glycyrrhizae Uralensis)
炙甘草 30g

Method: Grind the herbs into powder and form into 9-gram pills with honey. The dose is one pill 2-3 times daily. May also be decocted with a 90% reduction in dosage. When decocted, **zhi fu zi** is cooked for 30 minutes prior to the other herbs (*xian jian* 先煎), **lu rong** is taken separately or added to the strained decoction (*chong fu* 冲服). **Lu jiao jiao^** (Cornu Cervi Gelatinum) 鹿角胶 may be substituted for **lu rong** with a fourfold increase in dosage.

Patent medicines

Jin Kui Shen Qi Wan 金匮肾气丸 (Sexoton Pills)
Nan Bao 男宝 (Nan Bao Capsules)
Ba Ji Yin Yang Wan 巴戟阴阳丸 (Ba Ji Yin Yang Wan)
Cong Rong Bu Shen Wan 从容补肾丸 (Cong Rong Bu Shen Wan)
Wu Zi Yan Zong Wan 五子衍宗丸 (Wu Zi Yan Zong Wan)

Acupuncture

Bl.23 (*shen shu* +▲), Du.4 (*ming men* +▲), Ren.4 (*guan yuan* +▲), Sp.6 (*san yin jiao* +), Du.20 (*bai hui* ▲), Lu.7 (*lie que* +), Kid.7 (*fu liu* +). Needle sensation (*de qi*) on Ren.4 (*guan yuan*) should go to the tip of the penis. This can be achieved by needling 1½ cun deep angled inferiorly. Make sure the bladder is empty first.

Clinical notes

- Biomedical conditions that may present as Kidney *yang* deficiency type impotence include hypothyroidism, infertility, low sperm count, general debility and ageing.
- Persistent treatment will usually get satisfactory results in this pattern. Sometimes success is measured by the ability to impregnate a partner rather than the return of a rampant libido. During the first 2 or 3 months of treatment the patient should be advised to minimise or avoid ejaculation altogether. Modern drug therapy can be used in these patients to achieve erection, but an increase in fertility or return of libido will only be acheived by strengthening Kidney *yang*. Conditions like hypothyroidism can be difficult and may require a combination of Western medicine and TCM.

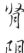
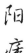

17.4 KIDNEY *YIN* DEFICIENCY

Pathophysiology
- Deficiency of Kidney *yin* generates Heat. This false Heat can create the appearance of sexual desire but because the Kidneys are actually weak, the ability to sustain sexual activity is reduced. Increasingly, depletion of Kidney *yin* is becoming a major cause of infertility in overworked men.

Clinical features
- Impotence or premature ejaculation, which is worse when the patient is stressed and fatigued. There may be frequent desire for sex but an inability to initiate or maintain an erection, or there may be erotic dreams with spontaneous emission.
- there may be increased numbers of abnormal sperm or low sperm count, scanty ejaculate
- soreness or weakness of the lower back and knees (which may be exacerbated by sex), heel pain
- dry mouth and throat
- insomnia, restlessness
- facial flushing, malar flush, nightsweats
- sensations of heat in the palms and soles ('five hearts hot')
- dizziness and tinnitus, more noticable after sex
- tendency to dry stools or constipation

T red and dry with little or no coat
P thready and rapid

Treatment principle
Nourish and strengthen Kidney *yin*

Prescription

LIU WEI DI HUANG WAN 六味地黄丸
(*Rehmannia Six Formula*) modified

shu di (Radix Rehmanniae Glutinosae Conquitae) 熟地	240g
shan zhu yu (Fructus Corni Officinalis) 山茱萸	120g
shan yao (Radix Dioscoreae Oppositae) 山药	120g
fu ling (Sclerotium Poria Cocos) 茯苓	90g
mu dan pi (Cortex Moutan Radicis) 牡丹皮	90g
ze xie (Rhizoma Alismatis Orientalis) 泽泻	90g
tu si zi (Semen Cuscutae Chinensis) 菟丝子	90g

Method: Grind herbs to powder and form into 9-gram pills with honey. The dose is one pill 2-3 times daily. May also be decocted with a dosage with a 90% reduction in dosage. (Source: *Shi Yong Zhong Yi Nei Ke Xue*)

Modifications

- With more severe Heat, add **zhi mu** (Rhizoma Anemarrhenae Asphodeloidis) 知母 60g and **huang bai** (Cortex Phellodendri) 黄柏 60g.
- With *yang* deficiency as well (pink or flabby tongue, aversion to cold, skin and extremities warm but feels cold inside), add **xian ling pi** (Herba Epimedii) 仙灵脾 60g and **ba ji tian** (Radix Morindae Officinalis) 巴戟天 60g.
- With night sweats, add **mu li**° (Concha Ostreae) 牡蛎 90g, **ma huang gen** (Radix Ephedra) 麻黄根 90g and **wu wei zi** (Fructus Schizandrae Chinensis) 五味子 40g.
- With restlessness and insomnia, add **long chi**° (Dens Draconis) 龙齿 90g and **suan zao ren** (Semen Zizyphi Spinosae) 酸枣仁 90g.
- With increased number of abnormal sperm, add **dan shen** (Radix Salviae Miltiorrhizae) 丹参 90g and **tao ren** (Semen Persicae) 桃仁 90g.
- For low sperm count, add **gou qi zi** (Fructus Lycii) 枸杞子 150g, **nu zhen zi** (Fructus Ligustri Lucidi) 女贞子 120g, **tu si zi** (Semen Cuscutae Chinensis) 菟丝子 180g, **wu wei zi** (Fructus Schizandrae Chinensis) 五味子 60 g, **he shou wu** (Radix Polygoni Multiflori) 何首乌 150g and **dang gui** (Radix Angelicae Sinensis) 当归 90g.
- For excessive sexual desire, add **gui ban**° (Plastri Testudinis) 龟板 90g, **mu li**° (Concha Ostreae) 牡蛎 150g and **bai zi ren** (Semen Biotae Orientalis) 柏子仁 150g.

Patent medicines

Liu Wei Di Huang Wan 六味地黄丸 (Liu Wei Di Huang Wan)
Tian Wang Bu Xin Dan 天王补心丹 (Tian Wang Bu Xin Dan)
   - Heart and Kidney *yin* deficiency
Zhi Bai Ba Wei Wan 知柏八味丸 (Zhi Bai Ba Wei Wan)
   - with more *yin* deficient Heat
Wu Zi Yan Zong Wan 五子衍宗丸 (Wu Zi Yan Zong Wan)

Acupuncture

Ren.4 (*guan yuan* +), Ht.6 (*yin xi* +), Kid.6 (*zhao hai* +), Bl.23 (*shen shu* +), Sp.6 (*san yin jiao* +), Ren.7 (*yin jiao*).
Needle sensation (*de qi*) on Ren.4 (*guan yuan*) should go to the tip of the penis. This can be achieved by needling 1½ *cun* deep angled inferiorly. Make sure the bladder is empty first.
   - with night sweats add SI.3 (*hou xi*)
   - with Heat add Kid.2 (*ran gu* -), Ht.8 (*shao fu* -), Du.4 (*ming men* -)

Clinical notes

- This pattern can be constitutional or a complication of chronic Liver *qi* stagnation that generates Heat, or lingering Damp Heat, both of

which may consume *yin*. It may develop in men who work long hours under significant pressure, or in men who have (or have a history of) excessive sexual activity or drug abuse. Marijuana and cocaine are particularly dangerous to Kidney *yin* and are implicated in infertility.
- As with all *yin* deficiency patterns, treatment needs to persist for months. Sexual activity, including masturbation, should be avoided or limited.
- Drugs that enable impotent men to have erections can prove counterproductive for men in this category. The excessive sexual desire they experience combined with the drug assisted ability to have frequent sexual intercourse can lead to further exhaustion of *yin*.
- Men who have had vasectomies reversed will benefit from taking herbs to increase the number of sperm and the percentage of these that are morphologically normal and have good motility. Where there are antisperm antibodies (not uncommon after a vasectomy) or a high proportion of abnormal forms, Blood regulating herbs are important, particularly **dan shen** (Radix Salviae Miltiorrhizae) 丹参, **tao ren** (Semen Persicae) 桃仁 and **hong hua** (Flos Carthami Tinctorii) 红». Other mild Blood movers are also suitable depending on the patient, for example **yu jin** (Tuber Curcumae) 郁金 with a tendency to Liver *qi* stagnation, **huai niu xi** (Radix Achyranthis Bidentatae) 怀牛膝 with rising *yang* etc. These should be combined with herbs to tonify Kidney *yin* or *yang* depending on the constitution (see also previous pattern).

17.5 HEART BLOOD AND SPLEEN *QI* DEFICIENCY

Pathophysiology
- In this pattern, there are two causes of impotence. The first is instability of the *shen* from Heart Blood deficiency–the weakened or scattered *shen* cannot lead *qi* to the penis, or if an erection occurs it can be easily lost. The second is simple insufficiency of *qi* and Blood to fill the penis.

Clinical features
- inability to get or maintain an erection, possibly associated with performance anxiety
- the impotence may also be worse with fatigue. These patients may be able to get erections during sleep or masturbation
- pale, lustreless complexion
- fatigue and low spirits
- abdominal distension, poor appetite
- insomnia, dream disturbed sleep
- palpitations with or without anxiety
- panic attacks, nervousness
- forgetfulness
- clammy palms

T pale with a thin white coat
P thready and weak

Treatment principle
Tonify and nourish Heart and Spleen
Support *yang*

Prescription

GUI PI TANG 归脾汤
(*Ginseng and Longan Combination*) modified

zhi huang qi (honey fried Radix Astragali Membranacei) 炙黄芪	15g
dang shen (Radix Codonopsis Pilosulae) 党参	12g
dang gui (Radix Angelicae Sinensis) 当归	9g
suan zao ren (Semen Zizyphi Spinosae) 酸枣仁	9g
yuan zhi (honey fried Radix Polygalae Tenuifoliae) 炙远志	6g
fu ling (Sclerotium Poria Cocos) 茯苓	9g
bai zhu (Rhizoma Atractylodes Macrocephalae) 白术	9g
long yan rou (Arillus Euphoriae Longanae) 龙眼肉	9g
mu xiang (Radix Aucklandiae Lappae) 木香	6g

zhi gan cao (honey fried Radix Glycyrrhizae Uralensis)
炙甘草 6g
shu di (Radix Rehmanniae Glutinosae Conquitae) 熟地 12g
du zhong (Cortex Eucommiae Ulmoidis) 杜仲 12g
gou qi zi (Fructus Lycii) 枸杞子 12g
shan zhu yu (Fructus Corni Officinalis) 山茱萸 12g
Method: Decoction. (Source: *Shi Yong Zhong Yi Nei Ke Xue*)

Patent medicines
Gui Pi Wan 归脾丸 (Gui Pi Wan)
Bai Zi Yang Xin Wan 柏子养心丸 (Bai Zi Yang Xin Wan)
Bu Nao Wan 补脑丸 (Cerebral Tonic Pills)
Yang Xin Ning Shen Wan 养心宁神丸 (Ning San Yuen Medical Pills)
Wu Zi Yan Zong Wan 五子衍宗丸 (Wu Zi Yan Zong Wan)

Acupuncture
Ren.4 (*guan yuan* +), Bl.15 (*xin shu* +), Bl.20 (*pi shu* +), Bl.23 (*shen shu* +), Ht.7 (*shen men* +), Ren.6 (*qi hai* +), Sp.6 (*san yin jiao* +), St.36 (*zu san li* +), *yin tang* (M-HN-3), Du.19 (*hou ding*), Du. 24 (*shen ting*).
Needle sensation (*de qi*) on Ren.4 (*guan yuan*) should go to the tip of the penis. This can be achieved by needling 1½ *cun* deep angled inferiorly. Make sure the bladder is empty first.
- with significant anxiety, add *yin tang* (M-HN-3)
- for insomnia, add *an mian* (M-HN-54)
- with abdominal distension, add St.25 (*tian shu*)

Clinical notes
- Biomedical conditions that may present as Heart Blood and Spleen *qi* deficiency type impotence include neuresthenia, chronic fatigue syndrome, convalescent stage of severe illness, anaemia and anxiety neurosis.
- If the psychological component is not exceedingly complex, this type of impotence will improve with treatment, although this may need to continue for several months until the reserve of *qi* and Blood is restored. Patients should be advised to avoid sexual relationships during the early stages of the treatment.

17.6 HEART AND GALL BLADDER *QI* DEFICIENCY

Pathophysiology
- Heart and Gall Bladder *qi* deficiency is also sometimes called 'fear and shock injuring Kidney *qi*' (the Chinese charaters to the left), because it can reflect profound damage to the *shen* and Kidney *zhi* manifesting as a chronically timid and disturbed personality. Such psychological imbalance can manifest in numerous ways, sexual dysfunction being one of them.
- As in the previous pattern (Heart and Spleen deficiency) the *shen* is unstable and easily scattered. The *shen* is unable to lead *qi* to the penis, or is unable to remain firm and thus easily scattered once there.

Clinical features
- inablity to get or maintain an erection
- the patient is anxious, timid, shy, easily startled and may appear very nervous, and may be very uneasy about intimate relationships
- palpitations
- insomnia

T thin greasy coat
P wiry and thready

Treatment principle
Benefit the Heart, Gall Bladder and Kidney, calm the *shen*
Support *yang*

Prescription

QI YANG YU XIN DAN 启阳娱心丹
(Arouse yang, Please the Heart Special Pill)

suan zao ren (Semen Zizyphi Spinosae) 酸枣仁	18g
fu shen (Sclerotium Poriae Cocos Pararadicis) 茯神	12g
bai shao (Radix Paeoniae Lactiflorae) 白芍	12g
tu si zi (Semen Cuscutae Chinensis) 菟丝子	12g
shen qu (Massa Fermenta) 神曲	9g
chai hu (Radix Bupleuri) 柴胡	9g
dang gui (Radix Angelicae Sinensis) 当归	9g
bai zhu (Rhizoma Atractylodes Macrocephalae) 白术	9g
ren shen (Radix Ginseng) 人参	6g
yuan zhi (Radix Polygalae Tenuifoliae) 远志	6g
shi chang pu (Rhizoma Acori Graminei) 石菖蒲	6g
chen pi (Pericarpium Citri Reticulatae) 陈皮	6g
sha ren (Fructus Amomi) 砂仁	6g
zhi gan cao (honey fried Radix Glycyrrhizae Uralensis)	

炙甘草 6g

Method: Grind herbs to powder and form into 9-gram pills with honey. The dose is one pill 2-3 times daily. May also be decocted, in which case **sha ren** is added towards the end of cooking (*hou xia* 后下). (Source: *Shi Yong Zhong Yi Nei Ke Xue*)

Patent medicines
Bu Nao Wan 补脑丸 (Cerebral Tonic Pills)
Gui Pi Wan 归脾丸 (Gui Pi Wan)
Bai Zi Yang Xin Wan 柏子养心丸 (Bai Zi Yang Xin Wan)
Yang Xin Ning Shen Wan 养心宁神丸 (Ning San Yuen Medical Pills)

Acupuncture
Bl.18 (*gan shu* +), Bl.19 (*dan shu* +), GB.34 (*yang ling quan* +),
Ren.4 (*guan yuan* +), Ren.6 (*qi hai* +), Liv.3 (*tai chong* -), Kid.4 (*da zhong*),
PC.5 (*jianshi*), Liv.12 (*ji mai*), *yin tang* (M-HN-3), Du.19 (*hou ding*),
Du. 24 (*shen ting*).

Needle sensation (*de qi*) on Ren.4 (*guan yuan*) should go to the tip of the penis. This can be achieved by needling 1½ *cun* deep angled inferiorly. Make sure the bladder is empty first.

Clinical notes
- Biomedical conditions that may present as Heart and Gallbladder *qi* deficiency type impotence include anxiety neurosis and post traumatic shock syndrome.
- As with the previous pattern, this pattern represents impotence of psychogenic origin, in this case, however, the constitution is not necessarily weak. Because the root of the *shen* disturbance is usually very deep, therapeutic results are less certain. While anxiety can certainly be ameliorated with acupuncture and herbs, the relationship and sexual dysfunction of this pattern may need to be addressed more directly in consultation with a sex therapist or counsellor.
- The use of impotence drugs that enable dilation of penile arteries may prove ineffective in this category since vascular disease is unlikely to be the underlying mechanism. In cases where such drugs do prove to have some effect, however, there may be a strong psychological benefit.

Appendix
NOCTURNAL SEMINAL EMISSION (*yi jing* 遺精)

Nocturnal seminal emission (NSE) is the spontaneous ejaculation of semen in the absence of tactile or sensual stimulation. It generally occurs during sleep and is divided into two types, that associated with dreams (wet dreams) and that which occurs without dreaming. In severe cases spontaneous emissions may occur while awake.

NSE may be physiological or pathological. In young and adolescent boys, a spontaneous emission once or twice per month is considered physiological; more than this is considered pathological.

In the Western world, practitioners are extremely unlikely to ever encounter a patient presenting with this condition, indeed in isolation from a clearly defined pathology it is not considered to be harmful at all. The Chinese, however, with their cultural emphasis on the preservation of *jing* feel that excessive NSE requires treatment. This section can also be used for the analysis of premature ejaculation. Biomedically, NSE may be associated with disorders such as prostatitis and neuresthenia.

AETIOLOGY

The most common cause of NSE is an excess of Heat in the system, stimulating a kind of pseudo-arousal (the Fire of *ming men* is the basis of normal physiological arousal). This Heat may be the result of chronic Damp Heat retention, stress and frustration giving rise to Liver Fire or *yin* deficiency. Frequently, the Heat is derived from inappropriate or excessive use of stimulating *yang* tonic herbs like red ginseng and deer horn.

Less frequently, Kidney *yang* fails to contain *jing*, which then 'leaks' out. In this case, there are usually no accompanying erotic dreams.

热湿热遗精

1. HEAT, DAMP HEAT

Pathophysiology
- When Damp Heat is present in the lower *jiao* it can force *jing* out, in much the same way as sweat is pushed to the surface by internal Heat.
- This pattern may occur as the result of prostatic irritation from an unresolved urinary tract infection.

Clinical features
- frequent NSE
- poor appetite, nausea
- bitter taste in the mouth
- thirst with little desire to drink
- irritability and restlessness
- tendency to constipation or alternating loose and sluggish stools
- concentrated urine
- heaviness and aching in the lower limbs
- lethargy, afternoon fatigue

T greasy yellow coat, especially over the root
P deep and slippery or soft and slippery, possibly rapid

Treatment principle
Clear Dampness and Heat

Prescription

CHENG SHI BEI XIE FEN QING YIN 程氏萆解分清饮
(*Tokoro Formula from the Cheng Clan*) modified

bei xie (Rhizoma Dioscoreae Hypoglaucae) 萆解	15g
fu ling (Sclerotium Poria Cocos) 茯苓	12g
bai jiang cao (Herba cum Radice Patriniae) 败酱草	12g
sheng di (Radix Rehmanniae Glutinosae) 生地	12g
che qian zi (Semen Plantaginis) 车前子	9g
chi shao (Radix Paeoniae Rubrae) 赤芍	9g
dan shen (Radix Salviae Miltiorrhizae) 丹参	9g
yan huang bai (salt fried Cortex Phellodendri) 盐黄柏	9g
bai zhu (Rhizoma Atractylodes Macrocephalae) 白术	9g
lian zi xin (Plumula Nelumbinis Nuciferae) 莲子心	6g
shi chang pu (Rhizoma Acori Graminei) 石菖蒲	6g
gan cao (Radix Glycyrrhizae Uralensis) 甘草	3g

Method: Decoction. (Source: *Zhong Yi Nei Ke Lin Chuang Shou Ce*)

Patent medicines
Ming Mu Shang Qing Pian 明目上清片 (Ming Mu Shang Ching Pien)
Long Dan Xie Gan Wan 龙胆泻肝丸 (Long Dan Xie Gan Wan)
Qian Lie Xian Wan 前列腺丸 (Prostate Gland Pills)
Chuan Xin Lian Kang Yan Pian 穿心连抗炎片
   (Chuan Xin Lian Antiphlogistic Tablets)

Acupuncture
Ren.3 (*zhong ji* -), Sp.9 (*yin lin quan* -), Sp.6 (*san yin jiao* -), Bl.22 (*san jiao shu* -), Lu.7 (*lie que*), GB.26 (*dai mai*)

肝火

2. LIVER FIRE

Pathophysiology
- This pattern occurs primarily in generally healthy young men who consume large or inappropriate quantities of *yang* tonic herbs, in a misguided effort to increase strength and virility. They are usually already hot headed individuals, often martial artists or competitive sportsmen. Therapy, in the case of tonic induced Heat, is purely educational and the Heat will quickly subside once the herbs are discontinued. If it continues, however, the Heat will deplete Kidney *yin*.
- As the Liver channel passes through the penis (the penis is considered the 'ancestral Tendon of the Liver'), Heat in the Liver can stimulate it and force the release of semen.

Clinical features
- frequent NSE
- quick temper, irritability
- hypochondriac tightness or pain
- red complexion
- distension, redness and pain in the eyes
- bitter taste in the mouth
- thirst, dry throat
- constipation
- scanty concentrated urine.

T red or with red edges and a thick dry yellow coat
P wiry, rapid and strong

Treatment principle
Clear the Liver and purge Liver Fire

Prescription

LONG DAN XIE GAN TANG 龙胆泻肝汤
(*Gentiana Combination*)

jiu long dan cao (wine fried Radix Gentianae Longdancao) 酒龙胆草	6-9g
huang qin (Radix Scutellariae Baicalensis) 黄芩	9g
shan zhi zi (Fructus Gardeniae Jasminoides) 山栀子	9g
sheng di (Radix Rehmanniae Glutinosae) 生地	9g
ze xie (Rhizoma Alismatis Orientalis) 泽泻	9g
che qian zi (Semen Plantaginis) 车前子	9g
dang gui (Radix Angelicae Sinensis) 当归	6g
mu tong (Caulis Mutong) 木通	6g
chai hu (Radix Bupleuri) 柴胡	6g
gan cao (Radix Glycyrrhizae Uralensis) 甘草	3g

Method: Decoction. (Source: *Shi Yong Zhong Yi Nei Ke Xue*)

Modifications

- If this condition has persisted for a period of time, the Fire may consume Liver and Kidney *yin*. If there is Liver Fire against a background of *yin* deficiency, delete **mu tong** (Caulis Mutong) 木通, **ze xie** (Rhizoma Alismatis Orientalis) 泽泻, **che qian zi** (Semen Plantaginis) 车前子 and **chai hu** (Radix Bupleuri) 柴胡, and add **he shou wu** (Radix Polygoni Multiflori) 何首乌 9g, **nu zhen zi** (Fructus Ligustri Lucidi) 女贞子 12g and **bai shao** (Radix Paeoniae Lactiflorae) 白芍 12g.

Patent medicines

Long Dan Xie Gan Wan 龙胆泻肝丸 (Long Dan Xie Gan Wan)
Ming Mu Shang Qing Pian 明目上清片 (Ming Mu Shang Ching Pien)
Qian Lie Xian Wan 前列腺丸 (Prostate Gland Tablets)
Chuan Xin Lian Kang Yan Pian 穿心连抗炎片
    (Chuan Xin Lian Antiphlogistic Pills)

Acupuncture

Liv.2 (*xing jian* -), Liv.5 (*li gou* -), Bl.18 (*gan shu* -), GB.34 (*yang ling quan* -), Liv.14 (*qi men* -), SJ.5 (*wai guan* -), GB.39 (*xuan zhong* -), Kid.6 (*zhao hai* +)
- with headaches, add GB.20 (*feng chi*), Liv.3 (*tai chong*)
- with constipation, substitute SJ.6 (*zhi gou*) for SJ.5 (*wai guan*)

3. KIDNEY *YIN* DEFICIENCY WITH FIRE

肾阴虚火

Pathophysiology
- In addition to the usual things that damage Kidney *yin*, this pattern can be generated by excessive masturbation and fantasising. Frequent ejaculation easily depletes *yin* and fantasising excessively is thought to create internal Heat, which can further damage *yin*.
- It can also follow any other pattern characterised by excess Heat, like the previous pattern, Liver Fire.

Clinical features
- prolific dreaming, with erotic dreams culminating in NSE
- soreness or weakness of the lower back and knees, heel pain
- sensations of heat in the palms and soles ('five hearts hot')
- dry mouth and throat
- irritability and restlessness
- insomnia
- facial flushing, malar flush
- afternoon fever, nightsweats
- dizziness
- tinnitus
- tendency to dry stools or constipation
- scanty concentrated urine

T red and dry with little or no coat
P thready and rapid

Treatment principle
Nourish *yin*, clear Fire
Calm the *shen*, consolidate *jing*

Prescription

ZHI BAI BA WEI WAN 知柏八味丸
(*Anemarrhena, Phellodendron and Rehmannia Formula*) modified

shu di (Radix Rehmanniae Glutinosae Conquitae) 熟地	18g
shan yao (Radix Dioscoreae Oppositae) 山药	12g
shan zhu yu (Fructus Corni Officinalis) 山茱萸	12g
zhi mu (Rhizoma Anemarrhenae Asphodeloidis) 知母	9g
huang bai (Cortex Phellodendri) 黄柏	9g
fu ling (Sclerotium Poria Cocos) 茯苓	9g
mu dan pi (Cortex Moutan Radicis) 牡丹皮	9g
ze xie (Rhizoma Alismatis Orientalis) 泽泻	9g
wu wei zi (Fructus Schizandrae Chinensis) 五味子	6g

    long guˆ (Os Draconis) 龙骨 15g
    mu liˆ (Concha Ostreae) 牡蛎 15g
    suan zao ren (Semen Zizyphi Spinosae) 酸枣仁 18g
    lian zi xin (Plumula Nelumbinis Nuciferae) 莲子心 6g
    gan cao (Radix Glycyrrhizae Uralensis) 甘草 6g
    Method: Decoction. (Source: *Shi Yong Zhong Yi Nei Ke Xue*)

Modifications
- If *qi* and *yin* are both deficient, add **ren shen** (Radix Ginseng) 人参 10g and **mai dong** (Tuber Ophiopogonis Japonici) 麦冬 15g.
- If the Heart is very active and restless, with lots of palpitations, dreaming and insomnia, delete **long gu**ˆ (Os Draconis), and add **long chi**ˆ (Dens Draconis) 龙齿 10g, **fu shen** (Sclerotium Poriae Cocos Pararadicis) 茯神 15g and **yuan zhi** (Radix Polygalae Tenuifoliae) 远志 6g.

Patent medicines
Liu Wei Di Huang Wan 六味地黄丸 (Liu Wei Di Huang Wan)
Zhi Bai Ba Wei Wan 知柏八味丸 (Zhi Bai Ba Wei Wan)
Zuo Gui Wan 左归丸 (Zuo Gui Wan)

Acupuncture
Bl.15 (*xin shu* +), Liv.2 (*xing jian* -), Kid.2 (*ran gu* -), Ht.7 (*shen men* -), PC.6 (*nei guan* -), Bl.52 (*zhi shi*), Bl.30 (*bai huan shu*), Kid.7 (*fu liu* +), Bl.23 (*shen shu* +), Ren.4 (*guan yuan* +)
- with insomnia, add *an mian* (N-HN-54)
- with dizziness, add Du.20 (*bai hui*)
- with night sweats, add SI.3 (*hou xi*) or Ht.6 (*yin xi*)

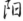

4. KIDNEY *YANG* (AND *YIN*) DEFICIENCY

Pathophysiology
- In this pattern the Kidney has lost its capacity to store and retain *jing*. This is a dual deficiency of the *yin* aspect (storage of *jing*) and the *yang* aspect (control of the urethra) of the Kidney, with the primary feature being *yang* deficiency.

Clinical features
- frequent NSE
- waxy pale complexion
- listlessness and fatigue
- aversion to cold, cold extremities
- lower abdominal distension
- urinary frequency or nocturia

- constipation or loose stools
- weak, cold and sore lower back and knees

T pale, wet and swollen
P deep and thready or slow and weak, particularly in the proximal positions

Treatment principle
Tonify the Kidney and consolidate *jing*

Prescription

YOU GUI WAN 右归丸
(*Eucommia and Rehmannia Formula*) modified

shu di (Radix Rehmanniae Glutinosae Conquitae) 熟地	240g
du zhong (Cortex Eucommiae Ulmoidis) 杜仲	120g
lu jiao jiao^ (Cornu Cervi Gelatinum) 鹿角胶	120g
shan yao (Radix Dioscoreae Oppositae) 山药	120g
gou qi zi (Fructus Lycii) 枸杞子	120g
tu si zi (Semen Cuscutae Chinensis) 菟丝子	120g
dang gui (Radix Angelicae Sinensis) 当归	90g
jin ying zi (Fructus Rosae Laevigatae) 金樱子	90g
long gu^ (Os Draconis) 龙骨	90g
mu li^ (Concha Ostreae) 牡蛎	90g
zhi fu zi* (Radix Aconiti Carmichaeli Praeparata) 制附子	60-180g
rou gui (Cortex Cinnamomi Cassiae) 肉桂	60-120g
zhi gan cao (honey fried Radix Glycyrrhizae Uralensis) 炙甘草	30g

Method: Grind the herbs into powder and form into 9-gram pills with honey. The dose is one pill 2-3 times daily. May also be decocted with a 90% reduction in doseage, in which case **zhi fu zi** is cooked for 30 minutes prior to adding the the other herbs (*xian jian* 先煎), and **rou gui** is added towards the end of cooking (*hou xia* 后下). (Source: *Zhong Yi Nei Ke Lin Chuang Shou Ce*)

Patent medicines

Jin Kui Shen Qi Wan 金匮肾气丸 (Sexoton Pills)
Ba Ji Yin Yang Wan 巴戟阴阳丸 (Ba Ji Yin Yang Wan)
You Gui Wan 右归丸 (You Gui Wan)
Jin Suo Gu Jing Wan 金锁固精丸 (Chin So Ku Ching Wan)
 - this last formula (which is primarily astringent) and one of the first three are generally taken together

Acupuncture

Du.20 (*bai hui* +), Ren.12 (*zhong wan* +), Ren.6 (*qi hai* +), Ren.4 (*guan yuan* +▲), Bl.23 (*shen shu* +▲), Bl.30 (*bai huan shu* +), Kid.3 (*tai xi* +) Du.4 (*ming men* +▲)

SUMMARY OF GUIDING FORMULAE FOR IMPOTENCE AND NOCTURNAL SEMINAL EMISSION

Impotence

Liver *qi* stagnation - *Xiao Yao San* 逍遥散
- In robust patients with restlessness and palpitations - *Chai Hu Jia Long Gu Mu Li Tang* 柴胡加龙骨牡蛎汤

Damp Heat - *Er Miao San* 二妙散
- with Liver Fire - *Long Dan Xie Gan Tang* 龙胆泻肝汤

Kidney *yang* deficiency
- *Wu Zi Yan Zong Wan* 五子衍宗丸 plus *Zan Yu Dan* 赞育丹

Kidney *yin* deficiency - *Liu Wei Di Huang Wan* 六味地黄丸

Heart Blood and Spleen *qi* deficiency - *Gui Pi Tang* 归脾汤

Heart and Gall Bladder *qi* deficiency - *Qi Yang Yu Xin Dan* 启阳娱心丹

Involuntary Seminal Emission

Damp Heat - *Cheng Shi Bei Xie Fen Qing Yin* 程氏萆解分清饮

Liver Fire - *Long Dan Xie Gan Tang* 龙胆泻肝汤

Kidney *yin* deficiency - *Zhi Bai Ba Wei Wan* 知柏八味丸

Kidney *yang* (and *yin*) deficiency - *You Gui Wan* 右归丸

Endnote

For more information regarding herbs marked with an asterisk*, an open circle° or a hat^, see the tables on pp.944-952.

Disorders of the Kidney

18. Tinnitus and Deafness

Excess patterns
Wind Heat
Liver *qi* stagnation
Liver Fire
Phlegm Heat
Stagnant Blood

Deficient patterns
Kidney deficiency
Spleen *qi* deficiency (with Phlegm Damp)
Qi and Blood deficiency

18 | TINNITUS AND DEAFNESS
er ming, er long 耳鸣, 耳聋

Tinnitus is the subjective experience of hearing a buzzing or ringing sound in one or both ears. Patients often describe it as 'ringing in the ears' though the sound described can vary considerably, from the sound of surf to a high pitched buzzing, or the sound of cicadas.

Deafness or loss of hearing may or may not be associated with tinnitus. The aetiology and pathophysiology of both tinnitus and hearing loss are essentially the same, although some patterns are more likely to cause one or the other. Tinnitus and deafness are traditionally included in the Kidney section because the ear is the sense organ associated with the Kidney. However, tinnitus and deafness can be the result not only of Kidney weakness but also of disorders of the Liver, Gall Bladder or Spleen, as well as trauma to the head and ears.

Tinnitus and deafness are common disorders and may be part of numerous biomedically defined conditions (see box). In cases where the cause is not obvious, referral to a specialist for investigation to exclude tumours and vascular malformations is recommended.

Some of the patterns described in this chapter cause 'earache' with tinnitus. Children (who are very prone to Wind Heat, Phlegm Heat and Spleen deficiency with Phlegm Damp patterns) will rarely complain of tinnitus, but often of earache. Similarly, children will not tend to notice loss of hearing. This deficit is usually detected by parents or teachers.

AETIOLOGY
Kidney deficiency
This is a common cause of chronic tinnitus and hearing loss, and some degree of pre-existing Kidney deficiency may also be involved in the excess categories of tinnitus and deafness. The Kidney 'opens into the ear', and intact Kidney *qi* is necessary for both the process of hearing and to protect the ear from pathogenic influence.

Tinnitus and deafness from Kidney deficiency is most frequently due to ageing, although other factors like stimulant drug use (which tends to damage Kidney *yin*), overwork (especially while under stress) and insufficient sleep may contribute. The Kidneys may also be damaged by excessive ejaculation or pregnancies close together. Kidney weakness may be the result of a congenital weakness or some prolonged or serious illness which has depleted *jing*. It seems Kidney *yin* deficiency is more likely to give rise to tinnitus, while Kidney *yang* deficiency is more likely to cause hearing loss.

External pathogens

Wind or Wind Heat can enter and disrupt the channels that surround and enter the ear (*san jiao*, Gall Bladder and Small Intestine), particularly in someone with a Kidney deficiency. As the Kidney and Urinary Bladder are internally/externally related, pathogenic Wind or Wind Heat penetrating the *tai yang* (Urinary Bladder and Small Intestine) channels can affect the Kidney.

Liver *qi* stagnation, Liver Fire

Anger, frustration, resentment and bitterness are all emotions that can damage the Liver and impede the free flowing nature of its *qi*. As the *qi* stagnates and the pressure increases, stagnant Heat is generated. At a certain point, the Heat is intense enough to become Fire which rises through the Gall Bladder channel to affect the ears. Liver Fire is exacerbated by a diet rich in fats and alcohol. Chronic Liver Fire will eventually consume Liver and Kidney *yin*, leading to a deeper and more recalcitrant type of tinnitus and hearing loss.

In the pure form, Liver *qi* stagnation and Fire are excess conditions. However, if persistent, Fire will eventually damage *yin*, and the condition will change to a mixed deficiency and excess condition. In the initial stages Liver Fire is more likely to cause tinnitus. As the condition progresses, the nature of the tinnitus may change from occasional loud tinnitus set off by emotions, to the softer, more persistent tinnitus and loss of hearing characteristic of Kidney deficiency.

BOX 18.1 SOME BIOMEDICAL CAUSES OF TINNITUS AND HEARING LOSS

External ear
- foreign body
- wax buildup

Middle ear
- otitis media (acute and chronic)
- eustachian catarrh
- glue ear
- perforated drum

Inner ear
- Meniere's disease
- cochlear degeneration
- post infectious (meningitis, measles, mumps, encephalitis and scarlet fever)
- labyrinthitis
- sound and physical trauma
- tumours

Drugs
- cannabis
- sodium salicylate
- kanamycin
- streptomycin
- gentamycin
- vancomycin
- quinine
- alcohol
- tobacco

Other
- anaemia
- hypertension
- altitude sickness
- temperomandibular joint dysfunction
- atherosclerosis
- aneurysm

> **BOX 18.2 KEY DIAGNOSTIC POINTS**
>
> - firstly always examine the inner ear for signs of infection, perforation or impacted wax
> - repeated courses of antibiotics (for ear infections) point to Spleen deficiency with Phlegm Damp
> - a history of head trauma (including exposure to loud noise) points to Blood stagnation
> - with exterior symptoms - Wind Heat (usually middle ear infection)
>
> **Aggravation**
> - with stress or anger - Liver *qi* stagnation or Liver Fire
> - with tobacco and alcohol - Liver Fire, Phlegm Heat
>
> **Amelioration**
> - with relaxation - Liver *qi* stagnation, Fire
> - with rest - Kidney or Spleen deficiency
>
> **Onset**
> - sudden - Wind Heat, Liver Fire, Phlegm Fire
> - gradual - Kidney deficiency, Spleen deficiency with Phlegm Damp

Phlegm Damp

Tinnitus and hearing loss may be caused by chronic stasis of Phlegm Damp in the channels around the ear, and within the ear itself. Phlegm Damp accumulates in those who have an excessively rich and oily diet, for example the typical Western diet heavy in dairy products and fried foods. Phlegm Damp can also be a product of the inefficient digestion that characterises Spleen deficiency. Repeated courses of antibiotics (often for recurrent middle ear or sinus infections) can, due to their cold nature, easily damage Spleen *qi*, allowing the generation and accumulation of Dampness and Phlegm.

Chronic stasis of Phlegm Damp can also generate Heat, which assists in elevating the Phlegm to the ear.

Stagnant Blood

Trauma, head injuries or long term stasis of *qi* can lead to Blood stagnation, which can prevent adequate circulation of *qi* to the ears. Exposure to loud noises may disrupt the channels of the ear sufficiently to cause stagnant *qi* and Blood, which in turn can damage the structures of the inner ear.

TREATMENT

Tinnitus is a common disorder and unfortunately one that is often difficult to treat successfully. Chronic cases are more difficult than acute or recent cases, and those due to exposure to loud noise generally do not respond very well. Having said this, prolonged therapy can be successful and results

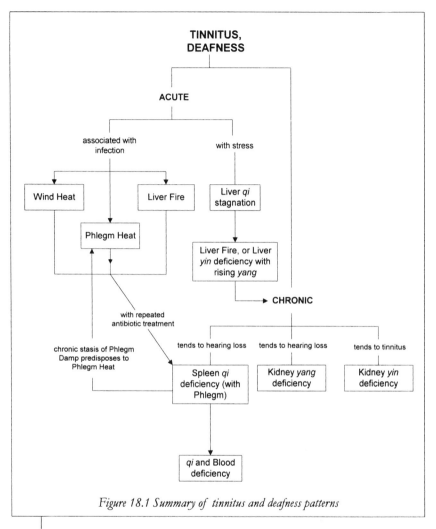

Figure 18.1 Summary of tinnitus and deafness patterns

are sometimes casually noted by patients being treated for some other condition—'now that I think about it I notice the buzzing in my ears is gone'. What this suggests is that a minimum of one or two courses of acupuncture (10-20 treatments), or several months of herbs should be given before making a judgement on whether the treatment is working or not.

Hearing loss is similar, and results of treatment in deficiency types are often subtle. In excess patterns the prognosis is better, especially the Phlegm type, where simple removal of the Phlegm can produce marked results.

18.1 WIND HEAT

Pathophysiology
- This pattern corresponds to an acute invasion of Wind Heat into the channels that surround the ear, and is associated with an infection of the inner ear.

Clinical features
- Unilateral tinnitus and/or hearing loss that is sudden and generally mild. It is often associated with a sensation of fullness, distension, blockage or persistent itching in the ear. There may also be pain in the ears or mastoid area, sometimes radiating into the jaw.
- possible purulent or bloody exudate from the ear
- headache
- fever
- muscle and joint aches
- cough
- thirst
- aversion to wind

T unremarkable or with thin white or yellow coat
P floating and rapid

Treatment principle
Disperse Wind and clear Heat
Open the ears

Prescription

YIN QIAO SAN 银翘散
(*Lonicera and Forsythia Formula*) modified

This prescription is selected if there is no suppuration or exudate from the ears.

jin yin hua (Flos Lonicerae Japonicae) 金银花	12g
jing jie (Herba Schizonepetae Tenuifoliae) 荆芥	12g
xia ku cao (Spica Prunellae Vulgaris) 夏枯草	12g
qing hao (Herba Artemisiae Annuae) 青蒿	12g
lian qiao (Fructus Forsythiae Suspensae) 连翘	9g
ju hua (Flos Chrysanthemi Morifolii) 菊花	9g
niu bang zi (Fructus Arctii Lappa) 牛蒡子	9g
jie geng (Radix Platycodi Grandiflori) 桔梗	6g
dan zhu ye (Herba Lophatheri Gracilis) 淡竹叶	6g
dan dou chi (Semen Sojae Praeparatum) 淡豆豉	6g
bo he (Herba Mentha Haplocalycis) 薄荷	3g

  gan cao (Radix Glycyrrhizae Uralensis) 甘草 3g
  shi chang pu (Rhizoma Acori Graminei) 石菖蒲 6g
Method: Decoction. Cook for 15-20 minutes maximum. **Qing hao** is added 5 minutes before the end of cooking (*hou xia* 后下). **Bo he** is added 1-2 minutes before the end of cooking (*hou xia* 后下). (Source: *Zhong Yi Er Bi Hou Ke Xue*)

MAN JING ZI SAN 蔓荆子散
(*Vitex Powder*)

This formula is selected if there is suppuration or exudate from the ears in addition to signs of Wind Heat.

  man jing zi (Fructus Viticis) 蔓荆子 12g
  sang bai pi (Cortex Mori Albae Radicis) 桑白皮 12g
  chi fu ling (Sclerotium Poria Cocos Rubrae) 赤茯苓 12g
  sheng di (Radix Rehmanniae Glutinosae) 生地 9g
  chi shao (Radix Paeoniae Rubrae) 赤芍 9g
  ju hua (Flos Chrysanthemi Morifolii) 菊花 9g
  mai dong (Tuber Ophiopogonis Japonici) 麦冬 9g
  qian hu (Radix Peucedani) 前胡 9g
  sheng ma (Rhizoma Cimicifugae) 升麻 6g
  mu tong (Caulis Mutong) 木通 6g
  zhi gan cao (honey fried Radix Glycyrrhizae Uralensis)
    炙甘草 3g
Method: Decoction. (Source: *Zhong Yi Er Bi Hou Ke Xue*)

FANG FENG TONG SHENG TANG 防风通圣汤
(*Siler and Platycodon Formula*)

This formula is selected if the Heat is relatively severe or the patient has pre-existing internal Heat, with constipation, strong fever and chills, red, sore eyes, bitter taste in the mouth, dark urine, a rapid pulse and a yellow tongue coat. The correct treatment is to dispel Wind and Heat, drain internal Heat and unblock the bowels.

  hua shi (Talcum) 滑石 90g
  gan cao (Radix Glycyrrhizae Uralensis) 甘草 60g
  shi gao (Gypsum) 石膏 30g
  huang qin (Radix Scutellariae Baicalensis) 黄芩 30g
  jie geng (Radix Platycodi Grandiflori) 桔梗 30g
  fang feng (Radix Ledebouriellae Divaricatae) 防风 15g
  ma huang* (Herba Ephedrae) 麻黄 15g
  jiu da huang (wine fried Radix et Rhizoma Rhei) 酒大黄 15g
  mang xiao (Mirabilitum) 芒硝 15g
  jing jie (Herba Schizonepetae Tenuifoliae) 荆芥 15g
  bo he (Herba Mentha Haplocalycis) 薄荷 15g

shan zhi zi (Fructus Gardeniae Jasminoidis) 山栀子 15g
lian qiao (Fructus Forsythiae Suspensae) 连翘 15g
chuan xiong (Radix Ligustici Chuanxiong) 川芎 15g
dang gui (Radix Angelicae Sinensis) 当归 15g
bai shao (Radix Paeoniae Lactiflorae) 白芍 15g
bai zhu (Rhizoma Atractylodes Macrocephalae) 白术 15g

Method: Grind into powder and take 6-9g as a draft twice daily. May also be prepared as decoction with a 30-90% reduction in dosage. If prepared as a decoction, **bo he** and **da huang** should be added towards the end of cooking (*hou xia* 后下), and **mang xiao** should be dissolved in the strained liquid (*chong fu* 冲服). (Source: *Zhong Yi Er Bi Hou Ke Xue*)

Modifications (apply to all three prescriptions)
- With high fever and ear pain, add **da qing ye** (Folium Daqingye) 大青叶 12g and **ban lan gen** (Radix Isatidis) 板蓝根 12g.
- With neck, shoulder and upper back stiffness, add **ge gen** (Radix Puerariae) 葛根 12g.

Patent medicines
Yin Qiao Jie Du Pian 银翘解毒片 (Yin Chiao Chieh Tu Pien)
Fang Feng Tong Sheng Wan 防风通圣丸 (Fang Feng Tong Sheng Wan)
Niu Huang Jie Du Pian 牛黄解毒片 (Peking Niu Huang Chieh Tu Pien)
Xiao Chai Hu Wan 小柴胡丸 (Xiao Chai Hu Wan)

Acupuncture
One or two of SI.17 (*tian rong* -), SI.19 (*ting gong* -), GB.2 (*ting hui* -), or SJ.21 (*er men* -) depending on tenderness, plus two or three of: Du.23 (*shang xing*), SJ.17 (*yi feng* -), LI.11 (*qu chi* -), LI.4 (*he gu* -), LI.5 (*yang xi* -), SJ.5 (*wai guan* -), GB.39 (*xuan zhong* -), GB.20 (*feng chi* -), SI.4 (*wan gu* -)
- with internal Heat add SJ.2 (*ye men* -) and Liv.2 (*xing jian* -)

Clinical notes
- Biomedical conditions that may present as Wind Heat type tinnitus or hearing loss include early stage of acute otitis media, measles, influenza and the common cold.
- This pattern will often present as an acute earache and is common in children. It generally responds well to correct and timely treatment with acupuncture and herbs.
- Acupuncture is very useful for removing local and acute obstruction in the channels around the ears, but may be poorly tolerated by sensitive individuals since the points are often quite tender and the *de qi* is strong.

肝气郁结

18.2 LIVER *QI* STAGNATION

Pathophysiology
- Liver *qi* stagnation, *qi* stagnation with stagnant Heat and Liver Fire are conditions with similar aetiology and of escalating severity. Typically, Liver *qi* stagnation precedes the development of Heat, which at a certain intensity is redefined as Fire. All stages involve emotional turmoil, especially anger, resentment and frustration as common aetiological features, with Liver Fire inflamed by a diet rich in alcohol and heating foods. Liver *qi* stagnation without Heat is less likely to cause hearing problems than that with Heat.
- Liver *qi* stagnation tends to gives rise to tinnitus rather than hearing loss. The obstructed *qi* seeks an alternate pathway and 'rebels' along the Gall Bladder channel disrupting the function of the ears.

Clinical features
- Mild intermittent tinnitus that is aggravated or initiated by emotional stress and improved with rest and relaxation. In women the tinnitus may be noticed premenstrually. There may be a sensation of pressure or fullness in the ears, but generally no pain or discharge.
- fullness in the chest, often described as difficulty getting a full breath, frequent sighing
- tension or discomfort beneath the ribs and in the neck or jaw
- headaches, tooth grinding
- mild dizziness
- loss of appetite or churning stomach
- irritability, depression
- occasional fatigue, which may be improved with exercise
- alternating constipation and diarrhoea
- irregular menstruation, premenstrual syndrome and breast tenderness

T normal or dark (*qing* 青)
P wiry and thready, or wiry and strong

Treatment principle
Soothe and invigorate the movement of Liver *qi*

Prescription

XIAO YAO SAN 逍遥散
(*Bupleurum and Dang Gui Formula*) modified

chai hu (Radix Bupleuri) 柴胡	9g
dang gui (Radix Angelicae Sinensis) 当归	9g
bai shao (Radix Paeoniae Lactiflorae) 白芍	9g
bai zhu (Rhizoma Atractylodes Macrocephalac) 白术	9g

fu ling (Sclerotium Poria Cocos) 茯苓 9g
man jing zi (Fructus Viticis) 蔓荆子 9g
xiang fu (Rhizoma Cyperi Rotundi) 香附 9g
pao jiang (roasted Rhizoma Zingiberis Offinalis) 炮姜 6g
shi chang pu (Rhizoma Acori Graminei) 石菖蒲 6g
zhi gan cao (honey fried Radix Glycyrrhizae Uralensis)
    炙甘草 6g
bo he (Herba Mentha Haplocalycis) 薄荷 3g
Method: Decoction. **Bo he** is added 1-2 minutes before the end of cooking time (*hou xia* 后下). (Source: *Zhong Yi Er Bi Hou Ke Xue*)

Modifications
- If the stagnant *qi* has generated some Heat (with facial flushing, reddish edges on the tongue, short temper, red eyes, feverishness), add **shan zhi zi** (Fructus Gardeniae Jasminoidis) 山栀子 9g and **mu dan pi** (Cortex Moutan Radicis) 牡丹皮 9g.

Patent medicines
Shu Gan Wan 舒肝丸 (Shu Gan Wan)
Xiao Yao Wan 逍遥丸 (Xiao Yao Wan)
Jia Wei Xiao Yao Wan 加味逍遥丸 (Jia Wei Xiao Yao Wan)

Acupuncture
One or two of (depending on tenderness) SI.19 (*ting gong*), GB.2 (*ting hui*), SJ.21 (*er men*) or SJ.17 (*yi feng*) plus two or three of: Liv.3 (*tai chong* -), LI.4 (*he gu* -), PC.6 (*nei guan*), BL.18 (*gan shu* -), GB.20 (*feng chi* -), SJ.6 (*zhi gou* -), *yin tang* (M-HN-3)

Clinical notes
- Biomedical conditions that may present as Liver *qi* stagnation type tinnitus include premenstrual syndrome, hypertension, stress related neck and jaw tension, TMJ syndrome and teeth grinding.
- Liver *qi* stagnation ear disorders generally respond well to correct treatment with acupuncture and herbs. Lifestyle changes are necessary for long term resolution, with stress management, exercise and relaxation techniques very useful. Acupuncture is often the treatment of choice for stagnation in the channels and will be used to great effect for tinnitus of this type, especially when there are points of tenderness around the neck and jaw. Physical work on the neck (such as osteopathic treatment or massage) may also be appropriate in those with significant neck tension.

肝火上扰

18.3 LIVER FIRE

Pathophysiology
- Liver Fire may progress from Liver *qi* stagnation if the stagnation creates sufficient Heat to engender Fire. When chronic Liver *qi* stasis together with diet are responsible for the development of Fire, the course is more prolonged. This appears in conditions such as hypertension and alcohol abuse. Liver Fire may also appear as an acute episode if external Heat penetrates through the *shao yang* channels, in which case an acute ear infection is the presenting symptom. In either case, Fire ascends through the Gall Bladder channel to the ear.
- Liver Fire tends to affect younger individuals. When prolonged, Liver *yin* is damaged and the pattern becomes one of mixed deficiency and excess (common in middle age), and ultimately deficiency (in the elderly).

Clinical features
- Sudden tinnitus and/or hearing loss, generally of short duration and clearly related to emotional upset, stress or overindulgence in alcohol, tobacco or Heat producing foods. The tinnitus is usually a high pitched buzzing. There may be ear pain and/or discharge.
- violent headaches or migraines, usually temporal, dizziness
- red complexion and eyes
- dry mouth and throat
- bitter taste in the mouth
- restlessness, extreme irritability
- insomnia
- hypochondriac pain
- constipation
- concentrated urine

T red or with red edges and a yellow coat
P wiry, rapid and strong

Treatment principle
Clear Heat from the Liver and Gall Bladder

Prescription

LONG DAN XIE GAN TANG 龙胆泻肝汤
(*Gentiana Combination*) modified

    long dan cao (Radix Gentianae Longdancao) 龙胆草 9g
    sheng di huang (Radix Rehmanniae Glutinosae) 生地黄 15g
    huang qin (Radix Scutellariae) 黄芩 12g
    shan zhi zi (Fructus Gardeniae Jasminoides) 山栀子 12g

che qian zi (Semen Plantaginis) 车前子 12g
ze xie (Rhizoma Alismatis Orientalis) 泽泻 9g
chai hu (Radix Bupleuri) 柴胡 9g
dang gui (Radix Angelicae Sinensis) 当归 6g
mu tong (Caulis Mutong) 木通 6g
shi chang pu (Rhizoma Acori Graminei) 石菖蒲 6g
gan cao (Radix Glycyrrhizae Uralensis) 甘草 6g

Method: Decoction. **Che qian zi** is cooked in a muslin bag (*bao jian* 包煎).
(Source: *Zhong Yi Er Bi Hou Ke Xue*)

Modifications
- With severe tinnitus, add **ci shi** (Magnetitum) 磁石 15g.
- With Phlegm or Phlegm Heat, add one or two of the following herbs: **quan gua lou** (Fructus Trichosanthis) 全栝楼 15g, **tian hua fen** (Radix Trichosanthis Kirilowii) 天花粉 12g, **zhe bei mu** (Bulbus Fritillariae Thunbergii) 浙贝母 9g or **zhu ru** (Caulis Bambusae in Taeniis) 竹茹 9g.
- With constipation, add **da huang** (Radix et Rhizoma Rhei) 大黄 6-9g.
- With purulent discharge, add **da qing ye** (Folium Daqingye) 大青叶 12g and **ban lan gen** (Radix Isatidis) 板蓝根 12g.
- With severe headache and sore red eyes, add **ju hua** (Flos Chrysanthemi Morifolii) 菊花 9g and **sang ye** (Folium Mori Albae) 桑叶 9g.
- If there are symptoms of Wind (tics, facial spasms, severe dizziness), add **gou teng** (Ramulus Uncariae cum Uncis) 钩藤 12g, **shi jue ming** (Concha Haliotidis) 石决明 15g and **ci shi** (Magnetitum) 磁石 15g.

Variations and additional prescriptions
- In chronic or recurrent cases (with internal causes), Liver (and Kidney) *yin* are gradually consumed, and the pattern changes. When *yin* deficiency is primary, see p.523. In many cases, there will be a mixture of *yin* deficiency and Liver *yang* rising. This is commonly seen in middle-aged patients with hypertension. The correct approach is to nourish *yin* and restrain *yang*. Suitable formulae include **TIAN MA GOU TENG YIN** (*Gastrodia and Gambir Formula* 天麻钩藤饮, p.670) and **ZHEN GAN XI FENG TANG** (*Sedate the Liver and Extinguish Wind Decoction* 镇肝熄风汤, p.655).

Patent medicines
Long Dan Xie Gan Wan 龙胆泻肝丸 (Long Dan Xie Gan Wan)
Ji Gu Cao Wan 鸡骨草丸 (Jigucao Pills)
Niu Huang Jie Du Pian 牛黄解毒片 (Peking Niu Huang Chieh Tu Pien)
  - with purulent discharge
Chuan Xin Lian Kang Yan Pian 穿心连抗炎片
  (Chuan Xin Lian Antiphlogistic Tablets)

- with purulent discharge

Tian Ma Gou Teng Wan 天麻钩藤丸 (Tian Ma Gou Teng Wan)
- *yin* deficiency with *yang* rising

Yang Yin Jiang Ya Wan 养阴降压丸 (Yang Yin Jiang Ya Wan)
- *yin* deficiency with *yang* rising

Acupuncture

SJ.17 (*yi feng* -), SJ.3 (*zhong zhu* -), SJ.5 (*wai guan* -), GB.40 (*qiu xu* -), GB.20 (*feng chi* -), GB.34 (*yang ling quan* -), Liv.3 (*tai chong* -), Liv.2 (*xing jian* -), LI.5 (*yang xi* -)
  • with *yin* deficiency and rising *yang* add Bl.18 (*gan shu* +), Bl.23 (*shen shu* +), Kid. 3 (*tai xi* +), Kid.1 (*yong quan*)

Clinical notes

• Biomedical conditions that may present as Liver Fire type tinnitus include hypertension, acute and chronic otitis media, alcohol toxicity, transient ischaemic attack and stress.

• Tinnitus from Liver Fire, especially with a short history, can often have a reasonably good prognosis if treatment and lifestyle changes can extinguish the Fire. Stimulating substances like coffee, alcohol, hot and spicy foods, cocaine and amphetamines should be strictly avoided. Stress management or relaxation techniques will be useful for some patients.

18.4 PHLEGM HEAT (FIRE)

Pathophysiology
- Phlegm Heat tinnitus often begins as an acute episode in patients who already have some Phlegm Damp accumulation in the ear. Such accumulation is usually seen in patients with rich, greasy or overly sweet diets, or in those with weak Spleen and Stomach function. Phlegm Damp easily causes stasis and the generation of Heat.
- Acute Phlegm Heat episodes are frequently treated with antibiotics which can weaken the Spleen, predisposing to more Phlegm Damp and the chronic tinnitus or hearing loss of Spleen deficiency with Phlegm Damp (p.526).
- This pattern often co-exists with Liver Fire.

Clinical features
- Tinnitus in one or both ears (with a sound like cicadas). There may be a feeling of blockage or pressure in the ears. This condition is often long term and deteriorates with time, with gradual loss of hearing.
- in some cases there will be a yellow purulent discharge, usually from one ear only and associated with earache
- fullness and heaviness in the head, woolly headedness
- fullness in the chest and epigastrium, nausea
- poor appetite, poor sense of taste or bitter taste in the mouth
- loose or sluggish stools
- recurrent clearing of the throat or coughing with yellow sputum

T red, with a thick greasy white or yellow coat
P wiry and slippery or slippery and rapid

Treatment principle
Clear Heat and transform Phlegm
Harmonise the Stomach and redirect turbidity downwards

Prescription

WEN DAN TANG 温胆汤
(*Bamboo and Hoelen Combination*) modified

zhu ru (Caulis Bambusae in Taeniis) 竹茹	12g
ban xia* (Rhizoma Pinelliae Ternatae) 半夏	9g
zhi shi (Fructus Immaturus Citri Aurantii) 枳实	9g
fu ling (Sclerotium Poria Cocos) 茯苓	9g
huang qin (Radix Scutellariae Baicalensis) 黄芩	9g
chai hu (Radix Bupleuri) 柴胡	9g
chen pi (Pericarpium Citri Reticulatae) 陈皮	6g
huang lian (Rhizoma Coptidis) 黄连	6g

痰火壅结

shi chang pu (Rhizoma Acori Graminei) 石菖蒲 6g
tong cao (Medulla Tetrapanacis Papyriferi) 通草 6g
sheng jiang (Rhizoma Zingiberis Officinalis) 生姜 3pce
Method: Decoction. (Source: *Zhong Yi Er Bi Hou Ke Xue*)

Modifications

- With Heat in the Liver or rising Liver *yang,* add one or two of the following herbs: **gou teng** (Ramulus Uncariae cum Uncis) 钩藤 12g, **shi jue ming^** (Concha Haliotidis) 石决明 15g and **ci shi** (Magnetitum) 磁石 15g or **ju hua** (Flos Chrysanthemi Morifolii) 菊花 9g.
- With a purulent discharge, add **da qing ye** (Folium Daqingye) 大青叶 12g and **ban lan gen** (Radix Isatidis) 板蓝根 12g.

Variations and additional prescriptions

Phlegm Fire

- In severe cases of tinnitus, accompanied by vertigo, a very thick yellow tongue coat, possible disturbances of consciousness and constipation, the correct treatment is to drain Fire and drive out Phlegm with **GUN TAN WAN** (*Vaporize Phlegm Pill* 滚痰丸).

　　duan meng shi (calcined Lapis Micae seu Chloriti) 煅礞石 ... 30g
　　jiu da huang (wine fried Radix et Rhizoma Rhei) 酒大黄 240g
　　huang qin (Radix Scutellariae Baicalensis) 黄芩 240g
　　chen xiang (Linum Aquilariae) 沉香 15g
　　Method: Grind herbs to a powder and form into small pills with water. The dose is 6-9 grams once or twice daily, with ginger tea. (Source: *Shi Yong Zhong Yi Nei Ke Xue*)

Residual Phlegm in the ear

- Following resolution of the Heat signs, or in between episodes of Phlegm Heat, there is usually residual or persistent Phlegm Damp. If there is little or no evidence of Heat, a formula such as **ER CHEN TANG** (*Citrus and Pinellia Combination* 二陈汤) modified, may be used for a lengthy period to dry the ear out and prevent reccurence.

　　ban xia* (Rhizoma Pinelliae Ternatae) 半夏 9g
　　fu ling (Sclerotium Poria Cocos) 茯苓 12g
　　chen pi (Pericarpium Citri Reticulatae) 陈皮 9g
　　zhi gan cao (honey fried Radix Glycyrrhizae Uralensis)
　　　　炙甘草 6g
　　shi chang pu (Rhizoma Acori Graminei) 石菖蒲 6g
　　tong cao (Medulla Tetrapanacis Papyriferi) 通草 6g
　　chai hu (Radix Bupleuri) 柴胡 6g
　　Method: Decoction.

- Other formula possibilities to prevent reccurence, include **BAN XIA BAI ZHU TIAN MA TANG** (*Pinellia and Gastrodia Combination* 半夏白术天麻汤, p.549) or **LIU JUN ZI TANG** (*Six Major Herbs Combination* 六君子汤, p.88), the former with dizziness and headaches or woolly headedness, the latter with Spleen *qi* deficiency.

Patent medicines
Qing Qi Hua Tan Wan 清气化痰丸 (Pinellia Expectorant Pills)
Hu Po Bao Long Wan 琥珀抱龙丸 (Po Lung Yuen Medical Pills)
Huang Lian Jie Du Wan 黄连解毒汤 (Huang Lian Jie Du Wan)
  - with much Heat and infection
Chuan Xin Lian Kang Yan Pian 穿心连抗炎片
    (Chuan Xin Lian Antiphlogistic Tablets) - in addition if there is purulent discharge

Acupuncture
one or two of SJ.21 (*er men* -), SI.19 (*ting gong* -), GB.2 (*ting hui* -), SJ.17 (*yi feng* -) plus two or three of: SJ.3 (*zhong zhu* -), St.40 (*feng long* -), GB.20 (*feng chi* -), PC.5 (*jian shi* -), Lu.7 (*lie que* -), Sp.4 (*gong sun* -), LI.4 (*he gu* -), Sp.9 (*yin ling quan* -)

Clinical notes
- Biomedical conditions that may present as Phlegm Heat type tinnitus include acute otitis media/externa, Meniere's disease and benign positional vertigo.
- If antibiotics are prescribed for this pattern (usually with ear pain) then treatment needs to be continued well past the end of the course of antibiotics to ensure the complete resolution of all Phlegm Damp. In small children (younger than three years old) prone to Phlegm, the patent medicine **BAO YING DAN** (*Protect the Child Special Pill* 保婴丹) is especially good for drying residual Phlegm and preventing the development of glue ear.
- Changes to diet are often necessary, especially reduction or exclusion of dairy products, raw food and undiluted juices.
- Children with chronic or recurrent ear infections and glue ear often present with this pattern or the Spleen deficiency pattern (p.526). In fact one can lead to the other - Phlegm Heat can occur as an acute episode in individuals with chronic Phlegm Damp, and recurrent episodes of Phlegm Heat that are treated with antibiotics or cooling herbs can predispose to accumulation of Phlegm Damp.

瘀阻宗脉

18.5 BLOOD STAGNATION

Pathophysiology
- Tinnitus and/or hearing loss due to stagnant Blood usually follows some traumatic head injury or injury to the ear, like exposure to loud noise or sudden pressure changes during flying or scuba diving. Alternatively, tinnitus from Blood stagnation may develop if other types of tinnitus become chronic or are unresolved.

Clinical features
- persistent tinnitus and/or hearing loss, possibly associated with a dark or black discharge from the ear, or dark matter mixed in with the ear wax
- possible earache or sharp pains
- dark complexion, dark rings under the eyes
- spider naevii on the face, neck and trunk
- chronic headaches
- hair loss, dizziness

T dark or purplish with brown or purple stasis spots and little or no coat
P wiry or choppy and thready

Treatment principle
Invigorate Blood, eliminate Blood stasis
Clear and open the ear

Prescription

TONG QIAO HUO XUE TANG 通窍活血汤
(*Unblock the Orifices and Invigorate Blood Decoction*)

This formula is designed for Blood stagnation affecting the senses, and is probably best when the stasis is largely confined to the head.

chi shao (Radix Paeoniae Rubrae) 赤芍 6g
chuan xiong (Radix Ligustici Chuanxiong) 川芎 6g
tao ren (Semen Persicae) 桃仁 9g
hong hua (Flos Carthami Tinctorii) 红花 9g
cong bai (Bulbus Allii Fistulosi) 葱白 3g
da zao (Fructus Zizyphi Jujubae) 大枣 7pce
sheng jiang (Rhizoma Zingiberis Officinalis) 生姜 9g
she xiang° (Secretio Moschus) 麝香 0.15g

Method: Decoction. **She xiang** is usually taken separately or added to the strained decoction (*chong fu* 冲服). (Source: *Shi Yong Zhong Yi Nei Ke Xue*)

Modifications
- If there are signs of Phlegm, add **zhe bei mu** (Bulbus Fritillariae Thunbergii) 浙贝母 9g, **hai zao** (Herba Sargassii) 海藻 12g and **kun bu**

(Thallus Algae) 昆布 12g.

XUE FU ZHU YU TANG 血府逐瘀汤
(*Achyranthes and Persica Combination*)

This formula is perhaps the most popular for all purpose removal of Blood stagnation. It is selected if there are more systemic signs of Blood stagnation.

tao ren (Semen Persicae) 桃仁	12g
hong hua (Flos Carthami Tinctorii) 红花	9g
chuan niu xi (Radix Cyathulae Officinalis) 川牛膝	9g
dang gui (Radix Angelicae Sinensis) 当归	9g
sheng di (Radix Rehmanniae Glutinosae) 生地	9g
chi shao (Radix Paeoniae Rubrae) 赤芍	6g
chuan xiong (Radix Ligustici Chuanxiong) 川芎	6g
zhi ke (Fructus Citri Aurantii) 枳壳	6g
jie geng (Radix Platycodi Grandiflori) 桔梗	6g
chai hu (Radix Bupleuri) 柴胡	6g
gan cao (Radix Glycyrrhizae Uralensis) 甘草	3g

Method: Decoction.

Patent medicines
Xue Fu Zhu Yu Wan 血府逐瘀丸 (Xue Fu Zhu Yu Wan)
Sheng Tian Qi Pian 生田七片 (Raw Tian Qi Ginseng Tablets)

Acupuncture
Local treatment is most important. Choose two or three of SJ.21 (*er men* -), SI.19 (*ting gong* -), SJ.17 (*yi feng* -), GB.2 (*ting hui* -) plus Sp.10 (*xue hai* -), BL.17 (*ge shu* -), GB.20 (*feng chi* -), Kid.3 (*tai xi*), GB.39 (*xuan zhong* -), SP.6 (*san yin jiao* -) as appropriate

Clinical notes
- Biomedical conditions that may present as Blood stagnation type tinnitus or hearing loss include auditory or cerebral tumours, traumatic head injury, inner ear damage, post concussion syndrome, migraine and TMJ problems.
- Can be difficult to treat, especially if long term or where there is structural damage to the inner ear.
- Patients exposed to loud noise (for example rock musicians, roadworkers and owners of walkmen) often fall into this pattern, but may have few (or none) of the classical signs and symptoms of Blood stagnation.

肾精亏损

18.6 KIDNEY DEFICIENCY

Pathophysiology
- Kidney deficiency tinnitus and/or hearing loss is typically seen in older patients. It may, however, occur in younger people if the Kidneys have been weakened by lifestyle factors or illness. Kidney *yin* deficiency tends to cause tinnitus, while Kidney *yang* deficiency tends to lead to hearing loss. The Kidneys influence hearing acuity, and some type of Kidney deficiency is thought to be at the root of most hearing disorders.

Clinical features
- gradual and progressive onset of tinnitus and/or hearing loss that is generally mild and constant, tending to be worse at night and when fatigued or after exertion (and ejaculation)
- the sound of the tinnitus is variable, sometimes high pitched, sometimes like holding a shell over the ear
- dizziness
- lower back weakness and pain
- poor memory
- loss of libido
- *yin* **deficiency:** flushing, insomnia, sensation of heat in the palms and soles ('five hearts hot'), night sweats, red, dry tongue with little or no coat, thready and rapid pulse
- *yang* **deficiency:** impotence, cold extremities, pale complexion, oedema or frequent urine or nocturia, pale swollen wet tongue, deep slow and thready pulse
- *qi* (*jing*) **deficiency:** if neither tending to *yin* or *yang* deficiency (that is, *qi* or *jing* deficiency) the tongue may be normal or pinkish and soft. The Kidney position on the pulse is deep and weak.

Treatment principle
Tonify and strengthen the Kidney (and Liver)
Benefit *yin* (or yang)

Prescription
18.6.1 Kidney *yin* deficiency

ER LONG ZUO CI WAN 耳聋左慈丸
(*Pill for Deafness that is Kind to the Left*)

shu di (Radix Rehmanniae Glutinosae Conquitae) 熟地	240g
shan yao (Radix Dioscoreae Oppositae) 山药	120g
shan zhu yu (Fructus Corni Officinalis) 山茱萸	120g
mu dan pi (Cortex Moutan Radicis) 牡丹皮	90g

fu ling (Sclerotium Poria Cocos) 茯苓	90g
ze xie (Rhizoma Alismatis Orientalis) 泽泻	90g
chai hu (Radix Bupleuri) 柴胡	90g
ci shi (Magnetitum) 磁石	90g
shi chang pu (Rhizoma Acori Graminei) 石菖蒲	60g
wu wei zi (Fructus Schizandrae Chinensis) 五味子	60g

Method: Grind herbs to powder and form into 9-gram pills with honey. The dose is one pill 2-3 times daily. May also be decocted with a 90% reduction in dosage.
(Source: *Zhong Yi Er Bi Hou Ke Xue*)

Modifications

- With Liver *yin* deficiency (dry eyes with blurring vision, irritability etc.), add **gou qi zi** (Fructus Lycii) 枸杞子 90g, **nu zhen zi** (Fructus Ligustri Lucidi) 女贞子 90g and **han lian cao** (Herba Ecliptae Prostratae) 旱连草 90g.

Patent medicines

Er Long Zuo Ci Wan 耳聋左磁丸 (Er Long Zuo Ci Wan)
Liu Wei Di Huang Wan 六味地黄丸 (Liu Wei Di Huang Wan)

18.6.2 Kidney *yang* (*qi*) deficiency

BU GU ZHI WAN 补骨脂丸
(*Psoraleae Pills*)

shu di (Radix Rehmanniae Glutinosae Conquitae) 熟地	180g
du zhong (Cortex Eucommiae Ulmoidis) 杜仲	120g
tu si zi (Semen Cuscutae Chinensis) 菟丝子	120g
bu gu zhi (Fructus Psoraleae Corylifoliae) 补骨脂	90g
hu lu ba (Semen Trigonellae Foeni-graeci) 葫芦巴	90g
bai zhi (Radix Angelicae Dahuricae) 白芷	90g
bai ji li (Fructus Tribuli Terrestris) 白蒺藜	90g
ci shi (Magnetitum) 磁石	90g
dang gui (Radix Angelicae Sinensis) 当归	90g
chuan xiong (Radix Ligustici Chuanxiong) 川芎	60g
shi chang pu (Rhizoma Acori Graminei) 石菖蒲	60g
chuan jiao (Pericarpium Zanthoxyli Bungeani) 川椒	50g
rou gui (Cortex Cinnamomi Cassiae) 肉桂	40g

Method: Grind herbs to powder and form into 9-gram pills with honey. The dose is one pill 2-3 times daily. May also be decocted with a 90% reduction in dosage.
(Source: *Zhong Yi Er Bi Hou Ke Xue*)

Patent medicines

Jin Kui Shen Qi Wan 金匮肾气丸 (Sexoton Pills)
You Gui Wan 右归丸 (You Gui Wan)

Ba Ji Yin Yang Wan 巴戟阴阳丸 (Ba Ji Yin Yang Wan)

Acupuncture
Kidney *yang* (*qi*) deficiency
BL.23 (*shen shu* +▲), Ren.4 (*guan yuan* +▲), Du.4 (*ming men* ▲), Kid.3 (*taixi* +), GB.2 (*ting hui* +), SJ.17 (*yi feng* +), St.36 (*zu san li* +), SI.3 (*hou xi*), SI.4 (*wan gu*), Bl.62 (*shen mai*)

Kidney *yin* deficiency
BL.23 (*shen shu* +), Kid.3 (*taixi* +), Kid.7 (*fu liu* +), SI.19 (*ting gong* +), GB.2 (*ting hui* +), Lu.7 (*lie que*), Kid.6 (*zhao hai*)

Clinical notes
- Biomedical conditions that may present as Kidney deficiency tinnitus and hearing loss include senile tinnitus/deafness, hypertension and chronic labyrinthitis.
- It is often difficult to obtain satisfactory results in this pattern, especially in older patients. Lengthy treatment is necessary before any results can be expected.
- Attention should be paid to aspects of lifestyle that influence the health of Kidney energy, such as sufficient sleep and rest, no lifting or excessive standing or sex.

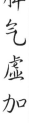

18.7 SPLEEN *QI* DEFICIENCY (WITH PHLEGM DAMP)

Pathophysiology
- Spleen *qi* deficient tinnitus and/or hearing loss occurs most commonly in those who have damaged the Spleen through overwork or poor dietary habits.
- This type may also be seen in people who have had repeated courses of antibiotics to treat middle ear or sinus infections. Frequent antibiotic use can damage Spleen *yang* predisposing to the buildup of fluids, Phlegm and Damp in the ear. This commonly happens in children, who often eventually need surgical implantation of grommets to drain the inner ear.

Clinical features
- Tinnitus and/or loss of hearing that is worse with fatigue and exertion, or on rising from sitting or lying. The sound is likened to cicadas or rushing water, and has a relatively low pitch. Occasionally the ear feels empty, cold, or wet. There may be recurrent or persistent sinus or eustachian tube congestion.
- fatigue and weakness
- poor appetite, picky eating
- abdominal distension after eating
- loose stools
- pale complexion and lips

T pale, with tooth marks and a thin white coat
P thready and weak

Treatment principle
Strengthen and tonify Spleen and Stomach *qi*
Raise *yang* and open the ears

Prescription

BU ZHONG YI QI TANG 补中益气汤
(*Ginseng and Astragalus Combination*) modified

This formula is selected when Phlegm is not excessive, and the patient sweats easily and catches frequent colds.

huang qi (Radix Astragali Membranacei) 黄芪	18g
dang shen (Radix Codonopsis Pilosulae) 党参	12g
bai zhu (Rhizoma Atractylodes Macrocephalae) 白术	12g
chai hu (Radix Bupleuri) 柴胡	9g
sheng ma (Rhizoma Cimicifugae) 升麻	6g
chen pi (Pericarpium Citri Reticulatae) 陈皮	6g
dang gui (Radix Angelicae Sinensis) 当归	6g

    shi chang pu (Rhizoma Acori Graminei) 石菖蒲 6g
    zhi gan cao (honey fried Radix Glycyrrhizae Uralensis)
    炙甘草 3g
    Method: Decoction. (Source: *Zhong Yi Er Bi Hou Ke Xue*)

LIU JUN ZI TANG 六君子汤
(Six Major Herbs Combination) modified

This formula is selected when Phlegm is copious. The patient may also have chronic sinus congestion, throat clearing and prominent digestive symptoms.

    ren shen (Radix Ginseng) 人参 9g
    bai zhu (Rhizoma Atractylodes Macrocephalae) 白术 12g
    fu ling (Sclerotium Poria Cocos) 茯苓 12g
    ban xia* (Rhizoma Pinelliae Ternatae) 半夏 9g
    chen pi (Pericarpium Citri Reticulatae) 陈皮 9g
    shi chang pu (Rhizoma Acori Graminei) 石菖蒲 6g
    yuan zhi (Radix Polygalae Tenuifoliae) 远志 6g
    cang zhu (Rhizoma Atractylodis) 苍术 6g
    gan cao (Radix Glycyrrhizae Uralensis) 甘草 3g
    Method: Decoction.

Modifications

- With weak Heart *qi* (palpitations, insomnia and anxiety), add **wu wei zi** (Fructus Schizandrae Chinensis) 五味子 6g, **suan zao ren** (Semen Zizyphi Spinosae) 酸枣仁 12g and **bai zi ren** (Semen Biotae Orientalis) 柏子仁 12g.
- With digestive weakness, loose stools and fluid retention, add **shan yao** (Radix Dioscoreae Oppositae) 山药 12g and **ze xie** (Rhizoma Alismatis Orientalis) 泽泻 9g.
- With Spleen *yang* deficiency, add **gan jiang** (Rhizoma Zingiber Officinalis) 干姜 6g, or use **FU ZI LI ZHONG WAN** (*Aconite, Ginseng and Ginger Formula* 附子理中丸, p.56) as guiding formula.

Patent medicines

Bu Zhong Yi Qi Wan 补中益气丸 (Bu Zhong Yi Qi Wan)
    - with frequent colds and easy sweating
Xiang Sha Liu Jun Zi Wan 香砂六君子丸 (Xiang Sha Liu Jun Wan)
Xiao Chai Hu Wan 小柴胡丸 (Xiao Chai Hu Wan)
    - especially good for children
Ren Shen Yang Ying Wan 人参养营丸 (Ginseng Tonic Pills)
    - with watery exudate from the ear and loose stools

Acupuncture
SJ.17 (*yi feng* +), SI.19 (*ting gong*), St.36 (*zu san li* +▲), St.40 (*feng long* +), BL.20 (*pi shu* +▲), GB.20 (*feng chi*), Ren.12 (*zhong wan* +▲), Sp.6 (*san yin jiao* +), Sp.9 (*yin ling quan* +), Lu.7 (*lie que*)

Clinical notes
- Biomedical conditions that may present as Spleen *qi* deficiency type tinnitus include glue ear and chronic otitis media.
- This condition may be the precursor to the Phlegm Heat pattern, or alternatively may be the result of repeated episodes of Phlegm Heat especially if these are treated with antibiotics.
- This pattern generally responds well to correct and prolonged treatment, however, dietary changes (low fat, sugar and dairy) will usually be necessary to maintain satisfactory results.

18.8 *QI* AND BLOOD DEFICIENCY

Pathophysiology
- *Qi* and Blood deficiency is typically a progression from, or a variation of, Spleen deficiency, where the Spleen fails to produce sufficient *qi* and Blood. The deficiency here is a degree more profound than that in the Spleen deficiency pattern (p.526). This pattern may also occur following haemorrhage or postpartum.

Clinical features
- Chronic tinnitus and/or hearing loss that tend to be intermittent and worse with fatigue. In some cases, the tinnitus may be loud enough to impair hearing.
- pale or sallow complexion, pale lips and nails
- fatigue and weakness
- dry skin and hair
- easily tired limbs
- light headedness or postural dizziness
- spots before the eyes
- poor appetite
- shortness of breath
- palpitations with anxiety and insomnia

T pale with a thin white coat
P thready and weak

Treatment principle
Tonify and nourish *qi* and Blood
Strengthen the Spleen

Prescription

SHI QUAN DA BU TANG 十全大补汤
(*Ginseng and Dang Gui Ten Combination*)

shu di (Radix Rehmanniae Glutinosae Conquitae) 熟地	15g
huang qi (Radix Astragali Membranacei) 黄芪	15g
dang shen (Radix Codonopsis Pilosulae) 党参	12g
bai zhu (Rhizoma Atractylodes Macrocephalae) 白术	9g
fu ling (Sclerotium Poria Cocos) 茯苓	9g
bai shao (Radix Paeoniae Lactiflorae) 白芍	9g
dang gui (Radix Angelicae Sinensis) 当归	9g
chuan xiong (Radix Ligustici Chuanxiong) 川芎	6g
rou gui (Cortex Cinnamomi Cassiae) 肉桂	3g
gan cao (Radix Glycyrrhizae Uralensis) 甘草	3g

Method: Decoction.

Modifications

- For a stronger Blood and *yin* generating action, add **lu jiao jiao**ˆ (Cornu Cervi Gelatinum) 鹿角胶 12g and **gui ban jiao**° (Plastrum Testudinis Gelatinum) 龟板胶 12g.
- With weak Heart Blood (insomnia, anxiety, palpitations), add **long yan rou** (Arillus Euphoriae Longanae) 龙眼肉 9g, **yi zhi ren** (Fructus Alpiniae Oxyphyllae) 益智仁 6g, **suan zao ren** (Semen Zizyphi Spinosae) 酸枣仁 12g and **mai dong** (Tuber Ophiopogonis Japonici) 麦冬 9g.
- With weak Liver Blood (muscular tics and spasms, blurred vision, pale conjunctive), add **mu gua** (Fructus Chaenomelis) 木瓜 6g, **nu zhen zi** (Fructus Ligustri Lucidi) 女贞子 12g and **han lian cao** (Herba Ecliptae Prostratae) 旱连草 12g.
- If the Blood deficiency generates some Heat (flushing, heat at night, red complexion), add **chai hu** (Radix Bupleuri) 柴胡 9g and **shan zhi zi** (Fructus Gardeniae Jasminoidis) 山栀子 9g.

Patent medicines

Shi Quan Da Bu Wan 十全大补丸 (Shi Quan Da Bu Wan)
Ba Zhen Wan 八珍丸 (Ba Zhen Wan)

Acupuncture

SJ.17 (*yi feng* +), GB.2 (*ting hui* +), St.36 (*zu san li* +▲), Sp.6 (*san yin jiao* +), Ren.4 (*guan yuan* +▲), BL.20 (*pi shu* +), BL.23 (*shen shu* +▲), BL.15 (*xin shu* +), Bl.17 (*ge shu*)

Clinical notes

- Biomedical conditions that may present as *qi* and Blood deficiency type tinnitus and hearing loss include anaemia, fatigue and overwork and neurosis.
- This pattern is generally difficult to treat, requiring lengthy treatment for any satisfactory result.

SUMMARY OF GUIDING FORMULAE FOR TINNITUS AND DEAFNESS

Excess patterns
Wind Heat - *Yin Qiao San* 银翘散
- with purulent exudate - *Man Jing Zi San* 蔓荆子散
- with strong internal Heat - *Fang Shen Tong Sheng Tang* 防风通圣汤

Liver *qi* stagnation - *Xiao Yao Wan* 逍遥丸

Liver Fire - *Long Dan Xie Gan Tang* 龙胆泻肝汤

Phlegm Heat - *Wen Dan Tang* 温胆汤
- After the acute episode with residual Phlegm - *Er Chen Tang* 二陈汤, or *Ban Xia Bai Zhu Tian Ma Tang* 半夏白术天麻汤

Blood stagnation - *Tong Qiao Huo Xue Tang* 通窍活血汤
- with systemic symptoms - *Xue Fu Zhu Yu Tang* 血府逐瘀汤

Deficient patterns
Kidney deficiency
- *yin* deficiency - *Er Long Zuo Ci Wan* 耳聋左慈丸
- *yang* deficiency - *Bu Gu Zhi Wan* 补骨脂丸

Spleen *qi* deficiency (with Phlegm Damp) - *Bu Zhong Yi Qi Tang* 补中益气汤
- with copious sticky Phlegm - *Liu Jun Zi Tang* 六君子汤

Qi and Blood deficiency - *Shi Quan Da Bu Tang* 十全大补汤

Endnote

For more information regarding herbs marked with an asterisk*, an open circle° or a hatˆ, see the tables on pp.944-952.

Disorders of the Liver

19. Dizziness and Vertigo

Excess patterns
Liver *qi* stagnation
Liver *yang* rising, Liver Fire
Phlegm Damp
Blood stagnation

Deficient patterns
Liver and Kidney *yin* deficiency with *yang* rising
Qi and Blood deficiency
Kidney deficiency

19 | DIZZINESS, VERTIGO
xuan yun 眩暈

The term *xuan yun* is used in Traditional Chinese Medicine to describe both dizziness and vertigo (Fig. 19.1), and is characterised by symptoms ranging from mild lightheadedness or giddiness, to severe loss of balance and equilibrium disturbance.

The mild end of the range, termed **dizziness**, may only occur on moving and last a few seconds. Occasionally, fainting may occur. It is frequently accompanied by blurring vision or spots in the visual field.

Vertigo is generally more severe, and is characterised by a sudden sensation of spinning, or the surroundings rotating. It may be described as 'head spinning', 'the room spinning', 'bedspins' or 'everything rocking and swaying'. Vertigo may or may not be precipitated by movement of the head, and may last for minutes or hours. Patients occasionally awake from sleep with vertigo. During episodes they usually become frightened and tend to remain immobile. Nausea, vomiting and tinnitus are often associated with vertigo.

In TCM, dizziness and vertigo are primarily due to either excess or deficiency affecting the head. In excess patterns, there is too much of some pathological entity in the head (*yang*, Wind, Phlegm, stagnant *qi*, Blood stasis), which hinders the normal flow of *yin*, *yang*, *qi*, and Blood. In the deficient patterns, there is too little of some physiological substance (Blood, *qi*, *yang*, *jing*) getting to the head.

AETIOLOGY

Liver *qi* stagnation, Liver *qi* stagnation with stagnant Heat, Liver Fire and Liver *yin* deficiency with *yang* rising

Frustration, anger, resentment, prolonged emotional turmoil, repressed emotions and stress disrupt the circulation of Liver *qi*. When *qi* stagnates for any

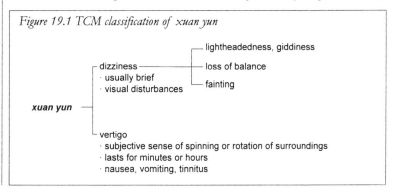

Figure 19.1 TCM classification of xuan yun

length of time, the resulting pressure can generate Heat. Depending on the intensity of the aetiological conditions, this can cause stagnant Heat, the more severe Fire or the eventual generation of internal Wind. *Qi* stagnation can give rise to Phlegm by damaging the Spleen and retarding the movement of fluids.

Qi stagnation, stagnant Heat and Fire are excess patterns. Once there is Heat, it can deplete and scorch the *yin*, giving rise to the more chronic *yin* deficiency with *yang* rising, or Liver Wind. The Wind that gives rise to dizziness is most frequently associated with Liver *yin* deficiency, although dizziness may be a symptom of all the patterns that can cause internal Wind (Box 19.2). The dizziness associated with Liver *qi* stagnation is generally quite mild (may be described as 'light-headedness') and due to poor distribution of *qi* and Blood. Dizziness severe enough to cause loss of balance or collapse is associated with rising Liver *yang* or Wind. See also Wind stroke, p.646.

Phlegm Damp

Phlegm Damp is generated by overindulgence in Phlegm or Damp producing foods and associated eating habits that weaken Spleen *qi*. Repeated courses of antibiotics can also damage Spleen *qi*, allowing the generation and accumulation of Dampness. Foods that can weaken the Spleen if consumed in excess include dairy products, fatty, sweet or raw foods, and alcohol. Once the Spleen is weak, inefficient digestion allows accumulation of Dampness, which over time congeals into Phlegm. In the presence of Heat, Damp may be condensed to form Phlegm in a shorter time.

BOX 19.1 SOME BIOMEDICAL CAUSES OF DIZZINESS AND VERTIGO

- motion sickness
- anxiety
- postural hypotension
- alcohol intoxication
- vertebrobasilar insufficiency
- benign positional vertigo
- ear infection, labyrinthitis
- vestibular neuronitis
- following head injury
- hyperventilation
- hypertension
- multiple sclerosis
- cardiac arrhythmia
- anaemia
- menopausal syndrome
- Meniere's disease
- epilepsy
- cerebellar degeneration
- ischaemia or infarction affecting the brain stem
- tumours, acoustic neuroma
- sternocleidomastoid trigger points

Drugs (vestibular nerve toxins)
- streptomycin
- kanamycin
- alcohol
- barbituates
- opiates
- nicotine
- caffeine
- salicylates
- quinine
- carbon monoxide

Others
- diuretics in large doses
- tranquillisers
- antihyperensive agents
- antidepressants

Poor fluid metabolism (due to Spleen, Lung or Kidney dysfunction) may cause stagnation, accumulation and thickening of physiological fluids into Phlegm. In addition, prolonged Liver *qi* stagnation can contribute, by weakening the Spleen and by retarding the movement of fluids, which gradually condense into Phlegm. Phlegm can fill the head, obstructing the 'clear *yang*' of the senses, and also obstruct the passage of *qi* and Blood to the head, causing relatively severe dizziness.

Stagnant Blood

Stagnant Blood type dizziness usually follows an injury to the head. It can also follow other long term pathologies, particularly stagnant *qi*, *yin* deficiency or Phlegm, all of which obstruct the circulation of *qi* and Blood.

Stagnant Blood type dizziness also appears to occur postpartum if the birth products and lochia are not completely expelled. If the complete downward discharge of *chong mai* is obstructed by stagnant Blood, *chong mai qi* will accumulate and rebel upwards to the head.

Qi and Blood deficiency

Overwork, excessive worry or mental activity, irregular dietary habits, excessive consumption of cold raw foods or prolonged illness can weaken Spleen *qi*.

BOX 19.2 MECHANISMS OF INTERNAL WIND

Yin deficiency

The body's *yin* is the anchor that secures *yang* and provides a counterweight to it's active and rising nature. At some critical point of deficiency, *yin* is unable to restrain Liver *yang*, which at a certain point of volatility and movement becomes Wind. This type of Wind can be sudden and catastrophic – it is the type of Wind that can cause severe dizziness, to the point of Wind stroke, leading to hemiplegia or death. It typically follows years of *yin* depletion.

Blood deficiency

This type of Wind is similar in aetiology to the previous type in that the Wind is generated by failure of the Blood to anchor *qi* – when *qi* moves without the grounding control of Blood, a mild form of Wind is generated. Blood deficient Wind is more likely to cause mild rhythmic tics, tremors and spasms. The dizziness associated with Blood deficiency is more likely to be mild and postural, and due to failure of Blood to reach the head.

Heat

Because Heat and movement are closely related physiologically, at a certain level of intensity, internal Heat can generate sufficient movement to become Wind. This most frequently manifests as the convulsions of a high fever.

> **BOX 19.3 KEY DIAGNOSTIC POINTS**
>
> **Aggravation**
> - with rising - *qi* and Blood deficiency
> - with stress or emotion - Liver *qi* stagnation, *yang* rising or Wind
> - with sexual activity - Kidney deficiency
>
> **Amelioration**
> - with rest - deficiency
>
> **Associated symptoms**
> - nausea or vomiting - Phlegm Damp
> - headache, blurring vision and facial flushing - *yin* deficiency with rising *yang* or Wind
>
> **Nature**
> - severe, as if the room is spinning - Phlegm Damp
> - mild dizziness or lightheadedness - deficiency

The Spleen (and Lungs) are the source of the body's *qi* and Blood, so weakness of these organs will inevitably lead to a decrease in production of *qi* and Blood. Other causes are acute or chronic haemorrhage, extended breast feeding and malnutrition (seen for example in vegetarians who consume too little protein). *Qi* and Blood are so closely related that deficiency of one often leads to deficiency of the other.

Kidney deficiency

Kidney deficiency can be either *jing*, *yang* or *yin* deficiency. Kidney deficiency may be inherited or may develop as a result of age, chronic illness or excessive sexual activity. Kidney *yang* or *qi* is particularly affected by prolonged exposure to cold conditions or excessive lifting or standing (particularly if this occurs in a cold environment). In younger people, Kidney *qi* may be weakened while Kidney *yang* remains intact, in which case the cold symptoms are not seen.

Kidney *yin* is damaged through overwork (especially while under stress), insufficient sleep, febrile disease, insufficient fluid replacement and by the use of some prescription and recreational drugs. Kidney *yin* may also be damaged by pregnancy or haemorrhage following childbirth.

DIFFERENTIAL DIAGNOSIS

Dizziness should be distinguished from the following disorders:
- ***Jue* syndrome** (*jue zheng* 厥证): *Jue* syndrome is characterised by sudden loss of consciousness accompanied by cold extremities, then a gradual regaining of consciousness with no residual paralysis, speech difficulties or sequelae. When dizziness is very severe, patients may fall over, however

there is no loss of consciousness. The sorts of disorders that are categorised as *jue* syndrome include hypoglycaemic coma, hysterical syncope, haemorrhagic or allergic shock.
- **Wind stroke** (*zhong feng* 中风): Wind stroke involves partial or total loss of consciousness with residual hemiplegia, slurring speech and/or facial paralysis. Patients suffering from Wind stroke will often feel dizzy, however the sequelae distinguishes Wind stroke from the TCM diagnosis of dizziness.
- **Epilepsy** (*xian zheng* 痫症): Epilepsy involves partial or total loss of consciousness, collapse and convulsions. Epileptic patients may experience dizziness as part of their aura or partial seizure, but the accompanying pattern makes discrimination clear. Upon regaining consciousness, epileptic patients are generally asymptomatic.

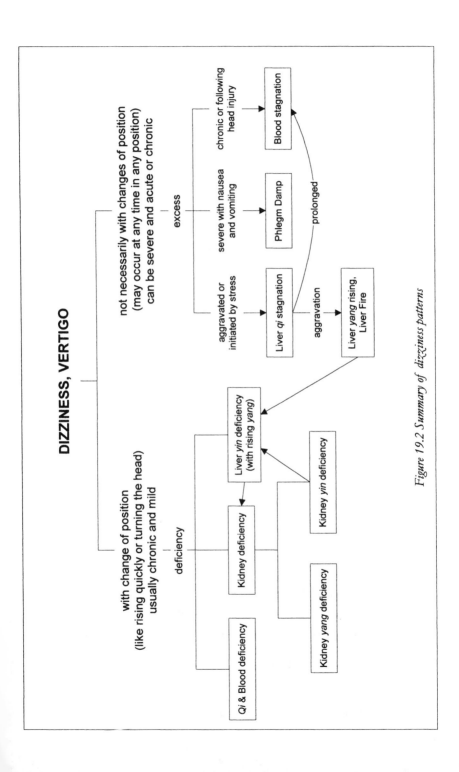

Figure 19.2 *Summary of dizziness patterns*

肝气郁滞

19.1 LIVER *QI* STAGNATION

Pathophysiology
- The Liver channel travels to the vertex of the head, so any obstruction of Liver *qi* may disrupt the distribution of *qi* and Blood to the head and cause dizziness. Liver *qi* stagnation can lead to an accumulation of *qi* in the head (and an excess type of dizziness), or the *qi* may be obstructed before it gets to the head, accumulating in the throat (causing 'plum stone *qi*') or in the chest. When *qi* fails to reach the head the dizziness is of a deficient type and usually mild.
- If Liver *qi* obstruction is persistent or severe, then Heat can be generated. Heat in the Liver causes Liver *yang* or Fire to rise. Over time the Heat can damage *yin*. The progression between Liver *qi* stagnation, *yang* rising, and *yin* deficiency is commonly observed clinically.

Clinical features
- dizziness that is worse with stress and generally not related to postural changes
- tightness or fullness in the chest, often described as difficulty in drawing a satisfying breath
- hypochondriac discomfort or tightness, frequent sighing
- headache or head distension
- occasional fatigue (although may feel better for activity or exercise)
- irritability or depression
- abdominal distension, flatulence and alternating constipation and diarrhoea
- women may experience irregular menstruation, pre-menstrual syndrome and breast tenderness
- all symptoms tend to be aggravated by stress

T normal or dark (*qing* 青) with a thin white or yellow coat
P wiry

Treatment principle
Soothe the Liver and regulate *qi*

Prescription

XIAO YAO SAN 逍遥散
(*Bupleurum and Dang Gui Formula*) modified

chai hu (Radix Bupleuri) 柴胡	9g
dang gui (Radix Angelicae Sinensis) 当归	9g
bai shao (Radix Paeoniae Lactiflorae) 白芍	9g
bai zhu (Rhizoma Atractylodes Macrocephalae) 白术	9g
fu ling (Sclerotium Poria Cocos) 茯苓	9g
wei jiang (roasted Rhizoma Zingiberis Officinalis) 煨姜	6g

bo he (Herba Mentha Haplocalycis) 薄荷 3g
sang ye (Folium Mori Albae) 桑叶 15g
ju hua (Flos Chrysanthemi Morifolii) 菊花 12g
zhi gan cao (honey fried Radix Glycyrrhizae Uralensis)
炙甘草 6g

Method: Decoction or pills. In decoction, **bo he** is added a few minutes before the end of cooking (*hou xia* 后下).

Modifications
- With stagnant Heat, add **mu dan pi** (Cortex Moutan Radicis) 牡丹皮 9g and **shan zhi zi** (Fructus Gardeniae Jasminoides) 山栀子 9g.
- Fullness and discomfort in the chest and hypochondrium, add **zhi xiang fu** (prepared Rhizoma Cyperi Rotundi) 制香附 6g, **yu jin** (Tuber Curcumae) 郁金 9g and **zhi ke** (Fructus Citri Aurantii) 枳壳 6g.
- If easily awoken, startled and frightened, add one or two of the following herbs: **zhen zhu mu**^ (Concha Margaritaferae) 珍珠母 30g, **long chi**^ (Dens Draconis) 龙齿 15g or **ci shi** (Magnetitum) 磁石 12g.

Variations and additional prescriptions
- Dizziness following an unresolved Wind attack, and accompanied by loss of appetite, fatigue, alternating fever and chills, bitter taste in the mouth, dry throat and wiry pulse, is *shao yang* syndrome. The correct treatment is to harmonise *shao yang* with **XIAO CHAI HU TANG** (*Minor Bupleurum Combination* 小柴胡汤, p.54).

Patent medicines
Xiao Yao Wan 逍遥丸 (Xiao Yao Wan)
Jia Wei Xiao Yao Wan 加味逍遥丸 (Jia Wei Xiao Yao Wan)
Chai Hu Shu Gan Wan 柴胡舒肝丸 (Chai Hu Shu Gan Wan)

Acupuncture
GB.20 (*feng chi*), Bl.18 (*gan shu*), Liv.3 (*tai chong* -), GB.43 (*xia xi* -), PC.6 (*nei guan*), GB.34 (*yang ling quan* -), *ah shi* points on the upper back, neck and superior sternocleidomastoid muscle

Clinical notes
- The dizziness in this pattern may be associated with the stress response, neuresthenia, hepatitis, anaemia or Meniere's disease.
- The dizziness of this pattern, particularly when it is due to stress, often has its origin in muscle spasm in the neck which constricts blood supply to the head. Needling the *ah shi* points on these muscles can relieve spasm and re-establish better blood flow.

肝阳上亢

19.2 LIVER *YANG* RISING, LIVER FIRE

Pathophysiology
- In their pure form these are excess patterns, and in younger individuals Liver *yang* rising or Liver Fire are a common cause of dizziness. However, the relationship between *qi* stagnation, rising Liver *yang* or Fire and Liver *yin* deficiency with rising *yang* is such that in many patients there are elements of all three.
- In this pattern, Liver *yang* rises when stagnant *qi* is suddenly released (like popping a cork). The relationship between *yang* rising and Fire in this pattern is one of degree. Both are the result of a sudden release of pent up *qi*, but Fire is hotter and drier and may cause haemorrhage. Liver Fire is more likely to develop if there is pre-existing internal Heat or severe aetiological conditions. Fire is exacerbated by a diet rich in heating foods and alcohol.

Clinical features
- dizziness and vertigo, which may be severe and initiated or aggravated by stress, anger or emotional upset
- headache or fullness and distension in the head and eyes
- blurring vision, red, sore, gritty eyes
- irritability, temper outbursts
- red complexion or facial flushing
- insomnia with much dreaming

T red edges with a thin yellow coat
P wiry and rapid

Treatment principle
Calm the Liver and subdue *yang*
Clear Heat and extinguish Wind

Prescription

TIAN MA GOU TENG YIN 天麻钩藤饮
(*Gastrodia and Gambir Formula*) modified

tian ma (Rhizoma Gastrodiae Elatae) 天麻	9g
gou teng (Ramulus Uncariae cum Uncis) 钩藤	9g
shi jue ming^ (Concha Haliotidis) 石决明	15g
xia ku cao (Spica Prunellae Vulgaris) 夏枯草	15g
fu shen (Sclerotium Poriae Cocos Pararadicis) 茯神	15g
ye jiao teng (Caulis Polygoni Multiflori) 夜交藤	15g
sang ji sheng (Ramulus Sangjisheng) 桑寄生	15g
du zhong (Cortex Eucommiae Ulmoidis) 杜仲	15g
niu xi (Radix Achyranthis Bidentatae) 牛膝	12g

ju hua (Flos Chrysanthemi Morifolii) 菊花 12g
shan zhi zi (Fructus Gardeniae Jasminoides) 山栀子 12g
huang qin (Radix Scutellariae Baicalensis) 黄芩 9g
Method: Decoction. **Shi jue ming** should be cooked for 30 minutes before the other herbs are added (*xian jian* 先煎), **gou teng** is added near the end of cooking (*hou xia* 后下). (Source: *Shi Yong Zhong Yi Nei Ke Xue*)

Modifications

- With Liver Fire, causing severe headache, red, sore, distended eyes, dark urine, severe irascibility, a red tongue with a thick, dry, yellow tongue coat and a wiry, rapid pulse, add **long dan cao** (Radix Gentianae Longdancao) 龙胆草 9g and **mu dan pi** (Cortex Moutan Radicis) 牡丹皮 12g, or use **LONG DAN XIE GAN TANG** (*Gentiana Combination* 龙胆泻肝汤, p.500) to clear the Liver and drain Fire.
- With constipation, add **da huang** (Radix et Rhizoma Rhei) 大黄 6-9g and **mang xiao** (Mirabilitum) 芒硝 6g, or combine with **DANG GUI LONG HUI WAN** (*Dang Gui, Gentiana Longdancao and Aloe Pill* 当归龙荟丸 p.771-772) to clear the Liver and bowels.
- With mild *yin* deficiency, add 2 or 3 of the following herbs: **mu li**ˆ (Concha Ostreae) 牡蛎 15g, **gui ban**° (Plastri Testudinis Gelatinum) 龟板 12g, **bie jia**° (Carapax Amydae Sinensis) 鳖甲 12g, **he shou wu** (Radix Polygoni Multiflori) 何首乌 12g or **sheng di** (Radix Rehmanniae Glutinosae) 生地 15g.
- With Liver Wind (severe dizziness and tinnitus, vomiting, numbness in the extremities, tics, tremors, fasiculations and spasms), add **long gu**ˆ (Os Draconis) 龙骨 15g, **mu li**ˆ (Concha Ostreae) 牡蛎 15g and **zhen zhu mu**ˆ (Concha Margaritaferae) 珍珠母 15g to calm the Liver and suppress Wind.

Variations and additional prescriptions

- If the Wind becomes the main concern, **LING YANG JIAO TANG** (*Antelope Horn Decoction* 羚羊角汤) modified, can be used to clear Liver Heat and extinguish Wind. See also Wind Stroke, p.661.

   ling yang jiao fen° (powdered Cornu Antelopis)
   羚羊角粉 4g
   gou teng (Ramulus Uncariae cum Uncis) 钩藤 12g
   shi jue mingˆ (Concha Haliotidis) 石决明 18g
   gui ban° (Plastri Testudinis Gelatinum) 龟板 15g
   xia ku cao (Spica Prunellae Vulgaris) 夏枯草 15g
   sheng di (Radix Rehmanniae Glutinosae) 生地 15g
   huang qin (Radix Scutellariae Baicalensis) 黄芩 9g
   niu xi (Radix Achyranthis Bidentatae) 牛膝 15g
   bai shao (Radix Paeoniae Lactiflorae) 白芍 15g

mu dan pi (Cortex Moutan Radicis) 牡丹皮 12g
Method: Decoction. **Ling yang jiao** powder is added to the strained decoction (*chong fu* 冲服), **gou teng** is added towards the end of cooking (*hou xia* 后下). (Source: *Shi Yong Zhong Yi Nei Ke Xue*)

Patent medicines
Tian Ma Gou Teng Wan 天麻钩藤丸 (Tian Ma Gou Teng Wan)
Yang Yin Jiang Ya Wan 养阴降压丸 (Yang Yin Jiang Ya Wan)
Long Dan Xie Gan Wan 龙胆泻肝丸 (Long Dan Xie Gan Wan)
 - Liver Fire
Hu Po Bao Long Wan 琥珀抱龙丸 (Po Lung Yuen Medical Pills)

Acupuncture
Bl.18 (*gan shu* -), Liv.3 (*tai chong* -), LI.4 (*he gu* -), LI.11 (*qu chi* -), GB.20 (*feng chi* -), GB.43 (*xia xi* -), St.8 (*tou wei*), Bl.23 (*shen shu* +), *yin tang* (M-HN-3)
- with Fire add Liv.2 (*xing jian* -)
- with hypochondriac pain add GB.34 (*yang ling quan* -) and SJ.6 (*zhi gou* -)

Clinical notes
- The dizziness of this pattern may be associated with hypertension, transitory ischaemic attacks (T.I.As), impending stroke, eclampsia, puerperal fever or Meniere's disease.
- Dizziness or vertigo of a *yang* rising or Fire type can represent a potentially dangerous condition or an impending catastrophe. Acupuncture with strong stimulation can be effective in the case of dangerously high blood pressure or impending stroke. Persistently high blood pressure that does not respond to TCM treatment should be thoroughly investigated medically.

肝肾阴虚阳上亢

19.3 LIVER AND KIDNEY *YIN* DEFICIENCY WITH *YANG* RISING

Pathophysiology
- Dizziness due to Liver and Kidney *yin* deficiency with rising *yang* is a mixed pattern of deficient *yin* leading to excess *yang*. The Liver and Kidney deficiency is the predominent pattern. Liver *yin* deficiency often follows chronic conditions involving rising Liver *yang* or Fire, or stagnant Heat. This pattern is more common in older individuals.
- The mechanism of rising *yang* in this category is different to that in the previous one. In simple *yang* rising, pent up *qi* eventually creates enough pressure to 'pop the cork'. In this pattern Liver and Kidney *yin* are deficient, and insufficient to anchor *yang* and provide a counterweight to its active and rising nature. When the anchoring *yin* reaches a critical point of deficiency, the *yang* loses its mooring and becomes excessively mobile, rising to the head. When rising *yang* reaches a certain level of intensity (sufficient to cause loss of balance or collapse), it may be redefined as Wind.

Clinical features
- dizziness which is generally mild, with occasional exacerbations in severity that may be triggered or aggravated by stress, overexertion, emotional upset, sexual activity or heating foods and alcohol
- blurring vision or visual disturbances, pressure behind the eyes
- irritability and restlessness
- headache, often temporal
- insomnia, or restless sleep with much dreaming
- facial flushing or malar flushing, night sweats
- sensation of heat in the palms and soles ('five hearts hot')
- tinnitus
- weakness, fatigue
- lower backache

T red and dry with little or no coat
P wiry, thready and rapid

Treatment principle
Nourish *yin*, sedate the Liver, anchor *yang* (subdue Wind)

Prescription

ZHEN GAN XI FENG TANG 镇肝熄风汤
(*Sedate the Liver and Extinguish Wind Decoction*)

This is an important formula for Liver and Kidney deficiency with *yang* rising hypertension and pre-stroke conditions. It is suitable for long term use, although a more specific Liver and Kidney *yin* tonic may be selected when the rising *yang* is sedated.

huai niu xi (Radix Achyranthis Bidentatae) 怀牛膝	30g
dai zhe shi (Haematitum) 代赭石	30g
long gu^ (Os Draconis) 龙骨	15g
mu li^ (Concha Ostreae) 牡蛎	15g
bai shao (Radix Paeoniae Lactiflorae) 白芍	15g
gui ban° (Plastri Testudinis Gelatinum) 龟板	15g
tian dong (Tuber Asparagi Cochinchinensis) 天冬	15g
xuan shen (Radix Scrophulariae) 玄参	15g
mai ya (Fructus Hordei Vulgaris Germinantus) 麦芽	12g
chuan lian zi* (Fructus Meliae Toosendan) 川楝子	6g
qing hao (Herba Artemesiae Annuae) 青蒿	6g
gan cao (Radix Glycyrrhizae Uralensis) 甘草	5g

Method: Decoction. (Source: *Shi Yong Zhong Yi Nei Ke Xue*)

Modifications

- For chronic headaches, add **dan shen** (Radix Salviae Miltiorrhizae) 丹参 15g and **chuan xiong** (Radix Ligustici Chuanxiong) 川芎 6g.
- With hypertension, add **xia ku cao** (Spica Prunellae Vulgaris) 夏枯草 15g, **gou teng** (Ramulus Uncariae cum Uncis) 钩藤 12g, **ju hua** (Flos Chrysanthemi Morifolii) 菊花 9g and **di long**^ (Lumbricus) 地龙 9g.
- With significant Kidney deficiency, add **shu di** (Radix Rehmanniae Glutinosae Conquitae) 熟地 18g and **shan zhu yu** (Fructus Corni Officinalis) 山茱萸 12g
- With constipation, delete **dai zhe shi** and add **chi shi zhi** (Halloysitum Rubrum) 赤石脂 15g.

Follow up treatment

- When the symptoms are under control, a *yin* nourishing patent formula like **QI JU DI HUANG WAN** (*Lycium, Chrysanthemum and Rehmannia Formula* 杞菊地黄丸, p.574) or **ZHI BAI BA WEI WAN** (*Anemarrhena, Phellodendron and Rehmannia Formula* 知柏八味丸, p.452) may be used to nourish Liver and Kidney *yin*.

Patent medicines

Qi Ju Di Huang Wan 杞菊地黄丸 (Lycium-Rehmannia Pills)
Zhi Bai Ba Wei Wan 知柏八味丸 (Zhi Bai Ba Wei Wan)
Ming Mu Di Huang Wan 明目地黄丸 (Ming Mu Di Huang Wan)
Er Long Zuo Ci Wan 耳聋左慈丸 (Er Long Zuo Ci Wan)
Tian Ma Gou Teng Wan 天麻钩藤丸 (Tian Ma Gou Teng Wan)
Yang Yin Jiang Ya Wan 养阴降压丸 (Yang Yin Jiang Ya Wan)

Acupuncture

Bl.23 (*shen shu* +), Kid.3 (*tai xi* +), Sp.6 (*san yin jiao* +), Liv.3 (*tai chong*), Bl.15 (*xin shu*), Kid.1 (*yong quan*), PC.6 (*nei guan*), GB.2 (*ting hui*)

Clinical notes

- The dizziness of this pattern may be associated with hypertension, menopausal syndrome or transitory ischaemic attacks.
- May respond well to correct and prolonged treatment, however unresponsive or persisent high blood pressure requires further investigation.

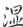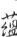

19.4 PHLEGM DAMP

Pathophysiology
- Dizziness caused by Phlegm Damp may present in two ways. The first is a pure excess of Phlegm Damp, the second presents as a mixture of Phlegm Damp and Spleen *qi* deficiency. In the excess pattern, overconsumption in general, particularly of fatty foods and dairy products, generates Phlegm Damp with little or no underlying deficiency. If the Phlegm persists the Spleen will eventually be weakened and will contribute to the ongoing production of Phlegm Damp (Fig. 19.3).
- Phlegm can cause dizziness by obstructing the passage of *qi* and 'clear *yang*' to the head, or by accumulating in the head and settling over the senses like a 'mist'. In the latter case, the Phlegm is often carried to the head with rising *yang* or Wind (Wind Phlegm), and indeed Phlegm frequently occurs with Liver *yang*. The pent up *yang* may be pre-existing, or the presence of Phlegm can cause stagnation and obstruct the *qi*, which at some point of critical intensity escapes and ascends as rising *yang*. In the head, Phlegm obstructs the ascent of 'clear *yang*' and the descent of 'turbid *yin*' leading to an imbalance in distribution of *yin* and *yang*, and relatively severe dizziness or vertigo.

Clinical features
- dizziness or vertigo, sometimes enough to make the patient fall over
- the dizziness may be triggered by movement of the head or strong smells, or have no obvious trigger; the sensation is sometimes likened to being on a ship, or having the world spin around–even in bed, there may be 'bedspins'
- tinnitus, usually during episodes of dizziness
- nausea or vomiting
- poor appetite
- poor concentration, woolly headedness, or a sensation of the head being 'wrapped in a wet cloth'
- frontal headaches
- fullness and discomfort in the chest and epigastrium
- heaviness in the body, lethargy
- frequent desire to sleep

T pale and swollen, with a greasy white coat
P slippery or soft and soggy

Treatment principle
Dry Dampness, transform Phlegm
Strengthen the Spleen and harmonise the Stomach

Prescription

BAN XIA BAI ZHU TIAN MA TANG 半夏白术天麻汤
(*Pinellia and Gastrodia Combination*)

ban xia* (Rhizoma Pinelliae Ternatae) 半夏	9g
bai zhu (Rhizoma Atractylodes Macrocephalae) 白术	12g
tian ma (Rhizoma Gastrodiae Elatae) 天麻	6g
chen pi (Pericarpium Citri Reticulatae) 陈皮	6g
fu ling (Sclerotium Poria Cocos) 茯苓	9g
gan cao (Radix Glycyrrhizae Uralensis) 甘草	3g
sheng jiang (Rhizoma Zingiberis Officinalis) 生姜	3pce
da zao (Fructus Zizyphi Jujubae) 大枣	3pce

Method: Decoction. (Source: *Shi Yong Fang Ji Xue*)

Modifications

- With severe dizziness and nausea, increase the dose of **tian ma** (Rhizoma Gastrodiae Elatae) 天麻 to 9g, and add one or two of the following herbs: **dai zhe shi** (Haematitum) 代赭石 15g, **xuan fu hua** (Flos Inulae) 旋复花 9g, **jiang can**^ (Bombyx Batryticatus) 僵蚕 9g or **dan nan xing*** (Pulvis Arisaemae cum Felle Bovis) 胆南星 6g.
- If the tongue coat is very thick, wet and greasy (indicating severe Dampness and fluid metabolism dysfunction), combine with **WU LING SAN** (*Hoelen Five Formula* 五苓散, p.50).
- With frontal headache, add **bai zhi** (Radix Angelicae Dahuricae) 白芷 9g
- With *qi* deficiency (shortness of breath, low voice, sweating during the day) add **dang shen** (Radix Codonopsis Pilosulae) 党参 15g and **huang qi** (Radix Astragali Membranacei) 黄芪 15g.
- With epigastric fullness and loss of appetite, add **bai dou kou** (Fructus Amomi Kravanh) 白豆蔻 6g and **sha ren** (Fructus Amomi) 砂仁 6g.
- If tinnitus is severe and persistent, add **shi chang pu** (Rhizoma Acori Graminei) 石菖蒲 6g.

Variations and additional prescriptions

Phlegm Heat

- Hot Phlegm is a frequent complication of Phlegm Damp, as the resulting obstruction easily generates Heat. The main features are flushing during episodes of dizziness, anxiety, palpitations, nausea, a slippery rapid pulse and greasy yellow tongue coat. The correct treatment is to resolve Hot Phlegm with **WEN DAN TANG** 温胆汤 (*Bamboo and Hoelen Combination*) modified.

zhu ru (Caulis Bambusae in Taeniis) 竹茹	6g
zhi shi (Fructus Immaturus Citri Aurantii) 枳实	6g
ban xia* (Rhizoma Pinelliae Ternatae) 半夏	6g

chen pi (Pericarpium Citri Reticulatae) 陈皮 6g
fu ling (Sclerotium Poria Cocos) 茯苓 6g
gan cao (Radix Glycyrrhizae Uralensis) 甘草 3g
sheng jiang (Rhizoma Zingiberis Officinalis) 生姜 3pce
huang qin (Radix Scutellariae Baicalensis) 黄芩 9g
shi chang pu (Rhizoma Acori Graminei) 石菖蒲 6g
huang lian (Rhizoma Coptidis) 黄连 6g
tian zhu huang (Concretio Silicea Bambusae Textillis)
   天竺黄 6g

Method: Decoction. (Source: *Shi Yong Zhong Yi Nei Ke Xue*)

Spleen deficiency with Phlegm Damp

♦ If Spleen deficiency is the source of the Phlegm, the correct treatment is to strengthen the Spleen to resolve Phlegm with **LIU JUN ZI TANG** (*Six Major Herbs Combination* 六君子汤) modified.

   chao bai zhu (dry fried Rhizoma Atractylodes Macrocephalae)
      炒白术 12g
   zhi huang qi (honey fried Radix Astragali Membranacei)
      炙黄芪 12g
   fu ling (Sclerotium Poria Cocos) 茯苓 12g
   ren shen (Radix Ginseng) 人参 9g
   ban xia* (Rhizoma Pinelliae Ternatae) 半夏 9g
   chen pi (Pericarpium Citri Reticulatae) 陈皮 6g

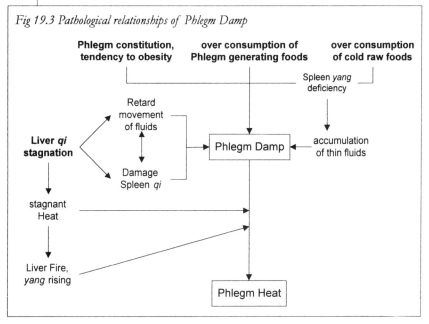

Fig 19.3 *Pathological relationships of Phlegm Damp*

19. DIZZINESS, VERTIGO

  zhu ru (Caulis Bambusae in Taeniis) 竹茹 6g
  dan nan xing* (Pulvis Arisaemae cum Felle Bovis)
   胆南星 6g
  bai jie zi (Semen Sinapsis Albae) 白芥子 6g
  zhi gan cao (honey fried Radix Glycyrrhizae Uralensis)
   炙甘草 6g
  Method: Decoction. (Source: *Shi Yong Zhong Yi Nei Ke Xue*)

Spleen yang deficiency with Phlegm Fluids

- Spleen *yang* deficiency can give rise to thin fluids causing dizziness, fullness in the chest and epigastrium, palpitations, shortness of breath, cough with thin sputum, a pale swollen tongue and a slippery pulse. The correct treatment is to warm and transform Phlegm and fluids, and strengthen the Spleen with **LING GUI ZHU GAN TANG** (*Atractylodes and Hoelen Combination* 苓桂术甘汤) modified.

  fu ling (Sclerotium Poria Cocos) 茯苓 12g
  bai zhu (Rhizoma Atractylodes Macrocephalae) 白术 9g
  gui zhi (Ramulus Cinnamomi Cassiae) 桂枝 6g
  zhi gan cao (honey fried Radix Glycyrrhizae Uralensis)
   炙甘草 3g
  gan jiang (Rhizoma Zingiberis Officinalis) 干姜 6g
  zhi fu zi* (Radix Aconiti Carmichaeli Praeparata) 制附子 3g
  bai jie zi (Semen Sinapsis Albae) 白芥子 6g
  Method: Decoction. Zhi fu zi is cooked for 30 minutes prior to the other herbs (*xian jian* 先煎). (Source: *Shi Yong Zhong Yi Nei Ke Xue*)

Patent medicines

 Er Chen Wan 二陈丸 (Er Chen Wan)
 Xiang Sha Liu Jun Zi Wan 香砂六君子丸 (Xiang Sha Liu Jun Wan)
  - Spleen deficiency with Phlegm
 Fu Zi Li Zhong Wan 附子理中丸 (Li Chung Yuen Medical Pills)

Acupuncture

 St.8 (*tou wei*), Ren.12 (*zhong wan*), Sp.5 (*shang qiu*), PC.6 (*nei guan*), PC.5 (*jian shi*), GB.40 (*qiu xu*), St.40 (*feng long* -), St.41 (*jie xi* -)
  • with Spleen deficiency add Bl.20 (*pi shu* +) and St.36 (*zu san li* +)

Clinical notes

- The dizziness or vertigo of this pattern may be associated with Meniere's disease, benign positional vertigo, hypertension or chronic congestion of the middle ear.
- This pattern can respond well to correct treatment and dietary modification.

LIVER

瘀血阻络

19.5 BLOOD STAGNATION

Pathophysiology
- Dizziness due to Blood stagnation may be acute or chronic. When acute, there will be a history of head trauma; when chronic, there is often a long history of Liver *qi* stagnation (and frequently depression). The presence of stagnant Blood obstructs the free movement of *qi* and Blood and the distribution of *yin* and *yang*.

Clinical features
- dizziness
- stubborn headache that is fixed and boring
- forgetfulness
- insomnia, restless sleep
- palpitations
- depression, low spirits, irritability, mood swings
- dark or purplish lips, complexion or sclera, dark rings under the eyes, or spider naevi on the cheeks and nose

T purplish or dark with brown or purple petichial spots
P wiry, choppy or thready

Treatment principle
Invigorate Blood, eliminate Blood stasis
Regulate *qi* and clear the channels

Prescription

XUE FU ZHU YU TANG 血府逐瘀汤
(*Achyranthes and Persica Combination*)

sheng di (Radix Rehmanniae Glutinosae) 生地	12g
tao ren (Semen Persicae) 桃仁	12g
hong hua (Flos Carthami Tinctorii) 红花	9g
chuan niu xi (Radix Cyathulae Officinalis) 川牛膝	9g
dang gui (Radix Angelicae Sinensis) 当归	9g
chi shao (Radix Paeoniae Rubrae) 赤芍	9g
chuan xiong (Radix Ligustici Chuanxiong) 川芎	6g
zhi ke (Fructus Citri Aurantii) 枳壳	6g
jie geng (Radix Platycodi Grandiflori) 桔梗	6g
chai hu (Radix Bupleuri) 柴胡	6g
gan cao (Radix Glycyrrhizae Uralensis) 甘草	3g

Method: Decoction. (Source: *Shi Yong Zhong Yi Nei Ke Xue*)

Modifications

- With *qi* deficiency (tiredness, easy sweating and shortness of breath), add **huang qi** (Radix Astragali Membranacei) 黄芪 24-30g to tonify *qi* and move Blood.
- With Cold, add **zhi fu zi*** (Radix Aconiti Carmichaeli Praeparata) 制附子 6g cooked for 30 minutes prior to the other herbs and **gui zhi** (Ramulus Cinnamomi Cassiae) 桂枝 9g.
- With bone steaming fever, delete **chai hu**, **jie geng** and **zhi ke**, and add **mu dan pi** (Cortex Moutan Radicis) 牡丹皮 9g, **zhi mu** (Rhizoma Anemarrhenae Asphodeloidis) 知母 9g and **huang bai** (Cortex Phellodendri) 黄柏 9g.

Variations and additional prescriptions

- Dizziness that occurs post partum (with signs of Blood stagnation) may be the result of obstruction to the complete discharge of *chong mai qi* downwards by retained birth products, causing the obstructed *qi* that accumulates in the lower *jiao* to rebel upwards towards the head. The correct approach is to gently move stagnant Blood and regulate *qi* and Blood with **QING HUN SAN** (*Clear the Hun Powder* 清魂散) modified.

ren shen (Radix Ginseng) 人参	9g
jing jie (Herba seu Flos Schizonepetae Tenuifolia) 荆芥	9g
ze lan (Herba Lycopi Lucidi) 泽兰	9g
dang gui (Radix Angelicae Sinensis) 当归	9g
yan hu suo (Rhizoma Corydalis Yanhusuo) 延胡索	9g
mo yao (Myrrha) 没药	6g
chuan xiong (Radix Ligustici Chuanxiong) 川芎	6g
gan cao (Radix Glycyrrhizae Uralensis) 甘草	3g

    Method: Decoction. (Source: *Shi Yong Zhong Yi Nei Ke Xue*)

Patent medicines

Xue Fu Zhu Yu Wan 血府逐瘀丸 (Xue Fu Zhu Yu Wan)

Acupuncture

Points of pain on the head (*ah shi*), Bl.17 (*ge shu*), Sp.6 (*san yin jiao* -), LI.4 (*he gu* -), Liv.4 (*zhong du* -), Liv.3 (*tai chong* -), SI.6 (*yang lao* -)

Clinical notes

- The dizziness of this pattern may be associated with post traumatic shock syndrome, post concussion syndrome, tumours, chronic depression or chronic migraines.
- Acute cases generally respond well depending on the severity of the trauma; chronic cases can be difficult to treat successfully.

气血亏虚

19.6 *QI* AND BLOOD DEFICIENCY

Pathophysiology
- There are two mechanisms that may contribute to dizziness in this pattern. First, *qi* and Blood can be weak or of poor quality, and thus unable to properly nourish the brain. Second, *qi* and Blood may fail to reach the head at all due to functional weakness of the Heart and Spleen–the *zang* primarily responsible for correct distribution of *qi* and Blood.

Clinical features
- dizziness that is usually mild and postural, worse with rising from sitting or lying down, or when fatigued
- palpitations with or without anxiety
- anxiety, phobias, panic attacks
- forgetfulness, poor memory
- blurring vision, spots before the eyes
- insomnia
- fatigue and lethargy
- low spirits or depression
- pale, sallow complexion, pale lips and nails
- poor appetite
- dry skin and hair
- heavy or prolonged menstrual periods, easy bruising

T pale and maybe swollen with little coat
P thready and weak

Treatment principle
Tonify *qi* and Blood
Strengthen the Spleen and Stomach

Prescription

GUI PI TANG 归脾汤
(*Ginseng and Longan Combination*)

zhi huang qi (honey fried Radix Astragali Membranacei) 炙黄芪	15g
suan zao ren (Semen Zizyphi Spinosae) 酸枣仁	12g
fu ling (Sclerotium Poria Cocos) 茯苓	12g
dang shen (Radix Codonopsis Pilosulae) 党参	12g
chao bai zhu (dry fried Rhizoma Atractylodes Macrocephalae) 炒白术	9g
dang gui (Radix Angelicae Sinensis) 当归	9g
long yan rou (Arillus Euphoriae Longanae) 龙眼肉	9g

> **yuan zhi** (Radix Polygalae Tenuifoliae) 远志 6g
> **mu xiang** (Radix Aucklandiae Lappae) 木香 5g
> **zhi gan cao** (honey fried Radix Glycyrrhizae Uralensis)
> 炙甘草 5g
> Method: Decoction. (Source: *Shi Yong Zhong Yao Xue*)

Modifications

- If the Spleen is particularly weak, with loose stools, abdominal bloating and loss of appetite, use **chao dang gui** (dry fried Radix Angelicae Sinensis) 炒当归, increase the dose of **mu xiang** to 9g, and add **shan yao** (Radix Dioscoreae Oppositae) 山药 12g and **shen qu** (Massa Fermentata) 神曲 9g.
- With Spleen *yang* deficiency (cold extremities, cold abdomen on palpation and a desire for warm drinks), add **rou gui** (Cortex Cinnamomi Cassiae) 肉桂 3g and **gan jiang** (Rhizoma Zingiberis Officinalis) 干姜 6g or use **FU ZI LI ZHONG WAN** (*Aconite, Ginseng and Ginger Formula* 附子理中丸, p.56) as guiding formula.
- With easy sweating and frequent colds, increase the dosage of **huang qi** to 24g, and add **ma huang gen** (Radix Ephedrae) 麻黄根 9g and **wu wei zi** (Fructus Schizandrae Chinensis) 五味子 6g, or use **BU ZHONG YI QI TANG** (*Ginseng and Astragalus Combination* 补中益气汤, p.394).
- With Blood deficiency (pale lips and nails, frequent dizziness, insomnia with anxiety and palpitations), add **shu di** (Radix Rehmanniae Glutinosae Conquitae) 熟地 15g and **e jiao^** (Gelatinum Corii Asini) 阿胶 9g the latter dissolved in the strained decoction.

Variations and additional prescriptions

- Other applicable formulae, depending on the mixture of deficiency, include **BA ZHEN TANG** (*Ginseng and Dang Gui Eight Combination* 八珍汤, p.726) and **SHI QUAN DA BU TANG** (*Ginseng and Dang Gui Ten Combination* 十全大补汤, p.529), the latter if there are cold signs.

Following a haemorrhage

- If the dizziness follows a haemorrhage (either postpartum or post traumatic), the correct approach is to first powerfully tonify *qi* and Blood with **DANG GUI BU XUE TANG** (*Tangkuei Decoction to Tonify the Blood* 当归补血汤).

> **huang qi** (Radix Astragali Membranacei) 黄芪 30g
> **dang gui** (Radix Angelicae Sinensis) 当归 6g
> Method: Decoction. (Source: *Formulas and Strategies*)

Patent medicines

Gui Pi Wan 归脾丸 (Gui Pi Wan)

- Heart and Spleen deficiency
Ba Zhen Wan 八珍丸 (Ba Zhen Wan)
 - *qi* and Blood deficiency
Shi Quan Da Bu Wan 十全大补丸 (Shi Quan Da Bu Wan)
 - *qi* and Blood deficiency with Cold
Bu Zhong Yi Qi Wan 补中益气丸 (Bu Zhong Yi Qi Wan)
 - Spleen *qi* sinking
Bu Nao Wan 补脑丸 (Cerebral Tonic Pills)
 - Heart and Kidney deficiency with *shen* disturbance
Dang Gui Ji Jing 当归鸡精 (Tang Kuei Essence of Chicken)
 - a liquid extract that is especially good postpartum

Acupuncture
Sp.6 (*san yin jiao* +▲), Bl.20 (*pi shu* +), St.36 (*zu san li* +▲), Ren.6 (*qi hai* +▲), Du.20 (*bai hui* +▲)
- with palpitations, add PC.6 (*nei guan*) and Bl.15 (*xin shu* +)
- with insomnia, add Ht.7 (*shen men* +) and *an mian* (N-HN-54)

Clinical notes
- The dizziness of this pattern may be associated with anaemia, thrombocytopoenia, hypotension and post-partum convalescence.
- In general, this pattern takes longer to treat satisfactorily than the excess patterns, but does respond well to correct and prolonged treatment.

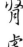

19.7 KIDNEY DEFICIENCY

19.7.1 Kidney *yin* deficiency
Pathophysiology
- Dizziness due to Kidney *yin* deficiency is a pure deficient pattern. In contrast to the previous pattern of Liver and Kidney *yin* deficiency with *yang* rising, characterised by severe episodic dizziness, Kidney *yin* deficiency dizziness is mild and occurs with exertion and fatigue.
- The type of dizziness described here is either a manifestation of deficient Heat rising to the head and disturbing the sensory orifices, or of inadequate Kidney *jing*. When *jing* is weak or insufficient, its function of producing Marrow is weakened, and this weakness leads to malnourishment of the 'sea of marrow', that is, the brain.

Clinical features
- mild dizziness that is worse with sex, overexertion and late nights
- low grade fever, afternoon feverishness
- sensation of heat in the palms and soles ('five hearts hot')
- malar or facial flushing
- forgetfulness and poor memory
- tiredness, fatigue
- insomnia
- tinnitus
- lower back soreness and weakness, heel pain
- tendency to constipation

T red with little or no coat
P thready and rapid

Treatment principle
Tonify and nourish Kidney *yin*

Prescription

ZUO GUI WAN 左归丸
(*Achyranthes and Rehmannia Formula*) modified

shu di (Radix Rehmanniae Glutinosae Conquitae) 熟地	240g
shan yao (Radix Dioscoreae Oppositae) 山药	120g
shan zhu yu (Fructus Corni Officinalis) 山茱萸	120g
gou qi zi (Fructus Lycii) 枸杞子	120g
tu si zi (Semen Cuscutae Chinensis) 菟丝子	120g
lu jiao jiaoˆ (Cornu Cervi Gelatinum) 鹿角胶	120g
gui ban jiao° (Plastri Testudinis Gelatinum) 龟板胶	120g
niu xi (Radix Achyranthis Bidentatae) 牛膝	90g

zhi mu (Rhizoma Anemarrhenae Asphodeloidis) 知母 90g
huang bai (Cortex Phellodendri) 黄柏 90g
dan shen (Radix Salviae Miltiorrhizae) 丹参 90g

Method: Grind the herbs to a powder and form into 9-gram pills with honey. The dose is one pill 2-3 times daily. May also be decocted with a 90% reduction in dosage. When decocted **lu jiao jiao** and **gui ban jiao** are melted before being added to the strained decoction (*yang hua* 烊化). (Source: *Shi Yong Zhong Yi Nei Ke Xue*)

Modifications
- If the dizziness is relatively severe, add **long gu**^ (Os Draconis) 龙骨 60g, **mu li**^ (Concha Ostreae) 牡蛎 60g and **ci shi** (Magnetitum) 磁石 60g.

Patent medicines
Liu Wei Di Huang Wan 六味地黄丸 (Liu Wei Di Huang Wan)
Zhi Bai Ba Wei Wan 知柏八味丸 (Zhi Bai Ba Wei Wan)
  - with deficient Heat
Er Long Zuo Ci Wan 耳聋左慈丸 (Tso-Tzu Otic Pills)
  - with tinnitus
Ming Mu Di Huang Wan 明目地黄丸 (Ming Mu Di Huang Wan)
  - with visual disturbances
Qi Ju Di Huang Wan 杞菊地黄丸 (Lycium-Rehmannia Pills)
  - Liver and Kidney *yin* deficiency

19.7.2 Kidney *yang* deficiency
Pathophysiology
- Kidney *yang* deficiency causes dizziness less frequently than *yin* deficiency. When Kidney *yang* is weak, the 'clear *yang*' (of consciousness) is unable to ascend fully to the head and invigorate the sensory orifices.

Clinical features
- dizziness that is generally mild and aggravated or initiated by exertion
- poor memory
- mental and physical fatigue
- loss of hearing acuity
- cold extremities, cold intolerance
- low libido
- fluid retention
- nocturia
- lower back and knees cold, sore and weak

T swollen and pale
P deep and thready

Treatment principle
Warm the Kidneys and support *yang*

Prescription

YOU GUI WAN 右归丸
(*Eucommia and Rehmannia Formula*)

shu di (Radix Rehmanniae Glutinosae Conquitae) 熟地	240g
chao shan yao (dry fried Radix Dioscoreae Oppositae) 炒山药	120g
du zhong (Cortex Eucommiae Ulmoidis) 杜仲	120g
gou qi zi (Fructus Lycii) 枸杞子	120g
tu si zi (Semen Cuscutae Chinensis) 菟丝子	120g
lu jiao jiao^ (Cornu Cervi Gelatinum) 鹿角胶	120g
shan zhu yu (Fructus Corni Officinalis) 山茱萸	90g
dang gui (Radix Angelicae Sinensis) 当归	90g
rou gui (Cortex Cinnamomi Cassiae) 肉桂	60-120g
zhi fu zi* (Radix Aconiti Carmichaeli Praeparata) 制附子	60-180g

Method: Grind the herbs to a powder and form into 9-gram pills with honey. The dose is one pill 2-3 times daily. May also be decocted with a 90% reduction in dosage, in which case **zhi fu zi** is cooked for 30 minutes prior to adding the other herbs (*xian jian* 先煎), and **lu jiao jiao** is melted before being added to the strained decoction (*yang hua* 烊化). (Source: *Shi Yong Zhong Yi Nei Ke Xue*)

Modifications

* If the *yang* is very weak, add two or three of the following herbs: **xian ling pi** (Herba Epimedii) 仙灵脾 90g, **xian mao** (Rhizoma Curculiginis Orchioidis) 仙茅 90g, **ba ji tian** (Radix Morindae Officinalis) 巴戟天 90g, or **rou cong rong** (Cistanches Deserticolae) 肉苁蓉 120g.
* If the dizziness is relatively severe, add **long gu^** (Os Draconis) 龙骨 60g, **mu li^** (Concha Ostreae) 牡蛎 60g and **ci shi** (Magnetitum) 磁石 60g.

Patent medicines

Jin Kui Shen Qi Wan 金匮肾气丸 (Sexoton Pills)
You Gui Wan 右归丸 (You Gui Wan)
Ba Ji Yin Yang Wan 巴戟阴阳丸 (Ba Ji Yin Yang Wan)
Zhuang Yao Jian Shen Pian 庄腰健肾片 (Zhuang Yao Jian Shen)

Acupuncture

Kidney *yin* deficiency
Bl.23 (*shen shu* +), Ren.4 (*guan yuan* +), Kid.3 (*tai xi* +), Kid.6 (*zhao hai*), Lu.7 (*lie que*), *tai yang* (M-HN-9), Bl.15 (*xin shu* +)

Kidney *yang* deficiency

Du.20 (*bai hui* ▲), Bl.23 (*shen shu* +▲), Ren.4 (*guan yuan* +▲), Du.4 (*ming men* +▲), SI.3 (*hou xi*), Bl.62 (*shen mai*), Kid.3 (*tai xi* +)

Clinical notes

- The dizziness of this pattern may be associated with chronic nephritis, diabetes mellitus, hypothyroidism, hyperthyroidism, hyperaldosteronism, pituitary hypofunction, hypertension or hypotension
- Dizziness related to Kidney deficiency patterns can respond well to treatment, although in general Kidney *yin* deficiency patterns require more prolonged treatment than *yang* deficiency patterns.

SUMMARY OF GUIDING FORMULAE FOR DIZZINESS

Excess patterns

Liver *qi* stagnation - *Xiao Yao Wan* 逍遥丸
  • following unresolved Wind invasion (*shao yang* syndrome) - *Xiao Chai Hu Tang* 小柴胡汤

Liver *yang* rising - *Tian Ma Gou Teng Yin* 天麻钩藤饮
  • Liver Fire - *Long Dan Xie Gan Tang* 龙胆泻肝汤
  • Liver Wind - *Ling Yang Jiao Tang* 羚羊角汤

Liver and Kidney *yin* deficiency with *yang* rising
  - *Zhen Gan Xi Feng Tang* 镇肝熄风汤

Phlegm Damp - *Ban Xia Bai Zhu Tian Ma Tang* 半夏白术天麻汤
  • with fluid metabolism dysfunction plus *Wu Ling San* 五苓散
  • Phlegm Heat - *Wen Dan Tang* 温胆汤
  • with predominant Spleen deficiency - *Liu Jun Zi Tang* 六君子汤
  • with thin fluids - *Ling Gui Zhu Gan Tang* 苓桂术甘汤

Blood stagnation - *Xue Fu Zhu Yu Tang* 血府逐瘀汤
  • post partum - *Qing Hun San* 清魂散

Deficient patterns

Qi and Blood deficiency - *Gui Pi Tang* 归脾汤
  • with cold - *Li Zhong Wan* 理中丸
  • predominant *qi* deficiency - *Bu Zhong Yi Qi Tang* 补中益气汤
  • following haemorrhage - *Dang Gui Bu Xue Tang* 当归补血汤

Kidney deficiency
  • *yin* deficiency - *Zuo Gui Wan* 左归丸
  • *yang* deficiency - *You Gui Wan* 右归丸

Endnote

For more information regarding herbs marked with an asterisk*, an open circle° or a hat^, see the tables on pp.944-952.

Disorders of the Liver

20. Hypochondriac Pain

Liver *qi* stagnation
Liver and Gall Bladder Damp Heat
Liver *yin* (Blood) deficiency
Blood stagnation

Appendix – Gallstones

20 | HYPOCHONDRIAC PAIN
xie tong 胁痛

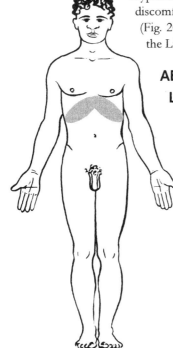

Figure 20.1 The hypochondriac region

Hypochondriac pain describes pain, aching or discomfort over and beneath the costal margin (Fig. 20.1). The area is primarily influenced by the Liver and Gall Bladder and their channels.

AETIOLOGY
Liver *qi* stagnation

Frustration, anger, resentment, prolonged emotional turmoil, repressed emotions and stress disrupt the circulation of Liver *qi*, which accumulates in the Liver causing pain. *Qi* stagnation is frequently complicated by a variety of other disorders that can also cause pain. Chronic *qi* stagnation can generate Heat, which, depending on duration and the intensity of the aetiological conditions, can develop into stagnant Heat or the more severe Fire. Long term *qi* stagnation can also lead to Blood stagnation. Stagnant Liver *qi* can disrupt the Spleen, weakening it and leading to the development of Dampness, which may then combine with any Heat in the system causing Damp Heat.

Damp Heat

There are two types of Damp Heat that cause hypochondriac pain - external and internal. The external variety of Damp Heat is a common seasonal pathogen in hot humid climates. Damp Heat has an affinity with several systems, particularly the Liver and Gall Bladder, Urinary Bladder and Intestines. In this case, the Liver and Gall Bladder are primarily affected, the presence of Damp Heat interrupting the circulation of *qi* and Blood at the level of the hypochondrium, causing pain. This type is usually acute and often follows symptoms of an external (*tai yang*) Wind attack.

Damp Heat is generated internally by simple overeating, or overconsumption of rich, greasy or spicy foods and especially alcohol, or by the accumulation of Dampness, which occurs if the Spleen is already weakened. Prolonged stagnation of Dampness easily produces Heat. This type is chronic and develops slowly.

Liver *yin* and Blood deficiency

Liver *yin* deficiency may be primary or, perhaps more commonly, secondary to Kidney *yin* deficiency. Liver *yin* deficiency may be an extension of Liver Blood deficiency, or follow any Liver Heat pattern, especially Liver Fire. Liver Blood deficiency can result from decreased production of Blood (due to Spleen *qi* deficiency), blood loss following trauma or childbirth, or overuse of the eyes. Long term stagnation of Liver *qi* can also damage Liver Blood, or, if stagnant Heat is generated, Liver *yin*.

BOX 20.1 SOME BIOMEDICAL CAUSES OF HYPOCHONDRIAC PAIN

- acute and chronic hepatitis
- cirrhosis of the liver
- cholecystitis
- gallstones
- intercostal neuralgia
- shingles
- parasitic diseases of the liver
- liver cancer
- gastric ulcer disease
- alcoholic liver disease
- leaking duodenal ulcer
- acute pancreatitis
- coronary thrombosis
- pyelonephritis
- renal colic
- trauma

Stagnant Blood

The stagnant Blood type hypochondriac pain may be acute or chronic. When acute, it is due to traumatic injury. When chronic, it is usually due to other prolonged Liver diseases such as Liver *qi* stagnation or Damp Heat that can secondarily lead to Blood stasis. Stagnant Blood is a common complicating feature of other prolonged Liver pathology.

BOX 20.2 KEY DIAGNOSTIC POINTS

Pain
- intermittent aching or distending pain, difficult to localise and clearly related to emotions - Liver *qi* stagnation
- fixed, stabbing pain that is easy to localise and is worse with pressure and at night - Blood stagnation
- dull ache, which is relieved by pressure and worse when stressed or fatigued - Liver *yin* deficiency
- continuous severe pain and fullness, worse for pressure - Damp Heat

Aggravation
- emotions and stress - Liver qi stagnation, *yin* (Blood) deficiency
- with palpation - Blood stagnation, Damp Heat, *qi* stagnation (up to a

肝气郁结胁痛

20.1 LIVER *QI* STAGNATION

Pathophysiology
- In this pattern Liver *qi* stagnation affects the distribution of *qi* and Blood through the hypochondriac region. *Qi* accumulates at the level of the Liver beneath the ribs, giving rise to the typical ache, fullness and distension associated with stagnant Liver *qi*.
- Liver *qi* stagnation is often complicated by Blood or *yin* deficiency. Prolonged *qi* stagnation can damage Liver Blood, first by weakening the source of Blood, namely the Spleen, and second by direct damage. The excess, in the form of stagnant *qi*, upsets the balance between the *yin* (that is the Blood) and *yang* (*qi*) of the Liver, with an excess of *yang* relative to *yin* and thus a relative deficiency of Liver Blood.
- Long term *qi* stagnation can generate Heat, which over time can damage Liver *yin*. The progression between Liver *qi* stagnation, stagnant Heat, and *yin* deficiency is commonly observed in the clinic.

Clinical features
- hypochondriac pain, ache, fullness or discomfort, usually on the right side, clearly related to the emotional state
- frequent sighing and belching
- fullness or tightness in the chest
- depression, irritability, moodiness
- dizziness
- headaches
- irregular menstruation, pre-menstrual breast tenderness
- shoulder and neck tension
- alternating constipation and loose stools, poor appetite

T normal or dark (*qing* 青)
P wiry

Treatment principle
Soothe the Liver and regulate *qi*

Prescription

CHAI HU SHU GAN SAN 柴胡疏肝散
(*Bupleurum and Cyperus Formula*)

This is an excellent formula for regulating and moving Liver *qi*, particularly when associated with muscular tension and pain. Its primary focus in this pattern is to 'soften' the Liver and relieve constraint.

    chai hu (Radix Bupleuri) 柴胡 9g
    cu bai shao (vinegar fried Radix Paeoniae Lactiflora)
        醋白芍 9g

xiang fu (Rhizoma Cyperi Rotundi) 香附 9g
zhi ke (Fructus Citri Aurantii) 枳壳 6g
chuan xiong (Radix Ligustici Chuanxiong) 川芎 6g
gan cao (Radix Glycyrrhizae Uralensis) 甘草 3g

Method: Decoction or as powder. (Source: *Shi Yong Zhong Yi Nei Ke Xue*)

YUE JU WAN 越鞠丸
(Escape Restraint Pill)

This elegant formula is particularly good for *qi* stagnation with depression. It is classically indicated for 'the six stagnations' (*liu yu* 六郁)–*qi*, Blood, Fire, food, Phlegm and Dampness. The base formula is altered depending on which of the six stagnations is prominent (see modifications below).

chuan xiong (Radix Ligustici Chuanxiong) 川芎 100g
xiang fu (Rhizoma Cyperi Rotundi) 香附 100g
cang zhu (Rhizoma Atractylodis) 苍术 100g
shen qu (Massa Fermentata) 神曲 100g
shan zhi zi (Fructus Gardeniae Jasminoides) 山栀子 ... 100g

Method: Grind the herbs to powder and form into 6-gram pills with water. The dose is one pill 2-3 times daily. May also be decocted with a 90% reduction in dosage. (Source: *Shi Yong Fang Ji Xue*)

Modifications (applicable to YUE JU WAN).
All doses 100g unless otherwise stated

- If general *qi* stagnation is predominant, add **yu jin** (Tuber Curcumae) 郁金, **mu xiang** (Radix Aucklandiae Lappae) 木香 and **wu yao** (Radix Linderae Strychnifoliae) 乌药.
- With Liver *qi* stagnation, add **chai hu** (Radix Bupleuri) 柴胡 and **bai shao** (Radix Paeoniae Lactiflora) 白芍.
- With Blood stagnation, add **tao ren** (Semen Persicae) 桃仁 and **hong hua** (Flos Carthami Tinctorii) 红花.
- With Damp stagnation, add **hou po** (Cortex Magnoliae Officinalis) 厚朴 and **fu ling** (Sclerotium Poria Cocos) 茯苓.
- With Fire, add **huang lian** (Rhizoma Coptidis) 黄连 60g and **qing dai** (Pulverata Indigo) 青黛 20g.
- With food stagnation, add **shan zha** (Fructus Crataegi) 山楂 and **mai ya** (Fructus Hordei Vulgaris Germinantus) 麦芽 150g.
- With fluid retention, add **ze xie** (Rhizoma Alismatis Orientalis) 泽泻, **che qian zi** (Semen Plantaginis) 车前子 and **fu ling** (Sclerotium Poria Cocos) 茯苓.
- With Phlegm, add **ban xia*** (Rhizoma Pinelliae Ternatae) 半夏, **dan nan xing*** (Pulvis Arisaemae cum Felle Bovis) 胆南星 60g and **gua lou** (Fructus Trichosanthis) 瓜楼.
- With Cold, add **wu zhu yu** (Fructus Evodiae Rutaecarpae) 吴茱萸 60g

and **gan jiang** (Rhizoma Zingiberis Officinalis) 干姜 60g.
- With severe fullness and distension, add **hou po** (Cortex Magnoliae Officinalis) 厚朴, **bing lang** (Semen Arecae Catechu) 槟榔, **zhi ke** (Fructus Citri Aurantii) 枳壳 and **qing pi** (Pericarpium Citri Reticulatae Viride) 青皮.

XIAO YAO SAN 逍遥散
(Bupleurum and Dang Gui Formula) modified

This very popular formula is used for cases of Liver *qi* stagnation with Spleen *qi* and Blood deficiency. It is a mild fomula and, in contrast to the previous two (with no tonifying aspects), it is suitable for prolonged use. Particularly good for patterns characterised by hypochondriac and breast pain, dizziness, irregular periods and a tongue with pale edges.

chai hu (Radix Bupleuri) 柴胡	9g
dang gui (Radix Angelicae Sinensis) 当归	9g
bai shao (Radix Paeoniae Lactiflorae) 白芍	9g
bai zhu (Rhizoma Atractylodes Macrocephalae) 白术	9g
fu ling (Sclerotium Poria Cocos) 茯苓	9g
xiang fu (Rhizoma Cyperi Rotundi) 香附	9g
fo shou (Fructus Citri Sarcodactylis) 佛手	9g
dan shen (Radix Salviae Miltiorrhizae) 丹参	12g
dang shen (Radix Codonopsis Pilosulae) 党参	12g
zhi gan cao (honey fried Radix Glycyrrhizae Uralensis) 炙甘草	6g

Method: Decoction or pills. (Source: *Formulas and Strategies*)

Modifications (applicable to all three above formulae, where not already included)

- When the pain is severe, add two or three of the following herbs: **chuan lian zi*** (Fructus Meliae Toosendan) 川楝子 9g, **yan hu suo** (Rhizoma Corydalis Yanhusuo) 延胡索 9g, **mo yao** (Myrrha) 没药 6g, **ru xiang** (Gummi Olibanum) 乳香 6g, **qing pi** (Pericarpium Citri Reticulatae Viride) 青皮 6g and **bai jie zi** (Semen Sinapsis Albae) 白芥子 6g.
- With nausea and vomiting, add **xuan fu hua** (Flos Inulae) 旋复花 9g, **ban xia*** (Rhizoma Pinelliae Ternatae) 半夏 9g and **sheng jiang** (Rhizoma Zingiberis Officinalis) 生姜 3pce.
- If there is Liver Heat disturbing the Stomach, with indeterminate gnawing hunger, acid reflux, vomiting, belching and bitter taste in the mouth, add **huang lian** (Rhizoma Coptidis) 黄连 6g and **wu zhu yu** (Fructus Evodiae Rutaecarpae) 吴茱萸 3g.
- With acid reflux, add **hai piao xiao**ˆ (Os Sepiae seu Sepiellae) 海螵蛸 9g and **mu li**ˆ (Concha Ostreae) 牡蛎 15g.

♦ When *qi* stagnation generates stagnant Heat with increased hypochondriac pain, irritability, facial flushing, dry mouth, red, sore eyes, a yellow tongue coat and a wiry, rapid pulse, add two or three of the following herbs: **mu dan pi** (Cortex Moutan Radicis) 牡丹皮 9g, **shan zhi zi** (Fructus Gardeniae Jasminoides) 山栀子 9g, **yu jin** (Tuber Curcumae) 郁金 9g, **chuan lian zi*** (Fructus Meliae Toosendan) 川楝子 9g, **ju hua** (Flos Chrysanthemi Morifolii) 菊花 9g or **gou teng** (Ramulus Uncariae cum Uncis) 钩藤 9g.

Variations and additional prescriptions

With Liver Fire
♦ Liver Fire can complicate long standing or severe Liver *qi* stagnation, causing intense hypochondriac pain, headache, constipation, concentrated urine, tinnitus, thirst, a rapid, full, wiry pulse and a red tongue. The correct treatment is to clear Liver Fire with **LONG DAN XIE GAN TANG** (*Gentiana Combination* 龙胆泻肝汤 p.571).

Following and unresolved Wind attack
♦ Hypochondriac pain following an unresolved Wind Cold invasion and accompanied by alternating fever and chills, dry throat, dizziness, irritability, nausea, anorexia and a wiry pulse is *shao yang* syndrome. The correct treatment is to harmonise *shao yang* with **XIAO CHAI HU TANG** (*Minor Bupleurum Combination* 小柴胡汤, p.54). This is also a very useful liver protecting formula for asymptomatic hepatitis, particularly Hepatitis C.

With gallstones
♦ If there are gallstones, combine with **SAN JIN TANG** (*Three Golden Herbs Decoction* 三金汤, p.583).

With Blood stagnation
♦ If there is some Blood stagnation (secondary to *qi* stagnation) and Spleen deficiency with intense hypochondriac pain, irritability, insomnia, fatigue, poor appetite, loose stools and epigastric fullness, the correct treatment is to spread Liver *qi*, regulate the Spleen, nourish and invigorate Blood with **SHU GAN LI PI TANG** (*Spread the Liver and Regulate the Spleen Decoction* 疏肝理脾汤).

    dang shen (Radix Codonopsis Pilosulae) 党参 15g
    chai hu (Radix Bupleuri) 柴胡 12g
    bai zhu (Rhizoma Atractylodes Macrocephalae) 白术 12g
    he shou wu (Radix Polygoni Multiflori) 何首乌 12g
    dan shen (Radix Salviae Miltiorrhizae) 丹参 12g
    xiang fu (Rhizoma Cyperi Rotundi) 香附 9g
    ze xie (Rhizoma Alismatis Orientalis) 泽泻 9g
    san qi fen (powdered Radix Notoginseng) 三七粉 3g

Method: Decoction. Powdered **san qi** is usually added to the strained decoction (*chong fu* 冲服). (Source: *Formulas and Strategies*)

With Spleen deficiency
- If the Spleen is predominantly weak, 'inviting' the invasion of Liver *qi*, which results in dull hypochondriac pain, fatigue, poor appetite, shortness of breath, low voice, abdominal distension, tightness in the epigastrium, a pale swollen tongue and a weak pulse, the correct approach is to strengthen the Spleen and regulate Liver *qi* with **SI JUN ZI TANG** (*Four Major Herbs Combination* 四君子汤) modified.

    ren shen (Radix Ginseng) 人参 9g
    bai zhu (Rhizoma Atractylodes Macrocephalae) 白术 9g
    fu ling (Sclerotium Poria Cocos) 茯苓 12g
    bai shao (Radix Paeoniae Lactiflorae) 白芍 12g
    chai hu (Radix Bupleuri) 柴胡 9g
    zhi gan cao (honey fried Radix Glycyrrhizae Uralensis)
    炙甘草 3g

Method: Decoction.

Patent medicines

Chai Hu Shu Gan Wan 柴胡舒肝丸 (Chai Hu Shu Gan Wan)
Xiao Yao Wan 逍遥丸 (Xiao Yao Wan)
Shu Gan Wan 舒肝丸 (Shu Gan Wan)
    - for *qi* stagnation with severe pain and no Heat
Long Dan Xie Gan Wan 龙胆泻肝丸 (Long Dan Xie Gan Wan)
    - Liver Fire
Xiang Sha Yang Wei Wan 香砂养胃丸 (Xiang Sha Yang Wei Wan)
    - with Spleen deficiency
Xiao Chai Hu Wan 小柴胡丸 (Xiao Chai Hu Wan)

Acupuncture

Liv.14 (*qi men* -), SJ.6 (*zhi gou* -), GB.34 (*yang ling quan* -), Liv.2 (*xing jian* -), PC.6 (*nei guan* -), GB.40 (*qiu xu* -)

Clinical notes

- Biomedical conditions that may present as *qi* stagnation hypochondriac pain include hepatitis, pleurisy, gastritis, chronic cholecystitis, gastric ulcers and stress.
- Acupuncture usually proves very effective in the treatment of hypochondriac pain related to simple *qi* stagnation. When Liver Blood or *yin* are damaged, herbs may need to be added.
- Stress management may be useful in recurrent cases.

20.2 LIVER AND GALL BLADDER DAMP HEAT
Pathophysiology
- Hypochondriac pain due to Damp Heat in the Liver and Gall Bladder may be due to an external or internally generated pathogen. The external pattern is mostly acute and due to invasion by pathogenic Damp Heat. In biomedical terms, it frequently corresponds to viral hepatitis. Invasion of Damp Heat may be associated with humid climates, but also describes transmission of Damp Heat through contaminated food and water, sexual intercourse, blood transfusion, and intravenous drug use.
- Internal Damp Heat may be acute, but is much more likely to be chronic and is usually the result of overindulgence in alcohol and rich heating foods. Whatever the origin of the Damp Heat, it lodges in the Liver/Gall Bladder, disrupting the circulation of *qi* and Blood.

Clinical features
- hypochondriac pain, usually right sided and worse for pressure
- fever, or fever and chills, or alternating fever and chills
- irritability, easily angered
- thirst, poor appetite, nausea, vomiting, bitter taste in the mouth
- fullness or stuffiness in the chest and abdomen
- possibly mild jaundice
- dark, concentrated or painful urination
- constipation or loose stools

T red with a thick, greasy yellow coat
P floating and rapid, or wiry and rapid

Treatment principle
Clear and drain Dampness and Heat, stop pain

Prescription

LONG DAN XIE GAN TANG 龙胆泻肝汤
(*Gentiana Combination*)

jiu long dan cao (wine fried Radix Gentianae Longdancao) 酒龙胆草	6-9g
huang qin (Radix Scutellariae Baicalensis) 黄芩	9g
shan zhi zi (Fructus Gardeniae Jasminoides) 山栀子	9g
ze xie (Rhizoma Alismatis Orientalis) 泽泻	9g
che qian zi (Semen Plataginis) 车前子	9g
sheng di (Radix Rehmanniae Glutinosae) 生地	9g
dang gui (Radix Angelicae Sinensis) 当归	6g
mu tong (Caulis Mutong) 木通	6g
chai hu (Radix Bupleuri) 柴胡	6g

肝胆湿热胁痛

gan cao (Radix Glycyrrhizae Uralensis) 甘草 6g
Method: Decoction. **Che qian zi** is decocted in a muslin bag (*bao jian*). (Source: *Shi Yong Zhong Yao Xue*)

Modifications

- With severe pain, add **chuan lian zi*** (Fructus Meliae Toosendan) 川楝子 10g and **yan hu suo** (Rhizoma Corydalis Yanhusuo) 延胡索 10g.
- With constipation, add **da huang** (Radix et Rhizoma Rhei) 大黄 6-9g and **mang xiao** (Mirabilitum) 芒硝 6g.
- With fever and jaundice, add **yin chen** (Herba Artemisiae Yinchenhao) 茵陈 30g and **huang bai** (Cortex Phellodendri) 黄柏 10g or select **YIN CHEN HAO TANG** (*Capillaris Combination* 茵陈蒿汤, p.594).
- Intermittent boring hypochondriac pain, possible vomiting of worms, jaundice and alternating fever and chills, suggests roundworm infestation and bile duct obstruction. Look for ascarid eggs in the stools. If present, combine with **DAN DAO QU HUI TANG** (*Decoction for Expelling Roundworms from the Bile Duct* 胆道驱蛔汤, p.602).
- If the Damp Heat is associated with gallstones, see p.581.

Patent medicines

Long Dan Xie Gan Wan 龙胆泻肝丸 (Long Dan Xie Gan Wan)
Ji Gu Cao Wan 鸡骨草丸 (Jigucao Wan)
Ji Gu Cao Chong Ji 鸡骨草冲剂 (Ji Gu Cao Infusion)
Xi Huang Cao 溪黄草 (Xi Huang Cao Chong Ji)
Li Dan Pian 利胆片 (Lidan Tablets)

Acupuncture

Liv.14 (*qi men* -), SJ.6 (*zhi gou* -), GB.34 (*yang ling quan* -), GB.24 (*ri yue* -), Liv.3 (*tai chong* -), GB.43 (*xie xi* -), Bl.18 (*gan shu* -), Bl.19 (*dan shu* -)
- with severe fever add Du.14 (*da zhui*)-) and LI.11 (*qu chi* -)
- alternating fever and chills, add SJ.5 (*wai guan* -) and GB.39 (*xuan zhong* -)
- with nausea add PC.6 (*nei guan* -)
- with jaundice add Du.9 (*zhi yang* -)

Clinical notes

- This pattern may be associated with acute viral hepatitis, alcholism, alcoholic hepatitis, acute cholecystitis, pancreatitis, gallstones, shingles and round worms in the bile duct.
- Acute external Damp Heat is relatively easy to cure and TCM treatment is very effective. Chronic Damp Heat is more difficult to resolve, and usually involves significant modifications to diet and lifestyle in addition to herbs for adequate results.

20.3 LIVER *YIN* (BLOOD) DEFICIENCY

Pathophysiology
- The hypochondriac pain due to Liver *yin* (Blood) deficiency is generally mild, and reflects a lack of nourishment of the Liver and Tendons. In addition, when Liver *yin* and Blood are deficient, Liver *qi* is relatively predominant and prone to stagnation. This causes two types of pain–a dull, aching background pain (from *yin* and Blood deficiency), and one that is occasionally severe and provoked by stress (*qi* stagnation).

Clinical features
- mild, dull, right sided hypochondriac pain aggravated or provoked by stress and relieved by pressure
- dry mouth and throat, thirst
- irritability and restlessness
- dizziness
- insomnia
- blurring vision; dry, red, sore eyes
- acid reflux

T red with little or no coat
P thready, wiry and rapid

Treatment principle
Nourish Liver *yin*, soothe the Liver

Prescription

YI GUAN JIAN 一贯煎
(*Linking Decoction*) modified

This is a particularly good formula for Liver *yin* deficiency with *qi* stagnation. Note that the *qi* moving herbs are mild and not very dispersing to either *qi* or *yin*.

sheng di (Radix Rehmanniae Glutinosae) 生地	18-45g
gou qi zi (Fructus Lycii) 枸杞子	9-18g
sha shen (Radix Adenophorae seu Glehniae) 沙参	9g
mai dong (Tuber Ophiopogonis Japonici) 麦冬	9g
dang gui (Radix Angelicae Sinensis) 当归	9g
chuan lian zi* (Fructus Meliae Toosendan) 川楝子	9g
he huan hua (Flos Albizziae Julibrissin) 合欢花	9g
bai ji li (Fructus Tribuli Terrestris) 白蒺藜	9g
mei gui hua (Flos Rosae Rugosae) 玫瑰花	6g

Method: Decoction. (Source: *Shi Yong Zhong Yi Nei Ke Xue*)

肝阴血不足胁痛

QI JU DI HUANG WAN 杞菊地黄丸
(*Lycium, Chrysanthemum and Rehmannia Formula*)

This formula is used when the Liver and Kidney *yin* deficiency is prominent, with little or no stagnation. The hypochondriac pain is mild, dull and in the background, and there will generally be deeper *yin* deficiency signs— night sweating, flushing, heat in the palms and soles, red dry eyes, lower back pain.

shu di (Radix Rehmanniae Glutinosae Conquitae) 熟地	240g
shan yao (Radix Dioscoreae Oppositae) 山药	120g
shan zhu yu (Fructus Corni Officinalis) 山茱萸	120g
fu ling (Sclerotium Poria Cocos) 茯苓	90g
ze xie (Rhizoma Alismatis Orientalis) 泽泻	90g
mu dan pi (Cortex Moutan Radicis) 牡丹皮	90g
gou qi zi (Fructus Lycii) 枸杞子	90g
ju hua (Flos Chrysanthemi Morifolii) 菊花	90g

Method: Grind the herbs to powder and form into 9-gram pills with honey. The dose is 2-3 pills daily. May also be decocted with a 90% reduction in dosage.

Modifications
- With severe pain, add **bai shao** (Radix Paeoniae Lactiflorae) 白芍 15g and **gan cao** (Radix Glycyrrhizae Uralensis) 甘草 6g.
- With irritability, add **suan zao ren** (Semen Zizyphi Spinosae) 酸枣仁 12g and **dan shen** (Radix Salviae Miltiorrhizae) 丹参 12g.
- With dizziness and blurred vision, add **sang zhi** (Ramulus Mori Albae) 桑枝 15g and **nu zhen zi** (Fructus Ligustri Lucidi) 女贞子 15g.

Variations and additional prescriptions
- If Blood deficiency is prominent (usually with Liver *qi* stagnation), the signs and symptoms are mild hypochondriac pain, dizziness, insomnia, depression, blurring vision, numbness in the extremities, fatigue, irregular menstruation, a pale tongue and thready, possibly wiry pulse. The correct treatment is to nourish Blood, strengthen the Spleen and move Liver *qi* with **XIAO YAO SAN** (*Bupleurum and Dang Gui Formula* 逍遥散, p.568).

Patent medicines
Qi Ju Di Huang Wan 杞菊地黄丸 (Lycium-Rehmannia Pills)
Ming Mu Di Huang Wan 明目地黄丸 (Ming Mu Di Huang Wan)
Er Long Zuo Ci Wan 耳聋左慈丸 (Er Long Zuo Ci Wan)

Acupuncture
Bl.23 (*shen shu* +), Bl.18 (*gan shu* +), Bl.17 (*ge shu* +), Liv.8 (*qu quan*), Liv.14 (*qi men* -), GB.43 (*xia xi* -), Liv.3 (*tai chong*), Kid.3 (*tai xi*)

Clinical notes
- The hypochondriac pain of this pattern may be associated with disorders like chronic hepatitis, chronic cholecystitis, cirrhosis, intercostal neuralgia or gastric ulcers.
- Care must be taken in this pattern (especially *yin* deficiency) to avoid using strong *qi* moving herbs as they can easily disperse *qi* and *yin* and cause aggravation of the symptoms.

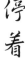

20.4 BLOOD STAGNATION

Pathophysiology
- Hypochondriac pain from Blood stagnation can be acute or chronic. The acute pattern is the direct result of a traumatic injury. The chronic pattern typically follows some other long term Liver pathology, such as prolonged Liver *qi* stagnation or Damp Heat. When chronic, it usually involves a fairly serious stage of Liver pathology, like liver cirrhosis or cancer.

Clinical features
- fixed, stabbing hypochondriac pain that is worse at night and with pressure
- dark or purplish spider naevi or broken vessels over the ribs, on the face and around the inner ankle and knee, especially around the Kid.3 (*tai xi*) and Sp.9 (*yin ling quan*) area
- mild feverishness at night, without sweating
- pain in the iliac fossae with palpation
- palpable masses under the ribs
- dry mouth and throat with no desire to drink
- dry, scaly skin
- dull, sallow or darkish complexion
- dark ring around the eyes
- dark or purplish lips and conjunctiva

T purplish or with purple or brown petechial spots with little or no coat
P thready and choppy

Treatment Principle
Invigorate Blood, eliminate Blood stagnation
Regulate *qi*, stop pain

Prescription

XUE FU ZHU YU TANG 血府逐瘀汤
(*Achyranthes and Persica Combination*)

This formula is excellent for general Blood (and *qi*) stagnation, especially in the chest and head. It is best for Blood stasis with signs of Heat.

tao ren (Semen Persicae) 桃仁 12g
dang gui (Radix Angelicae Sinensis) 当归 9g
sheng di (Radix Rehmanniae Glutinosae) 生地 9g
hong hua (Flos Carthami Tinctorii) 红花 9g
chuan niu xi (Radix Cyathulae Officinalis) 川牛膝 9g
zhi ke (Fructus Citri Aurantii) 枳壳 6g
chi shao (Radix Paeoniae Rubrae) 赤芍 6g

jie geng (Radix Platycodi Grandiflori) 桔梗 6g
chuan xiong (Radix Ligustici Chuanxiong) 川芎 6g
chai hu (Radix Bupleuri) 柴胡 6g
gan cao (Radix Glycyrrhizae Uralensis) 甘草 3g
Method: Decoction. (Source: *Shi Yong Fang Ji Xue*)

GE XIA ZHU YU TANG 膈下逐瘀汤
(*Drive Out Blood Stasis Below the Diaphragm Decoction*)

This formula is specific for *qi* and Blood stagnation in the area below the diaphragm, especially with severe pain and palpable masses.

chao wu ling zhi^ (dry fried Excrementum Trogopteri seu Pteromi) 炒五灵脂 9g
dang gui (Radix Angelicae Sinensis) 当归 9g
tao ren (Semen Persicae) 桃仁 9g
hong hua (Flos Carthami Tinctorii) 红花 9g
chi shao (Radix Paeoniae Rubrae) 赤芍 9g
xiang fu (Rhizoma Cyperi Rotundi) 香附 9g
wu yao (Radix Linderae Strychnifoliae) 乌药 9g
gan cao (Radix Glycyrrhizae Uralensis) 甘草 9g
chuan xiong (Radix Ligustici Chuanxiong) 川芎 6g
mu dan pi (Cortex Moutan Radicis) 牡丹皮 6g
zhi ke (Fructus Citri Aurantii) 枳壳 6g
cu yan hu suo (vinegar fried Rhizoma Corydalis Yanhusuo) 醋延胡索 6g
Method: Decoction. (Source: *Shi Yong Fang Ji Xue*)

Modifications (apply to the two previous formulae)
- With severe pain, add two or three of the following herbs: **yu jin** (Tuber Curcumae) 郁金 9g, **chuan lian zi*** (Fructus Meliae Toosendan) 川楝子 9g, **mo yao** (Myrrha) 没药 9g, **ru xiang** (Gummi Olibanum) 乳香 9g or **xie bai** (Bulbus Allii) 薤白 6g.
- With palpable masses beneath the ribs, or if the liver is enlarged and nodular, add **san leng** (Rhizoma Sparganii Stoloniferi) 三棱 9g, **e zhu** (Rhizoma Curcumae Ezhu) 莪术 9g and **di bie chong^** (Eupolyphaga seu Opisthoplatia) 地鳖虫 3g, or for severe cases combine with **DA HUANG ZHE CHONG WAN** (*Rhubarb and Eupolyphaga Pill* 大黄䗪虫丸, p.612) or **BIE JIA WAN** (*Turtle Shell Pills* 鳖甲丸).
   zhi bie jia° (honey fried Carapax Amydae Sinensis) 炙鳖甲 120g
   duan wa leng zi^ (calcined Concha Arcae) 煅瓦楞子 120g
   chao mai ya (dry fried Fructus Hordei Vulgaris Germinantus) 炒麦芽 60g

cu san leng (vinegar fried Rhizoma Sparganii Stoloniferi)
醋三棱 60g
cu e zhu (vinegar fried Rhizoma Curcumae Ezhu)
醋莪术 60g
di bie chong^ (Eupolyphaga seu Opisthoplatia) 地鳖虫 60g
zhi xiang fu (Rhizoma Cyperi Rotundi) 制香附 30g
qing pi (Pericarpium Citri Reticulatae Viride) 青皮 30g

Method: Grind herbs to a powder and form into 9-gram pills with honey. The dose is one pill 2-3 times daily. This is a useful formula for hepatosplenomegaly following hepatitis, cirrhosis and malaria. It may be combined with an appropriate tonic formula to protect *zheng qi* (Source: *Shi Yong Zhong Yao Xue*)

FU YUAN HUO XUE TANG 复元活血汤
(*Revive Health by Invigorating the Blood Decoction*)

This formula is selected for Blood stagnation hypochondriac pain following a traumatic injury. It is usually only used for a couple of weeks, depending on how acute the trauma is. Initially, the patient should experience loose stools or diarrhoea as the bruising and pain resolve.

jiu da huang (wine fried Radix et Rhizoma Rhei) 大黄 6-10g
chai hu (Radix Bupleuri) 柴胡 12g
dang gui (Radix Angelicae Sinensis) 当归 9g
tao ren (Semen Persicae) 桃仁 9g
tian hua fen (Radix Trichosanthes Kirilowii) 天花粉 9g
hong hua (Flos Carthami Tinctorii) 红花 6g
chuan shan jia° (Squama Manitis) 穿山甲 6g
gan cao (Radix Glycyrrhizae Uralensis) 甘草 3g

Method: Decoction. (Source: *Shi Yong Fang Ji Xue*)

Patent medicines

Xue Fu Zhu Yu Wan 血府逐瘀丸 (Xue Fu Zhu Yu Wan)
Nei Xiao Luo Li Wan 内消瘰疬丸 (Nei Xiao Luo Li Wan)
Gui Zhi Fu Ling Wan 桂枝茯苓丸 (Gui Zhi Fu Ling Wan)

Acupuncture

Liv.14 (*qi men* -), Liv.13 (*zhang men* -), Sp.21 (*da bao* -), SJ.6 (*zhi gou* -), GB.34 (*yang ling quan* -), Liv.3 (*tai chong* -), Bl.17 (*ge shu* -), Bl.18 (*gan shu* -)
- If post-traumatic, add points of tenderness (*ah shi*)
- With severe pain, add LI.4 (*he gu* -) and Liv.6 (*zhong du* -)

Clinical notes

- The hypochondriac pain of the pattern may be associated with disorders like cirrhosis, chronic hepatitis, liver cancer, trauma,

intercostal neuralgia, costochondritis, gastric ulcers, post herpetic neuralgia, chronic malaria, hepatosplenomegaly and post surgical pain (i.e. cholecystectomy, splenectomy etc.)
- Acute pain from trauma responds quickly to TCM treatment; chronic Blood stagnation pain can be difficult to treat successfully and prolonged and persistent treatment will be necessary. In cases of cancer, TCM should be combined with Western medicine.

SUMMARY OF GUIDING FORMULAE FOR HYPOCHONDRIAC PAIN

Liver *qi* stagnation - *Chai Hu Shu Gan San* 柴胡疏肝散
- with gallstones, plus *San Jin Tang* 三金汤
- Liver Fire - *Long Dan Xie Gan Tang* 龙胆泻肝汤
- with Spleen deficiency and Blood stasis
    - *Shu Gan Li Pi Tang* 疏肝理脾汤
- following unresolved Wind invasion (*shao yang* syndrome)
    - *Xiao Chai Hu Tang* 小柴胡汤
- predominant Spleen deficiency - *Si Jun Zi Tang* 四君子汤

Damp Heat in the Liver and Gall Bladder - *Long Dan Xie Gan Tang* 龙胆泻肝汤
- with roundworms - *Dan Dao Qu Hui Tang* 胆道驱蛔汤
- with gallstones, plus *San Jin Tang* 三金汤
- with jaundice plus *Yin Chen Hao Tang* 茵陈蒿汤

Liver *yin* deficiency - *Yi Guan Jian* 一贯煎

Blood stagnation - *Xue Fu Zhu Yu Tang* 血府逐瘀汤 or *Ge Xia Zhu Yu Tang* 膈下逐瘀汤
- with palpable masses plus *Da Huang Zhe Chong Wan* 大黄蛰虫丸 or *Bie Jia Wan* 鳖甲丸
- following trauma - *Fu Yuan Huo Xue Tang* 复元活血汤

Endnote

For more information regarding herbs marked with an asterisk*, an open circle° or a hat ˆ, see the tables on pp.944-952.

Appendix
GALLSTONES (*dan shi bing* 胆石病)

Gallstones are a common cause of hypochondriac and epigastric pain, and Chinese medicine describes some specific measures that can be applied to treat the stones directly. Gallstones may sit quietly in the gall bladder without causing any symptoms. They are often picked up during a routine ultrasound, and as many as 90% of such cases are asymptomatic, even with large or numerous gallstones.

However, once a stone moves and gets lodged in the neck of the gall bladder, the cystic duct or the common bile duct, it can cause pain and inflammation (Fig 20.2). Inflammation of the neck of the gall bladder or cystic duct, which can develop some hours after obstruction by a stone, is called cholecystitis. The pain is usually of sudden onset (typically after a big meal or at night) and is sustained for several hours. The person is restless, cannot get comfortable, may feel nauseous or vomit. The pain can be felt in the epigastrium or right hypochondrium, and may radiate to the tip of the shoulder. After the pain subsides there is tenderness in the right hypochondrium.

There are two common types of gallstones, classified according to their composition–cholesterol and pigment. Cholesterol stones account for

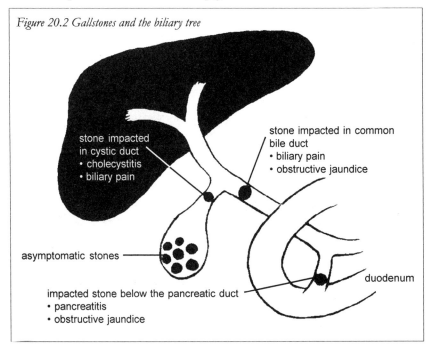

Figure 20.2 Gallstones and the biliary tree

approximately 75% of gallstones in the Western world. The pathophysiology of gallstone development is not clearly understood, but several factors seem to predispose people to stone formation. Gallstones are more common in patients of European origin, women, the obese and those over 40, hence 'fair, fat, female and forty - think gallstones'. Both types of stone appear to be amenable to TCM treatment, but some sources suggest cholesterol stones are easier to break down.

In TCM terms, the development of gallstones is due to prolonged Liver and Gall Bladder *qi* stagnation that causes poor excretion of bile from the gall bladder. The bile eventually condenses into stones. This process is facilitated by the presence of Heat and Dampness, either from a dietary source or from Spleen deficiency.

Acute or recurrent attacks of pain and inflammation from gallstones is usually due to Damp Heat. Less commonly the patient presents with a *shao yang* syndrome, or Liver *qi* stagnation. The *qi* stagnation pattern is seen in those with asymptomatic stones (those detected during routine screening) or in those with only vague and non specific symptoms.

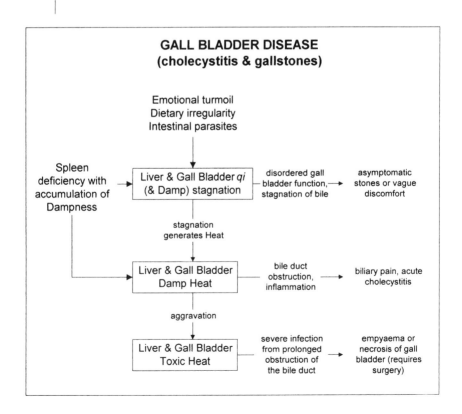

GENERAL TREATMENT

The basic approach, once gallstones have been identified, is to break up the stones (if large), and encourage their expulsion from the gall bladder. A treatment that is popular amongst the physicians of the Red Cross Hospital in Hangzhou, Zhejiang, is a two step program, first reducing the size of the stone or stones, then relaxing the bile duct and promoting contraction of the gall bladder. This treatment is done with the assistance of ultrasound measurement, as the second part of the treatment (the expulsion) should not proceed if the stones are too large (generally larger than 1cm). Once the stone or stones are estimated to be small enough, the risk of impaction in the common bile duct is reduced and the second part of the treatment can proceed.

First stage

In asymptomatic cases, only the following formula (which dissolves stones) is necessary. Where there is an accompanying pattern (usually either Damp Heat or *qi* stagnation), one of the constitutional formulae may be added to the stone dissolving formula. Ideally, the patient should have an ultrasound weekly, and as soon as the stones are small enough the second stage of the treatment can begin. Results can usually be expected within a few weeks.

Prescription

SAN JIN TANG 三金汤
(*Three Golden Herbs Decoction*)

jin qian cao (Herba Lysimachiae) 金钱草 30-60g
hai jin sha (Spora Lygodii Japonici) 海金砂 15g
ji nei jin fen^ (powdered Endothelium Corneum Gigeriae Galli) 鸡内金粉 6g

Method: Decoction. **Ji nei jin** powder is added to the strained decoction for stronger effect (*chong fu* 冲服), **hai jin sha** is decocted in a muslin bag (*bao jian* 包煎). (Source: *Zhong Yi Nei Ke Lin Chuang Shou Ce*)

Second stage

Once the stones are small enough (preferably smaller than 5mm) the second stage of the treatment can proceed. This stage uses herbs with three different actions. Acupuncture can assist at this stage (see below). Clinically, the three groups of herbs are combined and added to whatever other formula (if any) is applicable. If none is applicable they may be used alone. The patient should expect diarrhoea during the treatment, usually a maximum of a few days or until the stones are expelled and observed in the stools. The three groups of herbs are:

1. **wei ling xian*** (Radix Clematidis) 威灵仙 12g to relax the bile duct.

2. **di long^** (Lumbricus) 地龙 12g to stimulate gall bladder contraction.
3. **zhi da huang** (prepared Radix et Rhizoma Rhei) 制大黄 10g, **mang xiao** (Mirabilitum) 芒硝 12g and **gua lou** (Fructus Trichosanthis) 栝楼 30g to open and purge the *fu* (Gall Bladder and Intestines) to facilitate the passage of stones and clear the excess.

Acupuncture

This treatment stimulates the contraction of the gall bladder and relaxes the cystic duct. It is useful in cases of acute biliary pain where the stone or stones are already lodged in the cystic duct. In asymptomatic cases this treatment should only be attempted once the stones are shown to be small enough (smaller than 1cm diameter, ideally less than 0.5 cm) to be expelled safely, and without impaction. Ultrasound can be used to ensure the patient has no other stricture or obstruction further down the biliary tree.

Main points

dan nang xue (M-LE-23) - 1-2 *cun* below GB.34 (*yang ling quan*), GB.24 (*ri yue* -), Bl.19 (*dan shu* -), Liv.14 (*qi men* -), Liv.13 (*zhang men* -) Generally two points are connected to an electrical stimulator, for example, GB.24 (*ri yue*) and *dan nang xue* (M-LE-23) on the right side, and treated with a dense disperse wave. The other points may be selected on the basis of tenderness.
- with severe pain, add LI.4 (*he gu* -)
- with jaundice, add Du.9 (*zhi yang* -)
- with fever, add LI.11 (*qu chi* -)
- with vomiting, add PC.6 (*nei guan*)

Ear points: *shen men*, sympathetic, endocrine, liver, gall bladder, duodenum

1. Damp Heat
Pathophysiology
- The Damp Heat pattern is associated with gallstones accompanied by inflammation or infection in the gall bladder or bile duct. The Damp Heat is often accompanied by disruption of the *shao yang* level, characterised by alternating fever and chills. This often occurs in the early stages of inflammation.

Clinical features
- persisent hypochondriac or epigastric pain or fullness, worse with pressure
- bitter taste in the mouth, nausea, vomiting, aversion to fats, poor appetite

- fever, afternoon fever, or alternating fever and chills
- diarrhoea or constipation

T greasy yellow coat
P slippery or wiry and rapid

Treatment principle

Clear Damp Heat from the Gall Bladder
Promote expulsion of gallstones, clear the Intestines

Prescription

QING DAN XIE HUO TANG 清胆泻火汤
(*Clear the Gall Bladder and Drain Fire Decoction*) modified

This formula is excellent for clearing Damp Heat from the Gall Bladder. If the stones are still too large to attempt the second stage, delete the second stage herbs (the first five), and combine this formula with SAN JIN TANG (*Three Golden Herbs Decoction* 三金汤, p.583).

zhi da huang (prepared Radix et Rhizoma Rhei) 制大黄	10g
mang xiao (Mirabilitum) 芒硝	12g
gua lou (Fructus Trichosanthis) 栝楼	30g
wei ling xian* (Radix Clematidis) 威灵仙	12g
di long^ (Lumbricus) 地龙	12g
chai hu (Radix Bupleuri) 柴胡	15g
huang qin (Radix Scutellariae Baicalensis) 黄芩	15g
ban xia* (Rhizoma Pinelliae Ternatae) 半夏	9g
yin chen (Herba Artemisiae Yinchenhao) 茵陈	30g
shan zhi zi (Fructus Gardeniae Jasminoides) 山栀子	9g
long dan cao (Radix Gentianae Longdancao) 龙胆草	9g
yu jin (Tuber Curcumae) 郁金	9g
mu xiang (Radix Aucklandiae Lappae) 木香	6g
bai shao (Radix Paeoniae Lactiflorae) 白芍	15g
jin yin hua (Flos Lonicerae Japonicae) 金银花	30g
lian qiao (Fructus Forsythiae Suspensae) 连翘	15g

Method: Decoction. For a stronger purge, **da huang** is added towards the end of cooking (*hou xia* 后下). **Mang xiao** is added to the strained decoction (*chong fu* 冲服).

DA CHAI HU TANG 大柴胡汤
(*Major Bupleurum Combination*) modified

This formula can be used for patients with mixed patterns—some Dampness, some *qi* stagnation and a tendency to constipation.

chai hu (Radix Bupleuri) 柴胡	9g

huang qin (Radix Scutellariae Baicalensis) 黄芩 9g
ban xia* (Rhizoma Pinelliae Ternatae) 半夏 9g
bai shao (Radix Paeoniae Lactiflorae) 白芍 9g
zhi shi (Fructus Immaturus Citri Aurantii) 枳实 9g
da huang (Radix et Rhizoma Rhei) 大黄 6-9g
sheng jiang (Rhizoma Zingiberis Officinalis Recens) 生姜 9g
da zao (Fructus Zizyphi Jujubae) 大枣 5pce
Method: Decoction. (Source: *Zhui Xin Fang Ji Shou Ce*)

Modifications

- If there is already diarrhoea, a smaller dose of **da huang**~3g and **mang xiao**~3-6g should be used.
- With severe pain, add **chuan lian zi*** (Fructus Meliae Toosendan) 川楝子 12g and **yan hu suo** (Rhizoma Corydalis Yanhusuo) 延胡索 12g.

Patent medicines

Ji Gu Cao Wan 鸡骨草丸 (Jigucao Wan) or
Long Dan Xie Gan Wan 龙胆泻肝丸 (Long Dan Xie Gan Wan) plus
Li Dan Pian 利胆片 (Lidan Tablets)

Clinical notes

- The is pattern corresponds to disorders such as acute cholecystitis, pancreatitis and biliary colic due to gallstone obstruction.
- Dietary modification is important (see over).

2. Liver *qi* stagnation

Pathophysiology

- The Liver *qi* stagnation pattern involves gallstones without inflammation or infection. The function of the Gall Bladder is impaired and bile has stagnated and accumulated, forming gallstones. The following formula can be used to treat asymptomatic stones.

Clinical features

- If there are symptoms, they tend to be intermittent and mild. There will often be a history of indigestion, flatulence, belching and abdominal discomfort, hypochondriac ache or distension. There may be occasional upper right quadrant pain, which may radiate to the right shoulder.
- aversion to fats and oily food, occasional nausea, poor appetite, irregular bowel movements

T dark or slightly red with a thin white or yellow coat
P wiry, or deep and wiry

Treatment principle

Soothe the Liver, benefit the Gall Bladder
Regulate *qi*, move stagnation, dissolve stones

Prescription

CHAI HU SHU GAN SAN 柴胡疏肝散
(*Bupleurum and Cyperus Formula*) modified

If treating large stones (first stage) combine with SAN JIN TANG (*Three Golden Herbs Decoction* 三金汤, p.583). For second stage treatment combine with second stage herbs, p.584.

- **dan shen** (Radix Salviae Miltiorrhizae) 丹参 15-30g
- **mai ya** (Fructus Hordei Vulgaris Germinantus) 麦芽 12g
- **chai hu** (Radix Bupleuri) 柴胡 9g
- **yu jin** (Tuber Curcumae) 郁金 9g
- **zhi ke** (Fructus Citri Aurantii) 枳壳 9g
- **chi shao** (Radix Paeoniae Rubrae) 赤芍 9g
- **bai zhu** (Rhizoma Atractylodes Macrocephalae) 白术 9g
- **xiang fu** (Rhizoma Cyperi Rotundi) 香附 6g
- **qing pi** (Pericarpium Citri Reticulatae Viride) 青皮 6g
- **ze xie** (Rhizoma Alismatis Orientalis) 泽泻 6g

Method: Decoction. (Source: *Zhong Yi Nei Ke Lin Chuang Shou Ce*)

Modifications

- If there is Heat, with a bitter taste in the mouth, dry throat and thirst, delete **ze xie** and **bai zhu**, and add **long dan cao** (Radix Gentianae Longdancao) 龙胆草 6-9g, **dan zhu ye** (Herba Lophatheri Gracilis) 淡竹叶 6g, **tian hua fen** (Radix Trichosanthes Kirilowii) 天花粉 15g and **tai zi shen** (Radix Pseudostellariae Heterophyllae) 太子参 15g.
- If there is Spleen deficiency, with fatigue, abdominal distension, loose stools and anorexia, delete **xiang fu** and add **dang shen** (Radix Codonopsis Pilosulae) 党参 15g, **fu ling** (Sclerotium Poria Cocos) 茯苓 15g and **shen qu** (Massa Fermentata) 神曲 10g.

Follow up treatment

- Once the stones have resolved, a *qi* regulating formula such as **XIAO YAO SAN** (*Bupleurum and Dang Gui Formula* 逍遥散, p.139), should be given to consolidate the treatment and harmonise the Liver and Gall Bladder.

Patent medicines

Shu Gan Wan 舒肝丸 (Shu Gan Wan) or
Chai Hu Shu Gan Wan 柴胡舒肝丸 (Chai Hu Shu Gan Wan) plus
Li Gan Pian 利肝片 (Liver Strengthening Tablets)

Clinical notes

- This pattern corresponds to disorders such as asymptomatic gallstones or chronic cholecystitis.
- In all patients with gallstones, regulation of the diet is important. Foods to avoid or restrict are those richest in saturated fats and cholesterol–rich meat, dairy products, fried foods, eggs, peanuts and other nuts and seeds. Food items that are beneficial in softening gallstones and aiding the gall bladder are light and easily digested– grains, vegetables, fruits and pulses. Radish, apples, lemons and limes, seaweed, parsnip and tumeric are thought be be especially beneficial.[1]

---

1. from Pitchford P (1993) *Healing with Whole Foods*, North Atlantic Books, Berkely, Ca.

Disorders of the Liver

21. Jaundice

Yang jaundice
Damp Heat
Liver and Gall Bladder stagnant Heat
Toxic Heat

Yin jaundice
Cold Damp
Spleen *qi* and Blood deficiency
Blood stagnation

21 JAUNDICE
huang dan 黄疸

Jaundice is the yellow discolouration of the sclera, skin and mucous membranes resulting from increased concentration of bilirubin in body fluids. In mild cases, jaundice is most apparent in the sclera; in severe cases it can involve the whole body. True jaundice can be distinguished from yellowing of the skin due to other causes, like hypercarotenaemia, by the involvement of the sclera.

In TCM, there are a couple of theoretical mechanisms to account for jaundice, both involving Dampness. The first invokes the Five Phase (*wu xing* 五行) correspondence between earth, the colour yellow, and Dampness. Following this logic, simple accumulation of Dampness in the eyes and skin can lead to varying degrees of yellowing, depending on accompanying pathogens. Dampness plus Heat causes a brighter or orangey tinge to the yellowness, whereas Damp plus Cold causes a duller or 'dirtier' yellow. Cheng Ying-mao observes that "When Heat and Dampness intermingle and cannot find a way out, they will vaporise into yellowishness (jaundice)"...[1]

The second mechanism involves the bile, the 'pure' fluid stored in and excreted from the Gall Bladder. The relationship between bile and the Gall Bladder is very similar to that described in Western medicine, so it has been noted that "Damp Heat steams the Liver and Gall Bladder and forces bile to the surface and eyes, leading to jaundice in these areas"...[2]

The biomedical mechanisms of jaundice are summarised in Table 21.1.

AETIOLOGY

Acute jaundice is mostly due to Dampness and Heat, or in severe or epidemic cases Toxic Heat. The relative proportions of Dampness and Heat can vary, presenting with different clinical features and requiring different treatments. The source of the Damp Heat can be external (most common in acute cases) or internal. Acute jaundice is often described as *yang* jaundice.

If jaundice persists and becomes chronic, the patient is weakened and the pattern will change to one of deficiency or mixed excess and deficiency, usually Cold Damp, Spleen deficiency, *qi* and Blood stagnation or a mixture of all three. This is described as *yin* jaundice.

---

1. *Shang Han Lun* (Treatise on Febrile Diseases Caused by Cold, *c.*210AD) p.243, New World Press, Beijing, PRC
2. Clavey S (1995) *Fluid Physiology and Pathology in Traditional Chinese Medicine*, p.61, Churchill Livingstone, Edinburgh

Damp Heat

Damp Heat jaundice can be externally or internally generated. The external variety is due to invasion of Damp Heat that lodges in the Liver and Gall Bladder. Some commentators suggest that the Damp Heat 'steams' bile to the surface and eyes, others that Dampness and Heat alone are sufficient to produce jaundice. In either case, the end result is jaundice that develops quickly and exhibits a quite intense bright yellow or orange tinge. When external Damp Heat is very intense or epidemic, producing disturbances of consciousness or Wind, it is reclassified as Toxic Heat (see below).

Damp Heat can also be generated internally by overeating, or by overconsumption of alcohol and rich, greasy or spicy foods. Dampness may also develop as a result of Spleen deficiency. When Damp accumulates and stagnates, it can over time generate Heat, or combine with the Heat created by Liver *qi* stagnation to produce Damp Heat. This pattern is more insidious and slower to develop than external Damp Heat, sometimes taking years of steady overconsumption before becoming apparent. Prolonged Damp Heat (usually in combination with Liver *qi* stagnation) can congeal with bile into stones, which cause obstruction and the generation of more Heat.

> **BOX 21.1 SOME BIOMEDICAL CAUSES OF JAUNDICE**
> - acute and chronic hepatitis
> - cirrhosis of the liver
> - cholecystitis
> - gallstones
> - systemic lupus erythematosus
> - tumours of the bile duct
> - parasitic diseases of the liver
> - septicaemia
> - leptospirosis
> - alcoholic liver disease
> - malignancy (pancreatic carcinoma, bilary, hepatocellular, metastasis)
> - biliary atresia
> - haemolytic anaemia
> - sickle cell anaemia
> - pernicious anaemia
> - thalassaemia
> - malaria
> - syphilis
> - cytomegalovirus
> - Gilbert's disease
> - haemochromatosis
> - drug toxicity

Toxic Heat

Toxic Heat is an intense and concentrated variety of Heat or Damp Heat of external origin. It occasionally occurs in epidemics. Toxic Heat is characterised by the severity of the disease, the intense degree of Heat, disturbances of consciousness and the rapid deterioration of the patient.

Spleen deficiency

Deficient types of jaundice often occur if the excess patterns are unresolved or incorrectly treated. In this case, Spleen *qi* can be damaged by the unresolved and persistent Dampness lodged in the middle *jiao*. Spleen *qi* can also be damaged if the bitter cold herbs used to treat Damp Heat are applied over-

BOX 21.2 KEY DIAGNOSTIC POINTS

Duration
- acute, developing quickly – Damp Heat, Toxic Heat
- slow to develop – Cold Damp, Spleen deficiency

The colour of the jaundice
- bright, fresh clear yellow or yellow orange – Damp Heat or Toxic Heat
- dull, darkish yellow or matt yellow – Cold Damp, Spleen deficiency, *qi* and Blood stagnation

enthusiastically or inappropriately. If this occurs, in addition to the Spleen damage, Cold Dampness may be left obstructing the middle *jiao*, further damaging the body's *yang*.

Qi and Blood stagnation

Qi and Blood stagnation occur late in chronic Liver disease, and usually follow prolonged stasis of an unresolved pathogen, usually Damp Heat. At this point significant structural changes have occured in the Liver and associated organs, with the development of masses and swelling.

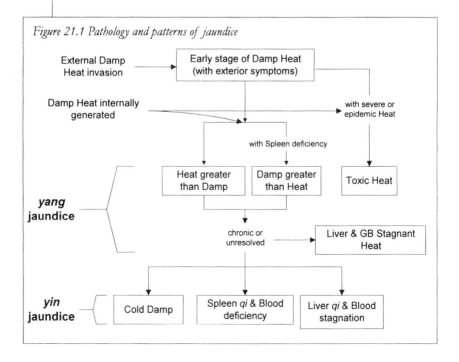

Figure 21.1 *Pathology and patterns of jaundice*

TREATMENT

Jaundice is always associated with Dampness, so the main therapeutic principle is to eliminate Dampness through diuresis. Herbs that clear Heat, or warm Spleen *yang*, are combined with the bland diuretic herbs. When urination increases, the Damp will be discharged downwards carrying Heat or Cold along with it. Clearing Toxic Heat is required in severe cases. Care must be taken when diagnosing acute Damp Heat jaundice to determine the relative degree of Dampness and Heat, so as to balance the mix of cooling and diuretic herbs correctly. Excessive Heat clearing can damage Spleen *yang* and lead to the development of *yin* jaundice; excessive diuresis can damage fluids. Once the Dampness and Heat are clearing, and the jaundice begins to subside, bitter cold herbs should be reduced and replaced by bitter warm parching and Spleen strengthening herbs. The treatment of chronic jaundice requires the Spleen to be strengthened to resolve Dampness, the *qi* and Blood to be tonified, and moving *qi* and Blood stasis.

Table 21.1. Biomedical mechanisms of jaundice

Type of jaundice	Mechanism	Representative diseases
Haemolytic	Results from the destruction of red blood cells & consequent liberation of haemoglobin into the plasma. The catabolic pathways for degradation of haemoglobin are overloaded & unconjugated bilirubin accumulates in the blood.	Systemic Lupus Erythematosus (SLE), haemolytic anaemia
Hepatic	Results from failure of bilirubin transport into the bile due to liver cell damage. When liver cells are damaged, by viral insult, drugs or alcohol, transport of bilirubin across cell membranes may be impaired, or the resulting inflammatory oedema may obstruct biliary canaliculi. Bilirubin backs up & accumulates in the blood.	hepatitis, alcohol toxicity, CCl_4 poisoning
Cholestatic, Post hepatic	Due to obstruction to the passage of bile between the liver hepatocytes & the duodenum. Cholestasis leads to dark urine & pale stools, as bile does not reach the intestine.	hepatitis, cirrhosis, or physical obstruction of the bile duct by gallstones, tumours, parasites, post surgical stricture or inflammation of surrounding structures

21.1 DAMP HEAT (HEAT GREATER THAN DAMPNESS)

热重于湿黄疸

Pathophysiology
- Jaundice due to Damp Heat may be external or internal. The external pattern is generally acute and due to invasion of pathogenic Damp Heat. In biomedical terms it often relates to viral hepatitis. Invasion of Damp Heat may be associated with humid climates, but also describes transmission of Damp Heat through contaminated food and water, sexual intercourse, blood transfusion, and intravenous drug use.
- Internal Damp Heat may be acute or have acute exacerbations, but is much more likely to be chronic and is usually the result of overindulgence in alcohol and rich heating foods. This pattern is also encountered in conditions like gallstones, cholecystitis, pancreatitis and alcoholism. Whatever the origin of the Damp Heat, it lodges in the Liver and Gall Bladder, 'steaming' bile out to the skin and eyes.

Clinical features
- jaundice that is a bright or orangey yellow, apparent in the sclera, mucous membranes or skin
- fever, or alternating fever and chills
- thirst (with desire to drink cold fluids)
- irritability and malaise
- an uncomfortable burning sensation in the chest and epigastrium
- concentrated scanty urination
- constipation or loose stools
- loss of appetite or indeterminate gnawing hunger
- nausea and vomiting
- aversion to cigarette smoke

T greasy, dryish yellow coat
P wiry and rapid, or slippery and rapid

Treatment principle
Clear Heat, eliminate Dampness (through the urine and stools)

Prescription

YIN CHEN HAO TANG 茵陈蒿汤
(*Capillaris Combination*) modified

yin chen (Herba Artemisiae Yinchenhao) 茵陈	30g
bai jiang cao (Herba cum Radice Patriniae) 败酱草	30g
lian qiao (Fructus Forsythiae Suspensae) 连翘	30g
shan zhi zi (Fructus Gardeniae Jasminoides) 山栀子	15g
che qian zi (Semen Plantaginis) 车前子	15g

sheng da huang (Radix et Rhizoma Rhei) 生大黄 10g
gan cao (Radix Glycyrrhizae Uralensis) 甘草 6g
Method: Decoction. Following adminstration of the formula the bowels should open vigorously at least 1-2 times daily, and in general be quite loose. If this does not occur increase the dose of **da huang** (or cook it less) until it does, and continue until the jaundice subsides. **Yin chen** and **da huang** are added towards the end of cooking (*hou xia* 后下), **che qian zi** is cooked in a cloth bag (*bao jian* 包煎). (Source: *Zhong Yi Nei Ke Lin Chuang Shou Ce*)

Modifications

* With nausea and vomiting, add **zhu ru** (Caulis Bambusae in Taeniis) 竹茹 15g and **ban xia*** (Rhizoma Pinelliae Ternatae) 半夏 10g.
* With epigastric and abdominal distension and fullness, add **zhi shi** (Fructus Immaturus Citri Aurantii) 枳实 12g and **hou po** (Cortex Magnoliae Officinalis) 厚朴 9g.
* With hypochondriac pain, add **chai hu** (Radix Bupleuri) 柴胡 10g, **yu jin** (Tuber Curcumae) 郁金 9g and **chuan lian zi*** (Fructus Meliae Toosendan) 川楝子 10g.
* With severe Heat (bitter taste in the mouth, severe thirst for cold fluids and rough dry yellow tongue coat, sore dry eyes and a flooding rapid pulse), add **long dan cao** (Radix Gentianae Longdancao) 龙胆草 9g, **ban lan gen** (Radix Isatidis seu Baphicacanthi) 板蓝根 15g and **hu zhang** (Radix et Rhizoma Polygoni Cuspidati) 虎杖 9g, or combine with **LONG DAN XIE GAN TANG** (*Gentiana Combination* 龙胆泻肝汤, p.571).
* With gallstones, combine with **SAN JIN TANG** (*Three Golden Herbs Decoction* 三金汤, p.583).
* Once the bowels have opened, the Heat has started to subside and the tongue coat has begun to thin, add some herbs to strengthen the Spleen and transform dampness, such as **bai zhu** (Rhizoma Atractylodis Macrocephalae) 白术 12g, **fu ling** (Sclerotium Poria Cocos) 茯苓 12g and **yi ren** (Semen Coicis Lachryma-jobi) 苡仁 18g. At the same time decrease the dosages (or eliminate some entirely) of the bitter cold herbs so as to protect Spleen *yang* and prevent the development of *yin* jaundice.

Patent medicines

Long Dan Xie Gan Wan 龙胆泻肝丸 (Long Dan Xie Gan Wan)
Ji Gu Cao Wan 鸡骨草丸 (Jigucao Wan)
Li Dan Pian 利胆片 (Lidan Tablets)
Xi Huang Cao 溪黄草 (Xi Huang Cao Chong Ji)
Ji Gu Cao Chong Ji 鸡骨草冲剂 (Ji Gu Cao Infusion)

Acupuncture

Du.9 (*zhi yang* -), SI.4 (*wan gu* -), Bl.19 (*dan shu* -), GB.34 (*yang ling quan* -), Sp.9 (*yin ling quan* -), Liv.3 (*tai chong* -)
- severe fever, add Du.14 (*da zhui* -) and LI.11 (*qu chi* -)
- with nausea, add PC.6 (*nei guan* -)
- with hypochondriac pain add Liv.14 (*qi men* -), SJ.6 (*zhi gou* -) and Liv.13 (*zhang men* -)

Clinical notes

- This type of jaundice may be associated with conditions such as acute infectious hepatitis, cholecystitis, gallstones, pancreatitis, leptospirosis, alcoholic or drug induced hepatitis.
- Acute Damp Heat jaundice (particulary the viral hepatitis group and cholecystitis) generally responds well to correct treatment. Once the jaundice has subsided the patient should be reassessed and another appropriate formula prescribed.
- Patients must avoid all alcohol, rich food and liver irritants, such as caffeine and non essential drugs.

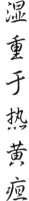

21.2 DAMP HEAT (DAMP GREATER THAN HEAT)

Pathophysiology
- This type of Damp Heat jaundice is similar to the previous Damp Heat pattern, however here the Dampness predominates. The Heat is 'wrapped' by the Damp and the hot manifestations are subdued. The predominance of Dampness also weakens the Spleen and Stomach, or occurs when there is pre-existing Spleen deficiency with internal Damp. Either way, this pattern exhibits a larger number of digestive symptoms than the previous one.

Clinical features
- jaundice
- usually there is no fever, or only mild fever
- the head is heavy and full ('like being wrapped in a wet cloth')
- a sensation of obstruction, fullness or discomfort in the chest and epigastrium
- loss of appetite
- nausea and vomiting
- abdominal distension, loose stools
- thirst with no desire to drink
- scanty concentrated urine
- aversion to cigarette smoke

T flabby with a thick yellow or whitish greasy coat
P soggy and moderate or wiry and slippery

Treatment principle
Eliminate Dampness and turbidity
Promote urination, clear Heat, reduce jaundice

Prescription

YIN CHEN WU LING SAN 茵陈五苓散
(*Capillaris and Hoelen Five Formula*) modified

yin chen (Herba Artemisiae Yinchenhao) 茵陈	30g
fu ling (Sclerotium Poria Cocos) 茯苓	15g
zhu ling (Sclerotium Polypori Umbellati) 猪苓	12g
ze xie (Rhizoma Alismatis Orientalis) 泽泻	12g
bai zhu (Rhizoma Atractylodis Macrocephalae) 白术	12g
huo xiang (Herba Agastaches seu Pogostemi) 藿香	10g
bai dou kou (Fructus Amomi Kravanh) 白豆蔻	6g
gui zhi (Ramulus Cinnamomi Cassiae) 桂枝	6g

Method: Decoction. **Yin chen** is added towards the end of cooking (*hou xia* 后下). (Source: *Zhong Yi Nei Ke Lin Chuang Shou Ce*)

Modifications

- With nausea and vomiting, add **ban xia*** (Rhizoma Pinelliae Ternatae) 半夏 9g and **chen pi** (Pericarpium Citri Reticulatae) 陈皮 9g.
- With food stagnation, add **shen qu** (Massa Fermentata) 神曲 10g, **shan zha** (Fructus Crataegi) 山楂 10g and **mai ya** (Fructus Hordei Vulgaris Germinantus) 麦芽 10g.
- If abdominal distension is relatively severe, add **da fu pi** (Pericarpium Arecae Catechu) 大服皮 10g and **mu xiang** (Radix Aucklandiae Lappae) 木香 6g
- With gallstones, combine with **SAN JIN TANG** (*Three Golden Herbs Decoction* 三金汤, p.583).

Patent medicines

Li Dan Pian 利胆片 (Lidan Tablets)
Ji Gu Cao Wan 鸡骨草丸 (Jigucao Wan)
Long Dan Xie Gan Wan 龙胆泻肝丸 (Long Dan Xie Gan Wan)
Xi Huang Cao 溪黄草 (Xi Huang Cao Chong Ji)
Ji Gu Cao Chong Ji 鸡骨草冲剂 (Ji Gu Cao Infusion)
Xing Jun San 行军散 (Xing Jun San, Five Pagodas Brand)
- This is a generic formula for acute Damp Heat in the digestive system. While not designed for jaundice, it is excellent for the nausea, vomiting and diarrhoea associated with this condition.

Acupuncture

Du.9 (*zhi yang* -), Bl.19 (*dan shu* -), GB.34 (*yang ling quan* -), Liv.3 (*tai chong* -), Sp.9 (*yin ling quan* -), Ren.12 (*zhong wan* -), St.36 (*zu san li* -), Bl.39 (*wei yang* -)
- with nausea, add PC.6 (*nei guan* -)
- with hypochondriac pain, add Liv.14 (*qi men* -), SJ.6 (*zhi gou* -) and Liv.13 (*zhang men* -)

Clinical notes

- This type of jaundice may be associated with conditions such as acute infectious hepatitis, liver cirrhosis, alcoholic or drug induced hepatitis, pancreatitis, chronic hepatitis
- Generally responds well to correct treatment, especially those cases due to viral infection.
- Patients must avoid all alcohol, rich food and liver irritants, such as caffeine and non essential drugs.

21.3 DAMP HEAT WITH EXTERIOR SYMPTOMS (EARLY STAGE EXTERNAL DAMP HEAT)

Pathophysiology
- In this pattern the jaundice is mild or may not yet be evident. Nevertheless, it is included in this chapter because early application of this treatment at times of hepatitis outbreaks may prevent the disease from becoming full blown.

Clinical features
- mild jaundice or no jaundice
- simultaneous fever and chills
- distension and heaviness of the head
- generalised myalgia
- fatigue and lethargy
- poor appetite
- epigastric fullness and discomfort
- concentrated urine
- aversion to cigarette smoke

T thin greasy coat
P floating and rapid or floating and wiry

Treatment principle
Clear Heat, eliminate Dampness
Clear the exterior, promote urination

Prescription

MA HUANG LIAN QIAO CHI XIAO DOU TANG
麻黄连翘赤小豆汤 (*Ma Huang, Forsythia and Aduki Bean Decoction*) plus
GAN LU XIAO DU DAN 甘露消毒丹
(*Sweet Dew Special Pill to Eliminate Toxin*)

yin chen (Herba Artemisiae Yinchenhao) 茵陈	24g
hua shi (Talcum) 滑石	18g
lian qiao (Fructus Forsythiae Suspensae) 连翘	12g
chi xiao dou (Semen Phaseoli Calcarati) 赤小豆	12g
huang qin (Radix Scutellariae Baicalensis) 黄芩	12g
sang bai pi (Cortex Mori Albae Radicis) 桑白皮	9g
xing ren* (Semen Pruni Armeniacae) 杏仁	9g
huo xiang (Herba Agastaches seu Pogostemi) 藿香	9g
she gan (Rhizoma Belamcandae) 射干	9g
bo he (Herba Mentha Haplocalycis) 薄荷	9g
bai dou kou (Fructus Amomi Kravanh) 白豆蔻	9g

ma huang* (Herba Ephedra) 麻黄 6g
shi chang pu (Rhizoma Acori Graminei) 石菖蒲 6g
chuan bei mu (Bulbus Fritillariae Cirrhosae) 川贝母 6g
mu tong (Caulis Mutong) 木通 6g
sheng jiang (Rhizoma Zingiberis Officinalis) 生姜 .... 3 pce
da zao (Fructus Zizyphi Jujubae) 大枣 .... 3 pce
gan cao (Radix Glycyrrhizae Uralensis) 甘草 3g

Method: Decoction. **Yin chen** and **bo he** are added towards the end of cooking (*hou xia* 后下). (Source: *Shi Yong Zhong Yi Nei Ke Xue*)

Modifications

◆ For infectious hepatitis, increase the dose of **yin chen** (Herba Artemisiae Yinchenhao) 茵陈 to 30g, and add **shan zhi zi** (Fructus Gardeniae Jasminoides) 山栀子 9g, **huang bai** (Cortex Phellodendri) 黄柏 9g and **da huang** (Radix et Rhizoma Rhei) 大黄 6g. Once the obvious exterior symptoms have gone delete **ma huang** and **bo he**.

Patent medicines

Ji Gu Cao Wan 鸡骨草丸 (Jigucao Wan)
Li Dan Pian 利胆片 (Lidan Tablets)
Long Dan Xie Gan Wan 龙胆泻肝丸 (Long Dan Xie Gan Wan)
Xi Huang Cao 溪黄草 (Xi Huang Cao Chong Ji)
Ji Gu Cao Chong Ji 鸡骨草冲剂 (Ji Gu Cao Infusion)
Huo Xiang Zheng Qi Pian 藿香正气片 (Huo Hsiang Cheng Chi Pien)

Acupuncture

Lu.6 (*kong zui* -), LI.4 (*he gu* -), Ren.12 (*zhong wan* -),
St.36 (*zu san li* -), SJ.6 (*zhi gou* -)
• if Dampness is severe, add Sp.9 (*yin ling quan* -)
• with fever, add Du.14 (*da zhui* -) and LI.11 (*qu chi* -)
• with diarrhoea, add St.25 (*tian shu* -) and *zhi xie* (N-CA-3)

Clinical notes

• This type of jaundice may be associated with conditions such as early stage of acute infectious hepatitis and leptospirosis.

21.4 LIVER AND GALL BLADDER STAGNANT HEAT (BILE DUCT OBSTRUCTION WITH HEAT)

Pathophysiology
- Jaundice caused by Liver and Gall Bladder stagnant Heat typically involves gallstones, cholecystitis or infestation by round worms (ascariasis). The typical presentation is an acute episode of a chronic or recurrent illness. Usually the patient will have been unwell for some time. See also Gallstones, p.581.

Clinical features
- the jaundice develops relatively quickly and is accompanied by severe, colicky, right sided, hypochondriac pain which may radiate to the right shoulder and upper back; the painful episodes are likely to be recurrent
- fever and chills, or alternating fever and chills
- bitter taste in the mouth
- dry throat and mouth
- nausea and poor appetite
- aversion to fats and oils
- abdominal distension
- pale sticky stools
- scanty concentrated urine, dysuria

T red with a thick yellow coat
P wiry and rapid

Treatment principle
Soothe the Liver and drain the Gall Bladder
Clear Heat and relieve fullness

Prescription

QING DAN XIE HUO TANG 清胆泻火汤
(*Clear the Gall Bladder and Drain Fire Decoction*) modified

yin chen (Herba Artemisiae Yinchenhao) 茵陈	30g
jin qian cao (Herba Lysimachiae) 金钱草	30g
chai hu (Radix Bupleuri) 柴胡	15g
huang qin (Radix Scutellariae Baicalensis) 黄芩	15g
ban xia* (Rhizoma Pinelliae Ternatae) 半夏	9g
shan zhi zi (Fructus Gardeniae Jasminoides) 山栀子	9g
long dan cao (Radix Gentianae Longdancao) 龙胆草	9g
mu xiang (Radix Aucklandiae Lappae) 木香	9g
yu jin (Tuber Curcumae) 郁金	9g
da huang (Radix et Rhizoma Rhei) 大黄	9g

肝胆瘀热黄疸

mang xiao (Mirabilitum) 芒硝 9g
Method: Decoction. **Da huang** is added towards the end of cooking (*hou xia* 后下) and **mang xiao** is dissolved in the strained decoction (*chong fu* 冲服).
(Source: *Formulas and Strategies*)

Modifications

- With Blood stasis (fixed sharp pain, spider naevi over the abdomen and hypochondrium), add **dan shen** (Radix Salviae Miltiorrhizae) 丹参 20g and use **chi shao** (Radix Paeoniae Rubrae) 赤芍 10g instead of **bai shao**.
- With severe Heat, add **jin yin hua** (Flos Lonicerae Japonicae) 金银花 15g, **lian qiao** (Fructus Forsythiae Suspensae) 连翘 9g and **pu gong ying** (Herba Taraxici Mongolici) 蒲公英 15g.
- With severe pain, add **yan hu suo** (Rhizoma Corydalis Yanhusuo) 延胡索 9g and **chuan lian zi*** (Fructus Meliae Toosendan) 川楝子 9g.
- Sudden jaundice, with alternating fever and chills, intermittent boring upper right quadrant pain, and possible vomiting of worms suggests roundworm infestation and bile duct obstruction. Look for ascarid eggs in the stools. Combine with **DAN DAO QU HUI TANG** (*Decoction for Expelling Roundworms from the Bileduct* 胆道驱蛔汤).

  shi jun zi (Fructus Quisqualis Indicae) 使君子 12g
  ku lian pi (Cortex Meliae Radicis) 苦楝皮 9g
  wu mei (Fructus Pruni Mume) 乌梅 9g
  bing lang (Semen Arecae Catechu) 槟榔 9g
  zhi ke (Fructus Citri Aurantii) 枳壳 6g
  mu xiang (Radix Aucklandiae Lappae) 木香 6g
  Method: Decoction. (Source: *Shi Yong Zhong Yao Xue*).

Patent medicines

Ji Gu Cao Wan 鸡骨草丸 (Jigucao Wan)
Li Dan Pian 利胆片 (Lidan Tablets)
Long Dan Xie Gan Wan 龙胆泻肝丸 (Long Dan Xie Gan Wan)
Da Chai Hu Wan 大柴胡丸 (Da Chai Hu Wan)
Chuan Xin Lian Kang Yan Pian 穿心莲抗炎片
  (Chuan Xin Lian Antiphlogistic Tablets)
Niu Huang Qing Huo Wan 牛黄清火丸 (Niu Huang Qing Huo Wan)
  - with severe Heat

Acupuncture

Bl.19 (*dan shu* -), GB.34 (*yang ling quan* -), GB.24 (*ri yue* -),
Liv.14 (*qi men* -), Du.9 (*zhi yang* -), SI.4 (*wan gu* -), Liv.3 (*tai chong* -)
- worms in the bile duct, needle LI.20 (*ying xiang*) through to St.2 (*si bai*)
- with fever, add Du.14 (*da zhui* -) and LI.11 (*qu chi* -)

- with alternating fever and chills, add SJ.5 (*wai guan*) and GB.41 (*zu lin qi*)
- with nausea, add PC.6 (*nei guan* -)

Clinical notes

- This type of jaundice may be associated with conditions such as acute cholecystitis, ascariasis and gallstones.

21.5 TOXIC HEAT

热毒炽盛黄疸

Pathophysiology
- Jaundice due to Toxic Heat is severe and most commonly caused by powerful external Damp Heat pathogens that quickly overwhelm the body's defenses. It typically affects many people and may be epidemic. Toxic Heat may also be seen in late stage liver failure.

Clinical features
- rapidly developing jaundice that quickly deepens in colour to orange or gold
- high fever
- restlessness and irritability
- thirst
- foul breath
- frequent vomiting
- abdominal distension and pain that is worse with pressure
- constipation
- scanty urine or anuria
- in severe cases there may be skin rashes, ecchymosis, epistaxis, haematemesis, bleeding gums, subcutaneous haemorrhages, confusion, delerium, muscular spasms or convulsions

T red or scarlet, or with red edges and a rough, dry, dirty coat
P wiry and rapid, or flooding and big, or wiry, thready and rapid (depending on the degree of damage to body fluids)

Treatment principle
Clear Heat and Toxins
Cool the Blood, support *yin*

Prescription

HUANG LIAN JIE DU TANG 黄连解毒汤
(*Coptis and Scute Combination*) plus
YIN CHEN HAO TANG 茵陈蒿汤 and
(*Capillaris Combination*)
WU WEI XIAO DU YIN 五味消毒饮
(*Five Ingredient Decoction to Eliminate Toxin*) modified

These three formulae combined drain Fire from the *san jiao*, cool the Blood and clear Toxic Heat. This prescription is suitable for less severe cases, those with mild skin eruptions and mental confusion.

    yin chen (Herba Artemisiae Yinchenhao) 茵陈 30g
    da huang (Radix et Rhizoma Rhei) 大黄 9g

shan zhi zi (Fructus Gardeniae Jasminoides) 山栀子	9g
huang qin (Radix Scutellariae Baicalensis) 黄芩	9g
huang bai (Cortex Phellodendri) 黄柏	6g
huang lian (Rhizoma Coptidis) 黄连	3g
jin yin hua (Flos Lonicerae Japonicae) 金银花	15g
pu gong ying (Herba Taraxici Mongolici) 蒲公英	15g
zi hua di ding (Herba cum Radice Violae Yedoensitis) 紫花地丁	15g
ye ju hua (Flos Chrysanthemi Indici) 野菊花	12g
zi bei tian kui (Herba Begoniae Fimbristipulatae) 紫北天葵	9g

Method: Decoction. (Source: *Shi Yong Zhong Yi Nei Ke Xue*)

XI JIAO SAN 犀角散
(*Rhinoceros Horn Powder*) modified

This prescription is suitable for severe cases with bleeding, confusion, convulsions or disturbances of consciousness.

xi jiao° (Cornu Rhinoceri) 犀角	3g
yin chen (Herba Artemisiae Yinchenhao) 茵陈	30g
da qing ye (Folium Daqingye) 大青叶	30g
jin yin hua (Flos Lonicerae Japonicae) 金银花	30g
lian qiao (Fructus Forsythiae Suspensae) 连翘	30g
sheng di (Radix Rehmanniae Glutinosae) 生地	30g
shan zhi zi (Fructus Gardeniae Jasminoides) 山栀子	15g
mu dan pi (Cortex Moutan Radicis) 牡丹皮	15g
xuan shen (Radix Scrophulariae) 玄参	15g
chi shao (Radix Paeoniae Rubrae) 赤芍	15g
huang lian (Rhizoma Coptidis) 黄连	9g
sheng ma (Rhizoma Cimicifugae) 升麻	9g
gan cao (Radix Glycyrrhizae Uralensis) 甘草	6g

Method: Decoction. **Shui niu jiao**^ (Cornu Bubali) 水牛角 is usually substituted for **xi jiao**, with a tenfold increase in dose and cooked for 30 minutes prior to adding the other herbs (*xian jian* 先煎). If the patient is confused or unable to ingest the medicine, the formula can be delivered via a nasogastric tube, or a resuscitation medicine can be given until consciousness is restored (see below). (Source: *Zhong Yi Nei Ke Lin Chuang Shou Ce*).

Variations and additional prescriptions

- If there is delirium, impaired consciousness and confusion, the patent medicines **AN GONG NIU HUANG WAN** (*Calm the Palace Pill with Cattle Gallstone* 安宫牛黄丸, p.914) or **ZHI BAO DAN** (*Greatest Treasure Special Pill* 至宝丹, p.660) are used to open the orifices and clear Heat. If the patient is unable to ingest the medicine, the dose is forced

into the mouth, blown into the nose, or given via a nasogastric tube until consciousness is restored.
- If there is constipation and muscular spasms or convulsions use **ZI XUE DAN** (*Purple Snow Special Pill* 紫雪丹, p.707). If the patient is unable to ingest the medicine, the dose is forced into the mouth or nose or given via a nasogastric tube until consciousness is restored. See also Convulsions, p.680.

Patent medicines
Huang Lian Jie Du Wan 黄连解毒丸 (Huang Lian Jie Du Wan)
Chuan Xin Lian Kang Yan Pian 穿心莲抗炎片
   (Chuan Xin Lian Antiphlogistic Tablets)
Niu Huang Qing Huo Wan 牛黄清火丸 (Niu Huang Qing Huo Wan)
An Gong Niu Huang Wan 安宫牛黄丸 (An Gong Niu Huang Wan)
   - with delirium or convulsions
Zi Xue Dan 紫雪丹 (Tzuhsueh Tan)
   - with delirium or convulsions
Wan Shi Niu Huang Qing Xin Wan 万氏牛黄清心丸
   (Wan Shi Niu Huang Qing Xin Wan) - with delirium or convulsions

Acupuncture
Bl.19 (*dan shu* -), GB.34 (*yang ling quan* -), Du.20 (*bai hui* -), Du.26 (*ren zhong* -), LI.11 (*qu chi* -), Liv.3 (*tai chong* -), GB.40 (*qiu xu* -), Bl.40 (*wei zhong* ↓)
   - With impaired conciousness, add *shi xuan* ↓ (M-UE-1)

Clinical notes
- This type of jaundice may be associated with conditions such as fulminant hepatitis, hepatic failure, hepatic encephalopathy or septicaemia.
- This pattern is a medical emergency and should be treated in hospital.
- The prognosis for fulminant hepatitis and hepatic failure is generally not good.

21.6 COLD DAMP

Pathophysiology
- Cold Damp jaundice is chronic and follows untreated or improperly treated *yang* jaundice, or occurs when weakness of *yang qi* enables Cold Dampness to accumulate and lodge in the middle *jiao*, obstructing the flow of bile. The main problem is the excess Damp, although as the pattern develops, Spleen weakness will become more prominent. This pattern will often overlap with the Spleen deficiency pattern (p.609).

Clinical features
- jaundice that is dull, matt or darkish yellow, and which may be hard to see in artificial light; it may be noticeable in the palms and palmar creases
- fatigue, malaise, lethargy
- cold intolerance
- poor appetite, nausea
- epigastric and abdominal fullness and distension
- loose stools or diarrhoea
- generalised pruritis

T pale and swollen with a greasy white coat
P deep, thready and slow, or soggy and moderate

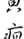

Treatment principle
Transform Dampness and promote urination
Warm the middle *jiao* and strengthen the Spleen

Prescription

YIN CHEN ZHU FU TANG 茵陈术附汤
(*Capillaris, Atractylodes and Aconite Combination*) modified

yin chen (Herba Artemisiae Yinchenhao) 茵陈	30g
fu ling (Sclerotium Poria Cocos) 茯苓	25g
chao bai zhu (dry fried Rhizoma Atractylodis Macrocephalae) 炒白术	15g
ze xie (Rhizoma Alismatis Orientalis) 泽泻	12g
gan jiang (Rhizoma Zingiberis Officinalis) 干姜	9g
zhi fu zi* (Radix Aconiti Carmichaeli Praeparata) 制附子	9g
gan cao (Radix Glycyrrhizae Uralensis) 甘草	3g

Method: Decoction. **Zhi fu zi** is cooked for 30 minutes prior to adding the other herbs (*xian jian* 先煎). (Source: *Zhong Yi Nei Ke Lin Chuang Shou Ce*)

Modifications
- With abdominal distension and a thick tongue coat, delete **bai zhu** and **gan cao**, and add **cang zhu** (Rhizoma Atractylodis) 苍术 10g and **hou**

po (Cortex Magnoliae Officinalis) 厚朴 6g.
- With *qi* deficiency, add **dang shen** (Radix Codonopsis Pilosulae) 党参 12g.
- With severe generalised pruritis, add two or three of the following herbs: **ai ye*** (Folium Artemisiae Argyi) 艾叶 9g, **cang er zi*** (Fructus Xanthii Sibirici) 苍耳子 9g, **qin jiao** (Radix Gentianae Qinjiao) 秦艽 10g or **di fu zi** (Fructus Kochiae Scopariae) 地肤子 15g.
- After the jaundice has resolved, the treatment principle is altered to strengthen the Spleen to transform Dampness. Appropriate formulae include **SHEN LING BAI ZHU SAN** (*Ginseng and Atractylodes Combination* 参苓白术散, p.925), **LIU JUN ZI TANG** (*Six Major Herbs Combination* 六君子汤, p.88), **BU ZHONG YI QI TANG** (*Ginseng and Astragalus Combination* 补中益气汤, p.394) and **HUANG QI JIAN ZHONG TANG** (*Astragalus Combination* 黄芪健中汤, p.609).

Patent medicines
Xi Huang Cao 溪黄草 (Xi Huang Cao Chong Ji) plus
Fu Zi Li Zhong Wan 附子理中丸 (Li Chung Yuen Medical Pills)

Acupuncture
Du.9 (*zhi yang* ▲), Sp.9 (*yin ling quan* ▲), Bl.20 (*pi shu* ▲),
Bl.19 (*dan shu* ▲), Ren.12 (*zhong wan* ▲), St.36 (*zu san li* ▲),
Sp.6 (*san yin jiao* ▲)

Clinical notes
- This type of jaundice may be associated with conditions such as biliary cirrhosis, chronic hepatitis or haemolytic anaemia.
- Even though this is considered an excess pattern (due to the predominance of Cold Damp) there is usually considerable Spleen *qi* or *yang* deficiency. Prescription should take this into account by altering the guiding principle from initially eliminating Dampness through diuresis to strengthening the Spleen with sweet warm and bitter warm parching herbs.

21.7 SPLEEN *QI* AND BLOOD DEFICIENCY

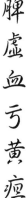

Pathophysiology
- This type of jaundice occurs when there is pre-existing or constitutional weakness of Spleen *qi*, or if Spleen *qi* is damaged by a chronic or persistant Damp Heat or Cold Damp condition, or by inappropriate treatment with excessive bitter cold herbs. Once the Spleen is weak, it is unable to generate sufficient Blood or clear residual Damp. The resulting withering of the Blood and development of Damp stagnation leads to a characteristic sallowness and lustrelessness of the skin.

Clinical features
- the face, eyes and skin are dull, lustreless yellow, or very pale, sickly or sallow
- lethargy and fatigue
- weakness in the extremities
- poor muscle tone
- palpitations
- shortness of breath
- loose stools or diarrhoea
- poor appetite

T pale and swollen, with a thin white coat
P soggy and thin

Treatment principle
Strengthen the Spleen, warm the middle *jiao*
Tonify *qi* and Blood

Prescription

HUANG QI JIAN ZHONG TANG 黄芪健中汤
(*Astragalus Combination*)

huang qi (Radix Astragali Membranacei) 黄芪	30g
yi tang (Saccharum Granorum) 饴糖	30g
bai shao (Radix Paeoniae Lactiflorae) 白芍	15g
gui zhi (Ramulus Cinnamomi Cassiae) 桂枝	9g
gan cao (Radix Glycyrrhizae Uralensis) 甘草	6g
sheng jiang (Rhizoma Zingiberis Officinalis) 生姜	3pce
da zao (Fructus Zizyphi Jujubae) 大枣	5pce

Method: Decoction. (Source: *Zhong Yi Nei Ke Lin Chuang Shou Ce*)

Modifications
- With severe *qi* deficiency, add **dang shen** (Radix Codonopsis Pilosulae) 党参 30g.

- With Blood deficiency, add **dang gui** (Radix Angelicae Sinensis) 当归 9g, **shu di** (Radix Rehmanniae Glutinosae Conquitae) 熟地 30g, **zhi he shou wu** (Radix Polygoni Multiflori) 制何首乌 15g.
- With *yang* deficiency and Cold, add **zhi fu zi*** (Radix Aconiti Carmichaeli Praeparata) 制附子 6-9g.
- With severe generalised pruritis, add one or two of the following herbs: **ai ye*** (Folium Artemisiae Argyi) 艾叶 9g, **cang er zi*** (Fructus Xanthii Sibirici) 苍耳子 9g or **di fu zi** (Fructus Kochiae Scopariae) 地肤子 15g.

Patent medicines
Wu Ji Bai Feng Wan 乌鸡白凤丸 (Wuchi Paifeng Wan)
Shi Quan Da Bu Wan 十全大补丸 (Shi Quan Da Bu Wan)
Dang Gui Ji Jing 当归鸡精 (Tang Kuei Essence of Chicken)
Bu Zhong Yi Qi Wan 补中益气丸 (Bu Zhong Yi Qi Wan)
  - if *qi* deficiency is prominent

Acupuncture
Bl.19 (*dan shu*), Du.9 (*zhi yang*), Bl.20 (*pi shu*), Ren.12 (*zhong wan*), St.36 (*zu san li*), Du.4 (*ming men* + ▲), Ren.6 (*qi hai* + ▲), Ren.4 (*guan yuan* + ▲)

Clinical notes
- This type of jaundice may be associated with conditions such as biliary cirrhosis, chronic hepatitis or haemolytic anaemia.

21.8 BLOOD STAGNATION

Pathophysiology
- Blood stagnation type jaundice is usually very chronic and follows years of unresolved liver disease, alcohol abuse or chronic jaundice. See also Ascites, p.730.

Clinical features
- chronic, darkish or dull yellow jaundice
- fixed, stabbing hypochondriac pain, worse at night and with pressure
- hepatosplenomegaly
- dark or purplish spider naevi over the ribs, face and around the inner ankle and knee–Kid.3 (*tai xi*) and Sp.9 (*yin ling quan*) area
- dark, ashen, sallow or purplish complexion, dark or purplish lips and conjunctiva, dark rings under the eyes
- easy bruising, purpura
- mild feverishness that is worse at night
- pain in the iliac fossae with palpation
- dry mouth and throat with no desire to drink
- dry, scaly skin, emaciation

T purplish or with purple or brown petechial spots with little or no coat
P thready and choppy

Treatment principle
Invigorate the circulation of Blood, eliminate stagnant Blood Alleviate jaundice and soothe the Liver

Prescription

GE XIA ZHU YU TANG 膈下逐瘀汤
(*Drive Out Blood Stasis Below the Diaphram Decoction*) modified

yin chen (Herba Artemisiae Yinchenhao) 茵陈	30g
mu dan pi (Cortex Moutan Radicis) 牡丹皮	15g
chao wu ling zhi^ (dry fried Excrementum Trogopteri seu Pteromi) 炒五灵脂	15g
dang gui (Radix Angelicae Sinensis) 当归	12g
chi shao (Radix Paeoniae Rubrae) 赤芍	12g
xiang fu (Rhizoma Cyperi Rotundi) 香附	12g
wu yao (Radix Linderae Strychnifoliae) 乌药	12g
cu yan hu suo (vinegar fried Rhizoma Corydalis Yanhusuo) 醋延胡索	9g
chuan xiong (Radix Ligustici Chuanxiong) 川芎	9g
tao ren (Semen Persicae) 桃仁	9g

肝郁血瘀黄疸

hong hua (Flos Carthami Tinctorii) 红花 9g
Method: Decoction. (Source: *Zhong Yi Nei Ke Lin Chuang Shou Ce*)

Modifications

* In severe cases, the primary prescription may be combined with either **BIE JIA JIAN WAN** (*Tortise Shell Decoction Pills* 鳖甲煎丸, p.915), a large and complex prepared medicine, or **DA HUANG ZHE CHONG WAN** (*Rhubarb and Eupolyphaga Pill* 大黄䗪虫丸).

    da huang (Radix et Rhizoma Rhei) 大黄 300g
    sheng di (Radix Rehmanniae Glutinosae) 生地 300g
    tao ren (Semen Persicae) 桃仁 120g
    xing ren* (Semen Pruni Armeniacae) 杏仁 120g
    bai shao (Radix Paeoniae Lactiflorae) 白芍 120g
    gan cao (Radix Glycyrrhizae Uralensis) 甘草 90g
    huang qin (Radix Scutellariae Baicalensis) 黄芩 60g
    meng chong^ (Tabanus) 虻虫 45g
    shui zhi^ (Hirudo seu Whitmania) 水蛭 45g
    qi cao^ (Holotrichia) 蛴螬 45g
    di bie chong^ (Eupolyphaga seu Opisthoplatia) 地鳖虫 30g
    gan qi^ (Lacca Sinica Exsiccatae) 干漆 30g
    Method: Grind herbs to a powder and form into 3-gram pills with honey. The dose is one pill, 1-2 times daily. (Source: *Shi Yong Zhong Yao Xue*)

Variations and additional prescriptions

* With Spleen weakness and anorexia, first use **HUANG QI JIAN ZHONG TANG** (*Astragalus Combination* 黄芪健中汤, p.609) plus **dan shen** (Radix Salviae Miltiorrhizae) 丹参 30g, **dang gui** (Radix Angelicae Sinensis) 当归 10g, **chuan xiong** (Radix Ligustici Chuanxiong) 川芎 6g and **ji nei jin**^ (Endothelium Corneum Gigeriae Galli) 鸡内金 15g to support Spleen *qi* and Blood before harsh Blood invigorating herbs are administered.

Patent medicines

Xue Fu Zhu Yu Wan 血府逐瘀丸 (Xue Fu Zhu Yu Wan)
Nei Xiao Luo Li Wan 内消瘰疬丸 (Nei Xiao Luo Li Wan)
Gui Zhi Fu Ling Wan 桂枝茯苓丸 (Gui Zhi Fu Ling Wan)

Acupuncture

Bl.20 (*pi shu*), Bl.19 (*dan shu* -), Bl.18 (*gan shu* -), GB.24 (*ri yue*), Sp.6 (*san yin jiao* -), Liv.14 (*qi men* -), Sp.10 (*xue hai* -), Bl.17 (*ge shu* -), Sp.7 (*lou gu*), LI.4 (*he gu* -)

Clinical notes

- This type of jaundice may be associated with conditions such as hepatic cirrhosis, liver cancer and chronic hepatitis.
- Difficult to treat, requiring persistence over a long time for any result.

SUMMARY OF GUIDING FORMULAE FOR JAUNDICE

Yang jaundice

Damp Heat
- Heat greater than Damp - *Yin Chen Hao Tang* 茵陈蒿汤
- Damp greater than Heat - *Yin Chen Wu Ling San* 茵陈五苓散
- Early stage with exterior symptoms - *Ma Huang Lian Qiao Chi Xiao Dou Tang* 麻黄连翘赤小豆汤 + *Gan Lu Xiao Du Dan* 甘露消毒丹
- with Liver Fire - *Long Dan Xie Gan Tang* 龙胆泻肝汤
- with gallstones, plus *San Jin Tang* 三金汤

Liver and Gall Bladder stagnant Heat - *Qing Dan Xie Huo Tang* 清胆泻火汤
- with roundworms, plus *Dan Dao Qu Hui Tang* 胆道驱蛔汤

Toxic Heat - *Huang Lian Jie Du Tang* 黄连解毒汤 + *Yin Chen Hao Tang* 茵陈蒿汤 and *Wu Wei Xiao Du Yin* 五味消毒饮
- in severe cases - *Xi Jiao San* 犀角散
- with delerium or impaired consciousness - *An Gong Niu Huang Wan* 安宫牛黄丸 or *Zhi Bao Wan* 至宝丸
- with spasms or convulsions - *Zi Xue Dan* 紫雪丹

Yin jaundice

Cold Damp - *Yin Chen Zhu Fu Tang* 茵陈术附汤

Spleen *qi* and Blood deficiency - *Huang Qi Jian Zhong Tang* 黄芪健中汤

Blood stagnation - *Ge Xia Zhu Yu Tang* 膈下逐瘀汤
- with palpable masses, plus *Da Huang Zhe Chong Wan* 大黄蛰虫丸 or *Bie Jia Wan* 鳖甲丸

For more information regarding herbs marked with an asterisk*, an open circle° or a hatˆ, see the tables on pp.944-952.

Disorders of the Liver

22. Shan Qi

Cold *shan qi*
Watery *shan qi*
Qi shan qi
Foxy *shan qi*
Phlegm and Blood stagnation *shan qi*

22 SHAN QI
shan qi 疝气

Shan qi is a collective term describing pain and swelling affecting the lower abdomen, groin and external genitalia, particularly the testicles and scrotum, that is, those parts of the body traversed by the Liver channel and thus strongly influenced by the Liver. *Shan qi* disorders appear primarily in males due to the peculiarities of the male anatomy.

Shan qi disorders are generally equated with various types of hernias (the term *shan qi* is often translated as hernial disorder[1]), however the term has broader connotations. While the *shan qi* category certainly describes true herniations, it also includes a number of other disorders exhibiting swelling and/or pain in the genital and groin region, such as varicocoele, hydrocoele, orchitis, testicular tumours, testicular torsion and filariasis.

There are five traditional categories of *shan qi*:

1 Cold (*han shan* 寒疝): characterised by coldness and firmness of the testicles.
2 Watery (*shui shan* 水疝): an accumulation of fluid in the scrotum (hydrocoele), or swollen veins in the scrotum (varicocoele), or eczema.
3 Qi (*qi shan* 气疝): distension and pain in the testicles and lower abdomen.
4 Foxy (*hu shan* 狐疝): where a portion of the intestine is intermittently squeezed through an aperture or weakness in the abdominal wall, usually through the inguinal canal into the testicles.
5 Hard (*tui shan*): a hard, solid mass with loss of testicular sensation.

AETIOLOGY
Cold Damp
This pattern is mostly due to prolonged exposure to external cold and damp, such as sitting on damp ground too long, wearing damp clothing or prolonged immersion in water. Cold Damp can also invade through the *yin* channels of the legs after prolonged standing on cold floors or exposure of the legs to cold and damp. People with underlying *yang* deficiency are especially vulnerable to such invasion.

Liver *qi* stagnation
Frustration, anger, resentment, prolonged emotional turmoil, repressed emotions, sexual anxiety and stress disrupt the circulation of Liver *qi*. Because the Liver channel is so intimately associated with the groin and genital region, stagnant *qi* easily influences this area.

---

1. Bensky D and Gamble A (1993) *Chinese Herbal Medicine: Materia Medica*, Eastland Press, Seattle, Washington

Damp Heat

Damp Heat causing *shan qi* can be due to an external Damp Heat pathogen that invades through the *taiyang* (Bladder) channel, the leg *yin* channels or the local *luo* channels.

Damp Heat can also be internally generated by excessive consumption of rich, greasy or spicy foods and alcohol, or by the interaction of *yin* deficiency, *qi* stagnation or Heat with any pre-existing Dampness. Damp Heat is heavy and tends to sink into the lower body.

Spleen *qi* deficiency

Overwork, excessive worry or mental activity, irregular dietary habits, excessive consumption of cold, sweet or raw foods or prolonged illness can weaken Spleen *qi*. When Spleen *qi* is weak, food and fluids are poorly processed, and Dampness may accumulate. These are *yin* pathogens and tend to sink into the lower *jiao*.

Weakness of Spleen *qi* can also lead to loss of muscle tone and prolapse of various structures–causing weakness of muscular apertures and consequent herniation of the intestines or other abdominal structures.

Phlegm and Blood stagnation

Phlegm and Blood stagnate as the result of other chronic disorders of the testicles. Fluid stagnation can eventually congeal into Phlegm. Cold easily obstructs the circulation of *qi* and Blood.

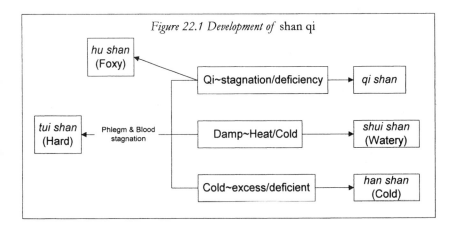

Figure 22.1 Development of shan qi

22.1 COLD SHAN QI

Pathophysiology
- In this pattern, Cold penetrates through the Liver channel, inhibiting the circulation of *qi* and Blood. The nature of Cold is to freeze and constrict, and exposed parts of the body are particularly vulnerable. Also known as Cold invading the Liver channel.
- There are two variants–excess Cold and deficient Cold. The excess Cold pattern most likely occurs in men with intact *qi* who are invaded by external Cold. The deficient pattern occurs in men with deficient *yang* and internal Cold.

22.1.1 Excess Cold
Clinical features
- swollen, firm, cold and retracted scrotum or testicles; in severe cases there is a stone like hardness
- testicular pain that is significantly improved with warmth
- cold intolerance

T white coat
P deep and wiry

Treatment principle
Warm the Liver (channel) and disperse Cold
Regulate *qi*, stop pain

Prescription

JIAO GUI TANG 椒桂汤
(*Sichuan Pepper and Cinnamon Decoction*)

gui zhi (Ramulus Cinnamomi Cassiae) 桂枝	9g
chuan jiao (Pericarpium Zanthoxyli Bungeani) 川椒	6g
gao liang jiang (Rhizoma Alpiniae Officinari) 高良姜	6g
chai hu (Radix Bupleuri) 柴胡	6g
xiao hui xiang (Fructus Foeniculi Vulgaris) 小茴香	6g
chen pi (Pericarpium Citri Reticulatae) 陈皮	6g
wu zhu yu (Fructus Evodiae Rutaecarpae) 吴茱萸	6g
qing pi (Pericarpium Citri Reticulatae Viride) 青皮	6g

Method: Decoction. (Source: *Shi Yong Zhong Yi Nei Ke Xue*)

Modifications
- With severe pain, add **li zhi he** (Semen Litchi Chinensis) 荔枝核 12g and **ju he** (Semen Citri Reticulatae) 橘核 9g.

22.1.2 Deficient Cold
Clinical features
- testicular coldness and distension
- lower abdominal coldness and pain which radiates through to the testicles, better for warmth
- cold intolerance, cold or numb extremities

T pale with a white coat
P deep, thready and slow

Treatment principle
Warm the Liver and Kidneys, move *qi*
Disperse Cold and stop pain

Prescription

NUAN GAN JIAN 暖肝煎
(*Warm the Liver Decoction*)

rou gui (Cortex Cinnamomi Cassiae) 肉桂	6g
xiao hui xiang (Fructus Foeniculi Vulgaris) 小茴香	6g
fu ling (Sclerotium Poria Cocos) 茯苓	15g
wu yao (Radix Linderae Strychnifoliae) 乌药	6g
gou qi zi (Fructus Lycii) 枸杞子	9g
dang gui (Radix Angelicae Sinensis) 当归	9g
chen xiang (Lignum Aquilariae) 沉香	3g
sheng jiang (Rhizoma Zingiberis Officinalis) 生姜	3pce

Method: Decoction.

Patent medicines
Shu Gan Wan 舒肝丸 (Shu Gan Wan) - Excess Cold
Shi Xiang Zhi Tong Wan 十香止痛丸 (Sap Heung Yuen Medical Pills) - Excess Cold
Li Zhong Wan 理中丸 (Li Zhong Wan) - Deficient Cold

Acupuncture (applicable to both types)
Liv.13 (*zhang men* +▲), Ren.6 (*qi hai* ▲), Kid.6 (*zhao hai* ▲), Liv.1 (*da dun* ▲)

Clinical notes
- This pattern may correspond to testicular tumours or herniae.
- The pain of this pattern generally responds well to treatment.

22.2 WATERY *SHAN QI*

Pathophysiology
- There are two patterns associated with watery *shan qi*, Cold Damp and Damp Heat. The Cold Damp type is associated with fluid filled cysts or hydrocoele. The Damp Heat type manifests as a moist eczema, or testicular inflammation or infection.

22.2.1 Cold Damp
Clinical features
- the scrotum is swollen and oedematous, or there is a unilateral, well defined fluid filled swelling which may or may not be painful
- dragging discomfort in testes
- watery splash when the lower abdomen is palpated
- scanty urination

T thin greasy coat
P wiry

Treatment principle
Expel pathogenic fluids and move *qi*
Aid the transformation of *qi*

Prescription

WU LING SAN 五苓散
(*Hoelen Five Formula*) modified

fu ling (Sclerotium Poria Cocos) 茯苓	25g
bai zhu (Rhizoma Atractylodes Macrocephalae) 白术	15g
ju he (Semen Citri Reticulatae) 橘核	15g
zhu ling (Sclerotium Polypori Umbellati) 猪苓	12g
ze xie (Rhizoma Alismatis Orientalis) 泽泻	12g
gui zhi (Ramulus Cinnamomi Cassiae) 桂枝	9g
mu xiang (Radix Aucklandiae Lappae) 木香	9g

Method: Decoction. (Source: *Zhong Yi Nei Ke Lin Chuang Shou Ce*)

Modifications
- With Cold, add **rou gui** (Cortex Cinnamomi Cassiae) 肉桂 6g, **xiao hui xiang** (Fructus Foeniculi Vulgaris) 小茴香 6g and **wu zhu yu** (Fructus Evodiae Rutaecarpae) 吴茱萸 6g.

Acupuncture
Liv.8 (*qu quan* ▲), St.28 (*shui dao* ▲), Sp.6 (*san yin jiao* -), Liv.1 (*da dun* -)

Patent medicines
Hai Zao Wan 海藻丸 (Hai Zao Wan)

Clinical notes
- This pattern may be associated with conditions such as hydrocoele, epididymal cyst, spermatocoele, varicocoele, haematocoele and testicular torsion.

22.2.2 Damp Heat
Clinical features
- the scrotum is red, swollen, painful or itchy with a watery yellow exudate from the skin
- may be fever
- concentrated urine
- irritability and restlessness

T greasy yellow coat
P wiry and rapid

Treatment principle
Clear Damp Heat

Prescription

DA FEN QING YIN 大分清饮
(Major Distinguishing Decoction)

This formula is selected when the Damp Heat is localised, and there are few systemic signs.

fu ling (Sclerotium Poria Cocos) 茯苓	12g
shan zhi zi (Fructus Gardeniae Jasminoides) 山栀子	9g
zhu ling (Sclerotium Polypori Umbellati) 猪苓	9g
ze xie (Rhizoma Alismatis Orientalis) 泽泻	9g
mu tong (Caulis Mutong) 木通	6g
zhi ke (Fructus Citri Aurantii) 枳壳	6g
che qian zi (Semen Plantaginis) 车前子	6g

Method: Decoction. **Che qian zi** is usually cooked in a muslin bag (*bao jian* 包煎).
(Source: *Shi Yong Zhong Yi Nei Ke Xue*)

LONG DAN XIE GAN TANG 龙胆泻肝汤
(Gentiana Combination) p.500

This formula is selected when Damp Heat is obviously affecting the Liver and sinking down through the Liver channel. There will be systemic symptoms reflecting the Liver's involvement–severe irritability, headaches, fullness in the chest and abdomen, constipation, dysuria etc.

Patent medicines
Long Dan Xie Gan Wan 龙胆泻肝丸 (Long Dan Xie Gan Wan)
Qian Lie Xian Wan 前列腺丸 (Prostate Gland Pills)
Chuan Xin Lian Kang Yan Pian 穿心连抗炎片
    (Chuan Xin Lian Antiphlogistic Tablets)

Acupuncture
Sp.9 (*yin ling quan* -), Liv.5 (*li gou* -), Ren.3 (*zhong ji* -),
Kid.6 (*zhao hai* -), Liv.1 (*da dun* -)

Clinical notes
- This pattern may be associated with conditions such as scrotal eczema, orchitis, orchitis associated with mumps, filariasis or testicular torsion.

22.3 LIVER *QI* STAGNATION *SHAN QI*

Pathophysiology
- This pattern of *shan qi* is due to disruption of Liver *qi* in the Liver channel. Liver *qi* stagnation can be the result of anger, smouldering resentment, frustration, repressed emotions or sexual anxiety. The Liver channel circulates through the genitals, therefore stasis of Liver *qi* can result in testicular symptoms.

Clinical features
- The scrotum is bilaterally or unilaterally swollen and distended, with distension or pain radiating from or to the lower abdomen and/or the lumbar region; the condition is aggravated or intiated by anger, stress or emotional upset, and is alleviated by relaxation.
- There may be other signs of *qi* stagnation, such as depression, irritability, sighing, headaches, menstrual problems, and so on.

T pale or normal with a white coat
P wiry

Treatment principle
Soothe the Liver and regulate *qi*

Prescription

TIAN TAI WU YAO SAN 天台乌药散
(*Top Quality Lindera Powder*) modified

wu yao (Radix Linderae Strychnifoliae) 乌药	15g
qing pi (Pericarpium Citri Reticulatae Viride) 青皮	15g
gao liang jiang (Rhizoma Alpiniae Officinari) 高良姜	15g
mu xiang (Radix Aucklandiae Lappae) 木香	15g
chao xiao hui xiang (dry fried Fructus Foeniculi Vulgaris) 炒小茴香	15g
li zhi he (Semen Litchi Chinensis) 荔枝核	12g
chuan lian zi* (Fructus Meliae Toosendan) 川楝子	9g
ju he (Semen Citri Reticulatae) 橘核	9g
bing lang (Semen Arecae Catechu) 槟榔	6g

Method: Powder and take as a draft with yellow wine or sake. The dose is 3 grams, 2-3 times daily. May also be decocted. (Source: *Shi Yong Zhong Yi Nei Ke Xue*)

Modifications
- With Cold, add **rou gui** (Cortex Cinnamomi Cassiae) 肉桂 6g and **wu zhu yu** (Fructus Evodiae Rutaecarpae) 吴茱萸 6g.

Patent medicines
Shu Gan Wan 舒肝丸 (Shu Gan Wan)
Chai Hu Shu Gan Wan 柴胡舒肝丸 (Chai Hu Shu Gan Wan)
Mu Xiang Shun Qi Wan 木香顺气丸 (Aplotaxis Carminative Pills)

Acupuncture
Ren.6 (*qi hai* -), Sp.6 (*san yin jiao* -), Liv.2 (*xing jian* -), GB.41 (*zu lin qi* -), Liv.3 (*tai chong* -)

Clinical notes
- This pattern may be associated with conditions such as inguinal hernia.

气虚疝

22.4 *QI* DEFICIENCY *SHAN QI*

Pathophysiology
- Weakness of Spleen *qi* leads to sinking of various suspended structures, and a general loss of muscle tone causing weakened abdominal apertures. This encourages abdominal contents (usually portions of the small intestine) to extrude, usually through the inguinal canal, affecting the testicles and scrotum, or in women, the region around St.30 (*qi chong*). This pattern is most common in elderly men.

Clinical features
- the scrotum is swollen, dropped or distended, usually unilaterally, with mild pain, discomfort or a dragging sensation, aggravated or initiated by fatigue, overwork, long hours standing and coughing
- frequent urination
- there will usually be signs of Spleen weakness, like abdominal distension, fatigue, poor appetite, fluid retention and loose stools

T pale and swollen with toothmarks and a thin coat
P weak or wiry (if there is pain)

Treatment principle
Tonify the Spleen to raise *qi*

Prescription

BU ZHONG YI QI TANG 补中益气汤
(*Ginseng and Astragalus Combination*) modified

huang qi (Radix Astragali Membranacei) 黄芪	15g
bai zhu (Rhizoma Atractylodes Macrocephalae) 白术	12g
dang shen (Radix Codonopsis Pilosulae) 党参	9g
dang gui (Radix Angelicae Sinensis) 当归	9g
ju he (Semen Citri Reticulatae) 橘核	9g
li zhi he (Semen Litchi Chinensis) 荔枝核	9g
chen pi (Pericarpium Citri Reticulatae) 陈皮	6g
gan cao (Radix Glycyrrhizae Uralensis) 甘草	6g
chai hu (Radix Bupleuri) 柴胡	6g
chao xiao hui xiang (dry fried Fructus Foeniculi Vulgaris) 炒小茴香	6g
sheng ma (Rhizoma Cimicifugae) 升麻	3g

Method: Decoction. (Source: *Shi Yong Zhong Yi Nei Ke Xue*)

Modifications
- With Kidney *qi* deficiency, add **ba ji tian** (Radix Morindae Officinalis)

巴戟天 9g, **xian ling pi** (Herba Epimedii) 仙灵脾 12g and **rou gui** (Cortex Cinnamomi Cassiae) 肉桂 6g.

Patent medicines
Bu Zhong Yi Qi Wan 补中益气丸 (Bu Zhong Yi Qi Wan)
Ba Ji Yin Yang Wan 巴戟阴阳丸 (Ba Ji Yin Yang Wan)
Zhuang Yao Jian Shen Pian 庄腰健肾片 (Zhuang Yao Jian Shen)

Acupuncture
Du.20 (*bai hui* ▲), St.36 (*zu san li* +▲), Ren.12 (*zhong wan* +▲), Bl.20 (*pi shu*), Liv.8 (*qu quan*), Sp.6 (*san yin jiao*)
- a useful technique for this condition (and lower abdominal prolapses in general) is to thread a 3-inch needle from Ren.6 (*qi hai*) to Ren.3 (*zhong ji*). The needle is twirled to anchor it, then raised towards the sternum creating a lifting sensation in the lower abdomen. It can be taped (in its lifted position) in place for the duration of the treatment.

Clinical notes
- This pattern may be associated with conditions such as inguinal hernia, varicocoele and hydrocoele.

22.5 FOXY *SHAN QI*

Pathophysiology
- This is a subcategory of *qi* stagnation or *qi* deficiency *shan qi*, clearly describing an inguinal or inguinoscrotal hernia. Termed 'foxy' because it appears and disappears (unexpectedly?) like a fox.

Clinical features
- a part of the small intestine intermittently descends into the groin or scrotum through the inguinal canal, disappearing when the patient lies flat or when manually reduced; it reappears when the patient stands, coughs or sneezes
- the hernia may be large or small, changing from time to time; when present there may or may not be distension and pain radiating into the testes

T no specific tongue
P no specific pulse, however if there is pain the pulse may be wiry or tight

Treatment principle
Soothe the Liver and regulate *qi*

Prescription

DAO QI TANG 导气汤
(*Conduct the Qi Decoction*) modified

chuan lian zi* (Fructus Meliae Toosendan) 川楝子	12g
xiao hui xiang (Fructus Foeniculi Vulgaris) 小茴香	10g
wu yao (Radix Linderae Strychnifoliae) 乌药	10g
yan hu suo (Rhizoma Corydalis Yanhusuo) 延胡索	10g
ju he (Semen Citri Reticulatae) 橘核	12g
qing pi (Pericarpium Citri Reticulatae Viride) 青皮	9g
mu xiang (Radix Aucklandiae Lappae) 木香	6g

Method: Decoction. (Source: *Zhong Yi Nei Ke Lin Chuang Shou Ce*)

Modifications
- With *qi* deficiency, add **dang shen** (Radix Codonopsis Pilosulae) 党参 15g, **huang qi** (Radix Astragali Membranacei) 黄芪 30g, **chai hu** (Radix Bupleuri) 柴胡 9g and **sheng ma** (Rhizoma Cimicifugae) 升麻 6g or combine with **BU ZHONG YI QI TANG** (*Ginseng and Astragalus Combination* 补中益气汤) modified, p.625).
- With Blood deficiency, add **dang gui** (Radix Angelicae Sinensis) 当归 9g and **bai shao** (Radix Paeoniae Lactiflorae) 白芍 12g.
- With Cold, add **rou gui** (Cortex Cinnamomi Cassiae) 肉桂 6g and **zhi**

fu zi* (Radix Aconiti Carmichaeli Praeparata) 制附子 6g.

Patent medicines

There are no specific patent medicines for this pattern, however, there are often signs of generalised *qi* deficiency, or sinking Spleen *qi* with poor muscle tone. Any of the *qi* and Blood tonics may be used, especially:

Bu Zhong Yi Qi Wan 补中益气丸 (Bu Zhong Yi Qi Wan)
Ren Shen Yang Ying Wan 人参养营丸 (Ginseng Tonic Pills)
Ba Zhen Wan 八珍丸 (Ba Zhen Wan)
Shi Quan Da Bu Wan 十全大补丸 (Shi Quan Da Bu Wan)

Acupuncture

St.29 (*gui lai*), St.30 (*qi chong*), Ren.4 (*guan yuan*), St.40 (*feng long*), Liv.12 (*ji mai*), Liv.1 (*da dun*), Liv.3 (*tai chong*)

- The vulnerable area (that is, the point of weakness in the abdominal wall) can be surrounded by needles inserted obliquely and shallowly, pointing towards the centre of the weakness.
- Three corner moxa (*san jiao jiu* 三角灸) is a technique recommended for this pattern. The points are the corners of an eqilateral triangle with the apex at Ren.8 (*shen que*) and the other two points the length of the patients smile (usually about 3-4 cun) inferolaterally. The points are warmed with a moxa stick.

Clinical notes

- Small hernias respond well to acupuncture and herbal treatment but large or recurrent hernias may need to be surgically corrected.
- Hernias can be dangerous if they are irreducible, quickly leading to necrosis and serious complications.

22.6 PHLEGM AND BLOOD STAGNATION *SHAN QI*

Pathophysiology
- Chronic Cold Dampness, *qi* stagnation, or other persistant pathogens gradually congeal (or allows fluids to congeal) into Phlegm, obstructing the circulation of Blood.

Clinical features
- the scrotum or testicles are swollen and hard with loss of testicular sensation

T pale or slightly purplish with a thin or greasy white coat
P deep

Treatment principle
Move *qi*, transform Phlegm
Soften hardness and disperse swelling

Prescription

JU HE WAN 橘核丸
(*Tangerine Seed Pill*)

ju he (Semen Citri Reticulatae) 橘核	30g
chuan lian zi* (Fructus Meliae Toosendan) 川楝子	30g
hai zao (Herba Sargassii) 海藻	30g
kun bu (Thallus Algae) 昆布	30g
hai dai (Herba Laminariae Japonicae) 海带	30g
tao ren (Semen Persicae) 桃仁	30g
mu xiang (Radix Aucklandiae Lappae) 木香	15g
yan hu suo (Rhizoma Corydalis Yanhusuo) 延胡索	15g
rou gui (Cortex Cinnamomi Cassiae) 肉桂	15g
mu tong (Caulis Mutong) 木通	15g
hou po (Cortex Magnoliae Officinalis) 厚朴	15g
zhi shi (Fructus Immaturus Citri Aurantii) 枳实	15g

Method: Powder and form into 9-gram pills with yellow wine or sake. The dose is 1-2 pills daily. May also be decocted with a 30% reduction in dose. (Source: *Shi Yong Zhong Yi Nei Ke Xue*)

Modifications
- For severe Blood stasis and pain, add **san leng** (Rhizoma Sparganii Stoloniferi) 三棱 15g and **e zhu** (Rhizoma Curcumae Ezhu) 莪术 15g.
- For predominance of Phlegm (rubbery, firm swelling, numbness), add **mu li^** (Concha Ostreae) 牡蛎 30g, **xuan shen** (Radix Scrophulariae Ningpoensis) 玄参 30g and **zhe bei mu** (Bulbus Fritillariae Thunbergii) 浙贝母 15g.

- If the stagnation generates Heat, causing redness and swelling of the scrotum, delete **rou gui**, and add **tu fu ling** (Rhizoma Smilacis Glabrae) 土茯苓 15g, **long dan cao** (Radix Gentianae Longdancao) 龙胆草 15g, **huang bai** (Cortex Phellodendri) 黄柏 15g and **huang qin** (Radix Scutellariae Baicalensis) 黄芩 15g.

Acupuncture

Liv.4 (*zhong du* -), Liv.5 (*li gou* -), Sp.9 (*yin ling quan* -), Ren.3 (*zhong ji* -), Liv.8 (*qu quan* -), St.29 (*gui lai* -), Bl.32 (*ci liao* -), Sp.6 (*san yin jiao* -), LI.4 (*he gu* -)

Patent medicines

Nei Xiao Luo Li Wan 内消瘰疬丸 (Nei Xiao Luo Li Wan)
Hai Zao Wan 海藻丸 (Hai Zao Wan)
Xue Fu Zhu Yu Wan 血府逐瘀丸 (Xue Fu Zhu Yu Wan)
Gui Zhi Fu Ling Wan 桂枝茯苓丸 (Gui Zhi Fu Ling Wan)

Clinical notes

- This pattern may be associated with conditions such as testicular cancer or chronic epididymo-orchitis.
- Any hard mass in the testicles should be thoroughly investigated.
- Acupuncture is of limited use in this pattern and in cases of cancer TCM treatment is generally supportive.

SUMMARY OF GUIDING FORMULAE FOR SHAN QI

Cold *shan qi*
- Excess Cold - *Jiao Gui Tang* 椒桂汤
- Deficient Cold - *Nuan Gan Jian* 暖肝煎

Watery *shan qi*
- Cold Damp - *Wu Ling San* 五苓散
- Damp Heat - *Da Fen Qing Yin* 大分清饮

Liver *qi* stagnation - *Tian Tai Wu Yao San* 天台乌药散

Qi deficiency - *Bu Zhong Yi Qi Tang* 补中益气汤

Foxy *shan qi* - *Dao Qi Tang* 导气汤
- with Spleen *qi* deficiency - *Bu Zhong Yi Qi Tang* 补中益气汤

Phlegm and Blood stagnation - *Ju He Tang* 橘核汤

Endnote

For more information regarding herbs marked with an asterisk*, an open circle° or a hatˆ, see the tables on pp.944-952.

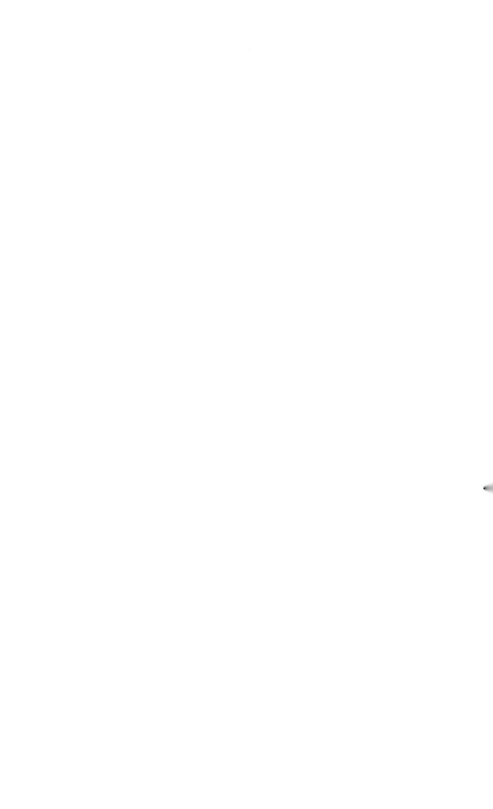

Disorders of the Liver

23. Tremors

Liver and Kidney *yin* deficiency
Qi and Blood deficiency
Phlegm Heat with Wind

23 | TREMORS
chan zheng 颤证

Tremors are involuntary muscular quivering or rhythmic movements of the extremities or head. In TCM, all such movement is due to the stirring of internal Wind. There are three main ways that internal Wind can be generated– Blood deficiency, *yin* deficiency and Heat (see also Box 19.2, p.536).

AETIOLOGY

Liver and Kidney *yin* deficiency

Liver and Kidney *yin* are damaged through ageing, excessive sexual activity, overwork (especially while under stress), insufficient sleep and febrile diseases Another common cause of *yin* depletion, especially in younger people, is abuse of recreational drugs. Liver *yin* deficiency can also be an extension of Liver Blood deficiency, or follow any Liver Heat pattern, especially Liver Fire. Prolonged Liver *qi* stagnation can also damage Liver *yin* by generating stagnant Heat. In tremor patterns, there are often mixtures of Phlegm Heat and *yin* deficiency.

Yin and Blood deficiency generate Wind in a similar way. *Yin* and Blood are the anchor that secures *yang* and provide a counterweight to its active and rising nature. When these stabilising elements reach a critical point of deficiency, *yang* (or *qi*) loses its mooring and becomes excessively mobile. This mobile and uncontrolled *yang* is Wind. Blood deficiency is relatively less severe than *yin* deficiency, and the resulting Wind tends to be milder and the tremors finer.

Yin deficiency can give rise to two degrees of Wind, the first milder and associated with the rhythmic tremors and spasms of diseases like Parkinson's disease or hyperthyroidism. The second, more severe, occurs when Liver *yang* suddenly (and disastrously) slips its mooring and becomes Wind, rushing towards the head to cause Wind stroke (see next chapter).

Phlegm Heat

Phlegm Heat can be generated in several ways. Excessive consumption of rich spicy foods and alcohol can directly generate Phlegm Heat. Any pre-existing Heat in the body (from Liver *qi* stagnation with stagnant Heat or Fire, *yin* deficiency or external invasion, etc), can thicken and congeal fluids into Phlegm, and subsequently Phlegm Heat. A weakness of Spleen *qi* or inappropriate consumption of cold natured foods can allow accumulation of Dampness and Phlegm, which can eventually become hot.

Phlegm Heat, at a certain point of intensity, can generate sufficient movement to be redefined as Wind. The variety of Wind associated with

Phlegm Heat type tremor is not severe enough to cause the convulsive Wind of extreme Heat or Fire. In this case the *yin* nature of the Phlegm restrains and modifies the intensity of the Heat's expression, and a milder form of Wind occurs. The Heat smoulders at just the right intensity to promote ongoing Wind, but is not severe enough to cause convulsions.

Qi and Blood deficiency

Overwork, excessive worry or mental activity, irregular dietary habits, excessive consumption of cold, raw foods or prolonged illness can weaken Spleen *qi*. As the Spleen (and Lungs) are the source of the *qi* and Blood of the body, weakness in these organs will inevitably lead to a decrease in production of *qi* and Blood. Other causes are acute or chronic haemorrhage, prolonged breast feeding and malnutrition (seen, for example in vegetarians who eat insufficient protein). *Qi* and Blood are so closely related that deficiency of one usually leads to deficiency of the other.

As noted previously, Blood deficiency can give rise to a mild form of Wind by failing to anchor *yang qi* securely. *Qi* (*yang*) deficiency may also contribute to the development of a type of Wind, one generated by the movement of *qi* to fill the vacuum formed by chronic deficiency. In the case of predominant *qi* deficiency, the Wind is more likely to manifest as chronic childhood convulsions (see Convulsions p.716).

BOX 23.1 SOME BIOMEDICAL CAUSES OF TREMOR

Physiological
- excitement/anxiety
- cold
- tension
- senile
- benign essential (familial) tremor

Pathological
- Parkinson's disease
- Wilson's disease
- Freidreich's ataxia
- hyperthyroidism
- multiple sclerosis
- Tourette's syndrome
- cerebellar disease
- frontal lobe tumours
- peripheral neuropathy
- hypoglycaemia
- liver failure
- uraemia

Drugs
- alcoholcaffeine
- salbutamol
- phenytoin
- lithium
- narcotic withdrawal

BOX 23.2 KEY DIAGNOSTIC POINTS

Tongue
- red and dry - *yin* deficiency
- pale - *qi* and Blood deficiency
- red with a thick yellow coat - Phlegm Heat

23.1 LIVER AND KIDNEY *YIN* DEFICIENCY

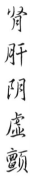

Pathophysiology
- Tremors due to Liver and Kidney *yin* deficiency occur in two ways. First, when there is a lack of *yin* (and Blood), the tendons will become dry from lack of nourishment and lubrication. Such dryness leads to intention tremor or difficult, jerky or shuffling movement. Second, when the *yin* becomes too weak to secure it, the *yang* will move uncontrollably, creating Wind and causing tremors and spasms. This pattern is characterised by generalised dryness and heat.

Clinical features
- usually long term tremor, typically of the hand, leg, jaw or tongue, usually in middle aged or elderly patients; in younger patients, however, it may manifest initially as a fine intention tremor
- some patients may be slow to initiate movement, with a slow and shuffling gait and blank stare
- poor memory, depression
- dizziness, tinnitus
- emaciation, dry skin, dried out look
- insomnia, dream disturbed sleep
- lower back soreness and weakness
- numbness or spasms in the extremities
- constipation
- night sweats, tidal fever, bone steaming fever

T red and dry or dark red and withered or moving, with little or no coat
P thready, wiry, rapid and deep

Treatment principle
Nourish and tonify the Liver and Kidney
Generate *yin*, extinguish Wind

Prescription

DA BU YIN WAN 大补阴丸
(*Great Tonify the Yin Pill*) plus
LIU WEI DI HUANG WAN 六味地黄丸
(*Rehmannia Six Formula*) modified

This formula is best when deficient Heat is strong, causing frequent night sweats, tidal fever and bone steaming.

shu di (Radix Rehmanniae Glutinosae Conquitae) 熟地 180g
sheng di (Radix Rehmanniae Glutinosae) 生地 180g
gui ban° (Plastri Testudinis) 龟板 180g

yan huang bai (salt fried Cortex Phellodendri)
盐黄柏 120g
yan zhi mu (salt fried Rhizoma Anemarrhenae Asphodeloidis)
盐知母 120g
shan yao (Radix Dioscoreae Oppositae) 山药 120g
shan zhu yu (Fructus Corni Officinalis) 山茱萸 120g
fu ling (Sclerotium Poria Cocos) 茯苓 90g
mu dan pi (Cortex Moutan Radicis) 牡丹皮 90g
xuan shen (Radix Scrophulariae) 玄参 90g
he shou wu (Radix Polygoni Multiflori) 何首乌 90g
gou teng (Ramulus Uncariae cum Uncis) 钩藤 90g
bai ji li (Fructus Tribuli Terrestris) 白蒺藜 90g
mu li^ (Concha Ostreae) 牡蛎 90g

Method: Grind herbs to powder and form into 9-gram pills with honey. The dose is 3 pills daily. May also be decocted with a 90% reduction in dosage. (Source: *Shi Yong Zhong Yi Nei Ke Xue*)

DA DING FENG ZHU 大定风珠
(Major Arrest Wind Pearl)

This formula nourishes *yin* and extinguishes Wind. It is not as cooling as the previous formula and is recommended in stubborn cases and in cases with muscle spasm.

sheng di (Radix Rehmanniae Glutinosae) 生地 18g
bai shao (Radix Paeoniae Lactiflorae) 白芍 18g
mai dong (Tuber Ophiopogonis Japonici) 麦冬 18g
mu li^ (Concha Ostreae) 牡蛎 12g
bie jia° (Carapax Amydae Sinensis) 鳖甲 12g
gui ban° (Plastri Testudinis) 龟板 12g
zhi gan cao (honey fried Radix Glycyrrhizae Uralensis)
炙甘草 12g
e jiao^ (Gelatinum Corii Asini) 阿胶 9g
huo ma ren (Semen Cannabis Sativae) 火麻仁 9g
wu wei zi (Fructus Schizandrae Chinensis) 五味子 6g
ji zi huang^ (egg yolk) 鸡子黄 2

Method: Decoction. The shells are decocted for 30 minutes prior to the other herbs (*xian jian* 先煎), **e jiao** and the eggs are added to the strained decoction (*yang hua* 烊化). (Source: *Shi Yong Zhong Yi Nei Ke Xue*)

Modifications (apply to both prescriptions)

- With poor appetite or digestive weakness, add **shen qu** (Massa Fermentata) 神曲 9(90)g and **shan zha** (Fructus Crataegi) 山楂 9(90)g.
- For severe night sweats, add **fu xiao mai** (Semen Tritici Aestivi Levis) 浮小麦 12(120)g and **ma huang gen** (Radix Ephedrae) 麻黄根 9(90)g.

Variations and additional prescriptions

Tremor associated with drug use
* Patients who have consumed large amounts of recreational drugs often have damaged *yin*. In particular, long term marijuana, cocaine or amphetamine use severely depletes Heart and Kidney *yin*. These patients often have a withered or dried out look, memory lapses, sleep disturbance and intention tremor. The correct treatment (in addition to stopping the drugs) is to nourish Heart and Kidney *yin* and calm the *shen* with **TIAN WANG BU XIN DAN** (*Ginseng and Zizyphus Formula* 天王补心丹, p.806)

Patent medicines
Zuo Gui Wan 左归丸 (Zuo Gui Wan)
Qi Ju Di Huang Wan 杞菊地黄丸 (Lycium-Rehmannia Pills)
Zhi Bai Ba Wei Wan 知柏八味丸 (Zhi Bai Ba Wei Wan)
Ming Mu Di Huang Wan 明目地黄丸 (Ming Mu Di Huang Wan)
Tian Wang Bu Xin Dan 天王补心丹 (Tian Wang Bu Xin Dan)

Acupuncture
Bl.23 (*shen shu* +), Bl.18 (*gan shu* +), Ren.4 (*guan yuan* +), Kid.3 (*tai xi* +), Liv.3 (*tai chong*), Liv.8 (*qu quan*), Kid.6 (*zhao hai*), Lu.7 (*lie que*), Ht.7 (*shen men*)
* with anxiety, add PC.6 (*nei guan*) and *yin tang* (M-HN-3)
* Scalp acupuncture may be useful

Clinical notes
* The tremors in this pattern may be associated with conditions such as Parkinson's disease, senile tremors, hyperthyroidism, anxiety and drug abuse.
* Tremors associated with drug abuse, anxiety and hyperthyroidism respond well to acupuncture and herbal treatment, although as always the degree of success depends on the degree of deficiency.
* Senile tremors and those associated with Parkinson's disease will require lengthy treatment with acupuncture and herbs to secure a satisfactory result, although delay of further deterioration is often the best result that can realistically be gained.
* Stimulant drugs (including caffeine) should be gradually withdrawn.
* Regular and sufficient rest and a minimum of mental stress is essential to allow the regeneration of *yin*.

23.2 *QI* AND BLOOD DEFICIENCY

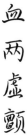

Pathophysiology
- Tremors due to *qi* and Blood deficiency tend to be a little milder than the tremors of the Liver and Kidney *yin* deficiency type, although there may be some overlap between the two. As with *yin* deficiency, Blood deficiency can cause tremors in two ways–by not lubricating and nourishing Tendons, and by not securing *yang qi*, thus generating Wind.

Clinical features
- mild tremor, head shaking, usually long term
- may be slow to initiate movement or has slow and shuffling gait
- numbness and weakness of the extremities
- sallow, lustreless complexion
- pale lips and nails
- lethargy and fatigue
- insomnia
- dizziness
- blurring vision
- spontaneous sweating

T pale or dark and swollen with tooth marks or purple stasis spots
P thready and weak

Treatment principle
Tonify *qi* and Blood
Extinguish Wind

Prescription

BA ZHEN TANG 八珍汤
(*Ginseng and Dang Gui Eight Combination*) plus
TIAN MA GOU TENG YIN 天麻钩藤饮
(*Gastrodia and Gambir Formula*) modified

shi jue ming^ (Concha Haliotidis) 石决明	18g
shu di (Radix Rehmanniae Glutinosae Conquitae) 熟地	15g
fu ling (Sclerotium Poria Cocos) 茯苓	12g
dang gui (Radix Angelicae Sinensis) 当归	12g
bai shao (Radix Paeoniae Lactiflorae) 白芍	12g
gou teng (Ramulus Uncariae cum Uncis) 钩藤	12g
chuan niu xi (Radix Cyathulae Officinalis) 川牛膝	12g
dan shen (Radix Salviae Miltiorrhizae) 丹参	12g
bai zhu (Rhizoma Atractylodes Macrocephalae) 白术	9g
ren shen (Radix Ginseng) 人参	9g

tian ma (Rhizoma Gastrodiae Elatae) 天麻 9g
du zhong (Cortex Eucommiae Ulmoidis) 杜仲 9g
sang ji sheng (Ramulus Sangjisheng) 桑寄生 9g
yi mu cao (Herba Leonuri Heterophylli) 益母草 9g
Method: Decoction. **Shi jue ming** is cooked for 30 minutes prior to the other herbs (*xian jian* 先煎), **gou teng** is added near the end of cooking (*hou xia* 后下). (Source: *Shi Yong Zhong Yi Nei Ke Xue*).

Modifications
- With Blood stagnation, add **tao ren** (Semen Persicae) 桃仁 9g, **chuan xiong** (Radix Ligustici Chuanxiong) 川芎 6g and **hong hua** (Flos Carthami Tinctorii) 红花 9g.
- With severe sweating, add **huang qi** (Radix Astragali Membranacei) 黄芪 15g and **mu li**^ (Concha Ostreae) 牡蛎 15g.
- With insomnia, add one or two of the following herbs: **wu wei zi** (Fructus Schizandrae Chinensis) 五味子 6g, **bai zi ren** (Semen Biotae Orientalis) 柏子仁 9g, **ye jiao teng** (Caulis Polygoni Multiflori) 夜交藤 30g, **he huan pi** (Cortex Albizziae Julibrissin) 合欢皮 9g.
- If there is abdominal and epigastric fullness and poor appetite, add **ban xia*** (Rhizoma Pinelliae Ternatae) 半夏 10g and **chen pi** (Pericarpium Citri Reticulatae) 陈皮 10g.

Variations and additional prescriptions
- Liver *qi* stagnation often precedes or accompanies Blood deficiency. In this case, the correct treatment is to move Liver *qi*, nourish Blood and extinguish Wind with **XIAO YAO SAN** (*Bupleurum and Dang Gui Formula* 逍遥散 p.139) plus **tian ma** (Rhizoma Gastrodiae Elatae) 天麻 9g, **gou teng** (Ramulus Uncariae cum Uncis) 钩藤 12g, **ban xia*** (Rhizoma Pinelliae Ternatae) 半夏 9g and **hou po** (Cortex Magnoliae Officinalis) 厚朴 9g.

Patent medicines
Ba Zhen Wan 八珍丸 (Ba Zhen Wan)
Bai Feng Wan 白凤丸 (Pai Feng Wan)
Dang Gui Ji Jing 当归鸡精 (Tang Kuei Essence of Chicken)
Shi Quan Da Bu Wan 十全大补丸 (Shi Quan Da Bu Wan)
Tian Ma Gou Teng Wan 天麻钩藤丸 (Tian Ma Gou Teng Wan)
 - combined with one of the patent medicines above

Acupuncture
St.36 (*zu san li* +▲), Sp.6 (*san yin jiao* +), Bl.20 (*pi shu* +▲), Ren.12 (*zhong wan* +▲), Ren.4 (*qi hai* +▲), Bl.23 (*shen shu* +▲), Liv.3 (*tai chong*), LI.10 (*shou san li* +▲).

- Scalp acupuncture may be useful

Clinical notes
- The tremors in this pattern may be associated with conditions such as Parkinson's disease, hyperthyroidism, benign familial tremors, anxiety and multiple sclerosis.
- Acupuncture can be useful to help control the Wind in this pattern but because it represents a profound deficiency of *qi* and Blood it will require long term treatment with herbs.
- A nourishing diet (with adequate protein) and sufficient rest are essential to rebuild Blood and *qi*.

23.3 PHLEGM HEAT GENERATING WIND

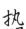

Pathophysiology
- Tremors due to Phlegm Heat with Wind can be mild to severe, yet do not result in the uncontrolled or convulsive tremors seen in the Wind stroke pattern (p.658). In this pattern, the *yin* congealing quality of the Phlegm restrains full expression of the *yang* Heat, which smoulders at an intensity sufficient to generate ongoing Wind, but insufficient to cause Wind stroke.

Clinical features
- mild or severe tremors of the head and extremities which can sometimes be stopped by conscious effort
- fullness and stuffiness in the chest and epigastrium
- dizziness, vertigo
- dry mouth
- sweating
- yellow sputum
- tendency to obesity

T greasy yellow coat
P wiry, slippery and rapid

Treatment principle
Clear Heat and transform Phlegm
Extinguish Wind

Prescription

DAO TAN TANG 导痰汤
(*Guide Out Phlegm Decoction*) plus
TIAN MA GOU TENG YIN 天麻钩藤饮
(*Gastrodia and Gambir Formula*) modified

shi jue ming^ (Concha Haliotidis) 石决明	18g
gou teng (Ramulus Uncariae cum Uncis) 钩藤	12g
chuan niu xi (Radix Cyathulae Officinalis) 川牛膝	12g
fu ling (Sclerotium Poria Cocos) 茯苓	12g
ban xia* (Rhizoma Pinelliae Ternatae) 半夏	9g
chen pi (Pericarpium Citri Reticulatae) 陈皮	9g
zhi shi (Fructus Immaturus Citri Aurantii) 枳实	9g
tian ma (Rhizoma Gastrodiae Elatae) 天麻	9g
shan zhi zi (Fructus Gardeniae Jasminoides) 山栀子	9g
huang qin (Radix Scutellariae Baicalensis) 黄芩	9g
dan nan xing* (Pulvis Arisaemae cum Felle Bovis) 胆南星	6g
gan cao (Radix Glycyrrhizae Uralensis) 甘草	3g

Method: Decoction. **Shi jue ming** is usually cooked for 30 minutes prior to the other herbs (*xian jian* 先煎), **gou teng** is added near the end of cooking (*hou xia* 后下). (Source: *Shi Yong Zhong Yi Nei Ke Xue*)

CUI GAN WAN 摧肝丸
(*Broken Liver Pills*)

This formula is recommended in cases with severe Liver Heat, Phlegm Heat and tremors.

dan nan xing* (Pulvis Arisaemae cum Felle Bovis) 胆南星	15g
gou teng (Ramulus Uncariae cum Uncis) 钩藤	15g
hua shi (Talcum) 滑石	15g
sheng tie luo (Frusta Ferri) 生铁落	15g
jiang can^ (Bombyx Batryticatus) 僵蚕	15g
tian ma (Rhizoma Gastrodiae Elatae) 天麻	15g
qing dai (Indigo Pulverata Levis) 青黛	10g
huang lian (Rhizoma Coptidis) 黄连	10g
zhu li (Succus Bambusae) 竹沥	10g
zhi gan cao (honey fried Radix Glycyrrhizae Uralensis) 炙甘草	10g
zhu sha* (Cinnabaris) 朱砂	5g

Method: Grind the herbs (except **zhu sha**) to powder and form into 6-gram pills with ginger juice. **Zhu sha** is used to coat the pills. The dose is 1-2 pills daily. (Source: *Shi Yong Zhong Yi Nei Ke Xue*).

Patent medicines

Hu Po Bao Long Wan 琥珀抱龙丸 (Po Lung Yuen Medical Pills) plus *Tian Ma Gou Teng Wan* 天麻钩藤丸 (Tian Ma Gou Teng Wan)

Acupuncture

St.40 (*feng long* -), Du.12 (*shen zhu* -), GB.13 (*ben shen*), Ren.15 (*jiu wei*), Liv.3 (*tai chong* -), St.25 (*tian shu*), PC.5 (*jian shi*)
- worse at night, add Kid.6 (*zhao hai*)
- worse during the day, add Bl.62 (*shen mai*)

Clinical notes

- The tremors in this pattern may be associated with conditions such as Meniere's disease, hypertension, epilepsy and multiple sclerosis.
- The tremors in this pattern, being excess rather than deficient, can resolve reasonably rapidly if the Phlegm can be cleared. Strong herbal treatment and dietary modifications are necessary to achieve this.

SUMMARY OF GUIDING FORMULAE FOR TREMORS

Liver and Kidney *yin* deficiency
- *Da Bu Yin Wan* 大补阴丸 + *Liu Wei Di Huang Wan* 六味地黄丸
- in stubborn cases - *Da Ding Feng Zhu* 大定风珠

Qi and Blood deficiency
- *Ba Zhen Tang* 八珍汤 + *Tian Ma Gou Teng Yin* 天麻钩藤饮
- with stagnant *qi* - *Xiao Yao San* 逍遥散

Phlegm Heat generating Wind
- *Dao Tan Tang* 导痰汤 + *Tian Ma Gou Teng Yin* 天麻钩藤饮
- severe cases - *Cui Gan Wan* 摧肝丸

Endnote

For more information regarding herbs marked with an asterisk*, an open circle° or a hatˆ, see the tables on pp.944-952.

Disorders of the Liver

24. Wind Stroke

Channel stroke
Channel emptiness with Wind invasion
Liver and Kidney *yin* deficiency with rising *yang* and Wind
Phlegm Heat with Wind Phlegm

Organ stoke
Closed syndrome
Flaccid collapse syndrome

Sequelae of Wind stroke
Hemiplegia
Dysphasia
Facial paralysis

24 | WIND STROKE
zhong feng 中风

The TCM classification of Wind stroke is closely analagous to the biomedically defined Cerebro-vascular accident (CVA). Brain damage as a result of a CVA is the third commonest cause of death in developed countries, and a significant contributor to morbidity, especially in those over 50 years.

About 50% of strokes are preceded by a transient ischaemic attack (TIA), which is a focal neurological dysfunction due to cerebral ischaemia lasting less than 24 hours, and in many cases only a few minutes. TIA's are characterised by transient vertigo, monocular blindness and confusion, double vision or ataxia. TIA's are important prognostic indicators for impending stroke. In TCM there are effective treatments for preventing stroke and alleviating the preconditions of hypertension, atherosclerosis and increased blood viscosity.

The mechanism of CVA is generally either haemorrhage from a burst aneurism, thrombosis due to partial or total atherosclerotic occlusion of vertebral or cerebral arteries, or embolism detached from a distant thrombus or atherosclerotic plaque. In all cases a portion of the brain is deprived of blood and oxygen and either dies or is damaged. The symptoms and extent of the condition depend on where in the brain the infarction occurs, and how extensive the damage is. Mild infarction or cerebral ischaemia is probably analagous to channel stroke (*feng zhong jing* 风中经), severe infarction to organ stroke (*feng zhong zang* 风中脏).

Wind stroke has long been thought to be one of the 'four major problems in internal medicine', and thus occupies a prominent place in traditional medical literature. Theories concerning Wind stroke have varied and developed over the centuries. Prior to the Tang dynasty (618-907AD), external Wind was thought to be the principle factor contributing to Wind stroke. Early physicians maintained that when *zheng* and *wei qi* were weak, the undefended channels were wide open to invasion by external Wind, and this Wind was sufficient to cause the characteristic symptoms of Wind stroke. The depth of Wind penetration could be determined by the severity of the symptoms and the level of the patient's consciousness. Early prescriptions were largely diaphoretic, aimed at expelling external Wind from the channels.

Centuries of clinical experience, however, demonstrated the shortcomings of this approach. Routine application of diaphoretic prescriptions was observed to be detrimental in some types of Wind stroke, and the standard formulae began to disappear from clinical records. Once physicians of the Song (960-1279AD) and Yuan (1271-1368AD) dynasties

> **BOX 24.1 TCM CLASSIFICATION OF WIND STROKE**
>
> - **Channel stroke**: a milder type that affects the channels only and does not cause loss of consciousness. The main problems are facial paralysis, dysphasia and hemiplegia. The general prognosis is good, or at least better than when consciousness is lost. There are two general categories:
> 1. Wind stroke with no internal predisposing factors: that is, sudden numbness, facial paralysis or motor dysfunction in an otherwise healthy individual. This is due to invasion of **external** Wind into the channels.
> 2. Wind Stroke with predisposing factors: usually in older people with the predisposing conditions of *yin* deficiency or Phlegm Heat. This is due to **internal** Wind, and is more common than the previous type.
>
> - **Organ (*zang fu*) stroke**: a serious disorder thought to involve serious damage to the internal organs. This type causes loss of consciousness as well as hemiplegia, facial paralysis and dysphasia. This type frequently leads to permanent disability or death. Preventitive treatment is strongly indicated for those at risk.
>
> - **Sequelae**: both channel and organ stroke have the same outcome (if the patient survives)–hemiplegia, facial paralysis, loss of vision, dysphasia etc. With channel stroke the damage is usually not so severe and the prognosis is better. With organ stroke the level of disability is usually greater and the prognosis poorer.

recognised that the regular Wind treatment was insufficient, and indeed sometimes dangerous, they proposed the existence of an internal Wind, a product of physiological imbalances. The internal Wind theory is now so predominant that the primary Wind stroke prescription of the 8th century, *Xiao Xu Ming Tang* (Minor Prolong Life Decoction 小续命汤) barely rates a mention in modern TCM texts, and has much reduced (although still useful), therapeutic indications.

AETIOLOGY

The aetiology of Wind stroke is usually complex and, with the exception of some types of channel stroke, it may take many years before the conditions are right for Wind to develop to the point where it is aggressive enough to cause a catastrophe. There are, however, several reasonably consistent features. Years of overindulgence in heating or Phlegm Damp generating foods, alcohol and tobacco are known to predispose people to Wind stroke. The most common predisposing conditions are Liver *yin* deficiency with rising *yang* and Phlegm Heat, both of which can generate Wind under the right conditions. Wind stoke of internal origin is thus usually a combination of *yin* deficiency, Heat, Phlegm and Wind, with Blood stagnation intervening in the sequelae phase.

Wind

As is clear from the chapter heading, Wind is implicated in all forms of Wind stroke. Regardless of the predisposing factors, it is Wind affecting the organs and lodging in the channels that ultimately does the damage. The evidence for this is the suddenness with which the symptoms appear, and the swift pathological change as a result, as if the patient has been 'hit by Wind' (*zhong feng* 中风). In general the Wind is of internal origin, that is, the byproduct of some physiological dysfuction involving *yin* or Blood deficiency, or Heat. The mechanisms of internal Wind are summarised in Box 24.2.

BOX 24.2 MECHANISMS OF INTERNAL WIND

Yin deficiency

The body's *yin* is the anchor that secures *yang* and provides a counterweight to its active and rising nature. At some critical point of deficiency, *yin* is unable to restrain Liver *yang*, which at a certain point of volatility and movement becomes Wind. This type of Wind can be sudden and catastrophic–it is the type of Wind that can cause Wind stroke leading to hemiplegia or death. It typically follows years of *yin* depletion.

Blood deficiency

This type of Wind is similar in aetiology to the previous type in that the Wind is generated by failure of the Blood to anchor *qi*–when *qi* moves without the grounding control of Blood, a mild form of Wind is generated. Blood deficient Wind is more likely to cause mild rhythmic tics, tremors and spasms.

Heat

Because Heat and movement are closely related physiologically, at a certain level of intensity, internal Heat can turn into Wind. This can manifest as the convulsions of a high fever, or in the case of Wind stroke, as a smouldering Heat that combines with and is contained by Phlegm (or congeals fluids into Phlegm). At some point the Heat breaks out and becomes Wind, carrying the Phlegm towards the head.

Some types of Wind stroke, especially those known as channel stroke (with no consciousness disturbance), may be due to external Wind. Indeed, the formulae designed for these patterns contain diaphoretic herbs to disperse external Wind rather than herbs to extinguish internal Wind.

Liver and Kidney *yin* deficiency

Liver and Kidney *yin* deficiency is an important predisposing factor in Wind stroke and can give rise to two degrees of Wind. The first is a mild variety that appears sporadically in the pre-stroke phase (as TIA's), and the second when Liver *yang* suddenly (and disastrously) slips its mooring and rushes towards the head causing full blown Wind stroke.

Liver and Kidney *yin* are damaged through ageing, excessive sexual activity, overwork (especially while under stress), insufficient sleep, febrile diseases and use of recreational drugs. Liver *yin* deficiency can also be an extension of Liver Blood deficiency, or follow any Liver Heat pattern, especially Liver Fire. Prolonged Liver *qi* stagnation can also damage Liver *yin* by generating stagnant Heat. Very often there are elements of Phlegm Heat associated with the *yin* deficiency patterns.

Phlegm Heat

The Phlegm Heat responsible for Wind stroke is usually created by overindulgence, particularly in rich, fatty foods and alcohol, although a constitutional tendency to Phlegm may be present. Phlegm Heat may also accumulate over time in individuals with Spleen *qi* deficiency and Liver *qi* stagnation. Phlegm Heat frequently combines with rising Liver *yang*. There are probably two reasons that Phlegm Heat can generate sufficient activity to generate Wind–the stagnating quality of Phlegm, which blocks the circulation of *qi* raising the pressure behind the obstruction (which can blow at some point), and the stimulating effects of the Heat. The resultant uncontrolled movement of *qi* can transform to Wind (usually in combination with exploding *yang*) when a critical intensity is reached.

Blood stagnation

Blood stagnation is the end result of Wind invasion, and persists long after the Wind has resolved. In the sequelae of Wind stroke, it tends to be localised to specific areas–the extremities, face and tongue.

TREATMENT

The treatment of Wind stroke can be divided into several phases:
- preventitive
- during the acute phase (during a stroke or in the first couple of weeks following a stroke, until the patient is stable)
- post acute treatment of the sequelae of the Wind stoke

Preventitive treatment is applied to patients with the warning signs of an impending stroke or those in a high-risk group. High-risk patients include the obese, those who smoke, and patients with chronic hypertension and hyerlipidaemia. In general, treatment at this phase involves both constitutional therapy (to nourish Liver and Kidney *yin*, extinguish Wind and/or transform Phlegm) and lifestyle modification. Acupuncture and herbs, with a sensible diet and exercise program can produce good results in restoring the patient to balance.

During the acute phase, treatment is focused on restoring consciousness, stopping bleeding and stabilising the patient. During the acute phase of an evolving Wind stroke, it can be difficult to determine whether a stroke is from a thrombus, embolus or haemorrhage, so a conservative approach is applied. Acupuncture moves *qi* and Blood, and so other than for resuscitation purposes, it is generally not used during the acute phase, as it can prolong bleeding from a leaking aneuysm[1]. Similarly, Blood invigorating herbs are avoided during this phase. The treatments that are applied at this time are directed towards relieving the vascular pressure in the head, usually through forcing the descent of *qi* through the 'big exit', (that is, the bowel, by purging) or by heavily weighing down *yang*. Ultimately, the main therapeutic principle is to allow the wild fluctuations in the patients *yin* and *yang* to settle, so they survive long enough and with the least disability to benefit from the final phase of treatment. During the acute phase patients should be managed in hospital.

The last phase is treatment of the sequelae of the Wind stroke. The treatment principle will vary somewhat depending on the chronicity of the disability. In general, the longer the paralysis the longer the treatment, but TCM really shines in the treatment of this phase. After the acute phase (about two weeks) acupuncture treatment can begin. After six months, treatment of hemiplegia and other paresis is difficult, although it is always worth a good go as different patients will respond (sometimes remarkably) differently. In the context of long term paralysis at least one course of acupuncture treatment (usually 10-12 sessions) or two months of herbal therapy should be attempted before making a judgement on whether the treatment is working or not.

DIFFERENTIAL DIAGNOSIS

- ***Jue* syndrome** (*jue zheng* 厥证): *Jue* syndrome is characterised by sudden loss of consciousness, then a gradual regaining of consciousness with no residual paralysis, speech difficulties or sequelae. The sorts of disorders that are categorised as *jue* syndrome include hypoglycaemic coma, hysterical syncope, haemorrhagic or allergic shock.
- **Epilepsy** (*dian xian* 癫痫): Epilepsy involves partial or total loss of consciousness, collapse, and convulsions. Upon regaining consciousness, epileptic patients are not left with any residual paralysis.

---

1. Acupuncture can be used, however, with complete safety for channel stroke patterns from external Wind (for example in conditions like Bell's palsy).

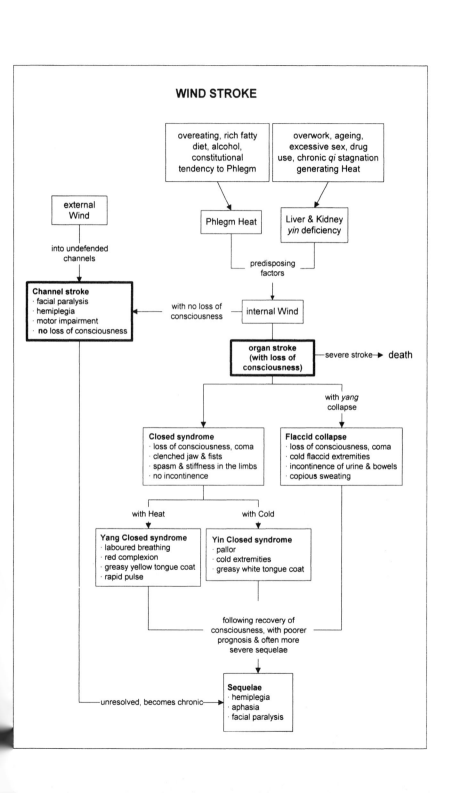

CHANNEL SYNDROMES

24.1 EMPTINESS OF THE CHANNELS WITH WIND INVASION

Pathophysiology
- There is still debate about the precise pathophysiology of this pattern, but the formulae recommended would suggest that the consensus falls in favour of external Wind. Therefore, this is most likely an invasion of external Wind into undefended channels. Once lodged in the channels, the circulation of *qi* and Blood is disrupted and the tissues are deprived of nourishment.
- The fundamental difference between this pattern and the patterns that follow is that here the predisposing factors for the development of internal Wind may be absent - it can occur in young and relatively healthy individuals.

Clinical features
- numbness or motor dysfunction of the extremities
- sudden facial paralysis
- dysphasia
- maybe fever and chills
- arthralgia
- no disturbance of consciousness

T thin white coat
P floating and wiry or wiry and thready

Treatment principle
Expel Wind (and Heat or Cold)
Nourish and invigorate *qi* and Blood and open the channels

Prescription

DA QIN JIAO TANG 大秦艽汤
(*Major Gentiana Qinjiao Decoction*)

This formula (and the next) are commonly used for acute facial paralysis, hemiplegia and Bell's Palsy where external Wind is the culprit. (The diaphoretic approach suggested here is not recommended, and in fact may be deleterious when the cause is internal Wind). This formula is suitable for the early and middle stages of channel stroke, and for cases with Heat.

qin jiao (Radix Gentianae Qinjiao) 秦艽	9g
dang gui (Radix Angelicae Sinensis) 当归	9g
bai shao (Radix Paeoniae Lactiflorae) 白芍	9g
chuan xiong (Radix Ligustici Chuanxiong) 川芎	6g
du huo (Radix Angelicae Pubescentis) 独活	6g
qiang huo (Rhizoma et Radix Notopterygii) 羌活	6g
fang feng (Radix Ledebouriellae Divaricatae) 防风	9g

24. WIND STROKE

xi xin* (Herba cum Radice Asari) 细辛 3g
huang qin (Radix Scutellariae Baicalensis) 黄芩 9g
shi gao (Gypsum) 石膏 12g
bai zhi (Radix Angelicae Dahuricae) 白芷 9g
bai zhu (Rhizoma Atractylodis Macrocephalae) 白术 9g
sheng di (Radix Rehmanniae Glutinosae) 生地 12g
shu di (Radix Rehmanniae Glutinosae Conquitae) 熟地 12g
fu ling (Sclerotium Poria Cocos) 茯苓 12g
gan cao (Radix Glycyrrhizae Uralensis) 甘草 6g

Method: Decoction. (Source: *Shi Yong Zhong Yi Nei Ke Xue*)

Modifications

- If there is no Heat, delete **shi gao** and **huang qin**.
- With Wind Heat, add **sang ye** (Folium Mori Albae) 桑叶 12g, **ju hua** (Flos Chrysanthemi Morifolii) 菊花 12g and **bo he** (Herba Mentha Haplocalycis) 薄荷 6g.
- With a stiff neck, add **ge gen** (Radix Puerariae) 葛根 12g.

XIAO XU MING TANG 小续命汤
(Minor Prolong Life Decoction)

This formula is selected when there are signs of Cold, and like the previous one, clear indications of an external Wind attack.

ma huang* (Herba Ephedra) 麻黄 3-6g
chuan xiong (Radix Ligustici Chuanxiong) 川芎 3-6g
guang fang ji* (Radix Aristolochiae Fangchi) 广防己 6-12g
xing ren* (Semen Pruni Armeniacae) 杏仁 9-12g
fang feng (Radix Ledebouriellae Divaricatae) 防风 9-12g
sheng jiang (Rhizoma Zingiberis Officinalis) 生姜 9-12g
ren shen (Radix Ginseng) 人参 3-6g
zhi fu zi* (Radix Aconiti Carmichaeli Praeparata)
    制附子 3-9g
rou gui (Cortex Cinnamomi Cassiae) 肉桂 3-6g
bai shao (Radix Paeoniae Lactiflorae) 白芍 6-12g
huang qin (Radix Scutellariae Baicalensis) 黄芩 4.5-9g
gan cao (Radix Glycyrrhizae Uralensis) 甘草 3-6g

Method: Decoction. **Zhi fu zi** is cooked for 30 minutes prior to the other herbs (*xian jian* 先煎). (Source: *Formulas and Strategies*)

QIAN ZHENG SAN 牵正散
(Lead to Symmetry Powder) modified

This formula is used when facial paralysis is the main feature and there are few (if any) other signs of external Wind.

jiang can^ (Bombyx Batryticatus) 僵蚕 12g
quan xie* (Buthus Martensi) 全蝎 10g
bai fu zi* (Rhizoma Typhonii Gigantei) 白附子 6g
jing jie (Herba seu Flos Schizonepetae Tenuifolia) 荆芥 10g
fang feng (Radix Ledebouriellae Divaricatae) 防风 10g
hong hua (Flos Carthami Tinctorii) 红花 10g
di long^ (Lumbricus) 地龙 10g
chi shao (Radix Paeoniae Rubrae) 赤芍 10g
gan cao (Radix Glycyrrhizae Uralensis) 甘草 6g

Method: Decoction or powder. When powdered, the dose is 3-grams, 2-3 times daily with hot wine. (Source: *Zhong Yi Nei Ke Lin Chuang Shou Ce*)

Patent medicines
Kang Wei Ling 亢痿灵 (Kang Wei Ling)
Hua Tuo Zai Zao Wan 华佗再造丸 (Hua Tuo Zai Zao Wan)
Bu Yang Huan Wu Wan 补阳还五丸 (Bu Yang Huan Wu Wan)

Acupuncture
Special method for Bell's Palsy
Threading technique with a 3-inch needle from St.6 (*jia che*) to St.4 (*di cang*) and St.7 (*xia guan*), and a 1.5-inch needle from St.2 (*si bai*) to St.4 (*di cang*) on the affected side. In addition LI.4 (*he gu*) and Lu.7 (*lie que*) may be treated with gentle electro-stimulation. Other points are added depending on the affected part:
- eye - GB.1 (*tong zi liao*), SJ.23 (*si zhu kong*)
- nose - LI.20 (*ying xiang*)
- tongue - Ren.23 (*lian quan*)
- lips - Du.26 (*ren zhong*), Ren.24 (*cheng jiang*)

Clinical notes
- This pattern may correspond to conditions such as Bell's palsy, facial paralysis and rheumatism.
- Modern TCM clinicians are generally of the opinion that the diaphoretic prescriptions recommended here are for use only in situations clearly related to external Wind, that is, in those with no obvious predisposing factors for internal Wind. If the Wind is of internal origin, application of these formualae can be detrimental. Their use is generally resticted to conditions like Bell's palsy and rheumatism.

24.2 LIVER AND KIDNEY *YIN* DEFICIENCY WITH RISING LIVER *YANG* AND WIND

Pathophysiology
- Wind stroke due to Liver and Kidney *yin* deficiency with rising Liver *yang* has two aspects to it, the prodrome and the catastrophe. The first is the background *yin* deficiency, which is a chronic disorder and the pre-condition for the sudden surge of *yang*. At a critical point of deficiency, Liver *yang* suddenly slips its mooring and surges towards the head. At a high level of intensity and mobility Liver *yang* is redefined as Wind, which in the prodome stage may cause vertigo, monocular blindness, double vision, confusion or ataxia. Swiftly applied treatment may subdue the Wind and avert the catastrophe. If the Wind is not constrained, however, it can wreak havoc in the channels causing loss of motor control and paralysis, or even loss of consciousness (see organ stroke p.660)

Clinical features
- dizziness, vertigo
- headache, often temporal or vertical
- tinnitus
- pressure behind the eyes, blurring vision, sudden loss of vision in one eye
- facial flushing
- irritability and restlessness
- insomnia or restless, dream disturbed sleep
- lower back ache
- progessive unilateral motor dysfunction, weakness, paralysis or numbness of the extremities, facial paralysis, dysphasia, which may develop over a period of a few hours to a few days
- hypertension

T red with little or no coat
P thready, wiry and rapid

Treatment principle
Sedate Liver *yang* and extinguish Wind
Nourish *yin* to anchor *yang*

Prescription

ZHEN GAN XI FENG TANG 镇肝熄风汤
(Sedate the Liver and Extinguish Wind Decoction)

This is an excellent formula for TIA's and the immediate sequelae of a CVA due to *yin* deficiency with *yang* rising, as well as for prevention of Wind stroke in hypertensive patients.

huai niu xi (Radix Achyranthis Bidentatae) 怀牛膝 30g
dai zhe shi (Haematitum) 代赭石 30g
long gu^ (Os Draconis) 龙骨 15g
mu li^ (Concha Ostreae) 牡蛎 15g
gui ban° (Plastri Testudinis) 龟板 15g
bai shao (Radix Paeoniae Lactiflorae) 白芍 15g
xuan shen (Radix Scrophulariae) 玄参 15g
tian dong (Tuber Asparagi Cochinchinensis) 天冬 15g
chuan lian zi* (Fructus Meliae Toosendan) 川楝子 6g
mai ya (Fructus Hordei Vulgaris Germinantus) 麦芽 6g
yin chen (Herba Artemisiae Yinchenhao) 茵陈 6g
gan cao (Radix Glycyrrhizae Uralensis) 甘草 6g

Method: Decoction. The mineral and shell ingredients are decocted for 30 minutes prior to the other herbs (*xian jian* 先煎). (Source: *Shi Yong Zhong Yi Nei Ke Xue*)

Modifications

- With copious Phlegm, delete **gui ban°** and add **dan nan xing*** (Pulvis Arisaemae cum Felle Bovis) 胆南星 6g and **zhu li** (Succus Bambusae) 竹沥 6g.
- With severe irritability, add **huang qin** (Radix Scutellariae Baicalensis) 黄芩 12g and **shi gao** (Gypsum) 石膏 18g.
- With severe headache, add **shi jue ming^** (Concha Haliotidis) 石决明 12g and **xia ku cao** (Spica Prunellae Vulgaris) 夏枯草 12g.
- If the tongue coat is greasy and yellow and the patient is constipated, add **quan gua lou** (Fructus Trichosanthis) 全栝楼 20g, **zhi shi** (Fructus Immaturus Citri Aurantii) 枳实 9g and **sheng da huang** (Radix et Rhizoma Rhei) 生大黄 6-9g.
- For slurred speech, add **shi chang pu** (Rhizoma Acori Graminei) 石菖蒲 6g, **tian nan xing*** (Rhizoma Arisaematis) 天南星 6g and **jiang can^** (Bombyx Batryticatus) 僵蚕 9g.
- For facial paralysis, add **bai fu zi*** (Rhizoma Typhonii Gigantei) 白附子 6g, **jiang can** (Bombyx Batryticatus) 僵蚕 9g and **quan xie*** (Buthus Martensi) 全蝎 3g.
- With numbness or paralysis of the limbs, add **di bie chong^** (Eupolyphaga seu Opisthoplatia) 地鳖虫 6g, **quan xie*** (Buthus Martensi) 全蝎 3g and **wu gong*** (Scolopendra Subspinipes) 蜈蚣 3g.
- If the tongue has a thick greasy coat, reduce the dose of some of the *yin* nourishing herbs - **xuan shen**, **tian dong**, **gui ban** and **bai shao**.

Patent medicines

All following formulae are suitable for prevention and treatment of Liver and Kidney *yin* deficiency and Phlegm Heat type stroke.

Yang Yin Jiang Ya Wan 养阴降压丸 (Yang Yin Jiang Ya Wan)
Tian Ma Gou Teng Wan 天麻钩藤丸 (Tian Ma Gou Teng Wan)
Xiao Shuan Zai Zao Wan 消栓再造丸 (Xiao Shuan Zai Zao Wan)

Acupuncture

There are two aspects to treatment–before a stroke (as preventitive) and treatment of the sequelae. Treatment of the sequelae are dealt with individually at the end of this chapter. Preventative treatment is applied to those individuals with the various warning signs of impending catastrophe–hypertension, obesity, dizziness, plethora, headaches, TIA's etc.

Appropriate points include Liv.3 (*tai chong*), LI.4 (*he gu*), LI.11 (*qu chi*), St.40 (*feng long*), GB.34 (*yang ling quan*), St.36 (*zu san li*), Liv.2 (*xing jian*), GB.20 (*feng chi*), an mian (N-HN-54), PC.6 (*nei guan*), SJ.5 (*wai guan*), GB.39 (*xuan zhong*), GB.41 (*zu lin qi*), GB.31 (*feng shi*), GB.21 (*jian jing*), *yin tang* (M-HN-3) depending on the symptom picture. Take care not to overstimulate points in patients with very high blood pressure.
Ear points: ear apex, lowering blood pressure groove (↓ to reduce blood pressure)

Caution In China acupuncture is generally not given (other than for rescusitation, see Organ syndromes) to **acute** stroke victims, as a bleeding aneurysm may continue to bleed with acupuncture stimulation. For the first two weeks following a stroke the treatment is with herbs until the patient is stable, then acupuncture is phased in.

Clinical notes

- This pattern may correspond to conditions such as hypertension, transient ischaemic attacks (TIA's) and cerebro-vascular accident.
- Strokes of this type are much easier to prevent than to treat, so identification of the warning signs is the key to a successful outcome.
- Lifestyle changes are very important as many patients with this pattern will be overworking, stressed and have poor dietary habits. Stress management and reduction of diary products, fats and oils and other Phlegm generating or Heat inducing substances is important.

24.3 PHLEGM HEAT WITH WIND PHLEGM

Pathophysiology
- Wind stroke due to Phlegm Heat with Wind has two aspects to it, like the previous Liver and Kidney deficiency pattern–the prodrome and the catastrophe. There may in fact be little to distinguish this from the previous pattern because Phlegm frequently combines with Liver *yang* in the genesis of Wind stroke. However, when Phlegm Heat is involved, treatment must quickly eliminate the accumulated Heat and Phlegm through the bowel, thereby reducing pressure in the head and increasing the prospects for survival.

Clinical features
- sudden heaviness, numbness or paralysis of the extremities on one side of the body, facial paralysis or dysphasia
- disordered consciousness
- dry stools or constipation
- may be dizziness, copious sputum and drooling

T stiff, quivering or deviated to one side, with a greasy yellow coat
P wiry and slippery

Treatment principle
Expel Phlegm and Heat through the bowels

Prescription

XING WEI CHENG QI TANG 星蒌承气汤
(*Fading Star Order the Qi Decoction*)

dan nan xing* (Pulvis Arisaemae cum Felle Bovis) 胆南星	6-10g
quan gua lou (Fructus Trichosanthis) 全栝楼	30-40g
sheng da huang (Radix et Rhizoma Rhei) 生大黄	10-15g
mang xiao (Mirabilitum) 芒硝	10-15g

Method: Decoction. Due to the large doses, the bowels should open vigorously within 10-15 minutes after which the symptoms should subside. (Source: *Shi Yong Zhong Yi Nei Ke Xue*)

Modifications
- After the bowels have vigorously opened, the dose of **da huang** and **mang xiao** should be reduced or deleted and the principle altered to clearing Phlegm Heat, invigorating the Blood and opening the channels with herbs like **dan nan xing*** (Pulvis Arisaemae cum Felle Bovis) 胆南星, **gua lou** (Fructus Trichosanthis) 栝楼, **dan shen** (Radix Salviae

Miltiorrhizae) 丹参, **chi shao** (Radix Paeoniae Rubrae) 赤芍 and **ji xue teng** (Radix et Caulis Jixueteng) 鸡血藤.
- If dizziness is severe, add **gou teng** (Ramulus Uncariae cum Uncis) 钩藤 12g, **ju hua** (Flos Chrysanthemi Morifolii) 菊花 12g and **zhen zhu mu^** (Concha Margaritaferae) 珍珠母 15g.

Patent medicines
see 24.2 Liver and Kidney *yin* deficiency with *yang* rising, p.657

Acupuncture
see 24.2 Liver and Kidney *yin* deficiency with *yang* rising, p.657

Clinical notes
- This pattern may correspond to conditions such as acute cerebro-vascular accident, cerebral haemorrhage and cerebral thrombosis.
- The principle of swiftly eliminating Phlegm and Heat through the 'big exit' is popular in China as an emergency treatment for a variety of serious conditions with consciousness disturbances[1]. This approach is most applicable when a full blown CVA has occured, and should only be used for a short period of time to drastically reduce pressure in the head, until symptoms settle down (in contrast to the previous formula [*Zhen Gan Xi Feng Tang*], which is best used as a stroke preventitive in hypertensive patients, and which can be used for lengthy periods of time).

---

1. Fruehauf, H. (1994) "Stroke and Post Stroke Syndrome". *Journal. Chin. Med.* 44:23-36

ORGAN STROKE SYNDROMES

These syndromes are characterised by partial or total loss of consciousness, preceded by, and in addition to, any of the symptoms listed for channel stroke. All are critical conditions and a high percentage of patients die or are left with serious debility. The main principle of treatment at this stage is the swift revival of the patient, as the sooner consciousness returns the less severe the aftermath.

24.4 CLOSED SYNDROMES

Closed syndrome is loss of consciousness characterised by pathogenic excess. The excess nature of this condition is reflected in the manifestations–the body being locked up tight and in spasm. The excess may be hot or cold. Differentiation of the closed and flaccid types is especially important because the therapeutic approaches are opposite. Closed (and Flaccid) syndromes are medical emergencies and management should include hospitalisation.

24.4.1 *Yang* Closed syndrome
Pathophysiology
- This syndrome is *yang* and hot, usually the progression of Phlegm Heat with Wind Phlegm channel stroke into full unconsciousness.

Clinical features
- loss of conciousness, coma
- clenched jaw and fists
- stiffness or spasm in the limbs
- no loss of bowel or bladder control
- laboured breathing
- red complexion

T greasy yellow coat
P wiry, slippery and rapid

Treatment principle
  Restore consciousness
  Clear Liver Heat and extinguish Wind

Prescription

ZHI BAO DAN 至宝丹
(Greatest Treasure Special Pill)

an xi xiang (Benzoinum) 安息香	45g
xi jiao° (Cornu Rhinoceri) 犀角	30g
dai mao° (Carapax Eretmochelydis Imbricatae) 玳瑁	30g

hu po (Succinum) 琥珀 30g
zhu sha* (Cinnabaris) 朱砂 30g
xiong huang (Realgar) 雄黄 30g
niu huang^ (Calculus Bovis) 牛黄 15g
bing pian (Borneol) 冰片 3g
she xiang° (Secretio Moschus) 麝香 3g

Method: Available in prepared form and a standard part of any TCM first aid kit, this pill is forced into the mouth or nose or given via a nasogastric tube until consciousness is restored. (Source: *Shi Yong Fang Ji Xue*)

Follow up treatment

♦ Once the patient is conscious, there are two general approaches. If Phlegm Heat is obvious, swift elimination through the bowel (see Phlegm Heat with Wind Phlegm, p.658) may be applied until some stability is restored. In the event of fluid depletion and Liver Heat (fever, deep red dry tongue with prickles, persistent spasm of the extremities), the alternative is to cool the Liver and extinguish Wind with **LING JIAO GOU TENG TANG** (*Antelope Horn and Uncaria Decoction* 羚角钩藤汤).

ling yang jiao fen° (powdered Cornu Antelopis) 羚羊角粉 .. 3g
gou teng (Ramulus Uncariae cum Uncis) 钩藤 15g
sheng di (Radix Rehmanniae Glutinosae) 生地 15g
zhu ru (Caulis Bambusae in Taeniis) 竹茹 15g
sang ye (Folium Mori Albae) 桑叶 12g
chuan bei mu (Bulbus Fritillariae Cirrhosae) 川贝母 9g
ju hua (Flos Chrysanthemi Morifolii) 菊花 9g
bai shao (Radix Paeoniae Lactiflorae) 白芍 9g
fu ling (Sclerotium Poria Cocos) 茯苓 9g
gan cao (Radix Glycyrrhizae Uralensis) 甘草 3g

Method: Decoction. **Ling yang jiao** powder is added to the strained decoction (3 grams in each dose, *chong fu* 冲服), **gou teng** is added towards the end of cooking (*hou xia* 后下). (Source: *Shi Yong Zhong Yao Xue*)

Patent medicines

Zhi Bao Dan 至宝丹 (Zhi Bao Dan)
 - this is the prefered medicine. In the event that it is unavailable, one of the following may be substituted, used only until consciousness is restored.

An Gong Niu Huang Wan 安宫牛黄丸 (An Gong Niu Huang Wan)
Zi Xue Dan 紫雪丹 (Tzuhsueh Tan)

Acupuncture

Du.26 (*ren zhong* -), *shi xuan* ↓ (M-UE-1), Liv.3 (*tai chong* -),
St.40 (*feng long* -), PC.8 (*lao gong* -), Kid.1 (*yong quan* -). Treat frequently until consciousness is restored.

24.4.2 *Yin* Closed syndrome
Pathophysiology

- The *yin* closed syndrome type Wind stroke is similar to the previous (*yang* closed syndrome) in that it is characterised by excess (spasm and tension), but differs by having signs of cold. It follows the same aetiological features, but may be the presentation of closed syndrome in a constitutionally *yang* deficient and cold individual.

Clinical features

- loss of consciousness, coma
- clenched jaw and fists
- stiffness or spasm in the limbs
- no loss of bowel or bladder control
- pale or ashen complexion
- cold extremities
- copious sputum

T greasy white coat
P deep, slippery and moderate

Treatment principle

Restore consciousness, warm and aromatically open the orifices
Eliminate Phlegm and extinguish Wind

Prescription

SU HE XIANG WAN 苏合香丸
(*Liquid Styrax Pill*)

su he xiang (Styrax Liquidis) 苏合香	30g
an xi xiang (Benzoinum) 安息香	60g
chen xiang (Lignum Aquilariae) 沉香	60g
she xiang° (Secretio Moschus) 麝香	60g
ding xiang (Flos Caryophylli) 丁香	60g
qing mu xiang* (Radix Aristolochiae) 青木香	60g
bai zhu (Rhizoma Atractylodes Macrocephalae) 白术	60g
xi jiao° (Cornu Rhinoceri) 犀角	60g
xiang fu (Rhizoma Cyperi Rotundi) 香附	60g
tan xiang (Lignum Santali Albi) 檀香	60g
zhu sha* (Cinnabaris) 朱砂	60g

he zi (Fructus Terminaliae Chebulae) 诃子 60g
bi ba (Fructus Piperis Longi) 荜拔 60g
bing pian (Borneol) 冰片 30g
ru xiang (Gummi Olibanum) 乳香 30g
Method: Like ZHI BAO DAN (*Greatest Treasure Special Pill* 至宝丹), this pill is a standard part of a TCM first aid kit. The pill is forced into the mouth or nose or given via a nasogastric tube until consciousness is restored. (Source: *Shi Yong Fang Ji Xue*)

Follow up treatment

♦ Once the patient is conscious **DI TAN TANG** (*Scour Phlegm Decoction* 涤痰汤) modified may be used to powerfully clear away Phlegm, open the orifices and tonify *qi*.

ban xia* (Rhizoma Pinelliae Ternatae) 半夏 9g
fu ling (Sclerotium Poria Cocos) 茯苓 9g
zhu ru (Caulis Bambusae in Taeniis) 竹茹 9g
dan nan xing* (Pulvis Arisaemae cum Felle Bovis) 胆南星 ... 6g
chen pi (Pericarpium Citri Reticulatae) 陈皮 6g
zhi shi (Fructus Immaturus Citri Aurantii) 枳实 6g
shi chang pu (Rhizoma Acori Graminei) 石菖蒲 6g
dang shen (Radix Codonopsis Pilosulae) 党参 12g
di long^ (Lumbricus) 地龙 9g
gou teng (Ramulus Uncariae cum Uncis) 钩藤 9g
gan cao (Radix Glycyrrhizae Uralensis) 甘草 3g
sheng jiang (Rhizoma Zingiberis Officinalis) 生姜 3pce
da zao (Fructus Zizyphi Jujubae) 大枣 4pce
Method: Decoction. (Source: *Shi Yong Zhong Yao Xue*)

Patent medicines

Su He Xiang Wan 苏合香丸 (*Liquid Styrax Pill*)

Acupuncture

Although the herbal approach differs between these two patterns, the same acupuncture can be applied, with the addition of moxa in this pattern. Treat frequently until consciousness is restored.

Du.26 (*ren zhong* -), *shi xuan* ↓ (M-UE-1), Liv.3 (*tai chong* -),
St.40 (*feng long* -), PC.8 (*lao gong* -), Kid.1 (*yong quan* - ▲)

Clinical notes

- Similar to shock, stroke, post cerebro-vascular accident or coma.
- Both these patterns are obvious medical emergencies and any TCM emergency treatment must be combined with appropriate paramedic attention and hospitalisation.

Table 24.1 Summary of acute phases of Wind stroke

Pattern				Features	Treatment principle	Guiding Formula
Channel stroke, with no loss of consciousness	external Wind			sudden facial paralysis, numbness or motor dysfunction of the extremities, fever & chills, arthralgia, floating pulse	Expel Wind & open the channels	DA QIN JIAO TANG
	Liver *yin* deficiency with *yang* rising & Wind			dizziness, headache, tinnitus, distension of the eyes, blurring vision, facial flushing, progressive motor dysfunction & paralysis, red tongue	Sedate Liver *yang*, extinguish Wind, nourish *yin*	ZHEN GAN XI FENG TANG
	Phlegm Heat with Wind Phlegm			sudden heaviness, numbness or paralysis on one side of the body, constipation, copious sputum, drooling, thick yellow tongue coat	Eliminate Phlegm Heat through the bowel	XING WEI CHENG QI TANG
Organ stroke, with loss of consciousness	Closed syndrome	Hot type		loss of consciousness, clenched fist & jaw, no incontinence, red face, yellow tongue coat	Restore consciousness, clear Heat & Wind	ZHI BAO DAN
		Cold type		loss of consciousness, clenched fist & jaw, no incontinence, pale or ashen face, cold extremities	Restore consciousness, warm & aromatically open orifices	SU HE XIANG WAN
	Flaccid syndrome			loss of consciousness, icy extremities, incontinence of urine & stools, copious sweating, imperceptible pulse	Rescue *yang* from collapse	SHEN FU TANG

脱证

24.5 FLACCID COLLAPSE SYNDROME

Pathophysiology
- This type of unconsciousness is due to sudden collapse of *yang*. This occurs when *yin* has been consumed to such an extent that physiological equilibrium is completely disrupted. *Yin* is unable to preserve and harness *yang*, which dissipates to the point of separation of *yin* and *yang* (that is, death). In contrast to the closed syndrome, where the *yang qi* is locked up tight in the body and needs to be vented, in this condition the *yang* is swiftly dissipating and has to be vigorously replaced.

Clinical features
- loss of consciousness, coma
- cold limbs
- incontinence of urine and stools
- pale or ashen complexion
- copious sweating
- flaccid extremities

T flaccid and pale
P minute or imperceptible

Treatment principle
Rescue and rescucitate *yang*

Prescription

SHEN FU TANG 参附汤
(*Ginseng and Prepared Aconite Decoction*)

ren shen (Radix Ginseng) 人参 10-15g
zhi fu zi* (Radix Aconiti Carmichaeli Praeparata)
制附子 10-15g

Method: Decoction. The decocted herbs may be administered via a nasogastric tube, enema, intramuscular injection or intravenous drip. (Source: *Shi Yong Zhong Yi Nei Ke Xue*)

Modifications
♦ With severe sweating, add two or three of the following herbs: **huang qi** (Radix Astragali Membranacei) 黄芪 20g, **long gu**^ (Os Draconis) 龙骨 20g, **mu li**^ (Concha Ostreae) 牡蛎 20g, **wu wei zi** (Fructus Schizandrae Chinensis) 五味子 9g or **shan zhu yu** (Fructus Corni Officinalis) 山茱萸 12g.

Acupuncture
1. Strong moxa on Ren.8 (*shen que*), usually on salt. Place a piece of thin

cloth over the navel and fill it with salt. Burn large cones of moxa on the salt. The cloth enables quick removal of the salt and prevents excessive burning. In addition, strong reinforcing needling on Ren.4 (*guan yuan* +) and St.36 (*zu san li* +)

2. A modern method for shock is strong needling on Du.25 (*su liao* -), Kid.1 (*yong quan* -) and PC.6 (*nei guan* -). Du.25 (*su liao*) is needled to 0.5-1 cun and manipulated continuously for 30 minutes. If these points are insufficient to elevate blood pressure add Du.26 (*ren zhong* -), LI.4 (*he gu* -) and St.36 (*zu san li*).

Clinical notes

- cerebro-vascular accident, shock, hypovolaemic shock, myocardial infarction
- The patient should be covered and have their legs elevated. This is a critical situation and paramedic attention should be sought immediately.

Table 24.2 Summary of Wind stroke sequelae

Sequelae	Pattern	Features		Guiding prescription
Hemiplegia	Qi deficiency with Blood stagnation	motor impairment, paralysis, numbness or loss of sensation on one side of the body	normal or low blood pressure, white tongue coat, moderate pulse	BU YANG HUAN WU TANG
	Liver yang rising with Blood stagnation		hypertension, dizziness, headache, red face & tongue, wiry slippery rapid pulse	ZHEN GAN XI FENG TANG
Dysphasia	Liver & Kidney yin & yang deficiency	stiffness or deviation of the tongue, slurred speech	weakness of the extremities, thready pulse, pale or red tongue	DI HUANG YIN ZI
	Wind Phlegm		greasy white tongue coat, wiry & slippery	JIE YU DAN
Facial paralysis	one sided facial paralysis, facial muscle spasms or tics			QIAN ZHENG SAN

SEQUELAE OF WIND STROKE
24.6 HEMIPLEGIA
- Hemiplegia is paralysis or motor dysfunction affecting one side of the body. The primary aetiological factor is Blood stagnation in the channels subsequent to their attack by Wind. Depending on the initial conditions and the duration of the hemiplegia, two presentations occur, *qi* deficiency with Blood stagnation (the most common) and Liver *yang* rising with Blood stagnation.

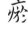

24.6.1 *Qi* deficiency with Blood stagnation
This presentation is the most common pattern following a stroke.

Clinical features
- motor impairment, paralysis, numbness or complete loss of sensation on one side of the body
- deviation of the eyes and mouth
- frequent urination or incontinence of urine
- blood pressure is low, normal, or only slightly elevated

T white coat
P moderate

Treatment principle
Tonify *qi* and invigorate Blood
Open the channels

Prescription

BU YANG HUAN WU TANG 补阳还五汤
(*Tonify the Yang to Restore Five Tenths Decoction*)

huang qi (Radix Astragali Membranacei) 黄芪	30-120g
dang gui wei (Radix Angelicae Sinensis) 当归尾	9g
chi shao (Radix Paeoniae Rubrae) 赤芍	9g
di long^ (Lumbricus) 地龙	9g
tao ren (Semen Persicae) 桃仁	9g
chuan xiong (Radix Ligustici Chuanxiong) 川芎	6g
hong hua (Flos Carthami Tinctorii) 红花	6g

Method: Decoction. (Source: *Shi Yong Zhong Yao Xue*)

Modifications
- Because **huang qi** may elevate blood pressure in patients with hypertension, some experts recommend the addition of a heavy mineral, like **shi gao** (Gypsum) 石膏 or **dai zhe shi** (Haematitum)

代赭石, to balance this unwanted effect.

- If hemiplegia is severe or chronic, add **chuan shan jia**° (Squama Manitis) 穿山甲 9g, **shui zhi**ˆ (Hirudo seu Whitmania) 水蛭 3g and **sang zhi** (Ramulus Mori Albae) 桑枝 12g or combine with the patent pill **XIAO HUO LUO DAN** (*Minor Invigorate the Collaterals Special Pill* 小活络丹, p.929).
- If speech is slurred, add **shi chang pu** (Rhizoma Acori Graminei) 石菖蒲 6g and **yuan zhi** (Radix Polygalae Tenuifoliae) 远志 6g.
- With visual disturbance or loss of vision, add **mi meng hua** (Flos Buddleiae Officinalis Immaturus) 蜜蒙花 9g, **gou qi zi** (Fructus Lycii) 枸杞子 12g and **jue ming zi** (Semen Cassiae) 决明子 9g (with the last herb be cautious where there is hypotension).
- With palpitations (on a background of *yang* deficiency), add **gui zhi** (Ramulus Cinnamomi Cassiae) 桂枝 9g and **zhi gan cao** (honey fried Radix Glycyrrhizae Uralensis) 炙甘草 9g.
- If the upper limbs are particularly affected, add **sang zhi** (Ramulus Mori Albae) 桑枝 12g and **gui zhi** (Ramulus Cinnamomi Cassiae) 桂枝 9g.
- If the lower limbs are particularly affected, add two or three of the following herbs: **sang ji sheng** (Ramulus Sangjisheng) 桑寄生 12g, **xu duan** (Radix Dipsaci Asperi) 续断 9g, **niu xi** (Radix Achyranthis Bidentatae) 牛膝 12g, **du zhong** (Cortex Eucommiae Ulmoidis) 杜仲 12g, **shu di** (Radix Rehmanniae Glutinosae Conquitae) 熟地 15g, **shan zhu yu** (Fructus Corni Officinalis) 山茱萸 12g or **rou cong rong** (Cistanches Deserticolae) 肉苁蓉 15g.
- With incontinence, add **sang piao xiao**ˆ (Ootheca mantidis) 桑螵蛸 9g and **yi zhi ren** (Fructus Alpiniae Oxyphallae) 益智仁 9g.
- With oedema, add **fu ling** (Sclerotium Poria Cocos) 茯苓 12g, **ze xie** (Rhizoma Alismatis Orientalis) 泽泻 9g and **mu tong** (Caulis Mutong) 木通 6g.
- With facial paralysis, add **bai fu zi*** (Rhizoma Typhonii Gigantei) 白附子 6g, **jiang can**ˆ (Bombyx Batryticatus) 僵蚕 9g and **quan xie*** (Buthus Martensi) 全蝎 3g.

Patent medicines

Xiao Huo Luo Dan 小活络丹 (Xiao Huo Luo Dan)
   - when chronic and cold
Bu Yang Huan Wu Wan 补阳还五丸 (Bu Yang Huan Wu Wan)
Hua Tuo Zai Zao Wan 华佗再造丸 (Hua Tuo Zai Zao Wan)

24.6.2 Liver *yang* rising with Blood stagnation

The second clinical presentation of hemiplegia is less common and occurs in the early days after the stroke when the blood pressure may still be quite high.

Clinical features
- motor impairment, paralysis, numbness or complete loss of sensation on one side of the body
- headache
- dizziness
- tinnitus
- facial flushing
- irritability
- hypertension

T red with little or no coat, or red and stiff or quivering
P wiry and slippery or wiry, thready and rapid

Treatment principle
Sedate Liver *yang* and extinguish Wind
Nourish *yin*, open the channels

Prescription

ZHEN GAN XI FENG TANG 镇肝熄风汤
(*Sedate the Liver and Extinguish Wind Decoction*) modified

huai niu xi (Radix Achyranthis Bidentatae) 怀牛膝	30g
dai zhe shi (Haematitum) 代赭石	30g
long gu^ (Os Draconis) 龙骨	15g
mu li^ (Concha Ostreae) 牡蛎	15g
gui ban° (Plastri Testudinis) 龟板	15g
bai shao (Radix Paeoniae Lactiflorae) 白芍	15g
xuan shen (Radix Scrophulariae) 玄参	15g
tian dong (Tuber Asparagi Cochinchinensis) 天冬	15g
ji xue teng (Radix et Caulis Jixueteng) 鸡血藤	15g
di long^ (Lumbricus) 地龙	9g
chuan lian zi* (Fructus Meliae Toosendan) 川楝子	6g
mai ya (Fructus Hordei Vulgaris Germinantus) 麦芽	6g
yin chen (Herba Artemisiae Yinchenhao) 茵陈	6g
gan cao (Radix Glycyrrhizae Uralensis) 甘草	3g

Method: Decoction. The mineral and shell ingredients are decocted for 30 minutes prior to the other herbs. (Source: *Shi Yong Zhong Yi Nei Ke Xue*)

肝阳上亢血瘀

TIAN MA GOU TENG YIN 天麻钩藤饮
(Gastrodia and Gambir Formula)

This is a popular formula for hypertension of a Liver *yang* rising type. It is similar to the primary formula, except it has less tonifying and anchoring elements and so is suitable for those with less underlying deficiency.

tian ma (Rhizoma Gastrodiae Elatae) 天麻	9g
gou teng (Ramulus Uncariae cum Uncis) 钩藤	12g
shi jue ming^ (Concha Haliotidis) 石决明	15g
ye jiao teng (Caulis Polygoni Multiflori) 夜交藤	15g
sang ji sheng (Ramulus Sangjisheng) 桑寄生	12g
huang qin (Radix Scutellariae Baicalensis) 黄芩	9g
shan zhi zi (Fructus Gardeniae Jasminoides) 山栀子	9g
yi mu cao (Herba Leonuri Officinalis) 益母草	9g
fu shen (Sclerotium Poriae Cocos Pararadicis) 茯神	9g
du zhong (Cortex Eucommiae Ulmoidis) 杜仲	9g
niu xi (Radix Achyranthis Bidentatae) 牛膝	9g

Method: Decoction. **Shi jue ming** should be cooked for 30 minutes before the other herbs are added (*xian jian* 先煎), **gou teng** is added near the end of cooking (*hou xia* 后下). (Source: *Shi Yong Zhong Yi Nei Ke Xue*)

Patent medicines

Yang Yin Jiang Ya Wan 养阴降压丸 (Yang Yin Jiang Ya Wan)
Tian Ma Gou Teng Wan 天麻钩藤丸 (Tian Ma Gou Teng Wan)
Xiao Shuan Zai Zao Wan 消栓再造丸 (Xiao Shuan Zai Zao Wan)

Acupuncture

The main points are selected from the *yang ming* channels (due to their 'abundance of *qi* and Blood'), *san jiao* and Gall Bladder channels. Gentle electro-stimulation may be used. Three or four points are selected for each treatment. In chronic hemiplegia (of more than a couple of months duration) points from the *yin* channels may be added.

Upper limb
LI.15 (*jian yu*), LI.11 (*qu chi*), LI.4 (*he gu*), SJ.5 (*wai guan*), SJ.14 (*jian liao*), SJ.4 (*yang chi*), SI.9 (*jian zhen*)

Lower limb
GB.30 (*huan tiao*), GB.31 (*feng shi*), GB.34 (*yang ling quan*), GB.39 (*xuan zhong*), St.36 (*zu san li*), St.41 (*jie xi*), Bl.60 (*kun lun*), Du.3 (*yao yang guan*)
- with *qi* deficiency add moxa
- with Liver *yang* excess add Liv.3 (*tai chong* -)

Clinical notes

- Combining acupuncture and herbs with physiotherapy, *tui na* or massage gives better results.
- Treatment is best given as soon as the patient is stable. After one month it becomes more difficult to treat, after six months results are often poor, nevertheless, treatment is always worth trying as some patients respond well even after long term disability.

24.7 DYSPHASIA

Dysphasia is the difficulty with talking due to stiffness, paralysis or deviation of the tongue. Depending on the initial conditions, there are two main presentations, Wind Phlegm and *yin* deficiency with *yang* rising.

24.7.1 Wind Phlegm

Clinical features
- stiffness of the tongue, slurred speech
- numbness of the extremities

T greasy white coat
P wiry and slippery

Treatment principle

Extinguish Wind and eliminate Phlegm
Open the orifices

Prescription

JIE YU DAN 解语丹
(*Relax the Tongue Special Pill*) modified

bai fu zi* (Rhizoma Typhonii Gigantei) 白附子	6g
shi chang pu (Rhizoma Acori Graminei) 石菖蒲	6g
yuan zhi (Radix Polygalae Tenuifoliae) 远志	6g
tian ma (Rhizoma Gastrodiae Elatae) 天麻	6g
qiang huo (Rhizoma et Radix Notopterygii) 羌活	6g
dan nan xing* (Pulvis Arisaemae cum Felle Bovis) 胆南星	6g
tian zhu huang (Concretio Silicea Bambusae Textillis) 天竺黄	6g
yu jin (Tuber Curcumae) 郁金	6g
mu xiang (Radix Aucklandiae Lappae) 木香	6g
gan cao (Radix Glycyrrhizae Uralensis) 甘草	3g
quan xie* (Buthus Martensi) 全蝎	1.5g

Method: Decoction. (Source: *Shi Yong Zhong Yi Nei Ke Xue*)

Modifications

- Both the Heart and Spleen channels have a strong influence on the tongue. If there are signs of Spleen involvement, add **cang zhu** (Rhizoma Atractylodis) 苍术 9g and **ban xia*** (Rhizoma Pinelliae Ternatae) 半夏 9g.
- With signs of Heart involvement, add **zhen zhu muˆ** (Concha Margaritaferae) 珍珠母 12g and **hu po** (Succinum) 琥珀 3g.

Acupuncture

Ht.5 (*tong li*), Ren.23 (*lian quan*), *shang liang quan* (M-HN-21), St.40 (*feng long*), LI.4 (*he gu*), LI.11 (*qu chi*), Sp.6 (*san yin jiao*), SJ.6 (*zhi gou*)

24.7.2 Liver and Kidney *yin* and *yang* deficiency

肝肾阴阳两虚

- This pattern represents a chronic stage of stroke sequelae, and involves decline of both *yin* and *yang*. It may present with signs of both *yin* or *yang* deficiency (in which case there are usually no obvious thermal disturbances), or with more heat (*yin* deficiency) or cold (*yang* deficiency) symptoms.

Clinical features
- slurred speech, stiffness or deviation of the tongue
- weakness, numbness or paralysis of the lower limbs
- weak, sore lower back and knees
- palpitations
- shortness of breath

T pale or red
P thready and weak, or deep, slow and thready

Treatment principle
Nourish and tonify Kidney *yin* and *yang*
Open the orifices, transform Phlegm

Prescription

DI HUANG YIN ZI 地黄饮子
(*Rehmannia Decoction*)

shu di (Radix Rehmanniae Glutinosae Conquitae) 熟地
shan zhu yu (Fructus Corni Officinalis) 山茱萸
rou cong rong (Cistanches Deserticolae) 肉苁蓉
ba ji tian (Radix Morindae Officinalis) 巴戟天
zhi fu zi* (Radix Aconiti Carmichaeli Praeparata) 制附子
rou gui (Cortex Cinnamomi Cassiae) 肉桂
shi hu (Herba Dendrobii) 石斛
mai dong (Tuber Ophiopogonis Japonici) 麦冬
shi chang pu (Rhizoma Acori Graminei) 石菖蒲
yuan zhi (Radix Polygalae Tenuifoliae) 远志
fu ling (Sclerotium Poria Cocos) 茯苓
wu wei zi (Fructus Schizandrae Chinensis) 五味子

Method: Grind equal amounts of all herbs into powder and take in 9-gram doses as a draft twice daily. (Source: *Formulas and Strategies*)

Modifications

- For predominance of *yin* deficiency, with little or no *yang* deficiency, delete **fu zi*** and **rou gui**.
- For predominance of *yang* deficiency, add **xian ling pi** (Herba Epimedii) 仙灵脾 and **xian mao** (Rhizoma Curculiginis Orchioidis) 仙茅.
- For severe dysphasia, add **mu hu die** (Semen Oroxyli Indici) 木蝴蝶 and **jie geng** (Radix Platycodi Grandiflori) 桔梗.

Acupuncture

Ht.5 (*tong li*), Ren.23 (*lian quan*), *shang liang quan* (M-HN-21), Kid.6 (*zhao hai*), Kid.3 (*tai xi*), Liv.3 (*tai chong*), Ren.4 (*guan yuan*), Bl.23 (*shen shu*), St.36 (*zu san li*)

Clinical notes

- These patterns are more difficult the longer they are left untreated.

24.8 FACIAL PARALYSIS

Facial paralysis may be the result of external Wind entering the channels, or internal Wind. In both cases treatment of the paralysis is the same. In the cases of internal Wind, lingering constitutional factors (*yin* deficiency or Phlegm) should also be addressed.

Clinical features
- one sided facial paralysis
- facial muscle spasms or tics

Treatment principle
Dispel Wind, transform Phlegm
Nourish and invigorate Blood, stop spasms

Prescription

QIAN ZHENG SAN 牵正散
(*Lead to Symmetry Powder*) modified

jiang can^ (Bombyx Batryticatus) 僵蚕	12g
quan xie* (Buthus Martensi) 全蝎	10g
bai fu zi* (Rhizoma Typhonii Gigantei) 白附子	6g
qiang huo (Rhizoma et Radix Notopterygii) 羌活	10g
fang feng (Radix Ledebouriellae Divaricatae) 防风	10g
hong hua (Flos Carthami Tinctorii) 红花	10g
di long^ (Lumbricus) 地龙	10g
chi shao (Radix Paeoniae Rubrae) 赤芍	10g
gan cao (Radix Glycyrrhizae Uralensis) 甘草	6g

Method: Decoction or powdered. When powdered, the dose is 3-grams 2-3 times daily with hot wine. (Source: *Zhong Yi Nei Ke Lin Chuang Shou Ce*). See also 24.1, p.652.

Modifications
- Herbs to nourish and activate Blood are commonly added, like **dang gui** (Radix Angelicae Sinensis) 当归 9g and **chuan xiong** (Radix Ligustici Chuanxiong) 川芎 6g because 'to treat Wind, first nourish Blood' and 'when Blood moves Wind has no place'.
- With spontaneous sweating, delete **qiang huo** and **fang feng**, and add **huang qi** (Radix Astragali Membranacei) 黄芪 18g and **gui zhi** (Ramulus Cinnamomi Cassiae) 桂枝 9g.
- With internal Heat, delete **qiang huo**, and add **xia ku cao** (Spica Prunellae Vulgaris) 夏枯草 15g, **huang qin** (Radix Scutellariae Baicalensis) 黄芩 9g and **ju hua** (Flos Chrysanthemi Morifolii) 菊花 9g.
- With severe tics and spasms, add **tian ma** (Rhizoma Gastrodiae Elatae)

天麻 9g, **gou teng** (Ramulus Uncariae cum Uncis) 钩藤 12g, **bai shao** (Radix Paeoniae Lactiflorae) 白芍 12g and **shi jue ming**^ (Concha Haliotidis) 石决明 12g.
- If the paralysis has persisted longer than two months delete **fang feng** and **qiang huo** and add **shui zhi** (Hirudo seu Whitmania) 水蛭 3g, **chuan shan jia**° (Squama Manitis) 穿山甲 9g, **bai jie zi** (Semen Sinapsis Albae) 白芥子 6g and **tian nan xing*** (Rhizoma Arisaematis) 天南星 6g.

Patent medicines
Xiao Huo Luo Dan 小活络丹 (Xiao Huo Luo Dan)
 - when chronic and cold
Kang Wei Ling 亢痿灵 (Kang Wei Ling)
Bu Yang Huan Wu Wan 补阳还五丸 (Bu Yang Huan Wu Wan)
Hua Tuo Zai Zao Wan 华佗再造丸 (Hua Tuo Zai Zao Wan)

Acupuncture
Special method
Threading technique with a 3-inch needle from St.6 (*jia che*) to St.4 (*di cang*) and St.7 (*xia guan*), and a 1.5-inch needle from St.2 (*si bai*) to St.4 (*di cang*) on the affected side. In addition, LI.4 (*he gu*) or Lu.7 (*lie que*) may be connected to one of the facial points and treated with gentle electro-stimulation.
Other points are added depending on the affected part:
- eye - SJ.23 (*si zhu kong*)
- nose - LI.20 (*ying xiang*)
- tongue - Ren.23 (*lian quan*)
- lips - Du.26 (*ren zhong*) and Ren.24 (*cheng jiang*).
- In chronic cases moxa may be added.

Clinical notes
- Corresponds to Bell's palsy or the sequelae of stroke.
- If treatment is prompt (with a day or two of Bell's palsy or as soon as the patient has stabilised following a CVA) the results are good. A complete cure is often the effected after a course of acupuncture. Ideally, treatment is applied every day or every other day.

SUMMARY OF GUIDING FORMULAE FOR WIND STROKE

Channel stroke
Emptiness of the channels with Wind invasion - *Da Qin Jiao Tang* 大秦艽汤
- with external Cold - *Xiao Xu Ming Tang* 小续命汤
- facial paralysis - *Qian Zheng San* 牵正散

Liver and Kidney *yin* deficiency with *yang* rising and Wind - *Zhen Gan Xi Feng Tang* 镇肝熄风汤

Phlegm Heat with Wind Phlegm - *Xing Wei Cheng Qi Tang* 星蒌承气汤

Organ syndromes
Closed syndrome
- *yang* closed syndrome - *Zhi Bao Wan* 至宝丸
- *yin* closed syndrome - *Su He Xiang Wan* 苏合香丸

Flaccid Collapse syndrome - *Shen Fu Tang* 参附汤

Sequelae of Wind stroke
Hemiplegia
- *Qi* and Blood deficiency with stagnant Blood - *Bu Yang Huan Wu Tang* 补阳还五汤
- Liver *yang* rising with stagnant Blood - *Zhen Gan Xi Feng Tang* 镇肝熄风汤

Dysphasia
- Wind Phlegm - *Jie Yu Dan* 解语丹
- Liver and Kidney *yin* and *yang* deficiency - *Di Huang Yin Zi* 地黄饮子

Facial paralysis
- *Qian Zheng San* 牵正散

Endnote

For more information regarding herbs marked with an asterisk*, an open circle° or a hat^, see the tables on pp.944-952.

Disorders of the Liver

25. Epilepsy

Seizure type
Yang seizures
Yin seizures

Underlying Pattern
Spleen deficiency with Phlegm
Liver Fire with Phlegm Heat
Liver and Kidney *yin* deficiency
Blood stagnation

25 EPILEPSY
dian xian 癫痫

Epilepsy is a disorder characterised by massive synchronous discharge of cerebral neurones. Seizures, hallucinations and incontinence occur as motor and sensory neurones discharge. Epilepsy is quite a common disease, affecting approximately 2 per cent of the population. There are two biomedical classifications of epilepsy, generalised and partial, defined by the type of seizure (Box 25.1).

The severity of epileptic seizures is highly variable. Some patients (mostly children) experience only mild 'absences' (*petit mal*)–brief lapses of awareness or sudden unresponsiveness lasting only a few seconds but sometimes reoccuring many times in one day. Other patients may be subject to frequent, violent and exhausting convulsive (*grand mal*, or 'tonic clonic') seizures. In between these two extremes there are varying degrees of partial seizure affecting a single limb, or sensory hallucinations. From a biomedical perspective, in many patients no cause can be found–this is primary or idiopathic epilepsy. There is some indication of a genetic link, as there is a family history in up to 40 per cent of patients with epilepsy. Secondary causes involve a variety of lesions of the brain–the sequelae of severe infections, head injury, tumours, abscesses and cysts, vascular malformations, aneurysms, infarction, as well as damage from both prescription or illicit drug and alcohol abuse. Epilepsy that begins in adults is particularly suspect, and appropriate investigation for conditions that may be dealt with surgically is indicated.

In TCM, seizures are classified as *yin* or *yang*, depending on frequency, severity, duration and accompanying manifestations. Violent convulsive seizures in a young, hot or robust patient are generally *yang* seizures; weak, mild partial seizures or absences are *yin*. The severity of the seizures is related to the relative strength of the *zheng qi* and the responsible pathogens (usually Wind and Phlegm, and possibly Heat). Seizures may begin infrequently, being mild and of short duration, as the *zheng qi* is intact and the pathogen held in check. As resistance declines with repeated episodes, or Phlegm accumulation increases, the condition deteriorates. In practice *yang* seizures can become *yin*, as underlying deficiency becomes more prominent. *Yin* seizures can also become *yang*, for example the *yin* absences of childhood often develop into *grand mal* seizures in adulthood.

AETIOLOGY
Wind and Phlegm
Wind and Phlegm are the primary aetiological factors for epilepsy that is not

caused by brain injury or trauma. Indeed, TCM texts note that 'without Phlegm there is no epilepsy'. Phlegm obstructs *qi* and pressure mounts behind the blockage. A sudden release of this pent up *qi* towards the head creates the Wind responsible for the seizure. If the Wind carries the Phlegm up with it, then the sensory orifices will be affected, causing altered perceptions and perhaps unconsciousness. The Phlegm in this disorder is frequently constitutional, or it may be produced by overconsumption of Phlegm

---

BOX 25.1 BIOMEDICAL CLASSIFICATION OF SEIZURE TYPES

Partial (or focal) seizures
In this type of seizure the locus of neuronal activity is limited to one part of the brain. Partial seizures can present with a variety of motor, sensory or visual symptoms and alteration of mood.
- Motor symptoms depend on the part of the brain affected and may begin in one part of the body and spread gradually to other parts. This is commonly known as Jacksonian epilepsy. Attacks vary in duration from seconds to hours.
- Sensory symptoms include tingling or electric sensations in one or more parts of the body.
- Visual symptoms include hallucinations of various types, from colours to fully detailed faces or scenes. There may also be auditory hallucinations, and altered smell and taste.
- Mood changes occur, and the patient may be unresponsive to stimuli.

Generalised seizures
1. ***Grand Mal*** **(or tonic clonic):** this type of seizure involves large areas of both hemispheres of the brain, loss of consciousness and tonic-clonic seizures. Tonic-clonic seizures have several phases (although not all phases occur in every seizure):
- the **prodrome**, with irritability and uneasiness hours or days prior to the seizure.
- the **aura**, with visual or auditory hallucinations, jerking of a limb or *déjà vu* for seconds or minutes before the seizure.
- the **tonic** phase with massive discharge of motor neurones causing tonic contraction of muscles, during which the arms are flexed and adducted and the legs extended. Spasm of the diaphram and respiratory muscles causes a cry as air is expelled (the origin of the ancient name 'goat Wind' *yang xian feng* 羊痫风). The patient loses consciousness. This phase lasts for about 30 seconds.
- the **clonic** phase, with spasmodic jerking of the limbs and incontinence lasting up to five minutes.
- the **recovery** phase where the patient is deeply unconscious and flaccid. Lasts from minutes to hours.

2. ***Petit Mal*** **(Absences):** seen mostly in children, this form of epilepsy involves sudden lapse of consciousness–the child stops activity and stares, blinks or rolls up the eyes, drops something or is completely unresponsive. Each episode may only last a few seconds but may reoccur many times in one day.

producing foods, or foods that weaken the Spleen, allowing the generation of Damp. Phlegm can also accumulate as a result of *qi* stagnation, causing poor fluid metabolism.

While Phlegm and Wind are the primary aetiological features, Heat or deficiency may complicate the picture in some acute and chronic patterns. As patients age, the excess (Wind and Phlegm) begins to be complicated by deficiency or Heat and other patterns emerge. These patterns will always have a component of Phlegm, even those where deficiency is primary.

Liver Fire

Liver Fire may occur alongside Wind Phlegm, creating a more complicated pattern. The Fire has its basis in emotions like frustration, anger, resentment and prolonged stress. These emotional states disrupt the circulation of Liver *qi*, which over time can give rise to stagnant Heat. At a certain intensity, this Heat becomes Fire. The presence of constitutional Phlegm will also contribute to stagnation of *qi* and aid the development of Fire. Alternatively, if Liver Fire is primary, it can give rise to Phlegm by heating and congealing fluids and stirring up internal Wind. This type of epilepsy often has a strong emotional component, or is triggered by emotional upset.

Liver and Kidney *yin* (*jing*) deficiency

The prolonged presence of Phlegm and Heat eventually consumes *yin* and weakens the Liver and Kidneys. Liver and Kidney deficiency is a common complication of other chronic forms of epilepsy, and is frequently found in older or weaker patients.

There is also a familial component in many cases of epilepsy, and therefore some weakness of *jing*. This inherited tendency may involve elements of both *jing* deficiency and Phlegm excess, as both may be inherited. When weakness of *jing* is involved, it appears mainly as a Liver and Kidney *yin* deficiency.

Spleen deficiency with Phlegm

A Spleen deficiency pattern of epilepsy may be constitutional, the result of poor dietary habits, such as excessive consumption of cold, raw foods, or the result of prolonged illness and overexertion. In addition, the anticonvulsant medications used to treat epilepsy are usually cold in nature[1] and prolonged use will often damage the Spleen and aggravate Phlegm accumulation. This pattern sometimes occurs in children following a febrile illness treated with antibiotics or a severe episode of vomiting or diarrhoea (see Convulsions p.716).

As the Spleen is the source of the *qi* and Blood of the body, weakness

---

1. Scott J P (1991) *Acupuncture in the Treatment of Children*. Eastland Press, Seattle

BOX 25.2 MANGEMENT DURING A SEIZURE
- Move the patient away from danger and possible injury while convulsing.
- After the convulsions cease, turn the patient on the side in the coma position and ensure the airway is clear.
- Paramedic aid should be summoned if the seizure continues longer than five minutes.

will inevitably lead to a decrease in production of *qi* and Blood. Blood deficiency can give rise to a mild form of Wind by failing to anchor *yang qi* securely. *Qi (yang)* deficiency may also contribute to the development of a type of Wind, one generated by the movement of *qi* to fill the vacuum formed by chronic deficiency.

Trauma
Birth trauma (such as forceps delivery or anoxia), head injury, cerebral infection, infarction or haemorrhage can trigger epilepsy. Trauma induced epilepsy can also result from any severe fright or shock the mother may have experienced during pregnancy. Trauma can damage *jing*, cause Blood stagnation, or both. This is the one type of epilepsy that does not necessarily involve Phlegm.

DIFFERENTIAL DIAGNOSIS
- **Wind stroke** (*zhong feng*): characterised by sudden or evolving facial paralysis, motor dysfunction, and in some cases unconsciousness. Following the episode, the patient may be left with residual disability. Wind stroke includes disorders like cerebro-vascular accident and Bell's palsy.
- ***Jue* syndrome** (syncope): *Jue* syndrome is characterised by sudden loss of consciousness with cold extremities, then a gradual regaining of consciousness, with no residual paralysis, speech difficulties or sequelae. The sorts of disorders that are categorised as *jue* syndrome include hypoglycaemic coma, hysterical syncope and haemorrhagic or allergic shock.

TREATMENT
Little can or need be done for a person during a major seizure other than the simple measures listed above in Box 25.2.

There are several factors that are known to trigger seizures in some patients, and these should be avoided as much as possible. They include lack of sleep, emotional stress, physical and mental exhaustion, drug or alcohol use, fever and flickering lights, such as television, strobe lighting and fluorescent tubes.

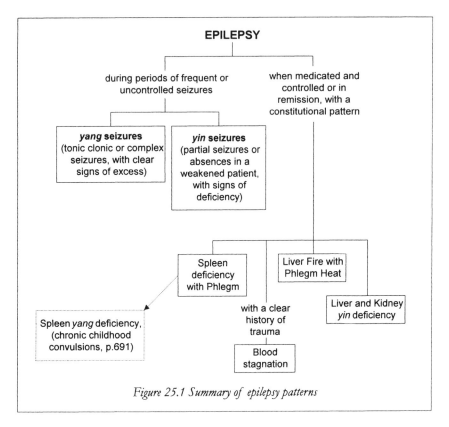

Figure 25.1 *Summary of epilepsy patterns*

TCM treatment of epilepsy is in two stages. For uncontrolled and frequent fits, strong, harsh treatments are applied between seizures. At this stage of the disorder, although the seizures may be classified as *yang* or *yin* (pp.685, 688), the emphasis of treatment will be the same–that is to eliminate Phlegm, extinguish Wind and regulate *qi*. As the disease comes under control and fits become less frequent (either as a result of the above or with the use of pharmaceutical drugs), treatment is then applied according to the patient's constitution (pp.690-698).

In practice there is considerable overlap between controlled presentations, and one pattern may transform into another in the same patient. For example, Liver Fire with Phlegm Heat damages *yin* and gradually *yin* deficiency becomes prominent; Phlegm Heat weakens Spleen *qi*, so Spleen *qi* deficiency with Phlegm becomes prominent. All patterns can cause *qi* and Blood stagnation. Often there will be elements of multiple patterns and it can be difficult to determine which is prominent. In such cases, prescription involves selecting appropriate elements of the various guiding formulae (and a degree of experimentation as the pattern changes).

25.1 *YANG* SEIZURES

Pathophysiology
- This pattern describes the classical *grand mal* seizure. The formula recommended is a strong treatment and is only suitable for periods where Phlegm has become predominant and has to be vigorously cleared. Most frequently this is a mixed deficiency and excess condition. There will often be signs of Heat in this pattern, and it may be the combination of Heat and Phlegm, both of which can cause Wind, that gives rise to the full blown tonic-clonic seizure.

Clinical features
- Hours or days before an attack begins there is often a prodrome, with irritability, mood alteration and a sense of unease.
- An 'aura' may occur just before an attack, with hallucinations, *déjà vu*, or jerking of a limb, followed by sudden collapse with tonic contraction of all the muscles of the body. The arms are flexed and adducted, legs extended and spasm of the diaphram causes an animal like cry as the air is forced from the lungs. This phase generally lasts 10-30 seconds
- The next (clonic) phase is characterised by spasmodic contractions of the muscles with jerking movements of the face, body and limbs. There may be incontinence of urine (often) or stools (rarely). This phase generally lasts 1-5 minutes.
- After the seizures have ceased, the patient is usually deeply unconscious. Following arousal there is drowsiness, headache, myalgia and weakness.
- not all phases occur in each episode

T greasy white or yellow coat
P wiry and rapid or wiry and slippery

Treatment principle
Clear and transform Phlegm
Extinguish Wind and stop seizures

Prescription

DING XIAN WAN 定闲丸
(*Arrest Seizures Pill*)

tian ma (Rhizoma Gastrodiae Elatae) 天麻	30g
chuan bei mu (Bulbus Fritillariae Cirrhosae) 川贝母	30g
ban xia* (Rhizoma Pinelliae Ternatae) 半夏	30g
fu ling (Sclerotium Poria Cocos) 茯苓	30g
fu shen (Sclerotium Poriae Cocos Pararadicis) 茯神	30g
dan nan xing* (Pulvis Arisaemae cum Felle Bovis) 胆南星	15g

shi chang pu (Rhizoma Acori Graminei) 石菖蒲	15g
quan xie* (Buthus Martensi) 全蝎	15g
jiang can^ (Bombyx Batryticatus) 僵蚕	15g
hu po (Succinum) 琥珀	15g
deng xin cao (Medulla Junci Effusi) 灯心草	15g
chen pi (Pericarpium Citri Reticulatae) 陈皮	21g
yuan zhi (Radix Polygalae Tenuifoliae) 远志	21g
dan shen (Radix Salviae Miltiorrhizae) 丹参	60g
mai dong (Tuber Ophiopogonis Japonici) 麦冬	60g
zhu sha* (Cinnabaris) 朱砂	9g

Method: Grind the herbs (except the **zhu sha**) into powder and form into 6 gram pills by decocting the powder with 120g of **gan cao** (Radix Glycyrrhizae Uralensis) 甘草, 100mls of **zhu li** (Succus Bambusae) 竹沥, 50 mls of ginger juice and sufficient water to form a thick paste. Use the **zhu sha** to coat the pills. The dose is one pill twice daily. (Source: *Formulas and Strategies*)

Modifications

♦ With obvious Heat, add **shan zhi zi** (Fructus Gardeniae Jasminoides) 山栀子 15g and **long dan cao** (Radix Gentianae Longdancao) 龙胆草 12g.

DIAN XIAN SAN 癫痫散
(*Epilepsy Powder*)

This is a strong formula with the same action as the primary formula, but without any tonifying herbs. **Ba dou shuang** is toxic and must be used with extra care. It is best reserved for severe and resistant cases.

yu jin (Tuber Curcumae) 郁金	90g
jiu xiang fu (wine fried Rhizoma Cyperi Rotundi) 酒香附	30g
wu gong* (Scolopendra Subspinipes) 蜈蚣	12g
quan xie* (Buthus Martensi) 全蝎	12g
ba dou shuang* (defatted Semen Croton Tiglii) 巴豆霜	4g

Method: Grind the herbs to a fine powder and form into 3-gram pills with water or honey. The adult dose is one pill daily, half dose (1.5g) for children. In serious cases the dose may be increased to 3 pills daily. (Source: *Shi Yong Zhong Yao Xue*)

Patent medicines

Hu Po Bao Long Wan 琥珀抱龙丸 (Po Lung Yuen Medical Pills)

Acupuncture

Du.12 (*shen zhu* -), GB.13 (*ben shen* -), Ren.14 (*jiu wei* -), St.40 (*feng long* -), Liv.3 (*tai chong* -), Du.20 (*bai hui*)

• If the fits occur at night, add Kid.6 (*zhao hai*)
• If the fits occur during the day, add Bl.62 (*shen mai*)

Clinical notes

- According to Chinese reports this pattern responds reasonably well to prolonged and correct TCM treatment.
- These formulae are used during periods of frequent or difficult to control seizures and it is recommended that they are gradually withdrawn one year after beginning therapy as the symptoms improve. Because of the harsh nature of these formulae, it may be appropriate to reduce the dose incrementally after there have been no seizures for one or two months (depending on how frequent the seizures were initially).
- The prescriptions described here must be used cautiously and monitored closely for possible side effects.

25.2 YIN SEIZURES

Pathophysiology
- This pattern describes partial or *petit mal* seizures, and chronic seizures in a weak or deficient patient. In children this pattern may appear as chronic convulsions following a cerebral or severe infection. In adults it follows frequent and long term *yang* seizures, which have significantly depleted Spleen and Kidney *yang*. It can present in a variety of ways, with or without loss of consciousness.

Clinical features
- during seizures the face is dark or sallow, with icy cold extremities, eyes half open, loss of consciousness with initial rigidity then quivering or twitching of the body or a limb, drooling, no cry, or weak cry
- May also present as an 'absence'–sudden blank, expressionless stare, upwards rolling of the eyes, unresponsiveness to sound. This pattern usually only lasts a few seconds but may occur many times in one day.

T pale with a thick greasy white coat
P deep and thready or deep and slow

Treatment principle
Warm *yang* and eliminate Phlegm
Soothe *qi* and stop seizures

Prescription

DING XIAN WAN 定闲丸 (see *yang* seizures p.685)
(*Arrest Seizures Pill*)

This formula is suitable for both *yin* and *yang* seizures, as the prime pathogen in both cases is Phlegm, which must be cleared before any other treatment is applied. Suitable modifications should be made according to individual presentations, bearing in mind that there are significant elements of deficiency in *yin* seizures. Combining this formula with one of the representitive deficiency formulae may be appropriate. As the formula contains some harsh ingredients, patients must be monitored closely during therapy.

Modifications
- With Liver Blood deficiency, add **dang gui** (Radix Angelicae Sinensis) 当归 15g and **bai shao** (Radix Paeoniae Lactiflorae) 白芍 15g.
- With Spleen deficiency, add **bai zhu** (Rhizoma Atractylodes Macrocephalae) 白术 30g and **dang shen** (Radix Codonopsis Pilosulae) 党参 30g.

- With Kidney deficiency, add **he shou wu** (Radix Polygoni Multiflori) 何首乌 30g and **tu si zi** (Semen Cuscutae Chinensis) 菟丝子 30g.

Patent medicines
Hu Po Bao Long Wan 琥珀抱龙丸 (Po Lung Yuen Medical Pills)

Acupuncture
Du.12 (*shen zhu* -), GB.13 (*ben shen* -), Ren.14 (*jiu wei* -), St.40 (*feng long* -), Liv.3 (*tai chong* -), Du.20 (*bai hui*)
- If the fits occur at night, add Kid.6 (*zhao hai*)
- If the fits occur during the day, add Bl.62 (*shen mai*)

Clinical notes
- *Yin* seizures correspond to conditions such as *petit mal* seizures, partial seizures and complex partial seizures.

25.3 SPLEEN DEFICIENCY WITH PHLEGM

Pathophysiology
- Spleen deficiency with Phlegm type epilepsy is a chronic condition and reflects a particular constitutional state in a medicated patient or one who's epilepsy is largely in remission. The patient will usually not be having seizures, or only very infrequent *yin* type seizures.

Clinical features
- long history of seizures or medication for epilepsy
- lethargy and fatigue, emaciation
- poor appetite, nausea or vomiting
- loose stools or diarrhoea
- pale or sallow complexion
- fullness and stuffiness in the chest and abdomen

T pale with a greasy white coat
P soft and slippery or thready, wiry and slippery

Treatment principle
Strengthen the Spleen and transform Phlegm

Prescription

LIU JUN ZI TANG 六君子汤
(*Six Major Herbs Combination*) modified

This formula is selected when Spleen deficiency and Phlegm are prominent.

ren shen (Radix Ginseng) 人参	10g
bai zhu (Rhizoma Atractylodes Macrocephalae) 白术	12g
fu ling (Sclerotium Poria Cocos) 茯苓	12g
ban xia* (Rhizoma Pinelliae Ternatae) 半夏	10g
chen pi (Pericarpium Citri Reticulatae) 陈皮	10g
shi chang pu (Rhizoma Acori Graminei) 石菖蒲	10g
yuan zhi (Radix Polygalae Tenuifoliae) 远志	10g
dan nan xing* (Pulvis Arisaemae cum Felle Bovis) 胆南星	10g
jiang can^ (Bombyx Batryticatus) 僵蚕	10g
zhi shi (Fructus Immaturus Citri Aurantii) 枳实	10g
zhi gan cao (honey fried Radix Glycyrrhizae Uralensis) 炙甘草	10g

Method: Decoction. May also be prepared as a powder or pills. (Source: *Zhong Yi Nei Ke Lin Chuang Shou Ce*)

AN SHEN DING ZHI WAN 安神定志丸
(Calm the shen, Settle the Emotions Pill)

This formula is selected when there are significant mental emotional aspects to the pattern, such as anxiety neurosis, fearfulness and inability to concentrate.

shi chang pu (Rhizoma Acori Graminei) 石菖蒲	15g
yuan zhi (Radix Polygalae Tenuifoliae) 远志	15g
long chi^ (Dens Draconis) 龙齿	15g
fu ling (Sclerotium Poria Cocos) 茯苓	15g
fu shen (Sclerotium Poriae Cocos Pararadicis) 茯神	15g
dang shen (Radix Codonopsis Pilosulae) 党参	30g
zhu sha* (Cinnabaris) 朱砂	5g

Method: Grind the herbs (except **zhu sha**) to a fine powder and form into 9-gram pills with water or honey. The **zhu sha** is used to coat the pills. The adult dose is 2 pills daily. (Source: *Shi Yong Zhong Yao Xue*)

Modifications

- In severe cases, add **quan xie fen*** (powdered Buthus Martensi) 全蝎粉 2g and **wu gong fen*** (powdered Scolopendra Subspinipes) 蜈蚣粉 2g to the strained decoction (*chong fu* 冲服).
- With nausea or vomiting, add **zhu ru** (Caulis Bambusae in Taeniis) 竹茹 12g and **xuan fu hua** (Flos Inulae) 旋复花 15g.
- With loose stools, add **yi ren** (Semen Coicis Lachryma-jobi) 苡仁 15g and **bian dou** (Semen Dolichos Lablab) 扁豆 15g.
- If there is a history of trauma (with Spleen deficiency predominant), add Blood moving herbs, **dan shen** (Radix Salviae Miltiorrhizae) 丹参 18g, **hong hua** (Flos Carthami Tinctorii) 红花 9g, **tao ren** (Semen Persicae) 桃仁 12g and **chuan xiong** (Radix Ligustici Chuanxiong) 川芎 9g.

Patent medicines

Fu Zi Li Zhong Wan 附子理中丸 (Li Chung Yuen Medical Pills)
Li Zhong Wan 理中丸 (Li Zhong Wan)

Acupuncture

Ht.5 (*tong li* +), St.40 (*feng long* + ▲), Bl.23 (*shen shu* + ▲), Du.20 (*bai hui* ▲), si shen cong (M-HN-1), GB.34 (*yang ling quan*), Sp.6 (*san yin jiao* + ▲), Du.8 (*jin suo* + ▲), St.36 (*zu san li* + ▲), Ren.12 (*zhong wan* + ▲), Du.26 (*ren zhong*)

Clinical notes

- This pattern corresponds to chronic epilepsy.

- In some cases, this pattern may follow a severe febrile disease that has drained Spleen *qi* or *yang* (or was treated with powerful antibiotics that damaged *yang*). The anti-convulsant drugs that may be given to treat the resulting seizures are generally cold in nature and may further exacerbate the deficiency. See also Convulsions, p.716.
- After several months of treatment as Spleen *yang* strengthens and the signs and symptoms of Spleen deficiency improve, epilepsy medication may be cautiously withdrawn. Treatment should continue for another 12 months or so to consolidate the result.

25.4 LIVER FIRE WITH PHLEGM HEAT

肝火痰热

Pathophysiology
- Epilepsy due to Liver Fire with Phlegm Heat reflects a particular constitutional state of a medicated patient, or one who's epilepsy is largely in remission. This pattern has a significant emotional component. The patient will not be having seizures, or only very infrequent *yang* type seizures induced by intense excitement or emotional triggers.

Clinical features
- seizures induced by worry, anxiety, anger and emotional stress
- after the seizure has ceased, the patient is still irritable and restless
- insomnia
- bitter taste in the mouth
- dry mouth, thirst
- constipation

T red with a yellow coat
P wiry and rapid

Treatment principle
Purge Liver Fire, transform Phlegm

Prescription

LONG DAN XIE GAN TANG 龙胆泻肝汤
(*Gentiana Combination*) plus
DI TAN TANG 涤痰汤
(*Scour Phlegm Decoction*) modified

long dan cao (Radix Gentianae Longdancao) 龙胆草	6-9g
shan zhi zi (Fructus Gardeniae Jasminoides) 山栀子	9g
huang qin (Radix Scutellariae Baicalensis) 黄芩	9g
ban xia* (Rhizoma Pinelliae Ternatae) 半夏	9g
mu tong (Caulis Mutong) 木通	6g
chen pi (Pericarpium Citri Reticulatae) 陈皮	6g
dan nan xing* (Pulvis Arisaemae cum Felle Bovis) 胆南星	6g
shi chang pu (Rhizoma Acori Graminei) 石菖蒲	6g

Method: Decoction. (Source: *Shi Yong Zhong Yi Nei Ke Xue*)

Modifications
- In severe cases, add **quan xie fen*** (powdered Buthus Martensi) 全蝎粉 and **wu gong fen*** (powdered Scolopendra Subspinipes) 蜈蚣粉, 2g each to the strained decoction (*chong fu* 冲服).
- When Phlegm Heat and constipation are severe or prominent combine

with **GUN TAN WAN** (*Vaporize Phlegm Pill* 滚痰丸).

    duan meng shi (Lapis Micae seu Chloriti) 礞石 30g
    jiu da huang (wine fried Rhizoma Rhei) 酒大黄 240g
    huang qin (Radix Scutellariae Baicalensis) 黄芩 240g
    chen xiang (Lignum Aquilariae) 沉香 15g

Method: Grind the herbs into powder and form into 9-gram pills with water. The dose is one pill 2-3 times daily. (Source: *Shi Yong Zhong Yao Xue*)

CHAI HU JIA LONG GU MU LI TANG 柴胡加龙骨牡蛎汤
(*Bupleurum and Dragon Bone Combination*) modified

This prescription may be useful in mild cases of Liver Fire with Phlegm type epilepsy. It is a very effective formula for *shen* disturbance in robust patients with Heat. It is widely used for disorders due to fright or shock and drug withdrawal, where palpitations, fullness in the chest and irritability are prominent

    dan shen (Radix Salviae Miltiorrhizae) 丹参 30g
    long gu^ (Os Draconis) 龙骨 24g
    mu li^ (Concha Ostreae) 牡蛎 24g
    fu ling (Sclerotium Poriae Cocos) 茯苓 12g
    chai hu (Radix Bupleuri) 柴胡 15g
    dang shen (Radix Codonopsis Pilosulae) 党参 9g
    ban xia* (Rhizoma Pinelliae Ternatae) 半夏 9g
    huang qin (Radix Scutellariae Baicalensis) 黄芩 9g
    gui zhi (Ramulus Cinnamomi Cassiae) 桂枝 6g
    da huang (Radix et Rhizoma Rhei) 大黄 6g
    sheng jiang (Rhizoma Zingiberis Officinalis) 生姜 3pce
    da zao (Fructus Zizyphi Jujubae) 大枣 5pce

Method: Decoction. (Source: *Formulas and Strategies*).

Patent medicines

Hu Po Bao Long Wan 琥珀抱龙丸 (Po Lung Yuen Medical Pills)
Long Dan Xie Gan Wan 龙胆泻肝丸 (Long Dan Xie Gan Wan)
Niu Huang Qing Huo Wan 牛黄清火丸 (Niu Huang Qing Huo Wan)

Acupuncture

Du.26 (*ren zhong*), Du.12 (*shen zhu* -), GB.13 (*ben shen* -), Du.20 (*bai hui*), PC.8 (*lao gong*), Ren.14 (*jiu wei* -), St.40 (*feng long* -), Liv.3 (*tai chong* -), Liv.2 (*xing jian* -), Bl.18 (*gan shu* -), *si shen cong* (M-HN-1)

Clinical notes

- Corresponds to conditions such as epilepsy, seizures, cerebral cysts or tumours.

- If Liver Fire is well controlled with acupuncture and herbs, then the trigger for the seizures is largely removed and they should become a rare occurence. Complete cure of the epilepsy requires removal of the internal Phlegm which may or may not be possible depending on the underlying physiological or neurological cause of the epilepsy (space occupying brain lesions are difficult to treat successfully with TCM alone).

25.5 LIVER AND KIDNEY *YIN* DEFICIENCY

肝肾阴虚

Pathophysiology
- Liver and Kidney *yin* deficiency type epilepsy is a chronic condition and reflects a particular constitutional state of a medicated patient or one who's epilepsy is largely in remission. The patient will not be having seizures, or only very infrequent seizures.

Clinical features
- long history of seizures
- vague or trance-like mental state
- dark complexion
- dizziness
- tinnitus
- dry, sore eyes
- withered ears
- insomnia and forgetfulness
- lower back and leg soreness and weakness
- dry stools or constipation

T red with little or no coat
P thready and rapid

Treatment principle
Nourish and tonify the Liver and Kidney

Prescription

DA BU YUAN JIAN 大补元煎
(*Great Tonify the Basal Decoction*) modified

shu di (Radix Rehmanniae Glutinosae Conquitae) 熟地	150-240g
chao shan yao (dry fried Radix Dioscoreae Oppositae) 炒山药	120g
shan zhu yu (Fructus Corni Officinalis) 山茱萸	120g
du zhong (Cortex Eucommiae Ulmoidis) 杜仲	90g
gou qi zi (Fructus Lycii) 枸杞子	90g
lu jiao jiao^ (Cornu Cervi Gelatinum) 鹿角胶	60g
gui ban jiao° (Plastri Testudinis Gelatinum) 龟板胶	60g
e jiao^ (Gelatinum Corii Asini) 阿胶	60g
mu li^ (Concha Ostreae) 牡蛎	60g
bie jia° (Carapax Amydae Sinensis) 鳖甲	60g

Method: Grind the herbs into powder and form into 9-gram pills with honey. The dose is one pill 2-3 times daily. May also be decocted with an 80% reduction in dosage. (Source: *Shi Yong Zhong Yi Nei Ke Xue*)

Modifications

- With severe irritability and restlessness, add **dan zhu ye** (Herba Lophatheri Gracilis) 淡竹叶 60g and **deng xin cao** (Medulla Junci Effusi) 灯心草 30g.
- With constipation, add **rou cong rong** (Cistanches Deserticolae) 肉苁蓉 90g, **dang gui** (Radix Angelicae Sinensis) 当归 60g and **huo ma ren** (Semen Cannabis Sativae) 火麻仁 60g.
- In severe cases, add **quan xie fen*** (powdered Buthus Martensi) 全蝎粉 20g and **wu gong fen*** (powdered Scolopendra Subspinipes) 蜈蚣粉 20g to the powder, or if decocted, 2g each to the strained decoction (*chong fu* 冲服).

Patent medicines

Ming Mu Di Huang Wan 明目地黄丸 (Ming Mu Di Huang Wan)
Zuo Gui Wan 左归丸 (Zuo Gui Wan)
Qi Ju Di Huang Wan 杞菊地黄丸 (Lycium-Rehmannia Pills)
Zhi Bai Ba Wei Wan 知柏八味丸 (Zhi Bai Ba Wei Wan)
Tian Wang Bu Xin Dan 天王补心丹 (Tian Wang Bu Xin Dan)

Acupuncture

Bl.23 (*shen shu* +), Bl.18 (*gan shu* +), Kid.3 (*tai xi* +), Liv.3 (*tai chong* +), Ren.4 (*guan yuan*), Kid.6 (*zhao hai*), *an mian* (N-HN-54), *si shen cong* (M-HN-1)

Clinical notes

- Corresponds to a type of chronic epilepsy.
- Prolonged treatment is necessary to secure any improvement.

25.6 BLOOD STAGNATION

Pathophysiology
- Blood stagnation type epilepsy may follow a traumatic injury, like a blow to the head, birth trauma or forceps delivery. It may also happen as a result of cerebral space occupying lesions, or may gradually occur as the result of another chronic pattern. The treatment described here is used when the seizures are largely controlled, although it may be useful in frequent seizures as an alternative to **DING XIAN WAN** (*Arrest Seizures Pill* 定痫丸, see *yang* seizures, p.685) where there is a clear association with head trauma.

Clinical features
- seizures with a clear relationship to some traumatic incident
- persistent insomnia with much dreaming and restlessness
- irritablity, anger, depression, mood swings
- low grade fever at night
- fixed sharp pains, particularly in the head and upper body
- dry, scaly skin
- broken vessels or spider naevi on the face, trunk, inner knee and ankle
- purplish lips, sclera, conjunctiva and nail beds
- dark rings around the eyes

T dark or purple with brown or purple stasis spots and a thin white coat
P choppy or wiry and thready

Treatment principle
Invigorate the circulation of Blood
Eliminate stagnant Blood, soothe *qi*

Prescription

XUE FU ZHU YU TANG 血府逐瘀汤
(*Achyranthes and Persica Combination*) modified

dan shen (Radix Salviae Miltiorrhizae) 丹参	20g
sheng di (Radix Rehmanniae Glutinosae) 生地	12g
tao ren (Semen Persicae) 桃仁	12g
dang gui (Radix Angelicae Sinensis) 当归	9g
hong hua (Flos Carthami Tinctorii) 红花	9g
chai hu (Radix Bupleuri) 柴胡	9g
niu xi (Radix Achyranthis Bidentatae) 牛膝	9g
zhi ke (Fructus Citri Aurantii) 枳壳	6g
chi shao (Radix Paeoniae Rubrae) 赤芍	6g
jie geng (Radix Platycodi Grandiflori) 桔梗	6g
chuan xiong (Radix Ligustici Chuanxiong) 川芎	6g

Method: Decoction. (Source: *Zhong Yi Nei Ke Lin Chuang Shou Ce*)

Modifications

- With Phlegm, add two or three of the following herbs: **tian nan xing*** (Rhizoma Arisaematis) 天南星 9g, **ban xia*** (Rhizoma Pinelliae Ternatae) 半夏 9g, **shi chang pu** (Rhizoma Acori Graminei) 石菖蒲 6g, **yuan zhi** (Radix Polygalae Tenuifoliae) 远志 6g, **zao jiao** (Fructus Gleditsiae Sinensis) 皂角 6g or **tian zhu huang** (Concretio Silicea Bambusae Textillis) 天竺黄 9g.
- With headache, add **tian ma** (Rhizoma Gastrodiae Elatae) 天麻 9g, **bai ji li** (Fructus Tribuli Terrestris) 白蒺藜 9g and **shi jue ming^** (Concha Haliotidis) 石决明 12g.
- With Cold, add **wu yao** (Radix Linderae Strychnifoliae) 乌药 9g, **xiao hui xiang** (Fructus Foeniculi Vulgaris) 小茴香 9g and **pao jiang** (quick fried Rhizoma Zingiberis Officinalis) 炮姜 6g.
- With *yang* deficiency, delete **chai hu**, and add **fu zi*** (Radix Aconiti Carmichaeli Praeparata) 制附子 6-9g and **gui zhi** (Ramulus Cinnamomi Cassiae) 桂枝 9g.
- Other herbs that are frequently added to the guiding prescription, depending on the severity of the condition, include **quan xie*** (Buthus Martensi) 全蝎 2g, **wu gong*** (Scolopendra Subspinipes) 蜈蚣 2g, **jiang can^** (Bombyx Batryticatus) 僵蚕 9g, **gou teng** (Ramulus Uncariae cum Uncis) 钩藤 12g, **tian ma** (Rhizoma Gastrodiae Elatae) 天麻 9g and **di long^** (Lumbricus) 地龙 6g.

TONG QIAO HUO XUE TANG 通窍活血汤
(*Unblock the Orifices and Invigorate Blood Decoction*) modified

This formula is recommended for Blood stagnation affecting the senses and head. It is stronger than the primary formula and suited to robust individuals.

dang gui (Radix Angelicae Sinensis) 当归	15g
chi shao (Radix Paeoniae Rubrae) 赤芍	15g
tao ren (Semen Persicae) 桃仁	10g
chuan xiong (Radix Ligustici Chuanxiong) 川芎	6g
hong hua (Flos Carthami Tinctorii) 红花	6g
bai zhi (Radix Angelicae Dahuricae) 白芷	6g
wu shao she^ (Zaocys Dhumnades) 乌梢蛇	6g
quan xie* (Buthus Martensi) 全蝎	3g
cong bai (Bulbus Allii Fistulosi) 葱白	3g
da zao (Fructus Zizyphi Jujubae) 大枣	7pce
sheng jiang (Rhizoma Zingiberis Officinalis) 生姜	9g
she xiang° (Secretio Moschus) 麝香	0.15g

Method: Decoction. **She xiang** and **quan xie** are usually powdered and taken separately or added to the strained decoction (*chong fu* 冲服). (Source: *Zhong Yi Nei Ke Lin Chuang Shou Ce*)

Patent medicines
Xue Fu Zhu Yu Wan 血府逐瘀丸 (Xue Fu Zhu Yu Wan)
Nei Xiao Luo Li Wan 内消瘰疬丸 (Nei Xiao Luo Li Wan)
Dan Shen Pian 丹参片 (Dan Shen Pills)

Acupuncture
Points of pain on the head (*ah shi*), Bl.17 (*ge shu* -), LI.4 (*he gu* -), Sp.6 (*san yin jiao* -), Liv.4 (*zhong du* -), Liv.3 (*tai chong*), SI.6 (*yang lao*), *si shen cong* (M-HN-1)

Clinical notes
• Corresponds to either acute or chronic epilepsy.

SUMMARY OF GUIDING FORMULAE FOR EPILEPSY

Uncontrolled or poorly controlled epilepsy
Yang seizures - *Ding Xian Wan* 定闲丸

Yin seizures - *Ding Xian Wan* 定闲丸

Constitutional patterns in controlled epileptics
Spleen deficiency with Phlegm - *Liu Jun Zi Tang* 六君子汤

Liver Fire with Phlegm Heat - *Long Dan Xie Gan Tang* 龙胆泻肝汤 + *Di Tan Tang* 涤痰汤
- with constipation + *Gun Tan Tang* 滚痰汤
- mild cases of Liver Fire with Phlegm - *Chai Hu Jia Long Gu Mu Li Tang* 柴胡加龙骨牡蛎汤

Liver and Kidney *yin* deficiency - *Da Bu Yuan Jian* 大补元煎

Blood stagnation - *Xue Fu Zhu Yu Tang* 血府逐瘀汤 or *Tong Qiao Huo Xue Tang* 通窍活血汤

Endnote

For more information regarding herbs marked with an asterisk*, an open circle° or a hatˆ, see the tables on pp.944-952.

Disorders of the Liver

26. Spasms and Convulsions

Febrile Convulsions
Wind Toxin Tetany (Muscular Tetany)
External pathogens
Phlegm obstruction
Blood stagnation
Qi and Blood deficiency

26 SPASMS AND CONVULSIONS
jing bing 痙病

The spasms and convulsions described in this chapter are the product of high fever, meningeal irritation, infection or cerebral space occupying lesions. They are characterised by the rhythmic or convulsive seizures accompanied by or following high fever, or muscular spasms of the extremities, neck and back, trismus or opisthotonos.

Convulsions are always due to the stirring of internal Wind, regardless of whether the Wind results from an excess or deficient pattern. Spasm of the muscles can be due to external or internal Wind, or from a lack of nutrition to the Tendons due to *yin* and/or Blood deficiency.

The patterns described in this chapter differ from epilepsy, in that *jing bing* usually have an immediate identifiable cause (like fever or a puncture wound), and once the basic cause is dealt with the patient gets better with no recurrence. Epilepsy on the other hand, is associated with deeply rooted Phlegm and often occurs without any identifiable precipitating event.

The disorders that fall into the *jing bing* category are a mixture of conditions characterised by muscular spasms or cramps and tetanic spasms or convulsions. The types of disorders that may be analysed using this chapter include febrile convulsions and numerous conditions that affect the central nervous system or irritate the meninges (like epidemic cerebrospinal meningitis or encephalitis, raised intracranial pressure, tumours and parasitic diseases of the brain), as well as tetanus and botulism. The most common reason for convulsions is high fever, usually related to diseases like meningitis or encephalitis, or in children a simple upper respiratory or urinary tract infection.

AETIOLOGY
Internal Wind
As with all involuntary body movement, internally generated Wind is the responsible pathogen. Wind can be generated in several ways, the common ones are summarised in Box 24.2 (p.648). Other mechanisms apply in certain unique situations, for example the Wind that results from Phlegm obstruction causing epilepsy (p.680), and the cold deficient Wind of chronic childhood convulsions. The latter is a mild form of Wind that occurs when *qi* moves to fill the vacuum formed by chronic deficiency.

The Wind that causes convulsions is most commonly derived from excess Heat, and manifests during a high fever. This excess type Wind can soon become Wind from deficiency as the Heat consumes *yin* and Blood–the nature of the convulsions changes from violent and convulsive, to milder jerking and muscle spasm.

External pathogens
External Wind, Cold Dampness or Heat can enter the channels and obstruct the circulation of *qi* and Blood, depriving the Tendons of nutrition. This affects the *tai yang* channels of the back and neck causing muscular spasm and pain. If a pathogen moves from the surface further into the body, it can become hot and, when severe, generate internal Wind giving rise to febrile convulsions with violent jerking of the limbs and body.

One exotic form of external Wind is that which combines with Toxins to cause muscular tetany (*po shang feng* 破伤风–tetanus). In this case the Wind enters through a puncture wound or an infected umbilicus and invades the channels and internal organs.

Blood stagnation
Traumatic injury, particularly affecting the head, can cause Blood stagnation type spasms or convulsions. Any chronic pathology will also eventually inhibit Blood circulation; for example long term *qi* stagnation and Cold or Phlegm obstruction directly block Blood circulation, while *yin* and *yang* deficiency increase Blood viscosity and slow circulation respectively. In practice, Blood stagnation that causes spasms or convulsions is a serious disorder, most likely involving a space occupying cerebral lesion, like a tumour, abscess, cyst or haemorrhage.

Phlegm
Spasms and convulsions caused by Phlegm often indicate the presence of a space occupying cerebral lesion. In this way, Phlegm obstruction is similar to Blood stagnation. The difference, however, is seen in the clinical features and signs which are indicative of systemic or constitutional Phlegm. In practice, Phlegm and Blood stagnation frequently co-exist. The Phlegm itself can be the product of overeating, overindulgence in Phlegm producing foods, Spleen deficiency and prolonged Damp stagnation, or *qi* stagnation that retards movement of fluids.

Qi and Blood deficiency
The *qi* and Blood deficiency of this pattern may follow fluid loss through haemorrhage or excessive sweating. It may also occur post partum, or following heatstroke. Spleen deficiency or chronic illness will lead to *qi* and Blood deficiency.

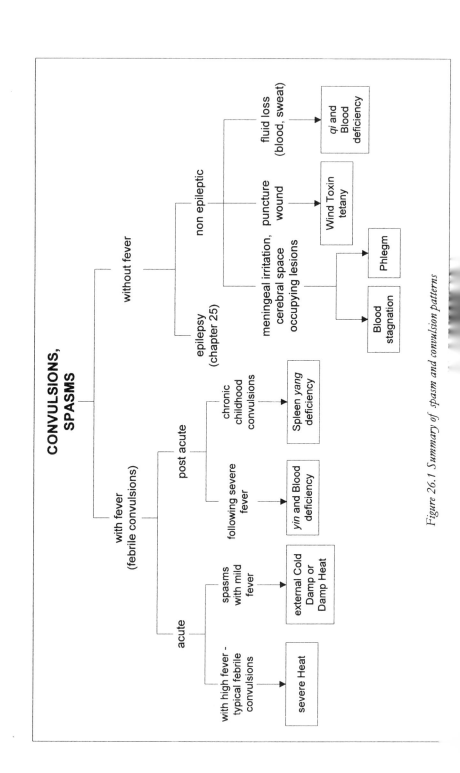

Figure 26.1 Summary of spasm and convulsion patterns

26.1 FEBRILE CONVULSIONS

26.1.1 ACUTE PHASE
Pathophysiology
- The convulsions, spasms or opisthotonos that characterise febrile convulsions are due to the stirring of internal Wind by severe Heat. As one commentator noted, 'as the severe winds of Summer are generated by the hottest of days, so, in the body, severe internal Wind is generated by an excess of Heat'.
- Febrile convulsions are most common in children and can occur in numerous biomedically defined disorders if the fever is high enough. Keep in mind that many of the diseases that can cause febrile convulsions are dangerous (commonly diseases like meningitis or encephalitis) and in most cases should be managed in hospital if possible.
- The main principle of treatment (for both adults and children) is to reduce the fever and stop the convulsion so as to minimise the possibility of brain damage. In some cases the convulsions can become chronic if the *qi*, *yang* or *yin* have been seriously damaged.
- The TCM treatment is fairly straightforward–administer an appropriate emergency medicine, followed by an appropriate decoction once the patient is stable and can take a liquid. The follow-up prescription depends on the type of fever.

Clinical features
- stiff neck, muscle spasms, opisthotonos or convulsions accompanied by high fever, malaise, headache, drowsiness, vomiting

Treatment principle
Clear Heat, eliminate Toxins
Extinguish Wind and stop convulsions

Prescription

ZI XUE DAN 紫雪丹
(*Purple Snow Special Pill*)

This is the standard formula for febrile convulsions and is widely available in patent medicine pill form for swift administration. It is one of the three treasures (*san bao* 三宝) of Chinese emergency medicine, the others being ZHI BAO DAN (*Greatest Treasure Special Pill* 至宝丹, p.660) and AN GONG NIU HUANG WAN (*Calm the Palace Pill with Cattle Gallstone* 安宫牛黄丸, p.914). These formulae are suitable for short term use. Once the patient is stable and the convulsions have ceased, a suitable formula based on the patient's febrile pattern should be commenced.

shi gao (Gypsum) 石膏 1500g
han shui shi (Calcitum) 寒水石 1500g
hua shi (Talcum) 滑石 1500g
ci shi (Magnetitum) 磁石 1500g
qing mu xiang* (Radix Aristolochiae Qingmuxiang)
    青木香 150g
chen xiang (Lignum Aquilariae) 沉香 150g
xuan shen (Radix Scrophulariae Ningpoensis) 玄参 500g
sheng ma (Rhizoma Cimicifugae) 升麻 500g
gan cao (Radix Glycyrrhizae Uralensis) 甘草 240g
ding xiang (Flos Caryophylli) 丁香 30g
mang xiao (Mirabilitum) 芒硝 5000g
huo xiao (Niter) 火硝 1000g
xi jiao° (Cornu Rhinoceri) 犀角 150g
ling yang jiao° (Cornu Antelopis) 羚羊角 150g
she xiang° (Secretio Moschus) 麝香 36g
zhu sha* (Cinnabaris) 朱砂 90g

Method: The quantities given here are for industrial preparation. Boil the first 4 mineral ingredients (crushed) in 37.5 litres of water and reduce to 30 litres, then discard the solids. In the remaining water boil the next 6 ingredients until reduced by two thirds, discard the solids and add the **mang xiao** and **huo xiao**, stirring continuously until the water has almost evaporated. Turn out into a flat dish and allow to dry. Add the **powdered horns**, the **musk** and **cinnabar** and sift to a fine powder. The dose for adults is 2 vials twice daily (in commercial preparations one vial is 0.8 grams). For children less than one year old, the dose is reduced to half a vial twice daily; for children over one year old, the dose is 1 vial twice daily.
(Source: *Shi Yong Fang Ji Xue*)

XIAO ER HUI CHUN DAN 小儿回春丹
(Childrens Return of Spring Special Pill)

This formula is prefered for febrile convulsions in children. It is available as pills or powder, with varying contents depending on the manufacturer. Also known as **HUI CHUN DAN** (*Return of Spring Special Pill* 回春丹).

niu huang^ (Calculus Bovis) 牛黄 3g
bing pian (Borneol) 冰片 4.5g
she xiang° (Secretio Moschus) 麝香 4.5g
zhu sha* (Cinnabaris) 朱砂 9g
qiang huo (Rhizoma et Radix Notopterygii) 羌活 9g
jiang can^ (Bombyx Batryticatus) 僵蚕 9g
tian ma (Rhizoma Gastrodiae Elatae) 天麻 9g
fang feng (Radix Ledebouriellae Divaricatae) 防风 9g
xiong huang (Realgar) 雄黄 9g
quan xie* (Buthus Martensi) 全蝎 9g
bai fu zi* (Rhizoma Typhonii Gigantei) 白附子 9g

tian zhu huang (Concretio Silicea Bambusae Textillis)
天竺黄 9g
chuan bei mu (Bulbus Fritillariae Cirrhosae) 川贝母 30g
dan nan xing* (Pulvis Arisaemae cum Felle Bovis) 胆南星 ... 60g
gou teng (Ramulus Uncariae) 钩藤 60g
gan cao (Radix Glycyrrhizae Uralensis) 甘草 30g

Method: Grind all ingredients (except the last two) to a fine powder. Boil the **gan cao** in 200 mls of water and reduce by half. Add the **gou teng** and boil for 15 minutes. Discard the solids. Use the remaining liquid to form the powder into small pills of about 0.1 gram each. The dose for infants less than one year old is one pill 2-3 times daily; over one year old two pills 2-3 times daily. (Source: *Shi Yong Fang Ji Xue*)

Follow-up treatment

After the patient is stable one of the following formulae may be selected to treat the underlying pattern.

LING JIAO GOU TENG TANG 羚角钩藤汤
(*Antelope Horn and Uncaria Decoction*) modified

This formula is selected when the pattern is Liver Heat stirring Wind. The main features are persistent high fever, irritability and restlessness, dizziness, vertigo, twitching, tics or spasms of the limbs, and in severe cases, clouding or loss of consciousness, a deep red, dry tongue with prickles and a wiry rapid pulse.

ling yang jiao fen° (powdered Cornu Antelopis)
羚羊角粉 4.5g
sang ye (Folium Mori Albae) 桑叶 12g
gou teng (Ramulus Uncariae) 钩藤 12g
chuan bei mu (Bulbus Fritillariae Cirrhosae) 川贝母 12g
sheng di (Radix Rehmanniae Glutinosae) 生地 15g
zhu ru (Caulis Bambusae in Taeniis) 竹茹 15g
ju hua (Flos Chrysanthemi Morifolii) 菊花 9g
bai shao (Radix Paeoniae Lactiflorae) 白芍 9g
fu ling (Sclerotium Poriae Cocos) 茯苓 9g
gan cao (Radix Glycyrrhizae Uralensis) 甘草 3g

Method: Decoction. **Ling yang jiao fen** is added as a powder to the strained decoction (*chong fu* 冲服), and **gou teng** is added towards the end of cooking (*hou xia* 后下). (Source: *Shi Yong Fang Ji Xue*)

BAI HU TANG 白虎汤
(*Anemarrhena and Gypsum Combination*)

This formula is used when external pathogenic Cold or Heat lodge at the *yang ming* level (of the six divisions). The features are high fever, sweating, severe thirst and a flooding or bounding pulse.

shi gao (Gypsum) 石膏	30g
zhi mu (Rhizoma Anemarrhenae Asphodeloides) 知母	9g
geng mi (Semen Oryzae) 梗米	9g
gan cao (Radix Glycyrrhizae Uralensis) 甘草	3g

Method: Decoction. (Source: *Shi Yong Fang Ji Xue*)

QING WEN BAI DU YIN 清瘟败毒饮
(Clear Epidemics and Overcome Toxin Decoction)

This formula is used for severe high fever due to epidemic Toxic Heat, with Fire at the *qi* and Blood levels. The pattern is characterised by fever, thirst, severe headache or stiff neck, delirium, febrile rashes or bleeding. The tongue is dark red and dry. The fever is usually associated with a severe infection like meningitis, encephalitis, scarlet fever or septicaemia.

shi gao (Gypsum) 石膏	30-60g
sheng di (Radix Rehmanniae Glutinosae) 生地	30g
huang qin (Radix Scutellariae Baicalensis) 黄芩	9g
shan zhi zi (Fructus Gardeniae Jasminoidis) 山栀子	9g
zhi mu (Rhizoma Anemarrhenae Asphodeloides) 知母	9g
chi shao (Radix Paeoniae Rubrae) 赤芍	9g
xuan shen (Radix Scrophulariae Ningpoensis) 玄参	9g
lian qiao (Fructus Forsythia Suspensae) 连翘	9g
mu dan pi (Cortex Moutan Radicis) 牡丹皮	9g
jie geng (Radix Platycodi Grandiflori) 桔梗	9g
dan zhu ye (Herba Lophatheri Gracilis) 淡竹叶	9g
xi jiao° (Cornu Rhinoceri) 犀角	1.5-3g
huang lian (Rhizoma Coptidis) 黄连	3g
gan cao (Radix Glycyrrhizae Uralensis) 甘草	3g

Method: Decoction. **Shi gao** is cooked first for 15 minutes (*xian jian* 先煎). **Shui niu jiao**^ (Cornu Bubali) 水牛角 is usually substituted for **xi jiao** with a tenfold increase in dosage. It is usually powdered and decocted for 30 minute before the other herbs are added (*xian jian* 先煎). (Source: *Shi Yong Fang Ji Xue*)

WU WEI XIAO DU YIN 五味消毒饮
(Five Ingredient Decoction to Eliminate Toxin)

This formula is used when localised Toxic Heat causes abscesses or boils that penetrate into the Blood. An excellent formula for all types of superficial suppurative sores and disorders like mastitis, lymphangitis, erysipelas and septicaemia.

jin yin hua (Flos Lonicera Japonicae) 金银花	15-30g
zi hua di ding (Herba cum Radice Violae Yedoensitis) 紫花地丁	15-30g

pu gong ying (Herba Taraxaci Mongolici cum Radice)
蒲公英 15-30g
ye ju hua (Flos Chrysanthemi Indici) 野菊花 12g
zi bei tian kui (Herba Begoniae Fimbristipulatae)
紫北天葵 9g
Method: Decoction. (Source: *Shi Yong Fang Ji Xue*)

BAI TOU WENG TANG 白头翁汤
(*Pulsatilla Decoction* 白头翁汤)

This formula is selected when a severe hot dysenteric disorder causes diarrhoea, high fever and muscle twitches and spasm. This is the guiding formula for bacterial and amoebic dysentery.

bai tou weng (Radix Pulsatillae Chinensis) 白头翁 12g
huang bai (Cortex Phellodendri) 黄柏 9g
huang lian (Rhizoma Coptidis) 黄连 9g
qin pi (Cortex Fraxini) 秦皮 9g
Method: Decoction. (Source: *Shi Yong Zhong Yi Nei Ke Xue*)

QING YING TANG 清营汤
(*Clear the Ying Decoction*)

This formula is used when Heat enters the *ying* and Blood levels causing high fever, delirium and febrile rashes.

xi jiao° (Cornu Rhinoceri) 犀角 3g
sheng di (Radix Rehmanniae Glutinosae) 生地 30g
xuan shen (Radix Scrophulariae Ningpoensis) 玄参 12g
mai dong (Tuber Ophiopogonis Japonici) 麦冬 12g
jin yin hua (Flos Lonicera Japonicae) 金银花 12g
lian qiao (Fructus Forsythia Suspensae) 连翘 9g
dan shen (Radix Salviae Miltiorrhizae) 丹参 9g
dan zhu ye (Herba Lophatheri Gracilis) 淡竹叶 6g
huang lian (Rhizoma Coptidis) 黄连 3g
Method: Decoction. **Shui niu jiao**^ (Cornu Bubali) 水牛角 is usually substituted for **xi jiao** with a tenfold increase in dose. It is usually powdered and decocted for 30 minutes before the other herbs are added (*xian jian* 先煎).

Acupuncture
shi xuan ↓ (M-UE-1), Du.14 (*da zhui* -), Bl.40 (*wei zhong* -↓),
GB.34 (*yang ling quan* -), LI.11 (*qu chi* -), Du.26 (*ren zhong*)

Clinical notes
• This pattern may correspond with disorders such as meningitis, encephalitis, scarlet fever, pneumonia, septicaemia, measles, eclampsia

and puerperal convulsions.
- Many of these conditions require management in hospital. In these cases herbs and acupuncture can be used as additional therapy to antibiotics where appropriate, or may be applied as a first line measure until other medical treatments are instituted.

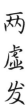

26.1.2 POST ACUTE PHASE (*YIN* AND BLOOD DEFICIENCY)

Pathophysiology
- Following a severe febrile disease (or in the late stages of a severe febrile disease), *yin* and Blood may be significantly damaged. This can give rise to continuing muscle spasms, cramps or convulsions. Improper treatment (either excessive diaphoresis or purgation) during a fever may also cause *yin* and Blood deficient spasms or convulsions. The pattern may also be associated with chronic *yin* and Blood deficiency, or follow a haemorrhage or other significant loss of body fluids.
- The spasms (in severe cases convulsions) are the result of a combination of Wind with *yin* and Blood deficiency (which cannot nourish and lubricate the Tendons).

Clinical features
- recurrent muscle spasms, cramps, twitches, quivering or alternating flexion and extension of the extremities
- sensation of heat in the palms and soles ('five hearts hot')
- low grade or relapsing fever, body feels hot to touch
- facial or malar flushing
- dry throat, thirst, parched lips
- emaciation
- irritability and fatigue
- dizziness, vertigo
- tinnitus, visual disturbances
- dry stools or constipation
- in severe cases disordered consciousness

T deep red and dry, with a scant or peeled coat
P thready, rapid and deficient

Treatment principle
 Nourish *yin*, clear Heat
 Anchor *yang*, extinguish Wind

Prescription

SAN JIA FU MAI TANG 三甲复脉汤
(*Three Shells Decoction to Restore the Pulse*)

This formula is selected when there is internal Wind and rising *yang* from *yin* and Blood deficiency, with the typical accompanying symptoms of relatively severe dizziness and tinnitus as well as spasms.

zhi gan cao (honey fried Radix Glycyrrhizae Uralensis)
炙甘草 18g
sheng di (Radix Rehmanniae Glutinosae) 生地 18g
bai shao (Radix Paeoniae Lactiflorae) 白芍 18g
mai dong (Tuber Ophiopogonis Japonici) 麦冬 15g
huo ma ren (Semen Cannabis Sativae) 火麻仁 9g
e jiao^ (Gelatinum Corii Asini) 阿胶 9g
mu li^ (Concha Ostreae) 牡蛎 15g
bie jia° (Carapax Amydae Sinensis) 鳖甲 24g
gui ban° (Plastri Testudinis Gelatinum) 龟板 30g

Method: Decoction. The shells are decocted for 30 minutes prior to the other herbs (*xian jian* 先煎), **e jiao** is melted before being added to the strained decoction (*yang hua* 烊化). (Source: *Formulas and Strategies*)

DA DING FENG ZHU 大定风珠
(*Major Arrest Wind Pearl*)

This formula is selected when the deficiency is prominent. It focuses primarily on the root of the disorder (the *yin* deficiency), rather than directly extinguishing the Wind.

sheng di (Radix Rehmanniae Glutinosae) 生地 18g
bai shao (Radix Paeoniae Lactiflorae) 白芍 18g
mai dong (Tuber Ophiopogonis Japonici) 麦冬 18g
mu li^ (Concha Ostreae) 牡蛎 12g
bie jia° (Carapax Amydae Sinensis) 鳖甲 12g
gui ban° (Plastri Testudinis Gelatinum) 龟板 12g
zhi gan cao (honey fried Radix Glycyrrhizae Uralensis)
炙甘草 12g
e jiao^ (Gelatinum Corii Asini) 阿胶 9g
huo ma ren (Semen Cannabis Sativae) 火麻仁 9g
wu wei zi (Fructus Schizandrae Chinensis) 五味子 6g
ji zi huang^ (egg yolk) 鸡子黄 2

Method: Decoction. The shells are decocted for 30 minutes prior to the other herbs (*xian jian* 先煎), **e jiao** is melted first and then added with the egg yolks to the strained decoction (*yang hua* 烊化). (Source: *Shi Yong Zhong Yi Nei Ke Xue*)

Modifications (applicable to both prescriptions)

- With *qi* deficiency, add **dang shen** (Radix Codonopsis Pilosulae) 党参 9g.
- With Blood stagnation, add **tao ren** (Semen Persicae) 桃仁 9g and **dan shen** (Radix Salviae Miltiorrhizae) 丹参 12g.
- For spontaneous sweating, add **long gu**^ (Os Draconis) 龙骨 15g, **dang shen** (Radix Codonopsis Pilosulae) 党参 9g and **fu xiao mai** (Semen Tritici Aestivi Levis) 浮小麦 15g.

- For palpitations, add **fu ling** (Sclerotium Poriae Cocos) 茯苓 12g, **dang shen** (Radix Codonopsis Pilosulae) 党参 9g and **fu xiao mai** (Semen Tritici Aestivi Levis) 浮小麦 15g.
- With severe Blood deficiency, add **dang gui** (Radix Angelicae Sinensis) 当归 9g, **shu di** (Radix Rehmanniae Glutinosae Conquitae) 熟地 18g and **chuan xiong** (Radix Ligustici Chuanxiong) 川芎 6g.

Acupuncture

Bl.18 (*gan shu* +), B.23 (*shen shu* +), Du.8 (*jin suo* -), Liv.8 (*qu quan* +), PC.6 (*nei guan*), Liv.3 (*tai chong*), Kid.3 (*tai xi* +), LI.4 (*he gu* -), LI.11 (*qu chi* -)

Patent medicines

Liu Wei Di Huang Wan 六味地黄丸 (Liu Wei Di Huang Wan)
Zhi Bai Ba Wei Wan 知柏八味丸 (Zhi Bai Ba Wei Wan)
 - with deficient Heat
Er Long Zuo Ci Wan 耳聋左慈丸 (Er Long Zuo Ci Wan)
 - with tinnitus
Ming Mu Di Huang Wan 明目地黄丸 (Ming Mu Di Huang Wan)
 - with visual disturbances
Qi Ju Di Huang Wan 杞菊地黄丸 (Lycium-Rehmannia Pills)
 - Liver and Kidney *yin* deficiency

Clinical notes

- This pattern may correspond with disorders such as encephalitis, meningitis and hypocalcaemia.
- This pattern superficially resembles the excess Heat type of spasms or convulsions, but the formulae given here are inappropriate for that condition. Clear differentiation from excess Heat stirring up internal Wind is important.
- This pattern is not as common as perhaps it once was because fevers nowadays are rarely allowed to persist long enough to seriously damage *yin* due to the widespread use of antibiotic and antipyretic medication.

26.1.3 POST ACUTE PHASE (CHRONIC CHILDHOOD CONVULSIONS DUE TO SPLEEN *YANG* DEFICIENCY)

Pathophysiology
- This chronic pattern occurs in children, either following a severe febrile disease, which has damaged Spleen *yang* (possibly also by the antibiotic medications used in the febrile pattern), or a bad episode of vomiting and/or diarrhoea (as in dysentery). The Wind in this pattern is the product of Cold and deficiency, and is generated by the movement of *qi* as it seeks to fill the vacuum created by the deficiency.
- This pattern can overlap with the Spleen deficiency with Phlegm type of epilepsy (see p.690).

Clinical features
- twitching, writhing or weak jerking of the limbs which is worse when the patient is fatigued or hungry; the movements are more choretic than convulsive in nature
- increased desire to sleep, possibly 'absences' (see pp.681, 688)
- watery vomiting and diarrhoea
- poor appetite or a very picky eater
- abdominal pains
- cold extremities
- sallow or pale complexion

T pale with a white coat
P deep and slow

Treatment principle
Warm the middle *jiao*, strengthen the Spleen
Stop convulsions

Prescription

LI ZHONG WAN 理中丸
(*Ginseng and Ginger Formula*) modified

ren shen (Radix Ginseng) 人参	9g
gan jiang (Rhizoma Zingiberis Officinalis) 干姜	9g
bai zhu (Rhizoma Atractylodes Macrocephalae) 白术	9g
zhi gan cao (honey fried Radix Glycyrrhizae Uralensis) 炙甘草	9g
tian ma (Rhizoma Gastrodiae Elatae) 天麻	9g

Method: Grind herbs to a fine powder and mix into the child's food or with honey. The dose is 3 grams daily. May also be decocted.

Modifications
- For severe internal Cold, add **zhi fu zi*** (Radix Aconiti Carmichaeli Praeparata) 制附子 6g cooked for 30 minutes prior to the other herbs
- In severe or resistant cases, add **wu gong*** (Scolopendra Subspinipes) 蜈蚣 1.5g and **quan xie*** (Buthus Martensi) 全蝎 1.5g to the strained decoction (*chong fu* 冲服), or take seperately as a powder.

Acupuncture
Ren.12 (*zhong wan* ▲), Ren.6 (*qi hai* ▲), St.25 (*tian shu* ▲), St.36 (*zu san li* ▲), Bl.20 (*pi shu* ▲), Du.14 (*da zhui* ▲)

Patent medicines
Fu Zi Li Zhong Wan 附子理中丸 (Li Chung Yuen Medical Pills)
Li Zhong Wan 理中丸 (Li Zhong Wan)

Clinical notes
- Children respond reasonably well to treatment, depending on how depleted the child is and the other pharmaceutical medications being administered.
- Children with chronic Cold convulsions may be diagnosed as epileptic and treated with anti-convulsant drugs. Anti-convulsants are usually cold in nature[1], and will aggravate the *yang* deficiency.

---

1. Scott J P (1991) *Acupuncture in the Treatment of Children.* Eastland Press, Seattle.

26.2 WIND TOXIN TETANY (MUSCULAR TETANY)

Pathophysiology
- This pattern corresponds primarily to tetanus, and is also known as 'incised wound tetany' (*jin chuang jing* 金创痉). It is due to Wind and Toxins that gain access to the channels and internal organs through an open wound.

Clinical features
- in the early stages there may be headache, fever, chills and malaise
- stiffness and spasm of the jaw
- deviation of the eyes
- muscle spasm, facial rictus
- opisthotonos or convulsions

P wiry and tight
T often unremarkable and may be difficult to see with the jaw in spasm

Treatment principle
Dispel Wind and Toxins, relieve spasm, stop pain

Prescription

YU ZHEN SAN 玉真散
(*True Jade Powder*) modified

tian nan xing* (Rhizoma Arisaematis) 天南星	10g
fang feng (Radix Ledebouriellae Divaricatae) 防风	10g
bai zhi (Radix Angelicae Dahuricae) 白芷	10g
tian ma (Rhizoma Gastrodiae Elatae) 天麻	10g
qiang huo (Rhizoma et Radix Notopterygii) 羌活	10g
bai fu zi* (Rhizoma Typhonii Gigantei) 白附子	10g
jiang can^ (Bombyx Batryticatus) 僵蚕	10g
quan xie* (Buthus Martensi) 全蝎	6g
wu gong* (Scolopendra Subspinipes) 蜈蚣	6g

Method: Grind all the herbs to a fine powder and take in 6-gram doses 2-3 times daily with warm yellow wine (*shao xing jiu* 绍兴酒). If the patient is unable to ingest the medicine, the herbs may be decocted and administered as a retention enema. (Source: *Shi Yong Fang Ji Xue*)

Modifications
- With Heat, add **huang lian** (Rhizoma Coptidis) 黄连 6g.
- With Phlegm, add **tian zhu huang** (Concretio Silicea Bambusae Textillis) 天竺黄 6g and **chuan bei mu** (Bulbus Fritillariae Cirrhosae) 川贝母 10g.

Patent medicines
Hu Po Bao Long Wan 琥珀抱龙丸 (Po Lung Yuen Medical Pills)

Acupuncture
Du.14 (*da zhui* -), Du.8 (*jin suo* -), Du.16 (*feng fu* -), LI.4 (*he gu* -), LI.11 (*qu chi* -), Du.3 (*yao yang guan* -), St.7 (*xia guan* -), St.6 (*jia che* -), Bl.60 (*kun lun* -), Bl.62 (*shen mai* -), Liv.3 (*tai chong* -)

Clinical notes
- This pattern may correspond with disorders such as tetanus and botulism.
- Tetanus anti-toxin must be given and the patient should be immediately referred to a hospital for intubation and ventilation (if necessary).

26.3 EXTERNAL COLD DAMP (DAMP HEAT)

Pathophysiology
- The spasms in this pattern are due to invasion of the *tai yang* channels by external Wind plus Cold, Damp or Damp Heat. It may appear as the early stage of a Warm disease (*wen bing* 温病).

Clinical features
- stiffness and spasms of the neck and back
- mild fever and chills
- headache
- no sweating or mild sweating
- aching and heaviness in the limbs
- trismus or spasms and contractures of the limbs

T unremarkable or with a thin white or greasy white coat
P floating and tight

Treatment principle
Expel Wind, disperse Cold Damp
Harmonise *ying*

Prescription

QIANG HUO SHENG SHI TANG 羌活胜湿汤
(*Notopterygium Decoction to Overcome Dampness*)

qiang huo (Rhizoma et Radix Notopterygii) 羌活	9g
du huo (Radix Angelicae Pubescentis) 独活	9g
gao ben (Rhizoma et Radix Ligustici) 藁本	6g
fang feng (Radix Ledebouriellae Divaricatae) 防风	6g
chuan xiong (Radix Ligustici Chuanxiong) 川芎	6g
man jing zi (Fructus Viticis) 蔓荆子	6g
zhi gan cao (honey fried Radix Glycyrrhizae Uralensis) 炙甘草	3g

Method: Decoction. (Source: *Shi Yong Zhong Yi Nei Ke Xue*)

Variations and additional prescriptions
Wind Cold
- If Cold is severe, with chills or rigors, stiffness and pain of the upper back and neck, no sweating, occipital headache, and spasms in the limbs or generalised myalgia, the correct treatment is to expel Cold, open the pores and relieve the muscles with **GE GEN TANG** (*Pueraria Combination* 葛根汤, p.7).

Damp Heat
- An invasion of Damp Heat into the channels causes afternoon fever, generalised muscle aches and spasm, headache, thirst with no desire to drink, scanty concentrated urine, fullness in the chest and abdomen, loss of appetite, nausea, a white tongue coat and a soggy pulse. The correct treatment is to clear Damp Heat and open the channels with **SAN REN TANG** (*Three Nut Decoction* 三仁汤) modified.

    yi ren (Semen Coicis Lachryma-jobi) 苡仁 18-30g
    hua shi (Talcum) 滑石 15g
    qin jiao (Radix Gentianae Qinjiao) 秦艽 15g
    wei ling xian* (Radix Clematidis) 威灵仙 15g
    si gua luo (Fasciculus Vascularis Luffae) 丝瓜络 15g
    xing ren* (Semen Pruni Armeniacae) 杏仁 12g
    ban xia* (Rhizoma Pinelliae Ternatae) 半夏 9g
    dan zhu ye (Herba Lophatheri Gracilis) 淡竹叶 9g
    bai dou kou (Fructus Amomi Kravanh) 白豆蔻 6g
    hou po (Cortex Magnoliae Officinalis) 厚朴 6g
    tong cao (Medulla Tetrapanacis Papyriferi) 通草 6g
    Method: Decoction.

Acupuncture

Du.20 (*bai hui* -), GB.20 (*feng chi* -), Du.16 (*feng fu* -), Bl.10 (*tian zhu* -), SJ.5 (*wai guan* -), Du.8 (*jin suo* -), Bl.18 (*gan shu* -), Bl.60 (*kun lun* -)

Patent medicines
Wind Cold
Gan Mao Ling 感冒灵 (Gan Mao Ling)
Gan Mao Qing Re Chong Ji 感冒清热冲剂 (Colds and Flu Tea)
Chuan Xiong Cha Tiao Wan 川芎茶调丸 (Chuan Xiong Cha Tiao Wan)
Yu Feng Ning Xin Wan 愈风宁心丸 (Headache and Dizziness Reliever)

Wind Damp
Huo Xiang Zheng Qi Pian 藿香正气片 (Huo Hsiang Cheng Chi Pien)
Xing Jun San 行军散 (Marching Powder, Five Pagodas Brand)

Clinical notes
- This pattern may correspond with disorders such as early stage of meningitis or encephalitis, influenza, dengue fever and fever of unknown origin.
- If the pattern is an early stage *wen bing*, then the patient may (if untreated or poorly treated) go on to exhibit full febrile convulsions.

26.4 PHLEGM OBSTRUCTION

Pathophysiology
- The spasms or convulsions in this pattern are due to Phlegm obstructing the channels. When the Tendons are poorly nourished by *qi* and Blood as a result of obstruction, spasms and cramps can occur. This category may overlap with some forms of epilepsy.

Clinical features
- spasms, cramps, stiffness in the limbs, neck and back or convulsions
- diffuse headache, heaviness, woolliness or fullness in the head
- dizziness, vertigo
- visual disturbances, double vision or loss of vision
- fullness and discomfort in the chest and epigastrium
- nausea, vomiting

T greasy, white coat
P soft, slippery and/or wiry

Treatment principle
Expel Wind, disperse Phlegm
Move *qi* and stop spasms

Prescription

QU FENG DAO TAN TANG 祛风导痰汤
(*Expel Wind and Guide Out the Phlegm Decoction*)

qiang huo (Rhizoma et Radix Notopterygii) 羌活	9g
fang feng (Radix Ledebouriellae Divaricatae) 防风	6g
fu ling (Sclerotium Poriae Cocos) 茯苓	12g
ban xia* (Rhizoma Pinelliae Ternatae) 半夏	9g
chen pi (Pericarpium Citri Reticulatae) 陈皮	6g
gan cao (Radix Glycyrrhizae Uralensis) 甘草	3g
tian nan xing* (Rhizoma Arisaematis) 天南星	6g
zhi shi (Fructus Immaturus Citri Aurantii) 枳实	9g
bai zhu (Rhizoma Atractylodes Macrocephalae) 白术	9g
zhu ru (Caulis Bambusae in Taeniis) 竹茹	6g
sheng jiang (Rhizoma Zingiberis Officinalis) 生姜	4pce

Method: Decoction. (Source: *Shi Yong Zhong Yi Nei Ke Xue*)

Modifications
- If there is Heat, substitute **dan nan xing*** (Pulvis Arisaemae cum Felle Bovis) 胆南星 for **tian nan xing**, and add **huang lian** (Rhizoma Coptidis) 黄连 3g, **huang qin** (Radix Scutellariae Baicalensis) 黄芩 9g

and **gua lou ren** (Semen Trichosanthis) 栝楼仁 12g.

Acupuncture
St.40 (*feng long* -), Sp.3 (*tai bai*), SI.3 (*hou xi* -), Bl.62 (*shen mai* -), GB.20 (*feng chi* -), Du.14 (*da zhui* -), Du.8 (*jin suo* -), Du.16 (*feng fu* -), Bl.20 (*pi shu* +), Du.20 (*bai hui*)

Patent medicines
Hai Zao Wan 海藻丸 (Hai Zao Wan)
Nei Xiao Luo Li Wan 内消瘰疬丸 (Nei Xiao Luo Li Wan)

Clinical notes
- This pattern may be due to meningeal irritation from a space occupying cerebral lesion, such as cerebral tumour, cyst or abscess, sarcoidosis, cysticercosis, echinococcosis.
- Once signs of Phlegm begin to clear the frequency of spasms and convulsions should subside. Tumours and other substantial lesions, however, are difficult to resolve with Chinese medicine alone and a combination of Western medicine and TCM should be used.

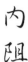

26.5 BLOOD STAGNATION

Pathophysiology
- The spasms or convulsions of this pattern are the result of stagnant Blood obstructing the circulation of *qi* and Blood through the channels, and consequent malnourishment of the Tendons. It may follow other chronic pathology or head injury. There may be an overlap with some forms of epilepsy.

Clinical features
- stiffness and spasms of the neck, back and occasionally extremities, torticollis, possible convulsions
- severe localised progressive headache
- visual disturbances, double vision or loss of vision
- dark, ashen, sallow or purple complexion, dark or purple lips and conjunctivae, dark rings around the eyes
- spider naevii, emaciation

T purple or with brown or purple stasis spots and little or no coat
P thready and choppy or wiry

Treatment principle
Invigorate the circulation of *qi* and Blood
Expel stagnant Blood, nourish the Tendons and stop spasms

Prescription

TONG QIAO HUO XUE TANG 通窍活血汤
(*Unblock the Orifices and Invigorate Blood Decoction*) modified

chi shao (Radix Paeoniae Rubrae) 赤芍	15g
dang gui (Radix Angelicae Sinensis) 当归	15g
tao ren (Semen Persicae) 桃仁	10g
hong hua (Flos Carthami Tinctorii) 红花	6g
chuan xiong (Radix Ligustici Chuanxiong) 川芎	6g
bai zhi (Radix Angelicae Dahuricae) 白芷	6g
wu shao she^ (Zaocys Dhumnades) 乌梢蛇	6g
quan xie* (Buthus Martensi) 全蝎	3g
cong bai (Bulbus Allii Fistulosi) 葱白	3g
da zao (Fructus Zizyphi Jujubae) 大枣	7pce
sheng jiang (Rhizoma Zingiberis Officinalis) 生姜	9g
she xiang° (Secretio Moschus) 麝香	0.15g

Method: Decoction. **She xiang** and **quan xie** are usually powdered and taken separately or added to the strained decoction (*chong fu* 冲服). (Source: *Zhong Yi Nei Ke Lin Chuang Shou Ce*)

Modifications
- With *qi* and Blood deficiency, add **huang qi** (Radix Astragali Membranacei) 黄芪 30g, **dang gui** (Radix Angelicae Sinensis) 当归 15g, **shu di** (Radix Rehmanniae Glutinosae Conquitae) 熟地 15g.
- With *yin* and *jing* deficiency, add **sheng di** (Radix Rehmanniae Glutinosae) 生地 20g, **shu di** (Radix Rehmanniae Glutinosae Conquitae) 熟地 20g, **gui ban**° (Plastri Testudinis Gelatinum) 龟板 15g, and **gou qi zi** (Fructus Lycii) 枸杞子 15g.

Acupuncture
GB.20 *(feng chi -)*, *ah shi* (points of pain on the head), Du.16 *(feng fu -)*, Du.8 *(jin suo -)*, Sp.10 *(xue hai -)*, Bl.18 *(gan shu -)*, Liv.14 *(qi men -)*, Bl.17 *(ge shu -)*, Liv.2 *(xing jian -)*, SI.3 *(hou xi -)*, Bl.62 *(shen mai -)*

Patent medicines
Xue Fu Zhu Yu Wan 血府逐瘀丸 (Xue Fu Zhu Yu Wan)
Nei Xiao Luo Li Wan 内消瘰疬丸 (Nei Xiao Luo Li Wan)

Clinical notes
- This patterns may correspnd to cerebral tumour, cyst or abscess, concussion, subdural haematoma, sarcoidosis, cysticercosis or echinococcosis.
- In general, most of these conditions are difficult to treat successfully with TCM alone. TCM treatment is supportive and palliative.

26.6 *QI* AND BLOOD DEFICIENCY

气血亏虚发痉

Pathophysiology
- Spasms due to *qi* and Blood deficiency may follow significant haemorrhage, sweating or other fluid loss, or some other chronic disease that damages the Spleen and consumes *qi* and Blood. The main factor is the Blood deficiency which fails to nourish the Tendons. An additional factor is the tendency of Liver *qi* to stagnate when Blood is deficient.

Clinical features
- stiffness, spasms or cramps of the muscles of the limbs, neck and back
- dizziness, light headedness
- spontaneous sweating
- lethargy, fatigue, weakness
- shortness of breath

T pale
P wiry and thready

Treatment principle
Tonify *qi* and Blood
Nourish the Tendons and ease spasms

Prescription

BA ZHEN TANG 八珍汤
(*Ginseng and Dang Gui Eight Combination*) modified

shu di (Radix Rehmanniae Glutinosae Conquitae) 熟地	12g
dang shen (Radix Codonopsis Pilosulae) 党参	12g
dang gui (Radix Angelicae Sinensis) 当归	9g
bai shao (Radix Paeoniae Lactiflorae) 白芍	9g
bai zhu (Rhizoma Atractylodes Macrocephalae) 白术	9g
fu ling (Sclerotium Poriae Cocos) 茯苓	9g
chuan xiong (Radix Ligustici Chuanxiong) 川芎	6g
gou teng (Ramulus Uncariae) 钩藤	12g
tian ma (Rhizoma Gastrodiae Elatae) 天麻	9g
zhi gan cao (honey fried Radix Glycyrrhizae Uralensis) 炙甘草	3g

Method: Decoction. **Gou teng** is added towards the end of cooking (*hou xia* 后下). (Source: *Shi Yong Zhong Yi Nei Ke Xue*)

Modifications
- With Liver *qi* stagnation, increase the dose of **bai shao** to 15g and add **xiang fu** (Rhizoma Cyperi Rotundi) 香附 9g and **mei gui hua** (Flos Rosea Rugosae) 玫瑰花 6g.

Patent medicines
Ba Zhen Wan 八珍丸 (Ba Zhen Wan)
Xiao Yao Wan 逍遥丸 (Xiao Yao Wan)
  - with Liver *qi* stagnation

Acupuncture
Bl.18 (*gan shu* +), Bl.17 (*ge shu* +), Sp.10 (*xue hai* +), Ren.12 (*zhong wan* +▲), Ren.6 (*qi hai* +▲), St.36 (*zu san li* +▲), Bl.20 (*pi shu* +▲), Du.20 (*bai hui* +), *ah shi* points of the upper back and neck

Clinical notes
- This pattern may correspond to disorders such as anaemia, stress, and chronic tension.
- This is a common pattern in overworked and stressed women who complain of chronic headaches or neck and upper back problems. When massaged, their muscles have a characteristic feel–tight and somewhat ropey at first, with a lack of tone at a deeper level.
- Spasms of this type respond well to acupuncture treatment, but lasting resolution of the condition requires long term tonification of *qi* and Blood with herbs, sensible diet and sufficient rest and relaxation.

SUMMARY OF GUIDING FORMULAE FOR CONVULSIONS AND SPASMS

Acute febrile convulsions - *Zi Xue Dan* 紫雪丹
- in children - *Xiao Er Hui Chun Dan* 小儿回春丹

Chronic convulsions
- *yin* and Blood deficiency - *San Jia Fu Mai Tang* 三甲复脉汤
- Spleen *yang* deficiency - *Li Zhong Wan* 理中丸

Muscular tetany - *Yu Zhen San* 玉真散

External Cold Damp - *Qiang Huo Sheng Shi Tang* 羌活胜湿汤
- with severe Cold - *Ge Gen Tang* 葛根汤
- with Damp Heat - *San Ren Tang* 三仁汤

Phlegm obstruction - *Qu Feng Dao Tan Tang* 祛风导痰汤

Blood stagnation - *Tong Qiao Huo Xue Tang* 通窍活血汤

Qi and Blood deficiency - *Ba Zhen Tang* 八珍汤

Endnote

For more information regarding herbs marked with an asterisk*, an open circle° or a hatˆ, see the tables on pp.944-952.

Disorders of the Liver

27. Ascites
(Drum like Abdominal Distension)

Excess patterns
Qi and Damp stagnation
Cold Damp
Damp Heat
Blood stagnation

Deficient patterns
Spleen and Kidney *yang* deficiency
Liver and Kidney *yin* deficiency

27 ASCITES (Drum Like Abdominal Distension)
gu zhang 臌脹

Gu zhang is fluid accumulation in the abdominal cavity, with a decrease in urinary output. *Gu zhang* is a serious disease, and occurs in such conditions as hepatic cirrhosis, congestive cardiac failure, abdominal and liver cancer, schistosomiasis, chronic malaria and tuberculous peritonitis. The name *gu zhang* (literally drum distension) derives from the the resemblance of the abdomen to a drum–firm and taut on the outside and empty within–the emptiness here referring to deficiency of the various *zang fu* involved.

In TCM terms, *gu zhang* is associated with severe disruption of fluid metabolism that causes fluids to accumulate in the middle and lower *jiao*. This fluid buildup may occur either from obstruction of fluid movement by some excess pathogen (*qi* or Blood stagnation, Cold Damp or Damp Heat), or from weakness and deficiency of the organs governing fluid metabolism (in this case the Spleen and Kidney). In practice, mixtures of deficiency and excess are the rule, with the deficiency generally more significant. What this suggests is that even though the manifestations are of an excess nature (the massive fluid accumulation), simple promotion of diuresis is inappropriate and may be harmful (see treatment), and therefore tonification and fluid drainage (or removal of excess pathogens) are always combined.

The main feature is swelling of the abdomen, in the early stages soft on palpation, gradually becoming harder and more drum like as the disease progresses. In the later stages the patient is very ill–with a sallow or yellow complexion, emaciation, jaundice, obvious blue veins snaking across the abdomen (caput medusae–the medusa's hair), numerous spider naevi, and other signs of severe Blood stagnation.

AETIOLOGY
Qi and Damp stagnation
Prolonged emotional repression, resentment, anger and frustration impair the Liver's ability to spread *qi*. Prolonged stasis of *qi* can both damage the Spleen and retard the normal movement of physiological fluids, causing accumulation of Dampness in the middle and lower *jiao*. Eventually Blood stagnation may complicate the *qi* stasis leading to the development of masses in the abdomen and Liver.

With moderate underlying *qi* or *yang* deficiency, the resulting Damp may accumulate as Cold Damp. Accumulation of Cold Damp is aided by irregular eating, excessive consumption of raw or cold food and beverages. Cold Dampness may also be the result of parasites in a cold or *yang* deficient individual.

Damp Heat
Chronic alcohol abuse and overconsumption of Damp or heating foods directly cause Damp Heat buildup, or weaken the Spleen sufficiently to cause Damp accumulation. Prolonged Damp Heat stagnation in the Liver and Spleen eventually leads to *qi* and Blood stasis and impaired fluid transport.

Chronic infection, with a variety of parasites and pathogens, like *Filaria* worms (schistosomiasis), *Plasmodia* (malaria) and hepatitis virus, can give rise to Damp Heat patterns. Prolonged stagnation of Damp Heat can eventually cause *qi* and Blood stagnation, and the development of abdominal masses.

Blood stagnation
Blood stagnation type ascites is the result of prolonged stagnation of *qi*, Dampness, Damp Heat or parasites. It indicates a fairly severe degree of damage to the Liver and/or the Spleen, and is associated with the development of abdominal masses or hepatosplenomegaly.

Spleen and Kidney *yang* deficiency
This pattern occurs when obstruction by *qi*, Damp or Blood has damaged the organs. In addition to the obstruction of fluid movement and metabolism by the excess pathogens, the Spleen and Kidneys become too weak to transform fluids which accumulate in the abdomen, compounding the ascites. Spleen and Kidney *yang* may also be damaged by overenthusiastic use of bitter cold herbs or drugs used to treat a Damp Heat pattern.

Liver and Kidney *yin* deficiency
Liver and Kidney *yin* deficiency can develop if inappropriate or excessive diuretic treatment is used early on. It can also occur when a Heat (or Damp Heat) pattern is prolonged, or incompletely cleared following treatment. It also represents a late development of Blood stagnation as *yin* is always damaged by long term disease.

DIFFERENTIAL DIAGNOSIS
Oedema (*shui zhong* 水肿): Oedema is fluid in interstitial tissues and affects the whole body, particularly the limbs. Ascites is fluid in the abdominal cavity.

Chang tan (肠覃): an ancient term describing a firm and moveable abdominal mass, small at first and gradually increasing in size until the abdomen resembles that during pregnancy. This term most likely refers to abdominal tumours, like fibroids or ovarian cysts.

TREATMENT

Ascites is invariably a chronic and complicated mixture of deficiency and excess, and correct treatment involves tonification at the same time as drainage of fluids, Heat clearing, Blood stasis elimination etc. Drastic catharsis is generally avoided (except under exceptional circumstances) as it has been observed for centuries that although draining fluids alone may dramatically reduce the ascites, it usually returns in a few days worse than before. Similarly, modern commentators stress that moving and draining fluid is only the first stage of ascites treatment. Once fluids are moving, more tonifying prescriptions (depending on the patient's constitution) should be selected and maintained for lengthy periods. This applies particularly to advanced cases that may have the appearance of excess, but in fact are significantly deficient. The nutritional status of the patient is extremely important (and often a major concern), and a nourishing, easily digested and low salt and protein diet is recommended.

27.1 *QI* AND DAMP STAGNATION

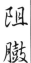

Pathophysiology
- *Qi* and Damp stagnation represents an early stage of ascites, as impeded circulation of *qi* retards fluid movement allowing accumulation of Dampness. At this stage the excess aspects of the pattern are dominant.

Clinical features
- swollen abdomen with tightly stretched skin that is not particularly firm or hard when palpated
- fullness, distension or pain beneath the ribs
- poor appetite
- epigastric and abdominal distension, worse after eating
- belching, flatulence
- irritability
- scanty urine
- sluggish stools

T greasy white coat
P wiry

Treatment principle
Soothe the Liver and regulate *qi*
Drain Dampness and reduce accumulation (of fluid)

Prescription

CHAI HU SHU GAN SAN 柴胡疏肝散
(*Bupleurum and Cyperus Formula*) plus
PING WEI SAN 平胃散
(*Magnolia and Ginger Formula*) modified

chai hu (Radix Bupleuri) 柴胡	9g
chi shao (Radix Paeoniae Rubrae) 赤芍	9g
chuan xiong (Radix Ligustici Chuanxiong) 川芎	6g
xiang fu (Rhizoma Cyperi Rotundi) 香附	9g
cang zhu (Rhizoma Atractylodis) 苍术	9g
hou po (Cortex Magnoliae Officinalis) 厚朴	9g
zhi ke (Fructus Citri Aurantii) 枳壳	6g
chen pi (Pericarpium Citri Reticulatae) 陈皮	6g

Method: Decoction. (Source: *Shi Yong Zhong Yi Nei Ke Xue*)

Modifications
- With very scanty urine, add **che qian zi** (Semen Plantaginis) 车前子 12g and **ze xie** (Rhizoma Alismatis Orientalis) 泽泻 12g.

- With vomiting of clear watery fluids, add **ban xia*** (Rhizoma Pinelliae Ternatae) 半夏 9g and **gan jiang** (Rhizoma Zingiberis Officinalis) 干姜 6g.
- For severe abdominal discomfort, add **mu xiang** (Radix Aucklandiae Lappae) 木香 6g, **bing lang** (Semen Arecae Catechu) 槟榔 9g and **sha ren** (Fructus Amomi) 砂仁 6g.
- With Spleen deficiency, add **fu ling** (Sclerotium Poria Cocos) 茯苓 12g, **bai zhu** (Rhizoma Atractylodes Macrocephalae) 白术 12g, **dang shen** (Radix Codonopsis Pilosulae) 党参 15g and **gan cao** (Radix Glycyrrhizae Uralensis) 甘草 6g.
- With Cold, add **zhi fu zi*** (Radix Aconiti Carmichaeli Praeparata) 制附子 6g cooked for 30 minutes prior to the other herbs, and **gan jiang** (Rhizoma Zingiberis Officinalis) 干姜 6g.
- With Heat, add **shan zhi zi** (Fructus Gardeniae Jasminoides) 山栀子 9g.
- With constipation, add **da huang** (Radix et Rhizoma Rhei) 大黄 6-9g.

Patent medicines
Mu Xiang Shun Qi Wan 木香顺气丸 (Aplotaxis Carminative Pills) plus
Wu Ling San 五苓散 (Hoelen Five Formula) or
Wu Pi Wan 五皮丸 (Wu Pi Wan)

Acupuncture
Ren.11 (*jian li* -), Ren.17 (*shan zhong*), Ren.6 (*qi hai* -), Liv.14 (*qi men* -), Liv.13 (*zhang men* -), PC.6 (*nei guan* -), St.36 (*zu san li* -), GB.34 (*yuang ling quan* -), Liv.3 (*tai chong* -), Ren.9 (*shui fen* ▲)

Clinical notes
- The ascite in this pattern may be associated with disorders such as early cirrhosis of the liver, chronic hepatitis and schistosomiasis.
- This pattern can respond well to correct treatment and modification of any contributing lifestyle factors, such as limiting alcohol intake.
- While ascites most often is a mixed excess and deficient condition, in this pattern the illness is at an early stage and the patient may still be relatively robust. Gentle movement of *qi* is appropriate for those patients with little underlying deficiency. Acupuncture is often the treatment of choice to achieve this. If signs of Dampness persist, herbs should be added.

27.2 COLD DAMP

寒湿凝聚臌胀

Pathophysiology
- Cold Damp type ascites can develop when Cold Damp accumulates in a patient with underlying Spleen *yang* deficiency. The Cold Damp obstructs the *yang* of the middle *jiao*, impairing fluid metabolism and transport. Pathological fluids accumulate, neither ascending or descending for elimination. The deficiency at this stage is a secondary consideration. The treatment principle is to first move fluids and clear the excess. Once the ascites is improving, the next step is to warm and tonify *yang*.

Clinical features
- swollen distended abdomen that feels like a bag of fluid on palpation
- heaviness in the body and head
- aversion to cold, the patient feels better with warmth on the abdomen
- oedema of the extremities, generally non-pitting
- scanty urine
- loose stools or diarrhoea

T greasy white coat
P soft and moderate or wiry and slow

Treatment principle
Transform Dampness and drain fluids
Warm *yang* and disperse Cold

Prescription

SHI PI YIN 实脾饮
(*Magnolia and Atractylodes Combination*) modified

This formula is excellent for warming *yang*, promoting diuresis and relieving the accumulation in the abdomen. It usually works quickly to clear accumulated fluids. Once fluids are moving well, a more tonifying prescription should be phased in.

fu ling (Sclerotium Poria Cocos) 茯苓	30g
da fu pi (Pericarpium Arecae Catechu) 大腹皮	30g
bai zhu (Rhizoma Atractylodes Macrocephalae) 白术	15g
mu gua (Fructus Chaenomelis) 木瓜	15g
zhi fu zi* (Radix Aconiti Carmichaeli Praeparata) 制附子	12g
gan jiang (Rhizoma Zingiberis Officinalis) 干姜	10g
yu jin (Tuber Curcumae) 郁金	10g
zhi ke (Fructus Citri Aurantii) 枳壳	10g
hou po (Cortex Magnoliae Officinalis) 厚朴	10g
mu xiang (Radix Aucklandiae Lappae) 木香	10g

zhi gan cao (honey fried Radix Glycyrrhizae Uralensis)
炙甘草 6g
sheng jiang (Rhizoma Zingiberis Officinalis) 生姜 3pce
da zao (Fructus Zizyphi Jujubae) 大枣 5pce

Method: Decoction. **Zhi fu zi** is cooked for 30 minutes prior to the other herbs (*xian jian* 先煎). (Source: *Zhong Yi Nei Ke Lin Chuang Shou Ce*)

Modifications

- With very scanty urine, add **rou gui** (Cortex Cinnamomi Cassiae) 肉桂 3g and **zhu ling** (Sclerotium Polypori Umbellati) 猪苓 10g.
- With abdominal pain, add **qing pi** (Pericarpium Citri Reticulatae Viridae) 青皮 10g, **xiang fu** (Rhizoma Cyperi Rotundi) 香附 6g and **yan hu suo** (Rhizoma Corydalis Yanhusuo) 延胡索 10g.
- As the patient improves, a more general Spleen *yang* strengthening prescription, such as **FU ZI LI ZHONG WAN** (*Aconite, Ginseng and Ginger Formula* 附子理中丸, p.56), may be phased in.

Patent medicines

Fu Zi Li Zhong Wan 附子理中丸 (Li Chung Yuen Medical Pills)

Acupuncture

Bl.20 (*pi shu* +), Ren.9 (*shui fen* ▲), Bl.23 (*shen shu* +▲), Sp.9 (*yin ling quan* -), Sp.6 (*san yin jiao* -), Bl.39 (*wei yang* -), Bl.22 (*san jiao shu* -)

Clinical notes

- The ascite in this pattern may be associated with disorders such as cirrhosis, chronic hepatitis, intestinal tuberculosis or chronic nephritis.
- This pattern may progress to Spleen or Kidney *yang* deficiency if unresolved or poorly treated.
- The patient should be advised to eat mild warming food only until Spleen *yang* recovers.

27.3 DAMP HEAT

湿热蕴结臌胀

Pathophysiology
- The fluid accumulation in this pattern results from obstruction to the movement and distribution of fluids by chronic retention of Dampness and Heat. The Damp Heat here is most frequently the result of chronic infection by parasites or viruses, or excessive alcohol consumption. It primarily affects the Liver, secondly the Spleen and Stomach.

Clinical features
- swollen, distended, firm abdomen that feels worse for pressure
- epigastric and/or abdominal pain, the abdomen is firm on the surface and painful when pressed
- feverishness, flushing
- bitter taste in the mouth
- thirst or dry mouth with little desire to drink
- scanty, concentrated urine
- constipation and/or diarrhoea
- there may be jaundice in some patients

T red tip and edges, with a greasy yellow or greyish black coat
P wiry and rapid

Treatment principle
Clear Heat and drain Dampness
Purge accumulation of fluid

Prescription

ZHONG MAN FEN XIAO WAN 中满分消丸
(*Separate and Reduce Fullness in the Middle Pill*) modified

fu ling (Sclerotium Poriae Cocos) 茯苓	30g
yin chen (Herba Artemisiae Yinchenhao) 茵陈	30g
zhu ling (Sclerotium Polypori Umbellati) 猪苓	15g
bai zhu (Rhizoma Atractylodes Macrocephalae) 白术	12g
ze xie (Rhizoma Alismatis Orientalis) 泽泻	12g
sha ren (Fructus Amomi) 砂仁	12g
zhi mu (Rhizoma Anemarrhenae Asphodeloidis) 知母	12g
hou po (Cortex Magnoliae Officinalis) 厚朴	10g
zhi ke (Fructus Citri Aurantii) 枳壳	10g
huang qin (Radix Scutellariae Baicalensis) 黄芩	9g
huang lian (Rhizoma Coptidis) 黄连	9g
ban xia* (Rhizoma Pinelliae Ternatae) 半夏	9g
chen pi (Pericarpium Citri Reticulatae) 陈皮	9g

jiang huang (Rhizoma Curcumae Longae) 姜黄 9g
da huang (Radix et Rhizoma Rhei) 大黄 6g
gan cao (Radix Glycyrrhizae Uralensis) 甘草 6g
Method: Decoction. (Source: *Zhong Yi Nei Ke Lin Chuang Shou Ce*)

Modifications
- Without obvious jaundice, delete **yin chen**.
- With diarrhoea, delete **da huang**.

Varriations and additional prescriptions
- In cases with very scanty urine or anuria, severe ascites and distension, drastic measures may be taken to swiftly reduce the ascites and purge fluid. The harsh cathartic pill **ZHOU CHE WAN** (*Vessel and Vehicle Pill* 舟车丸) may be given until the bowels open and urination increases, usually no more than 1-2 doses. This is a very harsh formula and must be monitored carefully.

    qian niu zi (Semen Pharbitidis) 牵牛子 120g
    gan sui* (Radix Euphorbiae Kansui) 甘遂 30g
    da ji* (Radix Euphorbiae seu Knoxiae) 大戟 30g
    yuan hua* (Flos Daphnes Genkwa) 芫花 30g
    da huang (Radix et Rhizoma Rhei) 大黄 60g
    chen pi (Pericarpium Citri Reticulatae) 陈皮 15g
    qing pi (Pericarpium Citri Reticulatae Viridae) 青皮 15g
    mu xiang (Radix Aucklandiae Lappae) 木香 15g
    bing lang (Semen Arecae Catechu) 槟榔 15g
    qing fen (Calomelas) 轻粉 3g
    Method: Grind the herbs to a fine powder and form into small pills with water. The dose is 2-3 grams at a time until drastic purgation occurs. (Source: *Shi Yong Fang Ji Xue*)

- In severe cases, the Heat can force the reckless movement of Blood and various types of bleeding may result. The treatment is to cool the Blood and stop bleeding with **XI JIAO SAN** 犀角散 (*Rhinoceros Horn Powder*) modified.

    xi jiao° (Cornu Rhinoceri) 犀角 3g
    yin chen (Herba Artemisiae Yinchenhao) 茵陈 30g
    da qing ye (Folium Daqingye) 大青叶 30g
    jin yin hua (Flos Lonicerae Japonicae) 金银花 30g
    lian qiao (Fructus Forsythiae Suspensae) 连翘 30g
    sheng di (Radix Rehmanniae Glutinosae) 生地 30g
    shan zhi zi (Fructus Gardeniae Jasminoides) 山栀子 15g
    mu dan pi (Cortex Moutan Radicis) 牡丹皮 15g
    xuan shen (Radix Scrophulariae) 玄参 15g

chi shao (Radix Paeoniae Rubrae) 赤芍 15g
sheng ma (Rhizoma Cimicifugae) 升麻 9g
huang lian (Rhizoma Coptidis) 黄连 9g
gan cao (Radix Glycyrrhizae Uralensis) 甘草 6g
Method: Decoction. If unconscious or confused, the formula can be delivered via a nasogastic tube until consciousness is restored. **Shui niu jiao^** (Cornu Bubali) 水牛角 is usually substituted for **xi jiao** with a tenfold increase in dosage.
(Source: *Zhong Yi Nei Ke Lin Chuang Shou Ce*)

• In some severe cases, or in those with an acute exacerbation of the chronic pattern, there may be delirium, impaired consciousness and confusion. **AN GONG NIU HUANG WAN** (*Calm the Palace Pill with Cattle Gallstone* 安宫牛黄丸, p.914) or **ZHI BAO DAN** (*Greatest Treasure Special Pill* 至宝丹, p.660) is selected to open the orifices and clear Heat. If the patient is unable to ingest the medicine, the dose is forced into the mouth or nose or given via a nasogastric tube until consciousness is restored.

Patent medicines
The patents listed here are for the extreme end of Damp Heat - with disturbance of consciousness or delirium.
An Gong Niu Huang Wan 安宫牛黄丸 (An Gong Niu Huang Wan)
Zi Xue Dan 紫雪丹 (Tzuhsueh Tan)
Wan Shi Niu Huang Qing Xin Wan 万氏牛黄清心丸
  (Wan Shi Niu Huang Qing Xin Wan)

Acupuncture
Bl.19 (*dan shu* -), Bl.18 (*gan shu* -), GB.34 (*yang ling quan* -), Liv.14 (*qi men* -), Liv.13 (*zhang men* -), *pi gen* (M-BW-16), Bl.20 (*pi shu* -), Bl.21 (*wei shu* -), LI.11 (*qu chi* -), Liv.3 (*tai chong* -), GB.40 (*qiu xu* -), Bl.40 (*wei zhong* ↓)
  • With impaired consciousness add *shi xuan* ↓ (M-UE-1) and Du.26 (*ren zhong* -)

Clinical notes
• The ascite in this pattern may be associated with disorders such as chronic hepatitis, schistosomiasis, chronic malaria or alcoholic cirrhosis.
• If untreated or unresolved, this pattern can develop into Blood stagnation and/or Liver and Kidney *yin* deficiency.
• Prognosis largely depends on the extent of Liver damage, and removal of aetiological factors. In many cases (especially those with an identifiable parasitic or avoidable cause) the prognosis is fair. If alcohol is involved, stopping consumption is of the utmost importance. Other factors like parasites may need to be dealt with specifically once the ascites has subsided (see also Malaria, Vol.3).

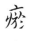
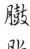

27.4 BLOOD STAGNATION

Pathophysiology
- This Blood stagnation pattern represents a serious and late stage of Liver and Spleen dysfunction. It usually overlaps with elements of *yin* deficiency and Spleen deficiency.

Clinical features
- swollen, distended, hard abdomen with obvious dilated blue green veins radiating out from the umbilicus (caput medusae)
- hypochondriac and abdominal pain
- dark, ashen, sallow or purplish complexion, dark or purplish lips and conjunctiva, dark rings under the eyes
- multiple vascular spiders on the face, neck, chest and trunk
- palmar erythema
- easy bruising, purpura
- black, tarry stools
- dry, scaly skin

T purplish or with purple or brown spots and little or no coat
P thready and choppy, or hollow if bleeding is significant

Treatment principle
Invigorate Blood and eliminate Blood stagnation
Move *qi* and drain fluids

Prescription

HUA YU TANG 化瘀汤
(*Transform Blood Stasis Decoction*) modified

dan shen (Radix Salviae Miltiorrhizae) 丹参	15g
mu li^ (Concha Ostreae) 牡蛎	15g
dang gui (Radix Angelicae Sinensis) 当归	12g
chuan shan jia° (Squama Manitis Pentadactylae) 穿山甲	12g
ze xie (Rhizoma Alismatis Orientalis) 泽泻	12g
hong hua (Flos Carthami Tinctorii) 红花	9g
tao ren (Semen Persicae) 桃仁	9g
mu dan pi (Cortex Moutan Radicis) 牡丹皮	9g
chi shao (Radix Paeoniae Rubrae) 赤芍	9g
bai zhu (Rhizoma Atractylodes Macrocephalae) 白术	9g
qing pi (Pericarpium Citri Reticulatae Viridae) 青皮	6g

Method: Decoction. (Source: *Shi Yong Zhong Yi Nei Ke Xue*)

Modifications
- With black stools, add **san qi fen** (powdered Radix Notoginseng) 三七粉 3g and **ce bai ye** (Cacumen Biotae Orientalis) 侧柏叶 12g.

Variations and additional prescriptions
- When the distension is severe, urination very scanty, the pulse strong and wiry and the patient's constitution strong enough, a dose of **ZHOU CHE WAN** (*Vessel and Vehicle Pill* 舟车丸 p.738) or, of the following formula, **SHI ZAO TANG** (*Ten Jujube Decoction* 十枣汤), may be given until the bowels open and urination increases, usually no more than 1-2 doses.
    gan sui* (Radix Euphorbiae Kansui) 甘遂
    da ji* (Radix Euphorbiae seu Knoxiae) 大戟
    yuan hua* (Flos Daphnes Genkwa) 芫花
    Method: Grind equal amounts of each herb into powder. The dose is 0.5-1 gram (in a gelatin capsule or wrapped in a date) on an empty stomach. Wash the capsule down with a decoction made from 10 pieces of **da zao** (Fructus Zizyphi Jujube) 大枣. This should produce abdominal discomfort and increased intestinal activity, followed by watery diarrhoea. Generally only one or two doses are taken. If watery diarrhoea persists it can be treated with cold rice porridge. (Source: *Formulas and Strategies*)

Patent medicines
Xue Fu Zhu Yu Wan 血府逐瘀丸 (Xue Fu Zhu Yu Wan) plus
Nei Xiao Luo Li Wan 内消瘰疬丸 (Nei Xiao Luo Li Wan)

Acupuncture
Sp.10 (*xue hai* -), Bl.17 (*ge shu* -), Liv.2 (*xing jian* -), Ren.3 (*zhong ji* -), Liv.13 (*zhang men* ▲), Liv.14 (*qi men* ▲), Bl.18 (*gan shu* -), *pi gen* (M-BW-16), Bl.20 (*pi shu* -), Bl.21 (*wei shu* -)

Clinical notes
- The ascite in this pattern may be associated with disorders such as severe hepatic cirrhosis, chronic malaria or liver cancer.
- This is obviously a severe condition and management options are limited, however there has been some reported benefit gained from prolonged treatment.
- Strong (smashing) Blood movers are not appropriate in this condition as they may exacerbate the patients weakness. Gradual transformation of stagnant Blood while strengthening the Spleen and supporting *qi* is the correct approach. Harsh treatments (other than those required for very short periods of time to manage particular features like anuria) are avoided. When fluids are moving and signs of Blood stasis are subsiding, a more *qi* and Blood tonifying approach should be adopted.

27.5 SPLEEN AND KIDNEY *YANG* DEFICIENCY

脾肾阳虚臌胀

Pathophysiology
- Spleen and Kidney *yang* deficiency reflects a late stage of ascites where the predominantly early stage excess patterns (*qi* and Cold Damp stagnation) have given way to significant deficiency. Instead of obstruction of fluids, weakness of fluid metabolism now predominates. The treatment principle is now more focused on warming *yang* to move fluids.

Clinical features
- swollen, distended abdomen, worse at the end of the day
- epigastric fullness and discomfort
- poor appetite
- sallow or waxy pale complexion
- aversion to cold, cold extremities
- lethargy and fatigue
- generalised oedema
- scanty urine

T pale or bluish and swollen with toothmarks
P deep and thready or wiry, big and forceless

Treatment principle
Warm Spleen and Kidney *yang*
Aid transformation of *qi* and drain fluids

Prescription

FU ZI LI ZHONG WAN 附子理中丸
(*Aconite, Ginseng and Ginger Formula*) plus
WU LING SAN 五苓散
(*Hoelen Five Formula*) modified

This prescription is selected if deficiency of Spleen *yang* is prominent, characterised by the prominence of digestive weakness. As fluid metabolism improves, the bland diuretic herbs may be reduced or omitted.

fu ling (Sclerotium Poriae Cocos) 茯苓	25g
zhu ling (Sclerotium Polypori Umbellati) 猪苓	15g
dang shen (Radix Codonopsis Pilosulae) 党参	15g
bai zhu (Rhizoma Atractylodes Macrocephalae) 白术	12g
ze xie (Rhizoma Alismatis Orientalis) 泽泻	12g
gan jiang (Rhizoma Zingiberis Officinalis) 干姜	12g
zhi fu zi* (Radix Aconiti Carmichaeli Praeparata) 制附子	9g
gan cao (Radix Glycyrrhizae Uralensis) 甘草	6g
rou gui (Cortex Cinnamomi Cassiae) 肉桂	6g

Method: Decoction. **Zhi fu zi** is cooked for 30 minutes prior to the other herbs (*xian jian* 先煎). (Source: *Shi Yong Zhong Yi Nei Ke Xue*)

JI SHENG SHEN QI WAN 济生肾气丸
(Kidney Qi Pill from Formulas to Aid the Living)

This prescription is prefered when Kidney *yang* deficiency is prominent, characterised by severe oedema in the lower body and lower backache.

shu di (Radix Rehmanniae Glutinosae Conquitae) 熟地	15g
shan zhu yu (Fructus Corni Officinalis) 山茱萸	30g
shan yao (Radix Dioscoreae Oppositae) 山药	30g
ze xie (Rhizoma Alismatis Orientalis) 泽泻	30g
fu ling (Sclerotium Poriae Cocos) 茯苓	30g
mu dan pi (Cortex Moutan Radicis) 牡丹皮	30g
rou gui (Cortex Cinnamomi Cassiae) 肉桂	15g
zhi fu zi* (Radix Aconiti Carmichaeli Praeparata) 制附子	15g
chuan niu xi (Radix Cyathulae Officinalis) 川牛膝	15g
che qian zi (Semen Plantaginis) 车前子	30g

Method: Grind herbs to a fine powder and form into 9-gram pills with honey. The dose is one pill 2-3 times daily. May also be decocted with an appropriate reduction in dosage. When decocted **zhi fu zi** is cooked for 30 minutes before the other herbs (*xian jian* 先煎) and **che qian zi** is decocted in a muslin bag (*bao jian* 包煎). (Source: *Shi Yong Zhong Yi Nei Ke Xue*)

Patent medicines

Fu Zi Li Zhong Wan 附子理中丸 (Li Chung Yuen Medical Pills)
  - Spleen *yang* deficiency

Jin Kui Shen Qi Wan 金匮肾气丸 (Sexoton Pills)
  - Kidney *yang* deficiency

Acupuncture

Bl.23 (*shen shu* +▲), Bl.20 (*pi shu* +▲), Bl.21 (*wei shu* +▲), Sp.6 (*san yin jiao*), Sp.9 (*yin ling quan*), St.36 (*zu san li* +▲), Ren.4 (*guan yuan* +▲), Ren.6 (*qi hai* +▲), Ren.9 (*shui fen* ▲)

Clinical notes

- The ascite in this pattern may be associated with disorders such as cirrhosis, chronic hepatitis, intestinal tuberculosis and chronic nephritis.
- Prolonged treatment and a warming, bland diet is advised.

27.6 LIVER AND KIDNEY YIN DEFICIENCY

肝肾阴虚臌胀

Pathophysiology
- Liver and Kidney *yin* deficiency corresponds to a late stage of ascites, particularly following patterns involving Damp Heat. At this stage there will usually also be a degree of Blood stasis. This pattern can also develop as a result of excessive or inappropriate use of diuretics herbs or drugs (which can damage *yin*) in early stage ascites.

Clinical features
- swollen, distended, hard abdomen with obvious distended blue green veins radiating out from the umbilicus (caput medusae)
- emaciation
- dark complexion, red purple lips
- dry mouth
- restlessness, irritability
- sensation of heat in the palms and soles ('five hearts hot')
- scanty concentrated urine
- may be various types of bleeding

T scarlet or crimson and dry with little or no coat
P wiry, thready and rapid

Treatment principle
Nourish and tonify Liver and Kidney *yin*
Cool the Blood, transform stagnation, drain fluids

Prescription

YI GUAN JIAN 一贯煎
(*Linking Decoction*) plus
XIAO YU TANG 消瘀汤
(*Eliminate Blood Stasis Decoction*) modified

sheng di (Radix Rehmanniae Glutinosae) 生地	18-45g
gou qi zi (Fructus Lycii) 枸杞子	9-18g
bie jia° (Carapax Amydae Sinensis) 鳖甲	12g
mu liˆ (Concha Ostreae) 牡蛎	12g
dang shen (Radix Codonopsis Pilosulae) 党参	12g
fu ling (Sclerotium Poriae Cocos) 茯苓	12g
chi shao (Radix Paeoniae Rubrae) 赤芍	12g
chai hu (Radix Bupleuri) 柴胡	9g
sha shen (Radix Adenophorae seu Glehniae) 沙参	9g
mai dong (Tuber Ophiopogonis Japonici) 麦冬	9g
dang gui (Radix Angelicae Sinensis) 当归	9g

chuan lian zi* (Fructus Meliae Toosendan) 川楝子 6g
qing pi (Pericarpium Citri Reticulatae Viridae) 青皮 6g
zhi ke (Fructus Citri Aurantii) 枳壳 6g
e zhu (Rhizoma Curcumae Ezhu) 莪术 6g
san leng (Rhizoma Sparganii Stoloniferi) 三棱 6g
ji nei jin^ (Endothelium Corneum Gigeriae Galli) 鸡内金 6g

Method: Grind herbs to a fine powder and form into 9-gram pills with honey. The dose is one pill 2-3 times daily. May also be decocted, in which cases **ji nei jin** is powdered and added to the strained decoction (*chong fu* 冲服). (Source: *Shi Yong Zhong Yi Nei Ke Xue*)

Modifications

* With afternoon fever, add **yin chai hu** (Radix Stellariae Dichotomae) 银柴胡 9g and **di gu pi** (Cortex Lycii Radicis) 地骨皮 12g.
* If urine is very scanty, add **zhu ling** (Sclerotium Polypori Umbellati) 猪苓 9g, **bai mao gen** (Rhizoma Imperatae Cylindricae) 白茅根 18g and **tong cao** (Medulla Tetrapanacis Papyriferi) 通草 6g.
* With bleeding, add **qian cao tan** (charred Radix Rubiae Cordifoliae) 茜草炭 12g, **mu dan pi** (Cortex Moutan Radicis) 牡丹皮 9g and **xian he cao** (Herba Agrimoniae Pilosae) 仙鹤草 12g.

Clinical notes

* The ascite in this pattern may be associated with disorders such as chronic liver cirrhosis and late stage of liver cancer.
* The long term prognosis is probably not very good, although reports from China suggest that even at this advanced stage there may be benefit from vigorous treatment. Stopping alcohol consumption (if appropriate) may help with quality of life.

SUMMARY OF GUIDING FORMULAE FOR ASCITES

Excess patterns (always with a degree of deficiency)

Qi and Damp stagnation
- *Chai Hu Shu Gan San* 柴胡疏肝散 plus *Ping Wei San* 平胃散

Cold Damp - *Shi Pi Yin* 实脾饮

Damp Heat - *Zhong Man Fen Xiao Wan* 中满分消丸
- with anuria + *Zhou Che Wan* 舟车丸
- with bleeding + *Xi Jiao San* 犀角散

Blood stagnation - *Hua Yu Tang* 化瘀汤

Deficient patterns

Spleen and Kidney *yang* deficiency
- *Fu Zi Li Zhong Wan* 附子理中丸 plus *Wu Ling San* 五苓散

Liver and Kidney *yin* deficiency
- *Yi Guan Jian* 一贯煎 plus *Xiao Yu Tang* 消瘀汤

Endnote

For more information regarding herbs marked with an asterisk*, an open circle° or a hatˆ, see the tables on pp.944-952.

Disorders of the Heart

28. Chest Pain

Heat scorching and knotting the chest
Phlegm obstruction
Qi stagnation
Cold congealing Heart Blood
Heart *yang* deficiency
Blood stagnation
Heart (Lung and Spleen) *qi* deficiency
Heart (and Kidney) *yin* deficiency

28 | CHEST PAIN
xiong bi 胸痹

Chest pain is pain, discomfort, fullness or a feeling of oppression affecting the area bounded by the lower costal margin below and the clavicles above. Chest pain is a common presentation of heart disease but not all chest pain involves the heart. The types that do involve the heart, however, often reflect serious underlying disease. In addition to pain of cardiac origin, chest pain frequently reflects disease of the lungs, musculoskeletal system or gastrointestinal system. The patterns described in this chapter correspond to numerous different biomedical conditions, including various cardiovascular and infectious diseases and emotional disorders. To clarify what can be a complex topic, some possible biomedical correlations are summarised in Figure 28.8.

In TCM terms, chest pain has numerous causes, although the basic mechanism that gives rise to pain is common to them all–obstruction to the circulation of *qi* and Blood (*bu tong ze tong* 不通则痛, where there is obstruction, there is pain). The Chinese name *xiong bi* literally translates as chest obstruction, the character for *bi* 痹 the same as is used in *bi zheng* (痹症)–Painful Obstruction Syndrome.

The mechanism of chest pain may be one of deficiency or excess. In the deficient patterns, the problem is weak propulsion of Blood with consequent pooling, or *yin* deficiency causing increased viscosity and stickiness of Blood. In excess patterns, a pathogenic substance blocks the circulation of *qi* and Blood.

The nature of the pain described in this chapter varies depending on the cause and clear identification of the pain quality can give valuable clues as to the origin of the pain. (See Key Diagnostic Points, Box 28.1)

In the Western world (as indeed in China) heart disease is a major cause of death, and for many sufferers the first symptom of a heart attack is pain. With improving education and more sophisticated diagnostic techniques, heart disease can be picked up at earlier stages and it is at these early stages that TCM is particularly useful. Because heart disease is so prevalent and a major cause of death, all practitioners should be familiar with emergency procedures. These are summarised in Box 28.2. It should be noted that while a man having a heart attack typically presents with the characteristic symptom of crushing retrosternal pain, women are just as likely to feel nausea or vague discomfort in the upper abdomen and back. Older women often get lots of little infarcts that may be symptomless but gradually cause more and more fatigue and reduced exercise tolerance.

All practitioners should be able to recognise pain or symptoms of cardiac origin, and differentiate them from symptoms arising from other structures. Clear identification of the pain origin and an understanding of the biomedical physiology involved not only aids prognosis and the correct lifestyle advice, but determines the necessity to bring in other forms of medical intervention. When in doubt, referral is strongly advised. The following descriptions will aid in distinguishing the origin of the chest pain.

DISTINGUISHING THE (BIOMEDICAL) ORIGIN OF THE CHEST PAIN

Pain of cardiac origin has some key characteristics that help distinguish it from other causes of chest pain:

- *Location* – cardiac pain is typically retrosternal or sometimes upper abdominal upper thoracic (Fig. 28.1, 28.2).
- *Radiation* – pain from cardiac ischaemia, especially if it is severe, may radiate to the throat, jaw, teeth and arms (particularly the left, Fig. 28.2).
- *Aggravation* – ischaemic cardiac pain is initiated by exertion and relieved by rest. Pain associated with a specific movement (twisting, bending, stretching) is likely to be myofacial in origin.
- *Character of the pain* – pain of cardiac origin is often described as squeezing, crushing, aching or heavy, however it may be experienced as indigestion or vague chest discomfort.

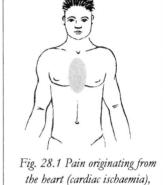

Fig. 28.1 Pain originating from the heart (cardiac ischaemia), typical site

- *Associated symptoms* – shortness of breath, palpitations, cyanosis, pallor, sweating, syncope, some patients report experiencing a 'sense of doom'.
- *Objective signs* – people with a predisposition to heart disease may develop a vertical or tangential crease on the ear lobes and a horozontal crease across the bridge of the nose; there will often be a deep narrow central crack on the tongue extending to

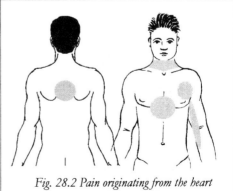

Fig. 28.2 Pain originating from the heart (cardiac ischaemia), other sites

the tip.
- *Other* – there may be a history of recurrent pain or medication for heart disease.

Pain of non cardiac origin can be distinguished by the following characteristics:

Gastro-intestinal pain
- Oesophageal (Fig 28.3) – burning or constricting retrosternal pain that may radiate to the jaw. It is aggravated or precipitated by eating, lying flat or bending over (especially after eating) and is relieved by antacids. Oesophageal spasm may also be initiated by stress.
- Gall bladder disease (Fig 28.4) – colicky or deep aching right hypochondriac pain. The pain may radiate to the scapula or right shoulder and is generally (but not always) related to fatty foods, and associated with flatulence and dyspepsia.
- Peptic ulcer – gnawing retrosternal pain, worse thirty minutes to three hours after eating, relieved by antacids.
- Hiatus hernia – retro-sternal pain which may be burning, associated with lying flat and eating.

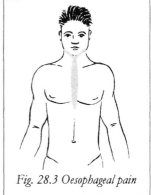
Fig. 28.3 Oesophageal pain

Lung disease
- Pleurisy – a pleural rub which varies with breathing, associated with fever and cough and focal pain that is worse with coughing and inspiration.
- Bronchitis – fever, cough, pain worse with coughing.
- Pneumonia – fever, cough and coloured sputum, pain worse with coughing.
- Pneumothorax (Fig 28.5) – sudden onset, asymmetric air entry, worse with inspiration.
- Pulmonary embolus or infarct – sudden onset with haemoptysis and shortness of breath.

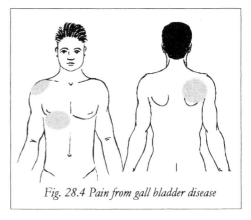
Fig. 28.4 Pain from gall bladder disease

Vascular
- Dissecting aortic aneurism – sudden, severe midline pain radiating to the abdomen and legs.

Pain of costal or spinal origin
- Vertebral dysfunction of the lower cervical or more commonly thoracic spine, typically T4-7 (usually costovertebral or facet joint dysfunction) – dull or aching pain, which is aggravated by exertion, certain body movements or deep breathing. Patients may be able to trace the pain along the affected segment. Pressure pain will be found at one or more spinal segments.
- Costochondritis – inflammation and focal pain associated with strain (or viral infection) at the costochondral or sternocostal junction.
- Rib fracture – following trauma or intense cough.

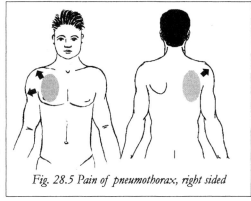

Fig. 28.5 Pain of pneumothorax, right sided

Myofacial pain
- Spasm or strain of muscles of the chest wall – chest pain with a predictable distribution. It tends to vary with posture or movement, can be brought on by exertion but is not quickly relieved by rest. Trigger points or points of tenderness (*ah shi*) over a rib or costal cartilage will be evident. Spasm of intercostal muscles can be severe and episodic, mimicking symptoms of myocardial infarction.

Other
- Shingles – 'nervy' pain along a neural pathway.

TCM AETIOLOGY

In TCM terms, the aetiology and manifestation of chronic or recurrent chest pain is invariably complex. In most cases there will be a mix of deficiency and excess–the root being deficient, the manifestation excess. Patterns frequently mingle, overlap or transform into one another. Care in diagnosis and flexibility in prescription are required for satisfactory results.

Some patterns, notably the exterior Heat pattern and some forms of the Liver *qi* stagnation pattern, are acute and reasonably straightforward to diagnose and treat. Keep in mind, however, that these patterns can overlap with other more chronic patterns as well.

Yang deficiency and Cold

Yang deficiency is at the root of much presenting chest pain, particularly that involving the Heart, and is the underlying condition for the severe excess conditions of Cold and Phlegm obstruction. Heart *yang* deficiency generally has its basis in Kidney or Spleen *yang* deficiency. When Heart (and Spleen or Kidney) *yang* is weakened it can give rise to chest pain in several ways:
1. From accumulation of Cold (which 'freezes and constricts' coronary vessels).
2. Due to weakness of the Heart's pumping action and subsequent pooling of Blood and development of Blood stasis.
3. From failure to mobilise and metabolise fluids which accumulate and congeal into Phlegm, which can then obstruct the coronary vessels.

Weakness of *yang* may be an inherited condition or may develop as a result of age, chronic illness, overexertion, too much exposure to cold environmental conditions or excessive lifting or standing. Kidney *yang* or *qi* may also be damaged by excessive ejaculation or, in women, by many pregnancies.

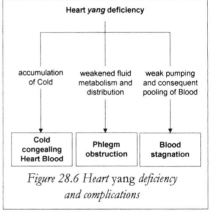

Figure 28.6 Heart yang *deficiency and complications*

The acute pattern of Cold congealing Heart Blood always has its root in *yang* deficiency - at a certain point enough Cold accumulates to cause the severe pain characteristic of constriction by Cold. Cold type chest pain can also be set off by external Cold, for example from invasion of pathogenic Cold, breathing cold air, or ingesting cold substances. This is usually only able to occur when there is an underlying *yang* deficiency.

Heat

The Heat that gives rise to chest pain is usually external. The Heart and Lungs are easily affected by Heat and other pathogens (see Acute Exterior Disorders pp.30, 48). The initial pathogen may be Hot, Cold or Damp, the latter two becoming Hot once lodged internally. The presence of pre-existing internal Heat from stagnant *qi*, *yin* deficiency or overconsumption of heating substances (including tobacco) can predispose patients to increased damage by external Heat. Once affected by Heat, Lung fluids and *yin* can be dried out and damaged. This can cause thickening of fluids into Phlegm, or increase the viscosity of Blood leading to stagnation of Blood.

> **BOX 28.1 KEY TCM DIAGNOSTIC POINTS**
>
> **Stuffy sensation, fullness and pain**
> - Stuffiness, generalised mild discomfort or fullness, which is aggravated by stress and emotional upset, and relieved by relaxation or sighing – *qi* stagnation.
> - Watery sputum or rattles in the chest, chest stuffiness or discomfort, which is worse on overcast or rainy days, and a greasy coat on the tongue – accumulation of Phlegm.
> - Mild pain and stuffiness, brought on by activity and accompanied by shortness of breath, palpitations or flutters – Heart *qi* deficiency.
>
> **Burning Pain**
> - Mostly due to some Hot pathogen. If accompanied by irritability, restlessness, a red tongue with a yellow coat and a rapid pulse without obvious signs of deficiency – pathogenic Heat or Fire penetrating into the Heart.
> - Stuffiness in the chest, paroxysmal burning pain, expectoration of thick sputum and a greasy yellow tongue coat – Phlegm Heat or Fire.
> - Burning pain with palpitations, dizziness and a red, dry tongue with little or no coat – deficient Fire from *yin* deficiency.
>
> **Sharp pain**
> - A sharp or stabbing pain, which is fixed in location, accompanied by a purple tongue indicates stagnant Blood.
> - Sharp pain may also be due to focal disorders of the chest wall, in which case it is usually aggravated by deep breathing or coughing.
>
> **Crushing, squeezing, twisting pain**
> - Feels like the Heart is being squeezed and crushed in a vice, or a weight is squashing the chest. Often accompanied by cold limbs, aversion to cold, and signs of *yang* deficiency. Mostly due to accumulation of *yin* Cold as a result of *yang* deficiency or invasion by external Cold.

Phlegm

Phlegm is a frequently implicated pathogen in chest pain. It can be the result of several factors. In the West, diet is a common cause of Phlegm accumulation. Overeating generally, which stresses the digestive system leading to inefficient digestion and a buildup of Dampness and Phlegm, is common. With its emphasis on dairy foods, sugar, fats and meat, the Western diet predisposes strongly to accumulation of Phlegm. Cold, raw foods can deplete Spleen *yang*. When the Spleen is weak, it produces Dampness which can congeal into Phlegm over time. *Yang* deficiency in general (affecting either or all of the Heart, Kidneys and Spleen) causes impaired fluid metabolism, with consequent accumulation and congealing of fluids into Phlegm.

Prolonged Liver *qi* stagnation may damage the Spleen and retard the movement of fluids, which then congeal into Phlegm. Phlegm and Liver *qi* stagnation are commonly seen together. Phlegm may also be congenital.

Liver *qi* stagnation

Emotional imbalance can affect the movement of *qi* in different organ systems and if these organ systems exert influence on the chest area then chest pain may result. The Liver system, including the Liver channel that traverses the chest, is the one most notably affected by emotional upsets, especially stress, frustration and anger. Obstruction of *qi* in other organs, such as the Heart or Lungs, can also cause chest pain, oppression, tightness, stuffiness, and difficulty getting a deep breath. Such pain may be precipitated by grief (a broken heart?), anxiety or overexcitment. Frequently, the pain associated with Liver *qi* stagnation is of a muscular type, that is, the muscles of the chest wall, oesophagus or diaphragm are in a state of chronic tension. This chronic tension can be exacerbated into tightness, discomfort and pain by increased stress.

Several complications of *qi* stagnation can also lead to chest pain. Prolonged *qi* stagnation can lead to Blood stagnation and the development of obstructive heart disease. *Qi* stagnation can generate Heat that ascends into the chest, or travels via the reverse controlling (*ke* 克, p.70) cycle to injure the Lungs or through the generative (*sheng* 生, p.70) cycle to the Heart. Liver *qi* stagnation may also damage the Spleen and retard fluid movement, causing accumulation of Dampness and congealing of fluids into Phlegm. The common feature of all types related to Liver *qi* stagnation is provocation or aggravation by emotional turmoil and stress.

Blood stagnation

Blood stagnation is often the end result of other prolonged disorders affecting the chest. Any pathology, excess or deficient, if long lasting enough, may lead to Blood stasis or involve elements of Blood stasis. Cold pathologies (Cold and *yang* deficiency) can cause stagnation by constricting the vessels and slowing circulation. Hot pathologies (Heat, Phlegm Heat and *yin* deficiency) can cause stagnation by 'evaporating' Blood and increasing the viscosity and stickiness of Blood. Blood stagnation frequently complicates *yang* deficiency, *yin* deficiency, Phlegm obstruction and prolonged Liver *qi* stagnation.

Heart and Kidney *yin* deficiency

Kidney *yin* becomes damaged through overwork (especially while under stress), late nights, shift work, insufficient sleep, and use of recreational drugs. Kidney *yin* may also be damaged by febrile illnesses, ageing and excessive sexual activity, or, in women, by many pregnancies.

Heart *yin* may be damaged by emotional trauma, shock or ongoing anxiety and worry. Heat affecting the chest and febrile illnesses also easily damage Heart *yin*. If Kidney *yin* is weak then Heart *yin* won't be supported—'Kidney Water fails to balance Heart Fire'. Once Heart *yin* has been damaged, circulation of Blood is impaired by increased Blood viscosity and by deficient Heat which smoulders in the chest. The Heat can also congeal fluids into Phlegm and the increased Blood viscosity can contribute to Blood stagnation. As well as complication by Phlegm and Blood stagnation, Heart *yin* deficiency is frequently complicated by other deficiencies, such as *qi* and Blood deficiency.

Qi (and Blood) deficiency

Overwork, excessive worry or mental activity, irregular dietary habits, excessive consumption of cold, raw foods or prolonged illness can weaken Spleen *qi*. As the Lungs and Spleen are the source of the *qi* and Blood of the body, weakness in these organs will inevitably lead to a decrease in production of *qi* and Blood. Other causes are acute or chronic haemorrhage and malnutrition. *Qi* and Blood are so closely related that deficiency of one often leads to deficiency of the other. Qi deficiency is often complicated by qi stagnation, Blood stagnation or Phlegm and fluid accumulation.

GENERAL APPROACH TO TREATMENT

There are several approaches to treatment depending on the severity of the symptoms and the mixture of excess and deficiency. The manifestations of chest pain are usually excess (Phlegm, Cold, Heat, *qi* or Blood stasis), while the underlying cause, the root, is deficient (*qi*, *yin*, *yang* or a mixture). What this implies is that in almost every case treatment must be twofold—both reducing (excess) and supplementing (deficiency).

During acute episodes with severe pain, TCM treatment addresses the manifestations and attempts to eliminate the responsible pathogen. In severe cases, emergency management may be necessary (Box 28.2). Treatment of an acute episode usually involves strong dispersing drugs with the potential to damage *zheng qi*, therefore, once the pain is under control, root treatments should be phased in.

In non acute cases, both the manifestation and the root can be treated together, although in general it is better to focus first on resolving the excess, and then when the patient's condition is improving, phase in the root tonifying treatment. This is primarily the case with herbal treatment, as excess removing herbs can aggravate deficiency and visa versa. The initial herbal approach is therefore weighted towards resolving Phlegm or Blood stasis, clearing Heat or warming and expelling Cold. Acupuncture treatment is slightly different, in that it is possible to tonify deficiency and remove excess effectively at the same time without causing any problems.

> **BOX 28.2 ACUTE CARDIAC EPISODE**
>
> Sudden severe chest pain, especially when accompanied by shortness of breath, sweating and arm or jaw pain, is cardiac in origin and must be treated as potentially fatal. Paramedic attention should be sought immediately.
>
> **Emergency management**
> - During an acute episode, emergency management may be necessary until paramedic assistance is available. If a pulse cannot be detected CPR should be started immediately. The principle of treatment is to improve circulation of *yang qi* in the chest.
>
> **TCM MANAGEMENT**
> **Main acupuncture points**
> - PC.6 (*nei guan*), PC.4 (*xi men*), Bl.15 (*xin shu*)
> - Huatuo Jiaji points around T4-T5, Ren.17 (*shan zhong*)
>
> All points are treated with strong reducing stimulation, with the needle sensation radiating up the arm or to the chest. The points can be needled or pressed with strong finger pressure or other appropriate instrument.
>
> **Secondary points**
> Select from
> - Ht.5 (*tong li*) - if palpitations are severe
> - PC.5 (*jian shi*) - stuffiness in the chest, sense of impending doom
> - St.36 (*zu san li*) - severe sweating, collapse
>
> **Patent medicines**
> *Guan Xin Su He Xiang Wan* 冠心苏合香丸 (Guan Xin Su Ho)

Many patients with pain of cardiac origin will be taking various conventional medications. The drug regime usually includes vasodilators like nitrogylcerine, which act by dispersing accumulated *qi*, as well as adrenaline blocking beta-blockers. Beta-blockers are thought to be Cold in nature[1], with an adverse long term effect on various organ systems. Cold drugs will damage *yang* and ultimately aggravate underlying *yang* deficiency. As treatment progresses, patients may wish to decrease their reliance on conventional medication. Any reduction of medication must be done **slowly and under supervision** over a period of months, as sudden withdrawal can precipitate an acute cardiac episode. Of course, this is only attempted as the patient's condition improves.

---

1. Gascoigne S (1995) *The Manual of Conventional Medicine for Alternative Practitioners*, Jigme Press, Dorking, Surrey

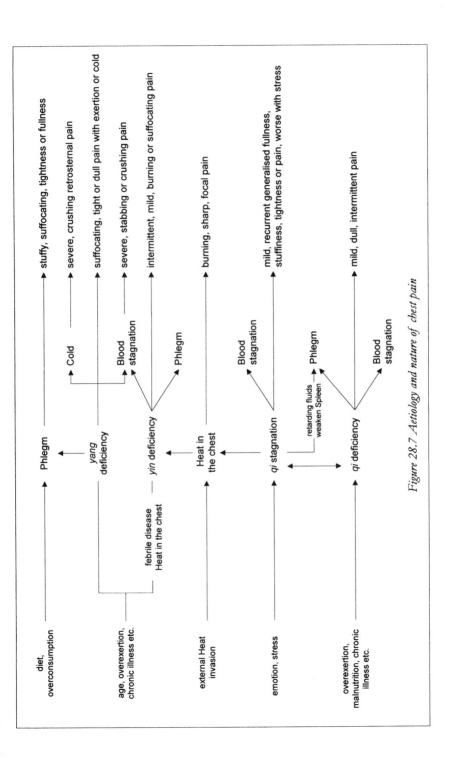

Figure 28.7 Aetiology and nature of chest pain

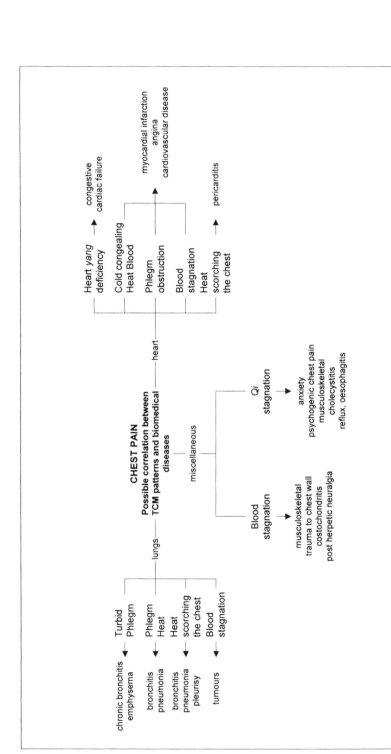

Figure 28.8 TCM patterns and possible biomedical correlations

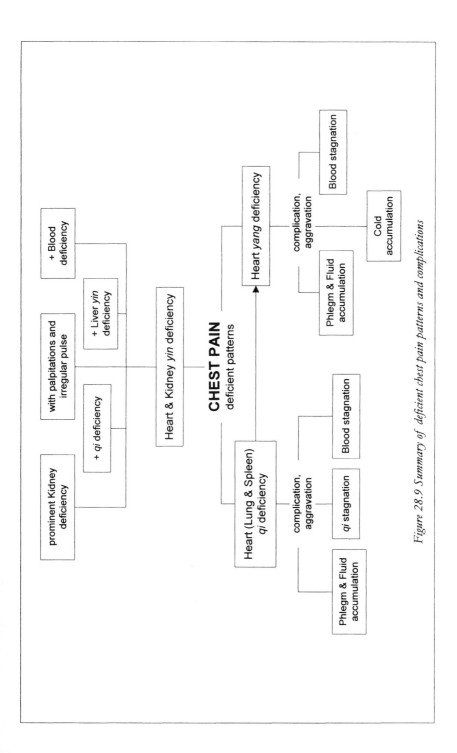

Figure 28.9 Summary of deficient chest pain patterns and complications

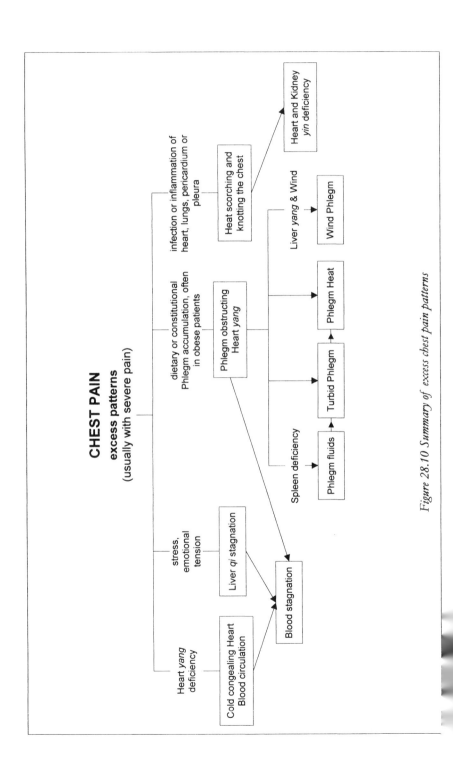

Figure 28.10 Summary of excess chest pain patterns

28.1 HEAT SCORCHING AND KNOTTING THE CHEST

火邪热结胸痹

Pathophysiology
- If external Heat penetrates through the Four Levels (see pp.30, 33) and settles in the Heart or Pericardium, the local *qi* is 'scorched and knotted' causing sharp burning pain in the chest. This pattern can also be associated with external Heat affecting the Lungs or be the result of internally generated Heat from *qi* stagnation or Heart or Liver Fire. External patterns tend to be acute (and associated with some sort of infection), while internally generated Heat tends to be a more chronic condition.

Clinical features
- burning, sharp, focal or retrosternal chest pain aggravated by cough, deep breathing, movement, exertion and swallowing
- fever
- irritability
- dry mouth and thirst
- rough laboured breathing
- cough with thick yellow mucus
- constipation

T red, with a yellow, rough coat
P rapid, or slippery and rapid

Treatment principle
Clear Heat, purge Fire
Invigorate Blood, disperse accumulation

Prescription

XIAO XIAN XIONG TANG 小陷胸汤
(*Minor Sinking Into the Chest Decoction*)

huang lian (Rhizoma Coptidis) 黄连	6g
ban xia* (Rhizoma Pinelliae Ternatae) 半夏	9-12g
gua lou (Fructus Trichosanthis) 栝楼	24-30g

Method: Decoction. (Source: *Shi Yong Zhong Yi Nei Ke Xue*)

Modifications
- If Heat or Fire affects the Heart causing insomnia, dream disturbed sleep, anxiety and tongue ulcers, add **sheng di** (Radix Rehmanniae Glutinosae) 生地 15g, **dan zhu ye** (Herba Lophatheri Gracilis) 淡竹叶 9g, **gan cao** (Radix Glycyrrhizae Uralensis) 甘草 6g and **mu tong** (Caulis Mutong) 木通 6g.
- With constipation, add **da huang** (Radix et Rhizoma Rhei) 大黄 6-9g,

zhi shi (Fructus Immaturus Citri Aurantii) 枳实 9g and **hou po** (Cortex Magnoliae Officinalis) 厚朴 9g.
- When cough is severe, see also pp.77, 84, 90.
- If the Heat has damaged fluids producing symptoms of dryness, add **xuan shen** (Radix Scrophulariae) 玄参 12g, **mai dong** (Tuber Ophiopogonis Japonici) 麦冬 12g and **sheng di** (Radix Rehmanniae Glutinosae) 生地 15g.
- With signs of Blood stasis (stabbing, burning pain, fixed pain), add herbs to invigorate Blood, remove Blood stasis and move *qi* like **mu dan pi** (Cortex Moutan Radicis) 牡丹皮 9g, **chi shao** (Radix Paeoniae Rubrae) 赤芍 12g, **pu huang** (Pollen Typhae) 蒲黄 9g, **yu jin** (Tuber Curcumae) 郁金 12g and **zhi shi** (Fructus Immaturus Citri Aurantii) 枳实 9g.

Variations and additional prescriptions

Heat affecting the Pericardium
- If the Heat sinks into the Pericardium, with fever, disorientation, delerium or impaired consciousness, the correct treatment is to clear Heat and Toxicity, and rescusitate with **ZHI BAO DAN** (*Greatest Treasure Special Pill* 至宝丹, p.660).

Other prescriptions for Heat in the chest
- See also pp.709-711 for other formulae designed to treat external Heat in the chest.

Stagnant Heat from Liver qi *stagnation*
- If the Heat is internally generated (most commonly by prolonged Liver *qi* stagnation), see also Liver *qi* stagnation, pp.770-771. With Liver Fire, the treatment is to clear Liver Fire with **LONG DAN XIE GAN TANG** (*Gentiana Combination* 龙胆泻肝汤, p.553) or **SANG DAN XIE BAI TANG** (*Mulberry Leaf and Moutan Decoction to Drain the White* 桑丹泻白汤, p.94).

Patent medicines

Huang Lian Jie Du Wan 黄连解毒丸 (Huang Lian Jie Du Wan)
  - general Heat clearing formula for Heat affecting the Heart or Lungs
Niu Huang Qing Huo Wan 牛黄清火丸 (Niu Huang Qing Huo Wan)
  - severe Heat with constipation
Chuan Xin Lian Kang Yan Pian 穿心连抗炎片
      (Chuan Xin Lian Antiphlogistic Tablets) - general Heat
Qing Fei Yi Huo Pian 清肺抑火片 (Ching Fei Yi Huo Pien)
  - Lung Heat

Long Dan Xie Gan Wan 龙胆泻肝丸 (Long Dan Xie Gan Wan)
- Liver Fire

Acupuncture
- for external Heat use LI.11 (*qu chi* -), Bl.13 (*fei shu* -), Lu.5 (*chi ze* -), PC.8 (*lao gong* -), Bl.15 (*xin shu* -), Du.14 (*da zhui* -), PC.3 (*qu ze* ↓), Ren.17 (*shan zhong* -)
- for Liver Heat use PC.5 (*jian shi*), PC.6 (*nei guan*), Bl.18 (*gan shu* -), Liv.2 (*xing jian* -), Liv.5 (*li gou* -), GB.34 (*yang ling quan* -), Liv.14 (*qi men* -),
- for hiatus hernia use St.36 (*zu san li*), St.44 (*nei ting* -), Ren.13 (*shang wan*), Ren.17 (*shan zhong* -), PC.6 (*nei guan*), Bl.21 (*wei shu*)
- for structural or focal pain use *ah shi* points and the metal and water points on the relevant channels

Clinical notes
- The chest pain in this pattern may correspond to disorders such as acute pericarditis, bronchitis, pneumonia, pleurisy, hiatus hernia, gastric reflux, peptic ulcer disease, psychogenic chest pain, costochondritis, stress related chest pain and smoke inhalation.
- In most cases, Heat type chest pain can respond reasonably well to correct treatment. Both external and internal Heat patterns occur in those who are overworked, often with a pre-existing Heart or Lung imbalance. Relapses occur at times of stress or overwork.
- Acute infections may need antibiotic therapy if the patient is elderly of frail or does not respond rapidly to herbal treatment.
- Costochondritis and hiatus hernia are treated very effectively with acupuncture (particularly applied to *ah shi* points), as is the pain associated with pericarditis and other inflammatory disorders.

28.2 PHLEGM OBSTRUCTION

Pathophysiology
- Phlegm obstruction can develop in those with *yang* or *qi* deficiency, *qi* stagnation, Heat in the chest and accumulation of Dampness and Phlegm. The symptom picture varies depending on the aetiology, and the relative mixture of underlying deficiency and Phlegm excess. Phlegm (and its variations) is a common cause of chest pain, and frequently complicates (or is complicated by) other patterns. The general rule of treatment, however, is to resolve Phlegm before dealing with other complicating patterns.
- Chest pain occurs when Phlegm obstructs the airways causing congestion and an oppressive feeling of discomfort and tightness. Alternatively, Phlegm obstructs the vessels of the Heart impeding Blood flow, creating a sense of pressure and pain.
- There are four subgroups of this pattern–Phlegm Fluids, Turbid Phlegm (which is somewhat thicker and stickier than Phlegm Fluids), Phlegm Fire and Wind Phlegm. They represent progressions from the initial condition of Phlegm Fluids.

Clinical features
Phlegm Fluids

This type frequently co-exists with Heart and Kidney *yang* deficiency. Following resolution of the Phlegm Fluids, tonifying treatments should be applied (see p.777).
- mild stuffiness, discomfort or tightness in the chest which is aggravated during wet or cold weather
- cough with thin watery sputum
- nausea and poor appetite
- lethargy
- loose stools

T pale with a greasy white coat
P slippery

Turbid Phlegm

This term describes Phlegm Fluids that have thickened and become more sticky and viscous.
- suffocating, tight or oppressive sensation in the chest, or chest pain radiating to the shoulders or upper back, aggravated during cloudy or rainy weather
- tendency to obesity
- feeling of heaviness in the body
- dizziness

- wheezing with thick white sputum

T greasy white coat
P slippery

Phlegm Heat (Fire)

If Phlegm stagnation generates Heat it is generally known as 'Phlegm Heat'. If pre-existing stagnant Heat, Fire or *yin* deficient Heat combines with Phlegm this is termed 'Phlegm Fire'. The greater the Heat signs the more 'Fire'.

- suffocating, tight, oppressive burning sensation or pain in the chest
- thick yellow sputum
- bitter taste in the mouth
- thirst
- irritability and restlessness, possible clouding of consciousness
- dry stools or constipation

T greasy yellow coat
P slippery rapid

Wind Phlegm

This is a combination of excess *yang* (usually rising Liver *yang*) and Phlegm, and is described in more detail in Wind Stroke, pp.658 and 672. See also Tremors, p.642.

- suffocating, tight sensation in the chest with occasional pain
- stiffness or retraction of the tongue
- speech impairment
- hemiplegia
- dizziness
- numbness and spasm in the limbs

T greasy coat
P wiry and slippery

Treatment principle

Open and unblock chest *yang*
 + warm and transform Phlegm Fluids
 + transform Turbid Phlegm
 + transform Phlegm and clear Heat (Fire)
 + extinguish Wind and transform Phlegm

Prescriptions
28.2.1 Phlegm Fluids

GUA LUO XIE BAI BAN XIA TANG 瓜楼薤白半夏汤
(*Trichosanthes, Bakeri and Pinellia Combination*) modified

gua lou (Fructus Trichosanthis) 栝楼	30g
xie bai (Bulbus Allii) 薤白	12g
ban xia* (Rhizoma Pinelliae Ternatae) 半夏	10g
hou po (Cortex Magnoliae Officinalis) 厚朴	10g
zhi shi (Fructus Immaturus Citri Aurantii) 枳实	10g
fu ling (Sclerotium Poriae Cocos) 茯苓	12g
gan jiang (Rhizoma Zingiberis Officinalis) 干姜	6g
xi xin* (Herba cum Radice Asari) 细辛	6g
gui zhi (Ramulus Cinnamomi Cassiae) 桂枝	6g

Method: Decoction. (Source: *Shi Yong Zhong Yi Nei Ke Xue*)

Modifications

- If pain radiates down the arm, add **jiang huang** (Rhizoma Curcumae Longae) 姜黄 10g and **chao bai shao** (dry fried Radix Paeoniae Lactiflora) 炒白芍 12g.
- If palpitations are severe, add **zhi gan cao** (honey fried Radix Glycyrrhizae Uralensis) 炙甘草 9g and **bai zi ren** (Semen Biotae Orientalis) 柏子仁 9g.
- With copious Phlegm, and wheezing or orthopnoea, add **ting li zi** (Semen Descurainiae seu Lepidii) 葶苈子 10g.
- In all the Phlegm patterns, Blood stagnation is a frequent complicating factor. Where there are signs of Blood stasis (secondary to a Phlegm pattern), herbs like **dan shen** (Radix Salviae Miltiorrhizae) 丹参 15g, **dang gui** (Radix Angelicae Sinensis) 当归 9g, **yi mu cao** (Herba Leonuri Heterophylli) 益母草 15g, **tao ren** (Semen Persicae) 桃仁 9g, **hong hua** (Flos Carthami Tinctorii) 红花 9g, **chi shao** (Radix Paeoniae Rubrae) 赤芍 9g, and **mu dan pi** (Cortex Moutan Radicis) 牡丹皮 9g are added as appropriate to invigorate Blood and clear stagnant Blood.

28.2.2 Turbid Phlegm

WEN DAN TANG 温胆汤
(*Bamboo and Hoelen Combination*) modified

ban xia* (Rhizoma Pinelliae Ternatae) 半夏	9g
chen pi (Pericarpium Citri Reticulatae) 陈皮	9g
fu ling (Sclerotium Poriae Cocos) 茯苓	15g
zhi shi (Fructus Immaturus Citri Aurantii) 枳实	9g
zhu ru (Caulis Bambusae in Taeniis) 竹茹	9g

gan cao (Radix Glycyrrhizae Uralensis) 甘草 3g
gua lou (Fructus Trichosanthis) 栝楼 30g
Method: Decoction. (Source: *Shi Yong Zhong Yi Nei Ke Xue*)

28.2.3 Phlegm Heat (Fire)

HUANG LIAN WEN DAN TANG 黄连温胆汤
(*Coptis Decoction to Warm the Gall Bladder*) modified

ban xia* (Rhizoma Pinelliae Ternatae) 半夏 9g
chen pi (Pericarpium Citri Reticulatae) 陈皮 9g
fu ling (Sclerotium Poriae Cocos) 茯苓 15g
zhi shi (Fructus Immaturus Citri Aurantii) 枳实 9g
zhu ru (Caulis Bambusae in Taeniis) 竹茹 9g
gan cao (Radix Glycyrrhizae Uralensis) 甘草 3g
huang lian (Rhizoma Coptidis) 黄连 6g
yu jin (Tuber Curcumae) 郁金 9g
gua lou (Fructus Trichosanthis) 栝楼 30g
Method: Decoction. (Source: *Shi Yong Zhong Yi Nei Ke Xue*).

Modifications

- With severe Phlegm Fire, or focal pain and distension, add **fu hai shi** (Pumice) 浮海石 9g and **hai ge ke**ˆ (Conchae Cyclinae Sinensis) 海蛤壳 9g.
- With irritability and insomnia, combine with **ZHU SHA AN SHEN WAN** (*Cinnabar Pill to Calm the Spirit* 朱砂安神丸, p.807).
- If the Heat damages fluids, add **sheng di** (Radix Rehmanniae Glutinosae) 生地 12g, **mai dong** (Tuber Ophiopogonis Japonici) 麦冬 9g and **xuan shen** (Radix Scrophulariae) 玄参 12g.
- With constipation, add **da huang** (Radix et Rhizoma Rhei) 大黄 6-9g or combine with **GUN TAN WAN** (*Vaporize Phlegm Pill* 滚痰丸, p.694).

28.2.4 Wind Phlegm

DI TAN TANG 涤痰汤
(*Scour Phlegm Decoction*)

ban xia* (Rhizoma Pinelliae Ternatae) 半夏 9g
chen pi (Pericarpium Citri Reticulatae) 陈皮 9g
fu ling (Sclerotium Poriae Cocos) 茯苓 9g
zhi shi (Fructus Immaturus Citri Aurantii) 枳实 9g
zhu ru (Caulis Bambusae in Taeniis) 竹茹 6g
dan nan xing* (Pulvis Arisaemae cum Felle Bovis)
胆南星 9g
shi chang pu (Rhizoma Acori Graminei) 石菖蒲 6g

ren shen (Radix Ginseng) 人参 6g
gan cao (Radix Glycyrrhizae Uralensis) 甘草 3g
Method: Decoction. (Source: *Shi Yong Zhong Yi Nei Ke Xue*)

Modifications
- To increase the Heat clearing, Phlegm transforming, Wind suppressing strength of the formula, other herbs, such as **tian zhu huang** (Concretio Silicea Bambusae Textillis) 天竺黄 6g, **zhu li** (Succus Bambusae) 竹沥 12g, **sheng jiang** (Rhizoma Zingiberis Officinalis) 生姜 9g, **jiang can^** (Bombyx Batryticatus) 僵蚕 9g, **di long^** (Lumbricus) 地龙 9g and **tian ma** (Rhizoma Gastrodiae Elatae) 天麻 9g, may be added as appropriate.

Patent medicines
Phlegm Fluids
Fu Zi Li Zhong Wan 附子理中丸 (Li Chung Yuen Medical Pills)

Turbid Phlegm
Er Chen Wan 二陈丸 (Er Chen Wan)
Ping Wei San 平胃散 (Ping Wei San)
Xiang Sha Liu Jun Zi Wan 香砂六君子丸 (Xiang Sha Liu Jun Wan)
 - Spleen deficiency with Phlegm

Phlegm Heat
Niu Huang Qing Huo Wan 牛黄清火丸 (Niu Huang Qing Huo Wan)

Wind Phlegm
Yang Yin Jiang Ya Wan 养阴降压丸 (Yang Yin Jiang Ya Wan)
Tian Ma Gou Teng Wan 天麻钩藤丸 (Tian Ma Gou Teng Wan)

Acupuncture
St.40 (*feng long* -), Ren.17 (*shan zhong* -), PC.6 (*nei guan*), PC.5 (*jian shi*), PC.4 (*xi men* -), Bl.13 (*fei shu*), Bl.15 (*xin shu*), Bl.14 (*jue yin shu*)
- with Phlegm Fluids add Lu.7 (*lie que*) and moxa to points on the trunk
- with Turbid Phlegm add Sp.3 (*tai bai*)
- with Phlegm Heat add PC.8 (*lao gong* -), Lu.6 (*kong zui* -) and Liv.2 (*xing jian* -)
- for Wind Phlegm see pp.657 and 673

Clinical notes
- Phlegm Fluids: cor pulmonale, angina, myocardial infarction, chronic bronchitis.

- Turbid Phlegm: atherosclerosis, coronary heart disease, myocardial infarction.
- Phlegm Heat: acute and chronic bronchitis, pneumonia, myocarditis, pericarditis.
- Wind Phlegm: CVA, hypertension.
- The Phlegm obstruction in this pattern often has its origin in the high fat diet popular in Western nations. While cholesterol status is still a controversial predictor of heart disease, it has been shown that diets rich in animal fats (low density lipoproteins) predispose to the development of atherosclerotic plaques in the coronary vessels. Atherosclerotic disease is often silent until it reaches the point where the obstruction causes ischaemia of cardiac muscle, resulting in the characteristic chest stuffiness or pain.
- Phlegm disorders require persistent treatment; herbs and their Phlegm dissolving properties being the treatment of choice. Phlegm dissolving herbs often have significant anti-cholesterol and anti-atherosclerotic action and their long term use (in conjuction with appropriate diet and lifestyle changes, especially stopping smoking) can begin to remove the atherosclerotic plaques from the artery walls. Acupuncture works well with herbs in these patterns, its *qi* moving abilities helping to dissolve Phlegm and relieve pain. Where there is serious organ damage, other forms of medical support will be necessary, and for bacterial infections in patients with weak constitutions, antibiotics may need to be taken in addition to or before treatment with herbs and acupuncture.

28.3 LIVER *QI* STAGNATION

肝气郁滞胸痹

Pathophysiology
- The Liver channel passes through the chest and thus influences the Heart and Lungs. Emotional stress constricts the *qi* in the Liver channel, and obstructs the free movement of *qi*, which accumulates in the chest. This pattern is frequently complicated by Phlegm, *qi* deficiency and/or Heat.

Clinical features
- mild, recurrent fullness, stuffiness, tightness or pain in the chest that is not localised, is provoked by emotional turmoil and relieved by sighing, belching and relaxation
- frequent sighing
- the patient may appear uptight, anxious, nervy or depressed
- dizziness, hyperventilation
- there may be epigastric distension and belching, after which the discomfort is relieved
- irregular menstruation, premenstrual syndrome and breast tenderness
- if Heat has been generated by the stagnation, there may be a dry mouth, irritability, quick temper, facial flushing and acid reflux

T unremarkable or dark (*qing* 青), or with red edges if there is Heat, or pale edges with Blood deficiency
P wiry

Treatment principle
Move and regulate Liver *qi*
Strengthen the Spleen and harmonise Blood

Prescription

CHAI HU SHU GAN SAN 柴胡疏肝散
(*Bupleurum and Cyperus Formula*)

chai hu (Radix Bupleuri) 柴胡	9g
chen pi (Pericarpium Citri Reticulatae) 陈皮	9g
bai shao (Radix Paeoniae Lactiflora) 白芍	12g
zhi ke (Fructus Citri Aurantii) 枳壳	9g
chuan xiong (Radix Ligustici Chuanxiong) 川芎	6g
xiang fu (Rhizoma Cyperi Rotundi) 香附	6g
zhi gan cao (honey fried Radix Glycyrrhizae Uralensis) 炙甘草	3g

Method: Decoction. (Source: *Shi Yong Zhong Yi Nei Ke Xue*)

Modifications

- If pain (rather than distension) is prominent, add two or three of the following herbs: **chuan lian zi*** (Fructus Meliae Toosendan) 川楝子 9g, **yan hu suo** (Rhizoma Corydalis Yanhusuo) 延胡索 9g, **mo yao** (Myrrha) 没药 6g, **ru xiang** (Gummi Olibanum) 乳香 6g, **qing pi** (Pericarpium Citri Reticulatae Viride) 青皮 6g and **bai jie zi** (Semen Sinapsis Albae) 白芥子 6g or **sheng pu huang** (Pollen Typhae) 生蒲黄 6g, or combine with **SHI XIAO SAN** (*Break Into a Smile Powder* 失笑散 p.782).
- With mild Blood stasis, add **san qi fen** (powdered Radix Notoginseng) 三七粉 3g, or combine with **DAN SHEN YIN** (*Salvia Decoction* 丹参饮, p.783).
- If anxious or nervous, add one or two of the following herbs: **zhen zhu mu**ˆ (Concha Margaritaferae) 珍珠母 30g, **long chi**ˆ (Dens Draconis) 龙齿 15g or **ci shi** (Magnetitum) 磁石 12g.
- With hysteria or hyperventilation, add **xiao mai** (Semen Triticum) 小麦 60g, and **da zao** (Fructus Zizyphi Jujubae) 大枣 6g.
- With nausea and vomiting, add **xuan fu hua** (Flos Inulae) 旋复花 9g, **ban xia*** (Rhizoma Pinelliae Ternatae) 半夏 9g and **sheng jiang** (Rhizoma Zingiberis Officinalis) 生姜 3pce.
- With Liver Heat disturbing the Stomach (indeterminate gnawing hunger, acid reflux, vomiting, belching and bitter taste in the mouth), add **huang lian** (Rhizoma Coptidis) 黄连 6g and **wu zhu yu** (Fructus Evodiae Rutaecarpae) 吴茱萸 3g.
- With acid reflux, add **hai piao xiao**ˆ (Os Sepiae seu Sepiellae) 海螵蛸 9g and **mu li**ˆ (Concha Ostreae) 牡蛎 15g.

Variations and additional prescriptions

With Spleen qi and Blood deficiency

- With significant digestive symptoms, or *qi* and Blood deficiency, **XIAO YAO SAN** (*Bupleurum and Dang Gui Formula* 逍遥散 p.139) may be used instead to soothe the Liver, move *qi*, regulate the Spleen and harmonise Blood, with any of the above modifications.

With stagnant Heat

- If chronic *qi* stagnation generates Heat, the correct treatment is to soothe *qi* and clear stagnant Heat with **DAN ZHI XIAO YAO SAN** (*Bupleurum and Paeonia Formula* 丹栀逍遥散 p.140).

With constipation

- With constipation due to stagnant Heat, combine with **DANG GUI LONG HUI WAN** (*Dang Gui, Gentiana Longdancao and Aloe Pill* 当归龙荟丸).

dang gui (Radix Angelicae Sinensis) 当归 30g
long dan cao (Radix Gentianae Longdancao) 龙胆草 30g
shan zhi zi (Fructus Gardeniae Jasminoides) 山栀子 30g
huang qin (Radix Scutellariae Baicalensis) 黄芩 30g
huang lian (Rhizoma Coptidis) 黄连 30g
huang bai (Cortex Phellodendri) 黄柏 30g
da huang (Radix et Rhizoma Rhei) 大黄 15g
lu hui* (Herba Aloes) 芦荟 15g
qing dai (Indigo Pulverata Levis) 青黛 15g
mu xiang (Radix Aucklandiae Lappae) 木香 6g
she xiang° (Secretio Moschus) 麝香 1.5g

Method: Grind the herbs to powder and form into 6-gram pills with honey. The dose is 1 pill twice daily, with ginger tea.

With prominent distension and fullness

• If distension and fullness in the lower chest and hypochondrium are prominent, with a continuous stuffy sensation which improves for pressure on the chest and warm drinks, **XUAN FU HUA TANG** (*Inula Flower Decoction* 旋复花汤) modified may be used.

xuan fu hua (Flos Inulae) 旋复花 12g
yu jin (Tuber Curcumae) 郁金 9g
xie bai (Bulbus Allii) 薤白 9g
tao ren (Semen Persicae) 桃仁 9g
cong bai (Bulbus Allii Fistulosi) 葱白 6pce
dang gui wei (tail of Radix Angelicae Sinensis) 当归尾 6g
hong hua (Flos Carthami Tinctorii) 红花 6g
gui zhi (Ramulus Cinnamomi Cassiae) 桂枝 6g
qian cao gen (Radix Rubiae Cordifoliae) 茜草根 3g
gua lou (Fructus Trichosanthis) 栝楼 15g

Method: Decoction. (Scource: *Zhong Yi Nei Ke Lin Chuang Shou Ce*)

Patent medicines

Chai Hu Shu Gan Wan 柴胡舒肝丸 (Chai Hu Shu Gan Wan)
Shu Gan Wan 舒肝丸 (Shu Gan Wan)
Xiao Yao Wan 逍遥丸 (Xiao Yao Wan)
  - with *qi* and Blood deficiency
Jia Wei Xiao Yao Wan 加味逍遥丸 (Jia Wei Xiao Yao Wan)
  - with stagnant Heat
Mu Xiang Shun Qi Wan 木香顺气丸 (Aplotaxis Carminative Pills)
Dan Shen Pian 丹参片 (Dan Shen Pills)
  - with mild Blood stasis

Acupuncture

Liv.14 (*qi men*), Liv.3 (*tai chong* -), PC.6 (*nei guan*), PC.5 (*jian shi*), Bl.18 (*gan shu*), Ren.17 (*shan zhong*), Lu.7 (*lie que*), *yin tang* (M-HN-3)
- with Heat add Liv.2 (*xing jian* -)
- with deficiency add St.36 (*zu san li* +), Sp.6 (*san yin jiao* +) and Bl.20 (*pi shu* +)

Clinical notes

- The chest pain in this pattern may correspond to disorders such as pleurisy, globus hystericus, psychogenic chest pain, angina pectoris, costochondritis, hiatus hernia, oesophagitis, oesophageal spasm or gastric reflux.
- This pattern generally responds well to correct treatment and appropriate stress management strategies. Liver *qi* stagnation probably only represents coronary heart disease when associated with Phlegm or if it leads to Blood stagnation. That stagnation of *qi* itself can precipitate a heart attack (where there already exists heart disease that may be associated with Phlegm and/or Blood stasis) was shown in a study conducted by the Mayo clinic. They found that the strongest predictor of a second heart attack was psychological stress. Similarly, the fact that Liver *qi* stagnation leading to Fire was dangerous in the presence of heart disease was shown by studies from Harvard University. They found the risk of having a second heart attack doubles after anger outbursts.

28.4 COLD CONGEALING HEART BLOOD CIRCULATION

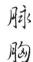

Pathophysiology
- Chest pain caused by obstruction of *qi* and Blood due to an accumulation of Cold is acute and intense and reflects a serious (and critical) heart condition. The priority of treatment must be to rapidly expel Cold and promote the circulation of *qi* and Blood. The Cold in this pattern usually develops from an underlying *yang* deficiency and there will usually be evidence of systemic Cold. Once the acute episode or emergency is stabilised, the *yang* deficiency should be addressed (see Heart *yang* deficiency, p.777).

Clinical features
- severe crushing or constricting retrosternal chest pain, which may be initiated or aggravated by cold weather or cold foods; the pain may radiate to the neck, jaw, left arm or through to the back
- shortness of breath, dyspnoea or orthopnoea
- palpitations
- aversion to cold, cold extremities
- in severe cases there may be cyanosis, pallor, sweating and vomiting

T normal, or pale with a thin white coat, or pale bluish or purple and swollen, with a white or greasy coat (depending on the degree of underlying *yang* deficiency)

P deep, slow, tight and maybe knotted or intermittent, or thready, slow and knotted or intermittent

Treatment principle
Warm and disperse Cold, invigorate Blood
Remove obstruction and promote circulation of Heart *yang*

Prescription

DANG GUI SI NI TANG 当归四逆汤
(*Dang Gui Decoction for Frigid Extremities*)

This prescription is suitable for relatively mild cases.
- **dang gui** (Radix Angelicae Sinensis) 当归 9g
- **gui zhi** (Ramulus Cinnamomi Cassiae) 桂枝 9g
- **bai shao** (Radix Paeoniae Lactiflora) 白芍 9g
- **xi xin*** (Herba cum Radice Asari) 细辛 6g
- **mu tong** (Caulis Mutong) 木通 6g
- **zhi gan cao** (honey fried Radix Glycyrrhizae Uralensis) 炙甘草 6g
- **da zao** (Fructus Zizyphi Jujubae) 大枣 4pce

Method: Decoction. (Source: *Shi Yong Zhong Yi Nei Ke Xue*)

WU TOU CHI SHI ZHI WAN 乌头赤石脂丸
(*Aconite and Halloysium Pills*) modified

This prescription is used in more severe cases, where pain is persistent and severe, radiating through to the back.

wu tou* (Radix Aconiti) 乌头 3g
zhi fu zi* (Radix Aconiti Carmichaeli Praeparata) 制附子 6-9g
chuan jiao (Pericarpium Zanthoxyli Bungeani) 川椒 6g
gan jiang (Rhizoma Zingiberis Officinalis) 干姜 9g
chi shi zhi (Halloysitum Rubrum) 赤石脂 15g

Method: Decoction. **Wu tou** is extremely toxic and rarely used today. It must be boiled for at least an hour to render it safe. Today, **rou gui** (Cortex Cinnamomi Cassiae) 肉桂 is usually substituted for **wu tou**. **Zhi fu zi** is boiled for 30 minutes prior to the other herbs (*xian jian* 先煎). (Source: *Shi Yong Zhong Yi Nei Ke Xue*)

Modifications

- With stagnant Blood (purple patches on the tongue, sharp pain, irregular pulse), add **dan shen** (Radix Salviae Miltiorrhizae) 丹参 30g, **chi shao** (Radix Paeoniae Rubrae) 赤芍 10g and **yu jin** (Tuber Curcumae) 郁金 10g.

- If there is significant wheezing and dyspnoea with thin sputum, add **sheng jiang** (Rhizoma Zingiberis Officinalis) 生姜 15g, **chen pi** (Pericarpium Citri Reticulatae) 陈皮 10g, **fu ling** (Sclerotium Poriae Cocos) 茯苓 15g, **xing ren*** (Semen Pruni Armeniacae) 杏仁 10g and **bai dou kou** (Fructus Amomi Kravanh) 白豆蔻 6g.

Variations and additional prescriptions

Collapse of Heart yang

- In severe cases the patient is cold and clammy, has cyanosis, extreme pallor, icy extremities and an imperceptible pulse indicating imminent collapse of Heart *yang*. The correct approach is to administer an emergency medicine such as **GUAN XIN SU HE XIANG WAN** (*Liquid Styrax Pills* for *Coronary Heart Disease* 冠心苏合香丸 - see below), and institute the emergency acupuncture techniques outlined in Box.28.2, p.756 until paramedic assistance arrives. An alternative approach used in hospitals in China is **SHEN FU TANG** (*Ginseng and Prepared Aconite Decoction* 参附汤, p.665) plus **long gu^** (Os Draconis) 龙骨 15-30g and **mu li^** (Concha Ostreae) 牡蛎 15-30g administered intravenously.

Patent medicines

Guan Xin Su He Xiang Wan 冠心苏合香丸 (Guan Xin Su Ho)
- usually given together with whichever prescription is applicable. This is a very popular pill and useful for patients with known cardiac disease to carry at all times.

Fu Zi Li Zhong Wan 附子理中丸 (Li Chung Yuen Medical Pills)
- good for warming *yang* generally

Xiao Huo Luo Dan 小活络丹 (Xiao Huo Luo Dan)
- a small dose of this very hot medicine may be useful in severe cases.

Acupuncture

Bl.15 (*xin shu* +▲), Bl.14 (*jue yin shu* +▲), Ren.17 (*shan zhong* +▲), Ren.15 (*jiu wei* +▲), Du.14 (*da zhui* +▲), St.36 (*zu san li* +▲), PC.6 (*nei guan* -), PC.4 (*xi men* -)

- treatment may be given frequently, every few hours in manageable cases
- in severe cases see Box 28.2, p.756
- in cases of collapse (with no available assistance), moxa can be burnt over Ren.8 (*shen que*). Spread a thin cloth over the navel and fill it with salt. Burn large moxa cones over the salt until consciousness is restored. The cloth enables swift removal of the salt if necessary.

Clinical notes

- The chest pain in this pattern may correspond to disorders such as myocardial infarction (if the pain persists for more than 15 minutes), angina pectoris, congestive cardiac failure, coronary artery disease
- While such an emergency as Cold congealing Heart Blood may be dealt with rapidly and effectively using herbs and acupuncture in combination with Western medicine in a Chinese hospital, it is unlikely that our patients in the West will be administered herbs before being taken to the casualty department. However, if the cardiac pain is unresponsive to Western treatment, there may be a place for the TCM management suggested here.
- For patients in a high risk group (previous transitory angina with *yang* deficiency), the patent medicine mentioned previously (*Guan Xin Su He Xiang Wan* 冠心苏合香丸) should be carried at all times.

28.5 HEART *YANG* DEFICIENCY

Pathophysiology
- Heart *yang* deficiency is usually a complication of either or both Spleen or Kidney *yang* deficiency and there will often be symptoms of deficiency affecting all three organs. When Heart *yang* (*zong qi* 宗气) is affected, the pumping power of the Heart is impaired and Blood begins to pool in the coronary vessels. Heart *yang* deficiency is at the root of several other pathologies, notably Phlegm (through weakened fluid metabolism), acute severe pain from Cold accumulation (see p.774), and Blood stagnation (from inadequate propulsion of Blood).

Clinical features
- a suffocating, tight or dull chest pain, or stuffiness in the chest, which is provoked or aggravated by exertion and exposure to cold
- shortness of breath with exertion, in severe cases (with pulmonary oedema) wheezing or orthopnoea
- cold intolerance and cold extremities
- palpitations
- listlessness and fatigue
- spontaneous sweating
- waxy pale complexion, with dark rings under the eyes and purple lips
- lower back soreness
- pitting oedema, worse in the lower limbs, with scanty urine

T pale bluish or purple and swollen, with a white or greasy coat
P deficient, thready, weak, slow or knotted and intermittent

Treatment principle
Warm and tonify *yang*
Warm and invigorate Heart *yang*

Prescription

LI ZHONG WAN 理中丸
(*Ginseng and Ginger Formula*) modified

This prescription is suitable for mild cases with signs of Heart and Spleen *yang* deficiency.

ren shen (Radix Ginseng) 人参	9g
gan jiang (Rhizoma Zingiberis Officinalis) 干姜	9g
bai zhu (Rhizoma Atractylodis Macrocephalae) 白术	9g
gui zhi (Ramulus Cinnamomi Cassiae) 桂枝	9g
fu ling (Sclerotium Poriae Cocos) 茯苓	9g

心阳亏虚胸痹

>   **zhi gan cao** (honey fried Radix Glycyrrhizae Uralensis)
>   炙甘草 9g
>   Method: Decoction. (Source: *Shi Yong Zhong Yi Nei Ke Xue*)

ZHEN WU TANG 真武汤
(*True Warrior Decoction*) modified

This prescription is selected when Heart and Kidney *yang* deficiency is causing generalised and pulmonary oedema (as in congestive cardiac failure), with dyspnoea, orthopnoea and frothy sputum. The correct treatment is to warm the *yang* and promote urination.

>   **zhi fu zi*** (Radix Aconiti Carmichaeli Praeparata) 制附子 9g
>   **chao bai zhu** (dry fried Rhizoma Atractylodis Macrocephalae)
>   炒白术 9g
>   **sheng jiang** (Rhizoma Zingiberis Officinalis) 生姜 9g
>   **bai shao** (Radix Paeoniae Lactiflora) 白芍 12g
>   **fu ling** (Sclerotium Poriae Cocos) 茯苓 12g
>   **che qian zi** (Semen Plantaginis) 车前子 12g
>   **ze xie** (Rhizoma Alismatis Orientalis) 泽泻 12g
>   Method: Decoction. **Zhi fu zi** should be decocted for 30 minutes before the other herbs (*xian jian* 先煎), **che qian zi** is usually cooked in a muslin bag (*bao jian* 包煎). (Source: *Shi Yong Zhong Yi Nei Ke Xue*). When fluids are moving, **LI ZHONG WAN** or the following prescription **JIN KUI SHEN QI WAN** should be selected, depending on the underlying pattern.

JIN KUI SHEN QI WAN 金匮肾气丸, p.874
(*Rehmannia Eight Formula*)

This is the representative Kidney *yang* strengthening formula, and is excellent as a general *yang* tonic. In cases of chest pain, it is used in between acute episodes of pain to strengthen both Heart and Kidney *yang*. It is particularly useful following resolution of the acute phase of pulmonary or generalised oedema.

Modifications (apply to all three prescriptions)

- If the Cold and chest pain are relatively severe, add two or three of the following herbs (where not already included): **lu rong pian**ˆ (sliced Cornu Cervi Parvum) 鹿茸片 3g, **chuan jiao** (Pericarpium Zanthoxyli Bungeani) 川椒 6g, **wu zhu yu** (Fructus Evodiae Rutaecarpae) 吴茱萸 6g, **bi ba** (Fructus Piperis Longi) 荜拔 3g, **gao liang jiang** (Rhizoma Alpiniae Officinari) 高良姜 9g, **xi xin*** (Herba cum Radice Asari) 细辛 6g, **zhi fu zi*** (Radix Aconiti Carmichaeli Praeparata) 制附子 6g or **chi shi zhi** (Halloysitum Rubrum) 赤石脂 15g.
- With *qi* and Blood stasis, add two or three of the following herbs: **cong**

bai (Bulbus Allii Fistulosi) 葱白 5pce, **chen xiang** (Lignum Aquilariae) 沉香 3g, **tan xiang** (Lignum Santali Albi) 檀香 9g, **xiang fu** (Rhizoma Cyperi Rotundi) 香附 9g, **ji xue teng** (Radix et Caulis Jixueteng) 鸡血藤 15g, **ze lan** (Herba Lycopi Lucidi) 泽兰 9g, **chuan xiong** (Radix Ligustici Chuanxiong) 川芎 6g, **tao ren** (Semen Persicae) 桃仁 9g, **hong hua** (Flos Carthami Tinctorii) 红花 9g, **yan hu suo** (Rhizoma Corydalis Yanhusuo) 延胡索 9g, **ru xiang** (Gummi Olibanum) 乳香 9g or **mo yao** (Myrrha) 没药 9g.

Variations and additional prescriptions
- In severe cases, see Box 28.2, p.756. The patient is cold and clammy, cyanotic, extremely pale with icy extremities and an imperceptible pulse indicating imminent collapse of Heart *yang*. The correct approach is to administer an emergency medicine such as **GUAN XIN SU HE XIANG WAN** (*Liquid Styrax Pills for Coronary Heart Disease* 冠心苏合香丸), and institute the emergency acupuncture techniques until paramedic assistance arrives. An alternative approach used in hospitals in China is **SHEN FU TANG** (*Ginseng and Prepared Aconite Decoction* 参附汤, p.665) plus **long gu^** (Os Draconis) 龙骨 15-30g and **mu li^** (Concha Ostreae) 牡蛎 15-30g administered intravenously.

Patent medicines
Jin Kui Shen Qi Wan 金匮肾气丸 (Sexoton Pills)
  - used inbetween episodes of pain to strengthen the constitution
Fu Zi Li Zhong Wan 附子理中丸 (Li Chung Yuen Medical Pills)
Xiao Huo Luo Dan 小活络丹 (Xiao Huo Luo Dan)
  - a small dose of this very hot medicine may be useful in severe cases.
Guan Xin Su He Xiang Wan 冠心苏合香丸 (Guan Xin Su Ho)
  - for acute or severe pain during an episode

Acupuncture
Bl.15 (*xin shu* ▲), Bl.14 (*jue yin shu* ▲), Bl.23 (*shen shu* ▲), Ren.6 (*qi hai* ▲), Ren.4 (*guan yuan* ▲)Ht.7 (*shen men*), PC.6 (*nei guan*), Ren.9 (*shui fen* ▲), St.36 (*zu san li*), Sp.6 (*san yin jiao*)
- in severe cases see Box 28.2, p.756

Clinical notes
- The chest pain in this pattern may correspond to disorders such as congestive cardiac failure, angina pectoris, myocardial infarction and coronary artery disease.
- In general, Heart *yang* deficiency is the predisposing pathology for more serious (and possibly fatal) cardiac episodes, but may respond

well to TCM treatment when applied before the severity of the pain indicates an impending critical event.
- In cases with obvious oedema, Cold and/or severe pain, **zhi fu zi*** (Radix Aconiti Carmichaeli Praeparata) 制附子 is the essential ingredient, and substitutes are inadequate.
- This pattern is frequently accompanied by severe Cold, Phlegm and/or Blood stagnation.

28.6 BLOOD STAGNATION

Pathophysiology
- Blood stagnation is most frequently encountered as a complication of another pathology. Elements of Blood stasis are found in most chronic cases of chest pain (and in some relatively acute types, see below). Blood stasis usually becomes prominent late in the course of a disease, and represents a serious and perhaps life threatening development. Blood stasis is a common feature of chronic chest pain patterns, and may involve some pathology of the coronary circulation or malignancy.
- Blood stagnation may also follow an acute external invasion of Wind Cold Damp to the Heart (as in rheumatic fever), or a trauma to the chest wall.

Clinical features
- relatively chronic and severe chest pain, which is stabbing or crushing, fixed in location and usually worse at night or with sudden excitement, anger, emotion or exertion
- palpitations, or sensations of the heart skipping beats during an attack
- stuffiness or fullness in the chest
- irritability, restlessness, easy anger or depression
- spider naevi on the chest and face
- purplish lips, nails, sclera, conjunctiva
- may be accompanying symptoms of Liver *qi* stagnation

T dark or red purple with brown or purple stasis spots and a thin white coat. Sublingual veins are distended and dark.
P deep and choppy or wiry, or intermittent

Treatment principle
Invigorate Blood and eliminate Blood stasis
Open the Heart vessels and stop pain

Prescription

XUE FU ZHU YU TANG 血府逐瘀汤
(*Achyranthes and Persica Combination*) modified

sheng di (Radix Rehmanniae Glutinosae) 生地	30g
dan shen (Radix Salviae Miltiorrhizae) 丹参	15g
tao ren (Semen Persicae) 桃仁	12g
dang gui (Radix Angelicae Sinensis) 当归	9g
hong hua (Flos Carthami Tinctorii) 红花	9g
chi shao (Radix Paeoniae Rubrae) 赤芍	9g
yan hu suo (Rhizoma Corydalis Yanhusuo) 延胡索	9g
zhi ke (Fructus Citri Aurantii) 枳壳	6g

chai hu (Radix Bupleuri) 柴胡 6g
chen xiang (Lignum Aquilariae) 沉香 6g
niu xi (Radix Achyranthis Bidentatae) 牛膝 6g
gan cao (Radix Glycyrrhizae Uralensis) 甘草 4g

Method: Decoction. (Source: *Zhong Yi Nei Ke Lin Chuang Shou Ce*)

Modifications (where not already included)

- As noted above, Blood stagnation is often a complication of other pathological conditions, frequently chronic Liver *qi* stagnation (see below), but also Cold, Phlegm, *yang* and *yin* deficiency etc., and prescription should take these mechanisms into account. For example, if Cold or *yang* deficiency is responsible for the slowing down and stasis of Blood, warm Blood invigorating herbs like **chuan xiong** (Radix Ligustici Chuanxiong) 川芎 9g, **yan hu suo** (Rhizoma Corydalis Yanhusuo) 延胡索 9g, **jiang huang** (Rhizoma Curcumae Longae) 姜黄 9g, **hong hua** (Flos Carthami Tinctorii) 红花 9g, **ru xiang** (Gummi Olibanum) 乳香 9g and **yue ji hua** (Flos et Fructus Rosae Chinensis) 月季花 9g should feature strongly in the selected prescription.

- When Heat or *yin* deficiency dry the Blood and increase its viscosity, Blood cooling and regulating herbs are indicated. Herbs such as **chi shao** (Radix Paeoniae Rubrae) 赤芍 9g, **sheng di** (Radix Rehmanniae Glutinosae) 生地 15-30g, **dan shen** (Radix Salviae Miltiorrhizae) 丹参 15g and **yu jin** (Tuber Curcumae) 郁金 9g are used.

- *Qi* and Blood deficiency should be addressed with Blood nourishing and regulating herbs, like **dang gui** (Radix Angelicae Sinensis) 当归 9g and **ji xue teng** (Radix et Caulis Jixueteng) 鸡血藤 15g.

- When Blood stagnation is combined with Phlegm, it is first necessary to distinguish Phlegm Fluids, Turbid Phlegm, Phlegm Heat or Wind Phlegm, and combine with formulae from that section or add appropriate herbs accordingly.

- If the pain is severe, add two or three of the following herbs: **chuan lian zi*** (Fructus Meliae Toosendan) 川楝子 9g, **yan hu suo** (Rhizoma Corydalis Yanhusuo) 延胡索 9g, **mo yao** (Myrrha) 没药 9g, **ru xiang** (Gummi Olibanum) 乳香 9g, **qing pi** (Pericarpium Citri Reticulatae Viride) 青皮 6g and **bai jie zi** (Semen Sinapsis Albae) 白芥子 6g, or combine with **SHI XIAO SAN** (*Break Into a Smile Powder* 失笑散).

sheng pu huang (Pollen Typhae) 生蒲黄 6g
wu ling zhi^ (Excrementum Trogopteri seu Pteromi) 五灵脂 6g

Method: Grind equal amounts of each herb into a fine powder. The dose is 6 grams of powder taken with the primary prescription or wine.

Variations and additional prescriptions
For mild cases
- In relatively mild cases, **DAN SHEN YIN** (*Salvia Decoction* 丹参饮) may be sufficient.
    dan shen (Radix Salviae Miltiorrhizae) 丹参 30g
    tan xiang (Lignum Santali Albi) 檀香 5g
    sha ren (Fructus Amomi) 砂仁 5g
    Method: Decoction.

Pain following trauma
- When associated with trauma (for example following a motor vehicle accident or broken rib), the formula of choice is **FU YUAN HUO XUE TANG** (*Revive Health by Invigorating the Blood Decoction* 复元活血汤, p.578). This formula is usually only used for a couple of weeks, depending on how serious the trauma is. Initially, the patient should experience loose stools or diarrhoea as the bruising and pain resolve. All the modifications noted above apply to this formula also.

In the post acute phase when qi *stagnation signs become obvious*
- Because *qi* and Blood stagnation occur so frequently together, after the main signs of Blood stasis have eased, *qi* stasis often becomes prominent. In this case (once the pain has been eased) use **XIAO YAO SAN** (*Bupleurum and Dang Gui Formula* 逍遥散 p.139) plus **dan shen** (Radix Salviae Miltiorrhizae) 丹参 30g, **zhi xiang fu** (prepared Rhizoma Cyperi Rotundi) 制香附 6g and **yu jin** (Tuber Curcumae) 郁金 10g.

Patent medicines
Xue Fu Zhu Yu Wan 血府逐瘀丸 (Xue Fu Zhu Yu Wan)
Dan Shen Pian 丹参片 (Dan Shen Pills)
Jian Kang Wan 健康丸 (Sunho Multi Ginseng Tablets)
Sheng Tian Qi Pian 生田七片 (Raw Tian Qi Ginseng Tablets)
Jin Gu Die Shang Wan 筋骨跌伤丸 (Chin Koo Tieh Shang Wan)
Guan Xin An Kou Fu Ye 冠心安口服液 (Guan Xin An Kou Fu Ye)
Fu Ke Wu Jin Wan 妇科乌金丸 (Woo Garm Yuen Medical Pills)

Acupuncture
Bl.15 (*xin shu* -), Bl.14 (*jue yin shu* -), Bl.17 (*ge shu* -), Bl.13 (*fei shu*),
hua tuo jia ji (M-BW-35) - from T3-T7 depending on tenderness,
PC.6 (*nei guan* -), PC.4 (*xi men* -), Ren.17 (*shan zhong*), Du.12 (*shen zhu*),
Du.10 (*ling tai*), Sp.10 (*xue hai* -)
- with *yang* deficiency add moxa
- with *qi* stagnation add Liv.3 (*tai chong* -)
- with Phlegm add St.40 (*feng long* -)

Clinical notes

- The chest pain in this pattern may correspond to disorders such as angina pectoris, myocardial infarction, coronary artery disease, cor pulmonale, trauma including contusions and rib or sternum fractures.
- Keep in mind that in most cases of chest pain, even though the manifestation is excess, the root is deficient (except in trauma). Most Blood invigorating herbs, especially those that 'smash stagnant Blood' (*po xue* 破血) are quite dispersing and prolonged use will damage *zheng qi*. Strong Blood movers should be used cautiously and reserved for short term use in severe cases.

28.7 HEART (LUNG AND SPLEEN) *QI* DEFICIENCY

Pathophysiology
- The primary mechanism in this pattern is weak Heart *qi* (*zong qi* 宗气), which is unable to propel Blood adequately, leading to pooling of Blood. Weakness of Lung *qi* contributes by allowing *qi* to accumulate in the chest instead of descending as it should.

Clinical features
- mild, dull, intermittent chest pain
- stuffiness in the chest
- shortness of breath or dyspnoea with exertion
- palpitations with anxiety
- fatigue and weakness
- easily flustered and panicky
- low voice or reluctance to speak
- pale or sallow complexion
- spontaneous sweating
- all symptoms initiated or aggravated by exertion
- when the Spleen is involved there will be digestive symptoms, like poor appetite, abdominal distension and loose stools

T pale and swollen with toothmarks and a thin coat
P weak, thready, moderate or intermittent

Treatment principle
Tonify Heart *qi*, invigorate *yang qi* in the chest

Prescription

BAO YUAN TANG 保元汤
(*Preserve the Basal Decoction*) modified

ren shen (Radix Ginseng) 人参	9g
huang qi (Radix Astragali Membranacei) 黄芪	9g
dan shen (Radix Salviae Miltiorrhizae) 丹参	9g
dang gui (Radix Angelicae Sinensis) 当归	9g
fu xiao mai (Semen Tritici Aestivi Levis) 浮小麦	12g
rou gui (Cortex Cinnamomi Cassiae) 肉桂	3g
da zao (Fructus Zizyphi Jujubae) 大枣	4pce
zhi gan cao (honey fried Radix Glycyrrhizae Uralensis) 炙甘草	3g

Method: Decoction. (Source: *Shi Yong Zhong Yi Nei Ke Xue*)

心脾气虚胸痹

YANG XIN TANG 养心汤
(*Nourish the Heart Decoction*)

This formula is selected if both the Spleen and Heart *qi* are equally weak.

huang qi (Radix Astragali Membranacei) 黄芪	12g
ren shen (Radix Ginseng) 人参	9g
fu ling (Sclerotium Poriae Cocos) 茯苓	9g
fu shen (Sclerotium Poriae Cocos Pararadicis) 茯神	9g
dang gui (Radix Angelicae Sinensis) 当归	9g
suan zao ren (Semen Zizyphi Spinosae) 酸枣仁	9g
chuan xiong (Radix Ligustici Chuanxiong) 川芎	6g
ban xia* (Rhizoma Pinelliae Ternatae) 半夏	6g
bai zi ren (Semen Biotae Orientalis) 柏子仁	9g
yuan zhi (Radix Polygalae Tenuifoliae) 远志	6g
wu wei zi (Fructus Schizandrae Chinensis) 五味子	6g
rou gui (Cortex Cinnamomi Cassiae) 肉桂	3g
zhi gan cao (honey fried Radix Glycyrrhizae Uralensis) 炙甘草	6g

Method: Decoction. (Source: *Shi Yong Zhong Yi Nei Ke Xue*)

Modifications (where not already included)

- With stuffiness in the chest, add **xuan fu hua** (Flos Inulae) 旋复花 9g.
- With insomnia, add **bai zi ren** (Semen Biotae Orientalis) 柏子仁 9g and **ye jiao teng** (Caulis Polygoni Multiflori) 夜交藤 30g.
- With spontaneous sweating, add **mu li**ˆ (Concha Ostreae) 牡蛎 15g, **ma huang gen** (Radix Ephedrae) 麻黄根 9g, **fu xiao mai** (Semen Tritici Aestivi Levis) 浮小麦 15g.
- With depression, add **he huan pi** (Cortex Albizziae Julibrissin) 合欢皮 12g.

Patent medicines

Gui Pi Wan 归脾丸 (Gui Pi Wan)
Bai Zi Yang Xin Wan 柏子养心丸 (Bai Zi Yang Xin Wan)

Acupuncture

Sp.6 (*san yin jiao* +), Ht.7 (*shen men* +), PC.6 (*nei guan*), Lu.7 (*lie que*), Ren.17 (*shan zhong*), Bl.15 (*xin shu* +), Bl.17 (*ge shu*), Bl.20 (*pi shu* +), St.36 (*zu san li* +)
- with insomnia add *an mian* (N-HN-54)

Clinical notes

- The chest pain in this pattern may correspond to disorders such as cardiac failure, coronary artery disease and weakness following illness.
- This pattern often combines with *qi* stagnation, Blood stagnation or Phlegm. The symptoms of deficiency are more noticeable between episodes of chest pain.

28.8 HEART (AND KIDNEY) YIN DEFICIENCY

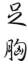

Pathophysiology
This pattern causes chest pain in two ways:
- First, deficient Heat can evaporate and concentrate body fluids making the Blood viscous and impeding its smooth circulation. This causes a feeling of fullness and pain, although at this stage the stagnation has usually not caused the degree of obstruction necessary to make the pain severe. Acute febrile disease (usually where Heat enters the Blood) can produce the same result, depending on the intensity of the fever.
- Second, deficient Heat may directly 'scorch and burn' the Heart and chest. This gives rise to a distinctive burning sensation in the chest.
- Heart *yin* anchors the *shen*. The anxiety that is characteristic of this pattern may be aggravated by fear of the disease itself, which intensifies the anxiety and tightness in the chest and so on, creating a self perpetuating cycle.

Clinical features
- intermittent, relatively mild chest pain, which may be burning or suffocating
- fullness and discomfort in the chest
- palpitations with anxiety
- restlessness, irritability and insomnia
- night sweats
- facial or malar flushing
- dry mouth and throat
- sensation of heat in the palms and soles ('five hearts hot')
- dizziness and tinnitus
- tendency to constipation
- weak or sore lower back and knees

T red, dry and thin with little or no coat or peeled patches in the coat; in severe or chronic cases there may be a deep narrow central crack that extends to to the tip of the tongue
P rapid and thready or intermittent

Treatment principle
Nourish Heart *yin* and calm the *shen*
Regulate Blood, clear Heat

Prescription

TIAN WANG BU XIN DAN 天王补心丹
(*Ginseng and Zizyphus Formula*)

This formula is selected when the *shen* signs (anxiety, insomnia, panic attacks) are strong. This is the main representative formula for Heart and Kidney *yin* deficiency.

sheng di (Radix Rehmanniae Glutinosae) 生地	120 (24)g
tian dong (Tuber Asparagi Cochinchinensis) 天冬	30 (12)g
mai dong (Tuber Ophiopogonis Japonici) 麦冬	30 (12)g
suan zao ren (Semen Zizyphi Spinosae) 酸枣仁	30 (12)g
xuan shen (Radix Scrophulariae) 玄参	15 (12)g
dan shen (Radix Salviae Miltiorrhizae) 丹参	15 (12)g
fu ling (Sclerotium Poriae Cocos) 茯苓	15 (12)g
dang gui wei (Extremitas Radicis Angelicae Sinensis) 当归尾	30 (9)g
wu wei zi (Fructus Schizandrae Chinensis) 五味子	30 (9)g
bai zi ren (Semen Biotae Orientalis) 柏子仁	30 (9)g
ren shen (Radix Ginseng) 人参	15 (9)g
jie geng (Radix Platycodi Grandiflori) 桔梗	15 (9)g
yuan zhi (Radix Polygalae Tenuifoliae) 远志	15 (6)g
zhi gan cao (honey fried Radix Glycyrrhizae Uralensis) 炙甘草	6 (6)g

Method: Grind herbs to a powder and form into 9-gram pills with honey. The dose is one pill 2 to 3 times daily. May also be decocted, with the dosage in brackets. (Source: *Shi Yong Zhong Yi Nei Ke Xue*)

HUANG LIAN E JIAO TANG 黄连阿胶汤
(Coptis and Ass-Hide Gelatin Decoction)

This formula is selected when the chest pain and *yin* deficiency follow a febrile disease (a kind of *shao yin* syndrome, with pain or a sensation of Heat in the chest, insomnia and irritability, palpitations, anxiety, sores in the mouth and on the tongue, a red tongue with a dry yellow coat and a thready rapid pulse). The correct treatment is to clear Fire, nourish *yin*, stop irritability and calm the *shen*.

huang lian (Rhizoma Coptidis) 黄连	12g
huang qin (Radix Scutellariae Baicalensis) 黄芩	6g
e jiao^ (Gelatinum Corii Asini) 阿胶	9g
bai shao (Radix Paeoniae Lactiflora) 白芍	6g
ji zi huang^ (egg yolk)	2 yolks

Method: Decoction. **E jiao** is melted in the hot strained decoction (*yang hua* 烊化). The egg yolks are stirred into the strained decoction. (Source: *Shi Yong Zhong Yi Nei Ke Xue*)

REN SHEN YANG YING TANG 人参养营汤
(Ginseng Nutritive Combination) plus
SHENG MAI SAN 生脉散
(Generate the Pulse Powder)

These formulae are combined when *qi* and *yin* are both deficient. The resulting pattern has characteristics of both deficiencies–increased Blood viscosity, weak propulsion of Blood and shallow breathing. The features are mild stuffiness and pain, shortness of breath, fatigue, palpitations, irritability, dry mouth, a swollen red or pink tongue with surface cracks and no coat, weak, thready and possibly slightly rapid pulse. The correct treatment is to tonify *qi* and nourish *yin*.

shu di (Radix Rehmanniae Glutinosae Conquitae) 熟地	12g
huang qi (Radix Astragali Membranacei) 黄芪	12g
ren shen (Radix Ginseng) 人参	12g
dang gui (Radix Angelicae Sinensis) 当归	9g
bai shao (Radix Paeoniae Lactiflora) 白芍	9g
bai zhu (Rhizoma Atractylodis Macrocephalae) 白术	9g
fu ling (Sclerotium Poriae Cocos) 茯苓	9g
mai dong (Tuber Ophiopogonis Japonici) 麦冬	9g
wu wei zi (Fructus Schizandrae Chinensis) 五味子	6g
yuan zhi (Radix Polygalae Tenuifoliae) 远志	6g
chen pi (Pericarpium Citri Reticulatae) 陈皮	6g
zhi gan cao (honey fried Radix Glycyrrhizae Uralensis) 炙甘草	6g
rou gui (Cortex Cinnamomi Cassiae) 肉桂	3g
sheng jiang (Rhizoma Zingiberis Officinalis) 生姜	3pce
da zao (Fructus Zizyphi Jujubae) 大枣	4pce

Method: Decoction. (Source: *Shi Yong Zhong Yi Xue*)

ZHI GAN CAO TANG 炙甘草汤
(Baked Licorice Combination)

This formula, also specific for *qi* and *yin* deficiency, is selected when palpitations and an intermittent or irregular pulse are prominent.

sheng di (Radix Rehmanniae Glutinosae) 生地	24g
zhi gan cao (honey fried Radix Glycyrrhizae Uralensis) 炙甘草	12g
ren shen (Radix Ginseng) 人参	6g
gui zhi (Ramulus Cinnamomi Cassiae) 桂枝	9g
mai dong (Tuber Ophiopogonis Japonici) 麦冬	9g
e jiao^ (Gelatinum Corii Asini) 阿胶	6g
huo ma ren (Semen Cannabis Sativae) 火麻仁	9g

sheng jiang (Rhizoma Zingiberis Officinalis) 生姜 9g
da zao (Fructus Zizyphi Jujubae) 大枣 5pce
Method: Decoction. **E jiao** is melted in the hot strained decoction (*yang hua* 烊化). A possible alternative to **huo ma ren** (if it is unavailable) is **da hu ma** (Semen Linum Usitatissimum) 大胡麻. (Source: *Shi Yong Zhong Yi Nei Ke Xue*)

YI GUAN JIAN 一贯煎
(*Linking Decoction*)

This formula is chosen when Liver and Kidney *yin* deficiency with *qi* stagnation give rise to chest and hypochondriac pain, epigastric and abdominal distension, dry mouth and throat, acid reflux, a red dry tongue and a thready wiry pulse. The correct treatment is to nourish *yin* and spread Liver *qi*.

sheng di (Radix Rehmanniae Glutinosae) 生地 18-45g
gou qi zi (Fructus Lycii) 枸杞子 9-18g
sha shen (Radix Adenophorae seu Glehniae) 沙参 9g
mai dong (Tuber Ophiopogonis Japonici) 麦冬 9g
dang gui (Radix Angelicae Sinensis) 当归 9g
chuan lian zi* (Fructus Meliae Toosendan) 川楝子 4.5g
Method: Decoction. (Source: *Formulas and Strategies*)

ZUO GUI YIN 左归饮
(*Restore the Left Decoction*)

This formula is selected as the guiding formula when Kidney *yin* deficiency is predominant.

shu di (Radix Rehmanniae Glutinosae Conquitae) 熟地 24g
fu ling (Sclerotium Poriae Cocos) 茯苓 12g
shan yao (Radix Dioscoreae Oppositae) 山药 9g
gou qi zi (Fructus Lycii) 枸杞子 9g
shan zhu yu (Fructus Corni Officinalis) 山茱萸 9g
zhi gan cao (honey fried Radix Glycyrrhizae Uralensis)
炙甘草 6g
Method: Decoction. (Source: *Shi Yong Zhong Yi Nei Ke Xue*)

SHENG MAI SAN 生脉散
(*Generate the Pulse Powder*) plus
DAN SHEN YIN 丹参饮
(*Salvia Decoction*) modified

This combination is selected when *yin* and Blood are both deficient, with chest pain, palpitations, shortness of breath, fatigue and weakness, postural dizziness, dry mouth and throat, insomnia, restlessness, forgetfulness, night sweats, a pale or pink dry tongue with a red dry tip and thready rapid pulse.

dan shen (Radix Salviae Miltiorrhizae) 丹参	30g
mai dong (Tuber Ophiopogonis Japonici) 麦冬	15g
gua lou (Fructus Trichosanthis) 栝楼	15g
yu jin (Tuber Curcumae) 郁金	10g
chi shao (Radix Paeoniae Rubrae) 赤芍	10g
ren shen (Radix Ginseng) 人参	9g
wu wei zi (Fructus Schizandrae Chinensis) 五味子	6g
sha ren (Fructus Amomi) 砂仁	6g
shi chang pu (Rhizoma Acori Graminei) 石菖蒲	6g
tan xiang (Lignum Santali Albi) 檀香	4g

Method: Decoction. **Sha ren** is added towards the end of cooking (*hou xia* 后下). (Source: *Zhong Yi Nei Ke Lin Chuang Shou Ce*)

The following modifications apply to all the preceding prescriptions, (where herbs mentioned below are not already included)

- With Blood stagnation, add two or three of the following herbs: **dang gui** (Radix Angelicae Sinensis) 当归 9g, **dan shen** (Radix Salviae Miltiorrhizae) 丹参 15g, **chuan xiong** (Radix Ligustici Chuanxiong) 川芎 6g, **mu dan pi** (Cortex Moutan Radicis) 牡丹皮 9g, **chi shao** (Radix Paeoniae Rubrae) 赤芍 9g, **yu jin** (Tuber Curcumae) 郁金 9g.

- With *yang* rising or deficient Heat (dizziness, blurring vision, facial flushing and numbness in the limbs), add two or three of the following herbs: **he shou wu** (Radix Polygoni Multiflori) 何首乌 12g, **nu zhen zi** (Fructus Ligustri Lucidi) 女贞子 12g, **gou teng** (Ramulus Uncariae) 钩藤 12g, **shi jue ming**^ (Concha Haliotidis) 石决明 15g, **mu li**^ (Concha Ostreae) 牡蛎 15g, **gui ban**° (Plastri Testudinis) 龟板 12g, **bie jia**° (Carapax Amydae Sinensis) 鳖甲 12g, **zhen zhu mu**^ (Concha Margaritaferae) 珍珠母 15g, **long gu**^ (Os Draconis) 龙骨 15g.

- With stagnant *qi*, herbs that gently regulate *qi* without warming or drying are selected. Add two or three of the following herbs: **gua lou** (Fructus Trichosanthis) 栝楼 24g, **yu jin** (Tuber Curcumae) 郁金 9g, **zhi shi** (Fructus Immaturus Citri Aurantii) 枳实 6g, **mei gui hua** (Flos Rosae Rugosae) 玫瑰花 6g, **he huan pi** (Cortex Albizziae Julibrissin) 合欢皮 12g, **chuan lian zi*** (Fructus Meliae Toosendan) 川楝子 6g or **yan hu suo** (Rhizoma Corydalis Yanhusuo) 延胡索 9g.

Patent medicines

Tian Wang Bu Xin Dan 天王补心丹 (Tian Wang Bu Xin Dan) - excellent for Heart *yin* deficiency with *shen* disturbance

Zuo Gui Wan 左归丸 (Zuo Gui Wan)

Sheng Mai Wan 生脉丸 (Sheng Mai Wan)

Liu Wei Di Huang Wan 六味地黄丸 (Liu Wei Di Huang Wan)
 - a general Kidney *yin* tonic formula
Zhu Sha An Shen Wan 朱砂安神丸 (Cinnabar Sedative Pills)
 - this pill can be combined with any other prescription (for a few weeks only) to treat Heart *yin* deficiency patterns with severe anxiety

Acupuncture

Bl.15 (*xin shu* +), Bl.14 (*jue yin shu* +), Bl.23 (*shen shu* +), Kid.3 (*tai xi* +), Ht.7 (*shen men*), Ht.5 (*tong li*), PC.6 (*nei guan*), Ren.17 (*shan zhong*), *yin tang* (M-HN-3), Lu.7 (*lie que*), Kid.6 (*zhao hai*)

Clinical notes

- The chest pain in this pattern may correspond to disorders such as angina pectoris, cardiac arrhythmia, convalescent stage of febrile disease and tuberculosis.
- *Yin* deficiency often combines with Blood stasis and/or Phlegm, both of which present a clinical challenge as Phlegm resolving and Blood stasis removing herbs can both damage *yin*. The mild end of both categories of herbs can be used, but should be monitored closely for unwanted effects. All patterns with *yin* deficiency generally require persistent and long term treatment.
- Herbs are generally better at replenishing *yin* than acupuncture, although the combination of both is best.

SUMMARY OF GUIDING FORMULAE FOR CHEST PAIN

Excess patterns

Heat scorching and knotting *qi* in the chest - *Xiao Xian Xiong Tang* 小陷胸汤

Phlegm obstructing Heart *yang*
- Phlegm Fluids - *Gua Lou Xie Bai Ban Xia Tang* 瓜楼薤白半夏汤
- Turbid Phlegm - *Wen Dan Tang* 温胆汤
- Phlegm Fire - *Huang Lian Wen Dan Tang* 黄连温胆汤
- Wind Phlegm - *Di Tan Tang* 涤痰汤

Qi stagnation - *Chai Hu Shu Gan San* 柴胡疏肝散
- with prominent stuffiness - *Xuan Fu Hua Tang* 旋复花汤

Cold congealing Heart Blood circulation
- mild cases - *Dang Gui Si Ni Tang* 当归四逆汤
- severe cases - *Wu Tou Chi Shi Zhi Wan* 乌头赤石脂丸
- with collapse of *yang* + *Guan Xin Su He Xiang Wan* 冠心苏合香丸

Blood stagnation - *Xue Fu Zhu Yu Tang* 血府逐瘀汤
- after trauma - *Fu Yuan Huo Xue Tang* 复元活血汤

Deficient patterns

Heart *yang* deficiency - *Li Zhong Wan* 理中丸
- Heart and Kidney *yang* deficiency with pulmonary oedema - *Zhen Wu Tang* 真武汤
- in convalescent stage, with Kidney deficiency - *Jin Kui Shen Qi Wan* 金匮肾气丸
- with collapse of *yang* + *Guan Xin Su He Xiang Wan* 冠心苏合香丸

Heart (Lung and Spleen) *qi* deficiency - *Bao Yuan Tang* 保元汤

Heart and Kidney *yin* deficiency - *Tian Wang Bu Xin Dan* 天王补心丹
- with *qi* and *yin* deficiency, with severe palpitations - *Zhi Gan Cao Tang* 炙甘草汤
- with Liver *yin* deficiency and *qi* stagnation - *Yi Guan Jian* 一贯煎
- predominant Kidney *yin* deficiency - *Zuo Gui Wan* 左归丸

Endnote

For more information regarding herbs marked with an asterisk*, an open circle° or a hatˆ, see the tables on pp.944-952.

Disorders of the Heart

29. Palpitations

Heart *qi* deficiency
Heart *yang* deficiency
Heart *yin* deficiency
Heart Blood and Spleen *qi* deficiency
Heart and Gall Bladder *qi* deficiency
Phlegm Heat
Spleen and Kidney *yang* deficiency
Blood stagnation

29 | PALPITATIONS
jing ji 惊悸, *zheng chong* 怔忡

Palpitations are an unpleasant and sometimes alarming awareness of the beating of the heart. The term palpitations includes not only an awareness of the heart racing (tachycardia), but also any sensation in the chest, such as 'pounding', 'flip flops', 'thumping', 'skipping', or 'fluttering'.
Chinese medicine describes two types of palpitations, with and without organic dysfunction. The first type (*zheng chong* 怔忡) is due to organic dysfunction of the heart or other organ system. *Zheng chong* palpitations are generally chronic, and brought on by even mild exertion, stress and fatigue. The other type (*jing ji* 惊悸) is primarily a disorder of the *shen* and is provoked by anxiety, fright or some other emotion. The patient suffering *jing ji* is generally in otherwise good health and the heart pathology is relatively benign.

The mechanisms of these two broad types of palpitations are quite different, although in practice there is often considerable overlap due to the intimate relationship between the Heart and *shen*. *Zheng chong* involves an actual weakness of the heart muscle or disordered signalling to the heart. The palpitations associated with this type may include irregularities in heart rate, tachycardia, bradycardia, fibrillation, missed beats and signs of circulatory disturbance. *Jing ji* on the other hand, is frequently a subjective palpitation, that is, the heart is perceived by the patient to be racing or skipping beats but objective examination may detect no abnormality. The most common sensation associated with *jing ji* is an awareness of accelerated heart rate, provoked by some emotion or fright. In *jing ji*, the *shen* is destabilised and becomes vulnerable and hypersensitive in the absence of a sound residence, namely the Heart.

Of the commonly recognised patterns associated with palpitations, Heart *qi* and *yang* deficiency, Spleen and Kidney *yang* deficiency and Blood stagnation are most often associated with organic heart disease–*zheng chong*. Heart *yin*

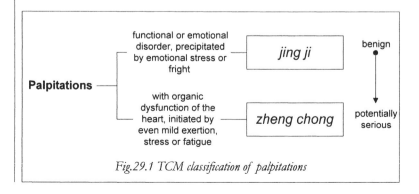

Fig.29.1 TCM classification of palpitations

deficiency, Heart Blood and Spleen deficiency, Heart and Gall Bladder deficiency and Phlegm Heat tend to give rise to palpitations through disturbance of the *shen–jing ji*. However, as noted above, because the Heart and *shen* are so closely related, disturbance of one can easily lead to disturbance of the other and the distinctions between the two types may be clinically blurred.

AETIOLOGY

Heart *yang* and *qi* deficiency

Kidney *yang* deficiency is often at the root of Heart *yang* deficiency, and Spleen *qi* deficiency is often at the root of Heart *qi* deficiency. In addition, Heart *qi* is easily dispersed by prolonged, excessive or unexpressed grief, sadness, anxiety or depression. Excessive coffee (bitter in taste) consumption appears to disperse Heart *qi*, especially when consumed in unusually large or unaccustomed quantities. Excessive sweating can also damage Heart *yang* and *qi*.

> **BOX 29.1 SOME BIOMEDICAL CAUSES OF PALPITATIONS**
> - anxiety/stress
> - fever
> - anaemia
> - hyperthyroidism
> - neuresthenia
> - myocarditis
> - myocardial infarction
> - paroxysmal supraventricular tachycardia
> - mitral stenosis
> - coronary ischaemia
> - heart failure
> - hypovolaemia
> - aortic incompetence
> - atrioventricular block
> - pulmonary embolism
> - pericarditis
> - sick sinus syndrome
> - rheumatic fever
> - hypokalaemia
> - menopause
> - hypercapnoea
>
> **Drugs**
> - caffeine
> - alcohol
> - amphetamines
> - salbutamol
> - tricyclic antidepressants
> - adrenaline
> - atropine

Heart *yin* deficiency (with Heat)

Heart *yin*, like Heart Blood, is depleted by ongoing emotional distress of any kind, but especially shock, anxiety or worry. Any factors that damage Kidney or Liver *yin* may also lead to depletion of Heart *yin*, due to lack of support through the generative (*sheng* 生, p.70) cycle. Heart *yin* can also be damaged by excessive sweating and by febrile diseases.

Heart Blood (and Spleen *qi*) deficiency

Heart Blood is most commonly depleted by prolonged worry or anxiety. The condition may also develop or be exacerbated if the Spleen is weak. In addition, if too much fluid is lost through haemorrhage or excessive sweating, then Heart Blood can be damaged. Finally, any factors that deplete Liver Blood will eventually also deplete Heart Blood.

Heart and Gall Bladder deficiency

This pattern describes a personality type that may be congenital or acquired. When congenital, it may be due to a significant shock that damaged the foetal *shen* during the mother's pregnancy. When acquired it is the result of some sudden and violent or extreme shock or fright, especially during childhood, as the *shen* is more unstable in the young. Often it is the combination of a congenital Heart and Gall Bladder weakness and some critical event that most effectively drain Heart and Gall Bladder *qi*. This pattern can occasionally be more acute, following a debilitating illnesses that drains *qi*.

Because the *shen* is so destabilised, it cannot cope easily with change and can be easily disturbed by trivial events. Palpitations may occur spontaneously and gradually worsen over time until they are constant. These patients are prone to anxiety, and worry about their health can set up a self perpetuating cycle–anxiety about their heart condition causes palpitations which in turn causes more anxiety and so on.

The involvement of the Gall Bladder here refers to the anxiety, timidity and 'lack of gall' (that is, fearfulness) to which these patients are prone. In the Chinese language (as in English) there is an implicit understanding of the relationship between the Gall Bladder and courage, indeed to be bold or courageous is to have a 'big Gall Bladder' (*da dan* 大胆).

Phlegm Heat

Phlegm Heat can be generated in several ways. First, the presence of Phlegm or Dampness due to Spleen weakness or overconsumption of Phlegm producing foods causes stagnation and Heat. Second, overconsumption of Phlegm Heat foods (rich, greasy, spicy food and alcohol) and tobacco can cause an accumulation of Phlegm Heat directly. Third, any pre-existing Heat in the body, due to Liver *qi* stagnation, *yin* deficiency or external invasion can congeal fluids into Phlegm, and subsequently Phlegm Heat. Phlegm Heat patterns are also observed in the convalescent stage of a febrile illness.

Spleen and Kidney *yang* deficiency

Failure of Spleen and Kidney *yang's* fluid transforming and metabolising action may lead to an accumulation of pathogenic fluids above the diaphragm. These accumulated fluids can disrupt Heart function. Spleen *yang* is weakened by excessive consumption of cold raw food and irregular eating habits, or by too many cold natured herbs (or antibiotics) in the treatment of a febrile disease. Excessive mental strain or prolonged concentration may deplete Spleen *qi*. The damage is aggravated when an irregular diet is combined with excessive mental activity (frequently seen in students and overworked executives).

Kidney *yang* deficiency may be an inherited condition, or may develop as a result of age, chronic illness, overexertion, overexposure to cold conditions, excessive lifting or standing, or in men by excessive ejaculation and in women by having many pregnancies.

Blood stagnation

Blood stagnation is usually a complication of some other Heart pathology, and typically occurs late in the course of an illness. The Heart 'rules the Blood', that is, it is responsible for physically moving Blood around the body. If it malfunctions, it is common to see symptoms of circulatory dysfunction and stagnation of Blood. Specifically, pooling of Blood in the vessels occurs if the pumping action of the Heart is weak (from Heart *qi* or *yang* deficiency), and congealing of the Blood due to increased viscosity can occur if there is a lack of fluids (Heart Blood or *yin* deficiency). In addition, circulation may be compromised by Cold (*yang* deficiency) or obstructed by Phlegm.

TREATMENT

The treatment of palpitations involves two approaches. In the cases of *zheng chong*, the disorder is likely to be chronic and the functional strength of the Heart is weakened. *Zheng chong* disorders are primarily deficiency patterns and treatment requires tonification of *yang*, *yin* or Blood. These patterns generally take longer to treat satisfactorily than the milder *jing ji* patterns.

Jing ji disorders, on the other hand, are primarily disorders of the *shen*. Treatment requires methods that settle, sedate and calm the *shen*. Acupuncture is particularly effective in calming the *shen*. In general, *jing ji* patterns respond quickly (with the exception of congenital Heart and Gall Bladder deficiency). Bear in mind when deciding upon treatment that *zheng chong* and *jing ji* patterns often overlap and a mixture of approaches including tonifying, Blood activating and *shen* calming may be required.

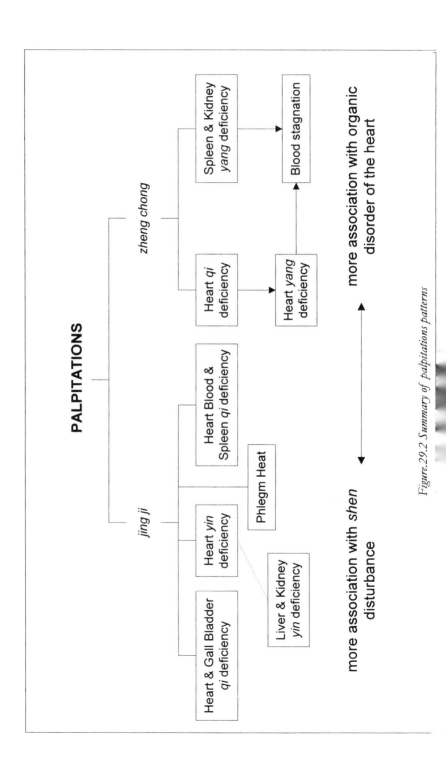

Figure 29.2 Summary of palpitations patterns

29.1 HEART *QI* DEFICIENCY

Pathophysiology
- Heart *qi* powers the regular and rhythmic contraction of the Heart. Weakened Heart *qi* leads to a disruption of the regularity and strength of contraction. This can give rise to missed beats, tachycardia, bradycardia or irregularity of rhythm.

Clinical features
- palpitations initiated or aggravated by exertion and relieved with rest
- fitful sleep, insomnia
- shortness of breath
- dizziness
- physical and mental fatigue
- pale complexion
- spontaneous sweating

T pale with a thin white coat
P thready and weak, possibly irregular

Treatment principle
Tonify and nourish Heart *qi*

Prescription

WU WEI ZI TANG 五味子汤
(*Schizandra Decoction*) modified

wu wei zi (Fructus Schizandrae Chinensis) 五味子	6g
mai dong (Tuber Ophiopogonis Japonici) 麦冬	9g
huang qi (Radix Astragali Membranacei) 黄芪	12g
ren shen (Radix Ginseng) 人参	9g
suan zao ren (Semen Zizyphi Spinosae) 酸枣仁	12g
bai zi ren (Semen Biotae Orientalis) 柏子仁	9g
he huan pi (Cortex Albizziae Julibrissin) 合欢皮	9g
gan cao (Radix Glycyrrhizae Uralensis) 甘草	3g

Method: Decoction. (Source: *Shi Yong Zhong Yi Nei Ke Xue*)

Modifications
- With severe *qi* deficiency, add **huang jing** (Rhizoma Polygonati) 黄精 12g, and increase the dose of **huang qi** to 24g.
- With copious sweating, add **mu li^** (Concha Ostreae) 牡蛎 18g, **ma huang gen** (Radix Ephedrae) 麻黄根 12g, **fu xiao mai** (Semen Tritici Aestivi Levis) 浮小麦 12g.
- With severe insomnia, add **ye jiao teng** (Caulis Polygoni Multiflori)

夜交藤 15g and **long chi**^ (Dens Draconis) 龙齿 10g.

Patent medicines
Gui Pi Wan 归脾丸 (Gui Pi Wan)
Sheng Mai Wan 生脉丸 (Sheng Mai Wan)
Bai Zi Yang Xin Wan 柏子养心丸 (Bai Zi Yang Xin Wan)
Ding Xin Wan 定心丸 (Ding Xin Wan)

Acupuncture
Bl.15 (*xin shu* +), PC.5 (*jian shi* +), Ht.7 (*shen men* +), Ht.5 (*tong li*), Ren.14 (*ju que* +), St.36 (*zu san li* +), Ren.6 (*qi hai* +)
- with spontaneous sweating, add Bl.43 (*gao huang shu*) and Du.14 (*da zhui* ▲)

Clinical notes
- The palpitations in this pattern may be associated with disorders such as anaemia, sinus tachycardia, premature ectopic beats, anxiety or sick sinus syndrome.
- This pattern is closely related to and often precedes the next pattern, Heart *yang* deficiency.
- This pattern generally responds well to correct TCM treatment.
- *Qi gong*, *tai chi*, yoga or a carefully monitored and graded exercise program can gradually build the *qi* and strengthen the Heart.

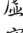

29.2 HEART *YANG* DEFICIENCY

Pathophysiology
- Heart *yang* deficiency is a more serious pathology than Heart *qi* deficiency, and is more likely to develop if there is constitutional or pre-existing Spleen and Kidney *yang* deficiency. The palpitations are generally more severe and the Heart is relatively weaker. In addition to the contractile weakness of the Heart, signs of Cold and fluid accumulation may appear. Heart *yang* deficiency is associated with *zheng chong*.

Clinical features
- palpitations initiated or aggravated by exertion and relieved with rest
- shortness of breath with exertion, in severe cases dyspnoea or orthopnoea
- stuffiness or discomfort in the chest
- listlessness and fatigue
- cold extremities, aversion to cold
- spontaneous sweating
- waxy pale complexion, dark rings under the eyes, purple lips, cyanosis
- pitting oedema, in which cases urine is scanty, or nocturia or frequent urination

T pale bluish or pale purple and swollen, with a white or greasy coat
P deficient, thready, weak, slow or knotted and intermittent

Treatment principle
Warm, tonify and strengthen Heart *yang*

Prescription

GUI ZHI GAN CAO LONG GU MU LI TANG 桂枝甘草龙骨牡蛎汤
(*Cinnamon, Licorice, Dragon Bone and Oyster Shell Decoction*) modified

gui zhi (Ramulus Cinnamomi Cassiae) 桂枝	6g
long gu^ (Os Draconis) 龙骨	15g
mu li^ (Concha Ostreae) 牡蛎	30g
ren shen (Radix Ginseng) 人参	9g
zhi fu zi* (Radix Aconiti Carmichaeli Praeparata) 制附子	9g
fu ling (Sclerotium Poriae Cocos) 茯苓	15g
zhi gan cao (honey fried Radix Glycyrrhizae Uralensis) 炙甘草	6g

Method: Decoction. **Zhi fu zi** should be cooked for 30 minutes before the other herbs are added (*xian jian* 先煎). (Source: *Zhong Yi Nei Ke Lin Chuang Shou Ce*)

ZHEN WU TANG 真武汤
(*True Warrior Decoction*) modified

This formula is selected if there is Heart and Kidney *yang* deficiency with generalised and pulmonary oedema, scanty urine, dyspnoea, orthopnoea and frothy sputum. The correct treatment is to warm the *yang* and promote urination until the fluid balance is controlled. When fluids are moving the original prescription or another suitable tonifying prescription should be selected.

zhi fu zi* (Radix Aconiti Carmichaeli Praeparata) 制附子	9g
chao bai zhu (dry fried Rhizoma Atractylodis Macrocephalae) 炒白术	9g
sheng jiang (Rhizoma Zingiberis Officinalis) 生姜	9g
bai shao (Radix Paeoniae Lactiflora) 白芍	12g
fu ling (Sclerotium Poriae Cocos) 茯苓	12g
che qian zi (Semen Plantaginis) 车前子	12g
ze xie (Rhizoma Alismatis Orientalis) 泽泻	12g

Method: Decoction. **Zhi fu zi** should be cooked for 30 minutes before the other herbs are added (*xian jian* 先煎), **che qian zi** is usually cooked in a muslin bag (*bao jian* 包煎). (Source: *Shi Yong Zhong Yi Nei Ke Xue*)

Modifications

♦ With Cold, add two or three of the following herbs: **lu rong pian**ˆ (sliced Cornu Cervi Parvum) 鹿茸片 3g, **chuan jiao** (Pericarpium Zanthoxyli Bungeani) 川椒 6g, **wu zhu yu** (Fructus Evodiae Rutaecarpae) 吴茱萸 6g, **bi ba** (Fructus Piperis Longi) 荜拔 3g, **gao liang jiang** (Rhizoma Alpiniae Officinari) 高良姜 9g, **xi xin*** (Herba cum Radice Asari) 细辛 6g or **chi shi zhi** (Halloysitum Rubrum) 赤石脂 15g.

Variations and additional prescriptions

With Kidney yang *deficiency*

♦ If Kidney *yang* is deficient, consider **JIN KUI SHEN QI WAN** (*Rehmannia Eight Formula* 金匮肾气丸, p.874) or **YOU GUI WAN** (*Eucommia and Rehmannia Formula* 右归丸, p.559) once the palpitations are under control. Both of these formulae are suitable for long term use.

Collapse of Heart yang

♦ In severe cases see Box 28.2, p.756. The patient is cold and clammy, cyanotic, pale and has icy extremities and a fibrillating pulse, indicating imminent collapse of Heart *yang*. The correct approach is to administer an emergency medicine such as **GUAN XIN SU HE XIANG WAN**

(*Liquid Styrax Pills for Coronary Heart Disease* 冠心苏合香丸), and institute the emergency acupuncture techniques outlined in Box.28.2 until paramedic assistance arrives. An alternative approach used in hospitals in China is **SHEN FU TANG** (*Ginseng and Prepared Aconite Decoction* 参附汤, p.665) plus **long gu**ˆ (Os Draconis) 龙骨 15-30g and **mu li**ˆ (Concha Ostreae) 牡蛎 15-30g administered intravenously.

Patent medicines

Jin Kui Shen Qi Wan 金匮肾气丸 (Sexoton Pills)

Fu Zi Li Zhong Wan 附子理中丸 (Li Chung Yuen Medical Pills)
  - good for warming *yang* generally, inclusing Heart *yang*

Xiao Huo Luo Dan 小活络丹 (Xiao Huo Luo Dan)
  - a small dose of this very hot medicine may be useful in severe cases.

Acupuncture

Bl.15 (*xin shu* +▲), Bl.14 (*jue yin shu* +▲), PC.6 (*nei guan* +), Ht.5. (*tong li*), Ht.7 (*shen men* +), Ren.4 (*guan yuan* +▲), St.36 (*zu san li* +▲)

Clinical notes

- The palpitations in this pattern may be associated with disorders such as congestive cardiac failure, atrial fibrillation or coronary artery disease.
- Symptoms of mild Heart *yang* deficiency may respond well to correct TCM treatment, fluid metabolism especially improves fairly quickly. Long term therapy is necessary to maintain the result. In severe cases it can be difficult to treat, especially patients presenting with Heart and Kidney *yang* deficiency. These patients are usually on the maximum dose of conventional medicine.
- In general, Heart *yang* deficiency is the predisposing pathology for more serious (and possibly fatal) cardiac episodes.

29.3 HEART *YIN* DEFICIENCY

Pathophysiology
- Heart *yin* deficiency can cause palpitations in two ways—by creating deficient Heat and by not stabilising and anchoring the *shen*. When there is *yin* deficiency, the false Heat that arises agitates the *shen* and Heart. When the *shen* is not anchored by *yin* (or Blood), the resulting instability causes the *shen* to be more vulnerable to sudden fright or shock, and palpitations easily ensue.

Clinical features
- palpitations, easily brought on by a start or fright
- insomnia, waking with palpitations or panic attacks and anxiety
- sensation of heat in the palms and soles ('five hearts hot')
- night sweats
- dry mouth and throat
- dizziness and tinnitus
- restlessness and fatigue
- poor concentration and memory, forgetfulness
- lower back ache
- dry stools or constipation
- possibly mouth or tongue ulcers

T red and dry with little or no coat
P thready and rapid

Treatment principle
Nourish Heart *yin*, calm the *shen*
Clear Heat

Prescription

TIAN WANG BU XIN DAN 天王补心丹
(*Ginseng and Zizyphus Formula*)

This is the basic Heart (and Kidney) *yin* deficiency formula, and is selected when the *shen* symptoms (anxiety, insomnia, panic attacks) are prominent.

- **sheng di** (Radix Rehmanniae Glutinosae) 生地 .... 120 (24)g
- **tian dong** (Tuber Asparagi Cochinchinensis) 天冬 .... 30 (12)g
- **mai dong** (Tuber Ophiopogonis Japonici) 麦冬 .... 30 (12)g
- **suan zao ren** (Semen Zizyphi Spinosae) 酸枣仁 .... 30 (12)g
- **xuan shen** (Radix Scrophulariae) 玄参 .... 15 (12)g
- **dan shen** (Radix Salviae Miltiorrhizae) 丹参 .... 15 (12)g
- **fu ling** (Sclerotium Poriae Cocos) 茯苓 .... 15 (12)g
- **dang gui** (Radix Angelicae Sinensis) 当归 .... 30 (9)g

wu wei zi (Fructus Schizandrae Chinensis) 五味子 .... 30 (9)g
bai zi ren (Semen Biotae Orientalis) 柏子仁 .... 30 (9)g
ren shen (Radix Ginseng) 人参 .... 15 (9)g
jie geng (Radix Platycodi Grandiflori) 桔梗 .... 15 (9)g
yuan zhi (Radix Polygalae Tenuifoliae) 远志 .... 15 (6)g
zhu sha* (Cinnabaris) 朱砂 (optional) .... 6 (0.5)g

Method: Grind herbs (except **zhu sha**) to a powder and form into 9-gram pills with honey. If used, coat the outside of the pills with the **zhu sha**. The dose is one pill 2-3 times daily. May also be decocted with the dosage in brackets. When decocted the **zhu sha** is taken as powder with the strained decoction. This is an excellent formula for long term use in treating *yin* deficiency with *shen* disturbance, in which case the **zhu sha** is deleted. (Source: *Shi Yong Zhong Yi Nei Ke Xue*)

SHENG MAI SAN 生脉散
(*Generate the Pulse Powder*) modified

This formula is selected if the palpitations occur following a febrile illness which has consumed Heart *qi* and *yin*. The signs and symptoms are a stifling sensation in the chest, shortness of breath, sweating, dry mouth and thirst, poor sleep, a pale red and dry tongue and a knotted or irregular pulse. This may occur following profuse sweating (as in heat stroke).

ren shen (Radix Ginseng) 人参 9-15g
mai dong (Tuber Ophiopogonis Japonici) 麦冬 9-12g
wu wei zi (Fructus Schizandrae Chinensis) 五味子 3-6g
gui zhi (Ramulus Cinnamomi Cassiae) 桂枝 6g
long gu^ (Os Draconis) 龙骨 15g
mu li^ (Concha Ostreae) 牡蛎 30g

Method: Decoction. (Source: *Formulas and Strategies*)

ZHU SHA AN SHEN WAN 朱砂安神丸
(*Cinnabar Pill to Calm the Spirit*)

This formula is selected when severe or continuous palpitations are accompanied by insomnia, anxiety and Heat. It is more sedative than the primary formula and designed to treat and control the symptoms quickly. Because it contains **zhu sha**, it is not suitable for prolonged use and once the condition is under control other more tonifying formulae should be used.

huang lian (Rhizoma Coptidis) 黄连 45g
zhu sha* (Cinnabaris) 朱砂 30g
dang gui (Radix Angelicae Sinensis) 当归 30g
sheng di (Radix Rehmanniae Glutinosae) 生地 30g
fu ling (Sclerotium Poriae Cocos) 茯苓 30g
suan zao ren (Semen Zizyphi Spinosae) 酸枣仁 30g
yuan zhi (Radix Polygalae Tenuifoliae) 远志 15g

zhi gan cao (honey fried Radix Glycyrrhizae Uralensis)
炙甘草 15g

Method: Grind herbs (except **zhu sha**) to a powder and form into 3-gram pills with honey. Coat the outside of the pills with the **zhu sha**. The dose is 1-2 pills daily. May also be decocted with a 60% reduction in dosage. **Huang lian** is reduced by 90%. If decocted the **zhu sha** (0.5g) is taken with the strained decoction (*chong fu* 冲服). (Source: *Shi Yong Zhong Yao Xue*)

HUANG LIAN E JIAO TANG 黄连阿胶汤
(*Coptis and Ass-Hide Gelatin Decoction*) modified

This formula is selected when Heart *yin* deficiency follows a febrile disease (a type of *shao yin* syndrome, with palpitations and anxiety, a sensation of heat in the chest, insomnia and irritability, sores in the mouth and tongue, a red tongue with a dry yellow coat and a thready rapid pulse). The correct treatment is to clear Fire, nourish *yin*, stop irritability and calm the *shen*.

huang lian (Rhizoma Coptidis) 黄连 12g
e jiao^ (Gelatinum Corii Asini) 阿胶 9g
huang qin (Radix Scutellariae Baicalensis) 黄芩 6g
bai shao (Radix Paeoniae Lactiflora) 白芍 6g
long chi^ (Dens Draconis) 龙齿 9-15g
mu li^ (Concha Ostreae) 牡蛎 15-30g
ji zi huang^ (egg yolk) .... 2 yolks

Method: Decoction. **E jiao** is melted in the hot strained decoction (*yang hua* 烊化). The egg yolks are stirred into the strained decoction. (Source: *Shi Yong Zhong Yi Nei Ke Xue*)

YI GUAN JIAN 一贯煎
(*Linking Decoction*) plus
SUAN ZAO REN TANG 酸枣仁汤
(*Zizyphus Combination*) modified

This formula is used when signs of Liver and Kidney *yin* deficiency are prominent. The Heat resulting from the deficiency can accelerate the Heart. Because Liver *yin* is weak, it is often complicated by *qi* stagnation. The main features are palpitations, insomnia, 'five hearts hot', night sweats, dizziness, tinnitus, irritability, lower back pain, dry eyes, blurred vision, photophobia, headaches, epigastric and abdominal distension, acid reflux and a thready or wiry and rapid pulse.

sheng di (Radix Rehmanniae Glutinosae) 生地 18-45g
gou qi zi (Fructus Lycii) 枸杞子 9-18g
sha shen (Radix Adenophorae seu Glehniae) 沙参 9g
mai dong (Tuber Ophiopogonis Japonici) 麦冬 9g
dang gui (Radix Angelicae Sinensis) 当归 9g
chuan lian zi* (Fructus Meliae Toosendan) 川楝子 4.5g

suan zao ren (Semen Zizyphi Spinosae) 酸枣仁 15g
zhi mu (Rhizoma Anemarrhenae Asphodeloidis) 知母 9g
fu ling (Sclerotium Poriae Cocos) 茯苓 15g
chuan xiong (Radix Ligustici Chuanxiong) 川芎 6g
gan cao (Radix Glycyrrhizae Uralensis) 甘草 3g
Method: Decoction. (Source: *Shi Yong Zhong Yi Nei Ke Xue*)

Patent medicines

Tian Wang Bu Xin Dan 天王补心丹 (Tian Wang Bu Xin Dan)
  - excellent for Heart *yin* deficiency with *shen* disturbance
Zuo Gui Wan 左归丸 (Zuo Gui Wan)
Sheng Mai Wan 生脉丸 (Sheng Mai Wan)
Liu Wei Di Huang Wan 六味地黄丸 (Liu Wei Di Huang Wan)
  - a general Kidney *yin* tonic formula
Suan Zao Ren Tang Pian 酸枣仁汤片 (Tabellae Suanzaoren)
Ci Zhu Wan 磁朱丸 (Ci Zhu Wan)
  - this pill is usually combined with one of the other formulae above

Acupuncture

Bl.23 (*shen shu* +), Bl.15 (*xin shu* -), Kid.3 (*tai xi* +), Ht.5 (*tong li*), Kid.6 (*zhao hai* +), Ht.7 (*shen men*), PC.6 (*nei guan*), PC.7 (*da ling*), Liv.3 (*tai chong* +), Bl.18 (*gan shu* +), Ren.17 (*shan zhong*)
  • with Fire add Ht.8 (*shao fu*)

Clinical notes

  • The palpitations in this pattern may be associated with disorders such as menopausal syndrome, neurasthenia, mitral stenosis, hyperthyroidism, anxiety neurosis, fever of unknown origin, convalescence following a febrile disorder or coronary artery disease.
  • The palpitations in this pattern often respond well to treatment although long term resolution may depend on the biomedical syndrome with which they are associated. For example, hyperthyroid conditions can be difficult to cure with TCM and may need to be controlled by drugs or surgery if TCM treatment is ineffective, before lasting results can be acheived.

29.4 HEART BLOOD AND SPLEEN *QI* DEFICIENCY

Pathophysiology
- Heart Blood and Spleen *qi* deficiency has elements of both *zheng chong* and *jing ji*, with *qi* deficiency contributing to weakness of Heart function, and Heart Blood deficiency failing to anchor and stabilise the *shen*. It occurs most commonly when Heart Blood is depleted by emotional distress and the Spleen is weak and unable to support the Heart. Prolonged overwork and worry in combination with irregular diet (commonplace in our modern society) easily deplete the Heart and Spleen. Sometimes this type of palpitations is seen as an acute episode following haemorrhage, especially uterine or postpartum.

Clinical features
- palpitations with or without anxiety, generally worse at night
- insomnia, with particular difficulty falling asleep (and switching off the mind) and dream disturbed sleep
- anxiety, phobias, panic attacks
- forgetfulness, poor memory, poor concentration
- postural dizziness
- blurring vision, spots in the visual field
- fatigue and weakness
- poor appetite, abdominal distension after eating
- sallow complexion
- easy bruising
- heavy or prolonged menstrual periods

T pale with a thin white coat
P thready and weak

Treatment principle
Strengthen and nourish the Heart and Spleen
Tonify *qi* and Blood, calm the *shen*

Prescription

GUI PI TANG 归脾汤
(*Ginseng and Longan Combination*)

This formula is selected when there is obvious digestive weakness and signs of *shen* disturbance.

  zhi huang qi (honey fried Radix Astragali Membranacei)
    炙黄芪 15g
  suan zao ren (Semen Zizyphi Spinosae) 酸枣仁 12g
  fu ling (Sclerotium Poria Cocos) 茯苓 12g

dang shen (Radix Codonopsis Pilosulae) 党参 12g
chao bai zhu (dry fried Rhizoma Atractylodis Macrocephalae)
炒白术 9g
dang gui (Radix Angelicae Sinensis) 当归 9g
long yan rou (Arillus Euphoriae Longanae) 龙眼肉 9g
yuan zhi (Radix Polygalae Tenuifoliae) 远志 6g
mu xiang (Radix Aucklandiae Lappae) 木香 6g
zhi gan cao (honey fried Radix Glycyrrhizae Uralensis)
炙甘草 6g

Method: Decoction. (Source: *Shi Yong Zhong Yi Nei Ke Xue*)

ZHI GAN CAO TANG 炙甘草汤
(*Baked Licorice Combination*)

This is an important formula for *qi* and Blood (or *yin*) deficiency type palpitations (or arrhythmias) that are brought on by activity and are accompanied by a knotted, intermittent or irregular pulse, the latter being an important indicator for the use of this formula. This pattern has elements of both *zheng chong* and *jing ji*.

sheng di (Radix Rehmanniae Glutinosae) 生地 24g
zhi gan cao (honey fried Radix Glycyrrhizae Uralensis)
炙甘草 12g
ren shen (Radix Ginseng) 人参 6g
gui zhi (Ramulus Cinnamomi Cassiae) 桂枝 9g
mai dong (Tuber Ophiopogonis Japonici) 麦冬 9g
e jiao^ (Gelatinum Corii Asini) 阿胶 6g
huo ma ren (Semen Cannabis Sativae) 火麻仁 9g
sheng jiang (Rhizoma Zingiberis Officinalis) 生姜 9g
da zao (Fructus Zizyphi Jujubae) 大枣 5pce

Method: Decoction. **E jiao** is melted in the hot strained decoction (*yang hua* 烊化). (Source: *Shi Yong Zhong Yi Nei Ke Xue*)

Modifications (applicable to both formulae, where the herbs are not already included)

- With severe palpitations, add **hu po** (Succinum) 琥珀 2g and **zhu sha*** (Cinnabaris) 朱砂 1g.
- If Heart Blood is very deficient, add **shu di** (Radix Rehmanniae Glutinosae Conquitae) 熟地 30-50g, **bai shao** (Radix Paeoniae Lactiflora) 白芍 15g and **e jiao^** (Gelatinum Corii Asini) 阿胶 15g.
- With Liver Heat, add **shan zhi zi** (Fructus Gardeniae Jasminoidis) 山栀子 9g and **chai hu** (Radix Bupleuri) 柴胡 6g.
- With severe insomnia, add one or two of the following herbs: **wu wei zi** (Fructus Schizandrae Chinensis) 五味子 6g, **bai zi ren** (Semen Biotae

Orientalis) 柏子仁 9g, **ye jiao teng** (Caulis Polygoni Multiflori) 夜交藤 30g, **he huan pi** (Cortex Albizziae Julibrissin) 合欢皮 9g, **long chi^** (Dens Draconis) 龙齿 10g, **mu li^** (Concha Ostreae) 牡蛎 30g.
- With abdominal and epigastric fullness, poor appetite, a greasy or glossy tongue coat, add **ban xia*** (Rhizoma Pinelliae Ternatae) 半夏 10g and **chen pi** (Pericarpium Citri Reticulatae) 陈皮 10g.
- With forgetfulness and poor concentration, add **shi chang pu** (Rhizoma Acori Graminei) 石菖蒲 6g.

Patent medicines
Gui Pi Wan 归脾丸 (Gui Pi Wan)
Bai Zi Yang Xin Wan 柏子养心丸 (Bai Zi Yang Xin Wan)
Dang Gui Ji Jing 当归鸡精 (Tang Kuei Essence of Chicken)
Bu Nao Wan 补脑丸 (Cerebral Tonic Pills)

Acupuncture
Sp.6 (*san yin jiao* +), St.36 (*zu san li* +), Ht.5 (*tong li* +), Bl.20 (*pi shu* +), *yin tang* (M-HN-3), Ht.7 (*shen men* +), Bl.15 (*xin shu* +), Bl.17 (*ge shu* +)
- with forgetfulness, add Du.20 (*bai hui*), Bl.52 (*zhi shi*)
- with much dreaming, add Bl.42 (*po hu*)
- with anxiety, add Du.19 (*hou ding*) and Du.24 (*shen ting*)

Clinical notes
- The palpitations in this pattern may be associated with disorders such as neurosis, anaemia, thrombocytopoenia, neuresthenia, chronic fatigue syndrome, post partum haemorrhage, sinus tachycardia, premature ectopic beats, sick sinus syndrome and arrhythmia.
- Heart and Spleen deficiency palpitations are generally very responsive to treatment, which should continue until it is clear the Spleen is strong enough to make sufficient Blood. Careful diet and eating patterns will enhance the result. A strictly regular bedtime routine should be adhered to.
- Acupuncture can be very effective at tonifying Spleen *qi* but if the patient is already very Blood deficient, herbs will probably be necessary as well.
- In women who lose blood (and thus Heart Blood) through heavy periods, Blood tonics and Blood replenishing and iron-rich foods should be taken after each period. Iron supplements are also useful.

29.5 HEART AND GALL BLADDER *QI* DEFICIENCY

Pathophysiology
- In Heart and Gall Bladder deficiency palpitations, the *shen* is congenitally unstable, or disrupted by a major shock or fright. The instability causes the patient to experience palpitations and anxiety with seemingly trivial events. In congenital cases there will usually be a long, often lifelong history of emotional timidity.

Clinical features
- palpitations, which may be initiated by anxiety or a fright
- apprehension, easily frightened and startled, timidity, anxiety
- insomnia, dream disturbed sleep, waking feeling anxious
- spontaneous sweating
- shortness of breath
- lethargy and fatigue

T normal or with a pale body and a thin white coat; in congenital or long standing cases there may be a deep narrow crack to the tip
P slightly weak, thready and rapid or thready and wiry

Treatment principle
Settle the mind, calm the *shen*
Nourish and tranquilise the Heart

Prescription

DING ZHI WAN 定志丸
(*Settle the Emotions Pill*) modified

This prescription is useful for palpitations and congenital *shen* instability in a frail and timid person. It is suited to long term use.

ren shen (Radix Ginseng) 人参	90g
fu ling (Sclerotium Poriae Cocos) 茯苓	90g
shi chang pu (Rhizoma Acori Graminei) 石菖蒲	60g
yuan zhi (Radix Polygalae Tenuifoliae) 远志	60g
long gu˘ (Os Draconis) 龙骨	60g
hu po (Succinum) 琥珀	30g

Method: Grind herbs to a powder and form into 9-gram pills with honey. The dose is 1 pill twice daily. May also be decocted with an 90% reduction in dosage.
(Source: *Formulas and Strategies*)

Modifications
- With Blood deficiency, add **dang gui** (Radix Angelicae Sinensis) 当归 60g and **bai shao** (Radix Paeoniae Lactiflora) 白芍 60g.

GUI ZHI JIA LONG GU MU LI TANG 桂枝加龙骨牡蛎汤
(Cinnamon and Dragon Bone Combination)

This formula is selected if following a major shock or trauma, there are palpitations with anxiety, insomnia and dream or nightmare disturbed sleep, hair loss, spontaneous sweating, loss of appetite, dizziness, depression, lack of motivation, a slightly pale tongue and a hollow slow pulse. This is typical of severed communication between the Heart and Kidneys due to shock.

> **gui zhi** (Ramulus Cinnamomi Cassiae) 桂枝 9g
> **bai shao** (Radix Paeoniae Lactiflora) 白芍 9g
> **long gu^** (Os Draconis) 龙骨 15-30g
> **mu li^** (Concha Ostreae) 牡蛎 15-30g
> **sheng jiang** (Rhizoma Zingiberis Officinalis) 生姜 9g
> **da zao** (Fructus Zizyphi Jujubae) 大枣 4pce
> **gan cao** (Radix Glycyrrhizae Uralensis) 甘草 6g
> Method: Decoction. (Source: *Formulas and Strategies*)

Patent medicines
Bu Nao Wan 补脑丸 (Cerebral Tonic Pills)
Ding Xin Wan 定心丸 (Ding Xin Wan)
Yang Xin Ning Shen Wan 养心宁神丸 (Ning San Yuen Medical Pills)

Acupuncture
Bl.15 (*xin shu* +), PC.6 (*nei guan*), Ht.5 (*tong li*), Ht.7 (*shen men* +), Ren.14 (*ju que*), Du.20 (*bai hui*), GB.40 (*qiu xu*), Bl.7 (*tong tian*), Ht.9 (*shao chong*), Du.19 (*hou ding*), Du.24 (*shen ting*)

Clinical notes
- The palpitations in this pattern may be associated with disorders such as anxiety neurosis, neuresthenia, involutional psychosis, premenstrual syndrome, sinus tachycardia, depression or panic attacks.
- This pattern, especially when congenital, can be difficult to treat and obtain a lasting result. Combining with psychotherapy of some sort may be useful. Acute palpitations with anxiety after shock or trauma is more responsive to treatment, especially when acupuncture treatment is given frequently. In these acute types, acupuncture is particularly useful.

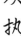

29.6 PHLEGM HEAT

Pathophysiology
- Phlegm Heat has both the cloying nature of Phlegm and the *shen* agitating quality of Heat. The Phlegm in this pattern (usually the insubstantial type), can 'obstruct (or mist) the orifices of the Heart'. This can lead to a disturbance of cardiac function or clouding of the *shen* and an exaggerated awareness of the Heart. The Heat component also agitates the *shen*. This pattern sometimes co-exists with Heart and Gall Bladder *qi* deficiency (p.813), and can follow a febrile illness that has congealed Fluids into Phlegm.

Clinical features
- palpitations with anxiety and nervousness
- dizziness and vertigo
- insomnia, with waking in the early hours, perhaps around 4am, unable to fall back to sleep
- irritability and restlessness
- nausea, vomiting or indeterminate gnawing hunger
- poor appetite
- belching
- acid reflux
- bitter taste in the mouth
- abdominal distension

T red tip or body and a greasy yellow coat
P rapid and slippery or wiry

Treatment principle
Clear Heat, transform Phlegm
Harmonize the Stomach, calm the *shen*

Prescription

WEN DAN TANG 温胆汤
(*Bamboo and Hoelen Combination*) modified

suan zao ren (Semen Zizyphi Spinosae) 酸枣仁	15g
fu ling (Sclerotium Poriae Cocos) 茯苓	12g
zhu ru (Caulis Bambusae in Taeniis) 竹茹	9g
zhi shi (Fructus Immaturus Citri Aurantii) 枳实	9g
ban xia* (Rhizoma Pinelliae Ternatae) 半夏	9g
chen pi (Pericarpium Citri Reticulatae) 陈皮	9g
yuan zhi (Radix Polygalae Tenuifoliae) 远志	6g
gan cao (Radix Glycyrrhizae Uralensis) 甘草	6g

Method: Decoction. (Source: *Shi Yong Zhong Yi Nei Ke Xue*)

Modifications

- If Heat is severe, add **huang lian** (Rhizoma Coptidis) 黄连 6g.
- With severe Phlegm Heat (thick yellow greasy coat, woolly headedness, dizziness), add **tian zhu huang** (Concretio Silicea Bambusae Textillis) 天竺黄 9g, **zhu li** (Succus Bambusae) 竹沥 10g and **dan nan xing*** (Pulvis Arisaemae cum Felle Bovis) 胆南星 6g. See also Variations and Additional Prescriptions, below.
- With severe palpitations, panic attacks, or if the patient is easily startled, add **zhen zhu mu**ˆ (Concha Margaritaferae) 珍珠母 30g, **long chi**ˆ (Dens Draconis) 龙齿 15g and **mu li**ˆ (Concha Ostreae) 牡蛎 15g.
- With food stagnation and obvious digestive disharmony, add two or three of the following herbs: **jiao shen qu** (baked Massa Fermentata) 焦神曲 10g, **jiao shan zha** (baked Fructus Crataegi) 焦山楂 10g, **chao mai ya** (dry fried Fructus Hordei Vulgaris Germinantus) 炒麦芽 10g or **chao lai fu zi** (dry fried Semen Raphani Sativi) 炒莱服子 15g.
- With constipation, add **da huang** (Radix et Rhizoma Rhei) 大黄 6-9g and **gua lou ren** (Semen Trichosanthis) 栝楼仁 15g.

Variations and additional prescriptions

Severe Phlegm Heat

- In very severe cases, with continuous palpitations, vertigo, tinnitus, a very thick yellow tongue coat and constipation, the correct treatment is to drain Fire and drive out Phlegm with **GUN TAN WAN** (*Vaporize Phlegm Pill* 滚痰丸).

> **duan meng shi** (calcined Lapis Micae seu Chloriti) 煅礞石 30g
> **jiu da huang** (wine fried Radix et Rhizoma Rhei) 酒大黄 240g
> **huang qin** (Radix Scutellariae Baicalensis) 黄芩 240g
> **chen xiang** (Linum Aquilariae) 沉香 15g
>
> Method: Grind herbs to a powder and form into small pills with water. The dose is 6-9 grams once or twice daily, with ginger tea. (Source: *Shi Yong Zhong Yi Nei Ke Xue*)

Phlegm Heat with Heart and Liver Fire

- Palpitations that occur at rest and that are accompanied by fullness in the chest and irritability, with constipation, heaviness in the body, difficulty twisting at the waist, a red tongue and wiry rapid pulse are due to Phlegm Heat and *qi* stagnation with Heart and Liver Fire. The correct treatment is to clear Phlegm Heat and Fire, move *qi* and calm the *shen* with **CHAI HU JIA LONG GU MU LI TANG** (*Bupleurum and Dragon Bone Combination* 柴胡加龙骨牡蛎汤).

> **chai hu** (Radix Bupleuri) 柴胡 9g
> **dang shen** (Radix Codonopsis Pilosulae) 党参 9g

ban xia* (Rhizoma Pinelliae Ternatae) 半夏 9g
huang qin (Radix Scutellariae Baicalensis) 黄芩 9g
long gu^ (Os Draconis) 龙骨 24g
mu li^ (Concha Ostreae) 牡蛎 24g
fu ling (Sclerotium Poriae Cocos) 茯苓 12g
gui zhi (Ramulus Cinnamomi Cassiae) 桂枝 6g
da huang (Radix et Rhizoma Rhei) 大黄 6g
sheng jiang (Rhizoma Zingiberis Officinalis) 生姜 3pce
da zao (Fructus Zizyphi Jujubae) 大枣 5pce

Method: Decoction. This is an extremely useful formula for *shen* disturbance in robust patients with Heat. It is widely used for disorders due to fright, shock or drug withdrawl, where palpitations, fullness in the chest, irritability and agitation are prominent. (Source: *Formulas and Strategies*)

Patent medicines

Er Chen Wan 二陈丸 (Er Chen Wan) plus *Huang Lian Jie Du Wan* 黄连解毒丸 (Huang Lian Jie Du Wan)

Hu Po Bao Long Wan 琥珀抱龙丸 (Po Lung Yuen Medical Pills)

Niu Huang Qing Huo Wan 牛黄清火丸 (Niu Huang Qing Huo Wan)
- severe cases

Chai Hu Jia Long Gu Mu Li San 柴胡加龙骨牡蛎散
(Bupleurum and Dragon Bone Combination) - for robust individuals with *qi* stagnation and Heat or Fire causing palpitations, extreme restlessness, fullness in the chest, agitation and insomnia

Acupuncture

Ht.5 (*tong li*), PC.4 (*xi men* -), Bl.13 (*fei shu* -), Lu.5 (*chi ze* -), St.40 (*feng long* -), GB.34 (*yang ling quan* -), PC.5 (*jian shi*)
- with insomnia add St.45 (*li dui*)
- with constipation add St.25 (*tian shu* -)
- with anxiety add Du.19 (*hou ding*) and Du.24 (*shen ting*)

Clinical notes
- The palpitations in this pattern may be associated with disorders such as anxiety neurosis, convalescence following a fever or early schizophrenia.
- The Phlegm Heat symptoms associated with this pattern generally respond well to correct treatment. When associated with schizophrenia the prognosis is much less reliable.
- This is a common pattern during the convalescent phase of a febrile disease.

29.7 SPLEEN AND KIDNEY *YANG* DEFICIENCY

Pathophysiology
- In this pattern Spleen and Kidney *yang* deficiency is the root of weakened Fluid metabolism and distribution. Phlegm Fluids (*tan yin* 痰饮) accumulate in the lower and middle *jiao* causing oedema in the lower body. Eventually the Phlegm Fluids back up from below and collect in the upper *jiao*, disrupting the Heart and Lungs, causing upper body oedema. Heart *yang* may be intact. The difference between this pattern and Heart *yang* deficiency is that here, the Spleen and Kidney *yang* deficiency is fundamental and reflected in the middle and lower *jiao* symptoms. *Yang* deficiency patterns are associated with *zheng chong* type palpitations.

Clinical features
- palpitations and shortness of breath, which are worse for exertion
- dizziness or vertigo
- chest and epigastric fullness and discomfort
- wheezing and coughing with thin watery sputum
- low voice, reluctance to speak
- nausea or vomiting
- poor appetite, abdominal distension, loose stools
- lower back cold and aching, cold extremities
- facial or eyelid oedema, or pitting leg and ankle oedema, with scanty or difficult urination, or nocturia and frequent urination

T pale and swollen, with a greasy white coat
P slippery and wiry or soggy, or deep, slow and possibly knotted or intermittent (if Heart *yang* is involved)

Treatment principle
Warm and Transform Phlegm Fluids
Strengthen the Spleen and resolve Damp

Prescription

LING GUI ZHU GAN TANG 苓桂术甘汤
(*Atractylodes and Hoelen Combination*)

This formula is suitable for relatively mild cases.
fu ling (Sclerotium Poriae Cocos) 茯苓 30g
bai zhu (Rhizoma Atractylodis Macrocephalae) 白术 15g
gui zhi (Ramulus Cinnamomi Cassiae) 桂枝 9g
gan cao (Radix Glycyrrhizae Uralensis) 甘草 6g
Method: Decoction. (Source: *Zhong Yi Nei Ke Lin Chuang Shou Ce*)

Modifications

- With nausea and vomiting, add **ban xia*** (Rhizoma Pinelliae Ternatae) 半夏 10g.
- With epigastric and abdominal distension, and loss of appetite, add **hou po** (Cortex Magnoliae Officinalis) 厚朴 10g, **shen qu** (Massa Fermentata) 神曲 10g, **dang shen** (Radix Codonopsis Pilosulae) 党参 15g.
- With obvious Kidney *yang* deficiency and Cold (cold extremities, cold intolerance, bluish lips), add two or three of the following herbs: **hu lu ba** (Semen Trigonellae Foeni-graeci) 葫芦巴 10g, **ba ji tian** (Radix Morindae Officinalis) 巴戟天 10g, **rou gui** (Cortex Cinnamomi Cassiae) 肉桂 6g or **xian ling pi** (Herba Epimedii) 仙灵脾 10g.
- If sweating is severe, add two or three of the following herbs: **ren shen** (Radix Ginseng) 人参 9g, **zhi gan cao** (honey fried Radix Glycyrrhizae Uralensis) 炙甘草 6g, **wu wei zi** (Fructus Schizandrae Chinensis) 五味子 6g, **duan long gu**ˆ (calcined Os Draconis) 煅龙骨 15g or **duan mu li**ˆ (calcined Concha Ostreae) 煅牡蛎 15g.

ZHEN WU TANG 真武汤, p.778
(*True Warrior Decoction*)

This formula is used in severe cases, when the palpitations are associated with wheezing and coughing, dyspnoea or orthopnoea, scanty urine and relatively severe oedema. These symptoms indicate that Kidney *yang* is seriously failing to eliminate fluids that are backing up and affecting the Heart. The correct treatment is to powerfully warm *yang* to move fluids. When fluids are moving, a more tonifying formula should be used.

Follow up treatment

- Once the palpitations have subsided and fluid metabolism is improving, a basic Spleen and/or Kidney *yang* strengthening formula may be phased in. Consider **JIN KUI SHEN QI WAN** (*Rehmannia Eight Formula* 金匮肾气丸, p.874), **YOU GUI WAN** (*Eucommia and Rehmannia Formula* 右归丸, p.559), **FU ZI LI ZHONG WAN** (*Aconite, Ginseng and Ginger Formula* 附子理中丸, p.873) depending on the combination of Spleen and Kidney deficiency.

Patent medicines

Jin Kui Shen Qi Wan 金匮肾气丸 (Sexoton Pills) plus
Fu Zi Li Zhong Wan 附子理中丸 (Li Chung Yuen Medical Pills) or
Li Zhong Wan 理中丸 (Li Zhong Wan)

Acupuncture
Bl.15 (*xin shu* +▲), Bl.20 (*pi shu* +▲), Bl.22 (*san jiao shu* +▲), Bl.23 (*shen shu* +▲), Bl.13 (*fei shu* +▲), Ren.9 (*shui fen* +▲), PC.4 (*xi men*), St.40 (*feng long* -), St.28 (*shui dao* -), Du.4 (*ming men* +▲)

Clinical notes
- The palpitations in this pattern may be associated with disorders such as congestive cardiac failure, chronic nephritis, chronic bronchitis, angina pectoris or coronary artery disease.
- Spleen and Kidney *yang* deficiency symptoms generally respond well to correct treatment. Once Fluid metabolism improves and the accumulated fluids are moving, the palpitations should improve. Herbal medicine may be the treatment of choice to warm *yang* and move Fluids, although intensive acupuncture and moxibustion will certainly enhance the result.

29.8 BLOOD STAGNATION

Pathophysiology
- Blood stagnation type palpitations are chronic and usually follow some other long term pathology that affects the Heart or chest, typically *yang* deficiency, Phlegm or *qi* stagnation. Palpitations from Blood stagnation may also follow an external invasion of Wind Cold Damp to the Heart (as occurs in rheumatic fever). Stagnant Blood obstructs the channels of the Heart disrupting the smooth flow of *qi* and Blood and consequently Heart function, so irregular beats and pain may occur. This pattern is clearly associated with *zheng chong*.

Clinical features
- palpitations and occasional chest pain that are worse at night
- stuffiness or fullness in the chest
- irritability, restlessness, easy anger or depression
- purplish lips, nails, sclera, conjunctiva
- spider naevi on the chest and face
- possibly signs of stagnant Liver *qi*

T dark or red purple with brown or purple stasis spots and a thin white coat; sublingual veins are distended and dark

P deep and choppy or wiry, or intermittent

Treatment principle
Invigorate the circulation of Blood, expel stagnant Blood
Regulate *qi* and open the channels

Prescription

XUE FU ZHU YU TANG 血府逐瘀汤
(*Achyranthes and Persica Combination*)

tao ren (Semen Persicae) 桃仁	12g
sheng di (Radix Rehmanniae Glutinosae) 生地	9g
hong hua (Flos Carthami Tinctorii) 红花	9g
chuan niu xi (Radix Cyathulae Officinalis) 川牛膝	9g
dang gui (Radix Angelicae Sinensis) 当归	9g
chi shao (Radix Paeoniae Rubrae) 赤芍	9g
chuan xiong (Radix Ligustici Chuanxiong) 川芎	6g
zhi ke (Fructus Citri Aurantii) 枳壳	6g
jie geng (Radix Platycodi Grandiflori) 桔梗	6g
chai hu (Radix Bupleuri) 柴胡	6g
gan cao (Radix Glycyrrhizae Uralensis) 甘草	3g

Method: Decoction. (Source: *Shi Yong Zhong Yi Nei Ke Xue*)

Modifications

- With Heat, add **dan shen** (Radix Salviae Miltiorrhizae) 丹参 12g and **huang qin** (Radix Scutellariae Baicalensis) 黄芩 9g.
- With Heat in the Liver, add **yu jin** (Tuber Curcumae) 郁金 9g.
- With chest pain, add **yan hu suo** (Rhizoma Corydalis Yanhusuo) 延胡索 9g, **mo yao** (Myrrha) 没药 6g, **ru xiang** (Gummi Olibanum) 乳香 6g.
- With insomnia or depression, add **he huan pi** (Cortex Albizziae Julibrissin) 合欢皮 12g.
- With headache, add **man jing zi** (Fructus Viticis) 蔓荆子 9g and **bai ji li** (Fructus Tribuli Terrestris) 白蒺藜 9g.
- With Heart *qi* deficiency, delete **chai hu**, **jie geng** and **zhi ke**, and add **dang shen** (Radix Codonopsis Pilosulae) 党参 30g, **huang jing** (Rhizoma Polygonati) 黄精 12g, and **huang qi** (Radix Astragali Membranacei) 黄芪 30g.
- With *yang* deficiency, delete **chai hu** and **jie geng**, and add **zhi fu zi*** (Radix Aconiti Carmichaeli Praeparata) 制附子 6g, **rou gui** (Cortex Cinnamomi Cassiae) 肉桂 3g, **xian ling pi** (Herba Epimedii) 仙灵脾 12g and **ba ji tian** (Radix Morindae Officinalis) 巴戟天 9g.
- With *yin* deficiency, delete **chai hu**, **jie geng**, **chuan xiong** and **zhi ke**, and add **mai dong** (Tuber Ophiopogonis Japonici) 麦冬 10g, **yu zhu** (Rhizoma Polygonati Odorati) 玉竹 10g, **nu zhen zi** (Fructus Ligustri Lucidi) 女贞子 10g and **han lian cao** (Herba Ecliptae Prostratae) 旱连草 10g.
- With Blood deficiency, add **shu di** (Radix Rehmanniae Glutinosae Conquitae) 熟地 15g, **gou qi zi** (Fructus Lycii) 枸杞子 15g and **he shou wu** (Radix Polygoni Multiflori) 何首乌 15g.

Patent medicines

Xue Fu Zhu Yu Wan 血府逐瘀丸 (Xue Fu Zhu Yu Wan)
Dan Shen Pian 丹参片 (Dan Shen Pills)
Jian Kang Wan 健康丸 (Sunho Multi Ginseng Tablets)
Sheng Tian Qi Pian 生田七片 (Raw Tian Qi Ginseng Tablets)
Jin Gu Die Shang Wan 筋骨跌伤丸 (Chin Koo Tieh Shang Wan)
Guan Xin An Kou Fu Ye 冠心安口服液 (Guan Xin An Kou Fu Ye)
Fu Ke Wu Jin Wan 妇科乌金丸 (Woo Garm Yuen Medical Pills)

Acupuncture

Bl.15 (*xin shu -*), Bl.17 (*ge shu -*), Bl.14 (*jue yin shu -*), PC.4 (*xi men -*), PC.5 (*jian shi -*), PC.6 (*nei guan -*), Sp.6 (*san yin jiao -*), LI.4 (*he gu -*), Ht.5 (*tong li -*), Sp.10 (*xue hai -*)

Clinical notes

- The palpitations in this pattern may be associated with disorders such as rheumatic heart disease, angina pectoris, coronary artery disease or mitral stenosis.
- The diagnosis of Blood stagnation may occasionally be one of exclusion; if in a case of chronic palpitations all other treatments have failed, then a provisional diagnosis of stagnant Blood may be made, even in the absence of other objective signs.
- Blood stagnation symptoms can respond reasonably well to correct and prolonged treatment and the palpitations should improve (although if the underlying pathology is too deep, that is, there is excessive tissue damage already, then the results are much less certain).
- Long term use of Blood stagnation removing formulae alone is not advisable in frail or elderly patients. An appropriate tonic formula may need to be added to prevent excessive dispersal of *qi* and Blood.

SUMMARY OF GUIDING FORMULAE FOR PALPITATIONS

Heart *qi* deficiency - *Wu Wei Zi Tang* 五味子汤

Heart *yang* deficiency - *Gui Zhi Gan Cao Long Gu Mu Li Tang* 桂枝甘草龙骨牡蛎汤
- Heart and Kidney *yang* deficiency with pulmonary oedema - *Zhen Wu Tang* 真武汤
- Kidney *yang* predominant - *Jin Kui Shen Qi Wan* 金匮肾气丸

Heart *yin* deficiency - *Tian Wang Bu Xin Dan* 天王补心丹
- following a febrile disease - *Huang Lian E Jiao Tang* 黄连阿胶汤
- with anxiety and insomnia - *Zhu Sha An Shen Wan* 朱砂安神丸
- Liver and Kidney *yin* deficiency predominant - *Yi Guan Jian* 一贯煎 + *Suan Zao Ren Tang* 酸枣仁汤

Heart Blood and Spleen *qi* deficiency - *Gui Pi Tang* 归脾汤
- with *qi* and *yin* deficiency, with severe palpitations and an irregular pulse - *Zhi Gan Cao Tang* 炙甘草汤

Heart and Gall Bladder *qi* deficiency - *Ding Zhi Wan* 定志丸
- as a result of shock - *Gui Zhi Jia Long Gu Mu Li Tang* 桂枝加龙骨牡蛎汤

Phlegm Heat - *Wen Dan Tang* 温胆汤

Spleen and Kidney *yang* deficiency - *Ling Gui Zhu Gan Tang* 苓桂术甘汤
- with severe fluid accumulation - *Zhen Wu Tang* 真武汤

Blood stagnation - *Xue Fu Zhu Yu Tang* 血府逐瘀汤

Endnote

For more information regarding herbs marked with an asterisk*, an open circle° or a hatˆ, see the tables on pp.944-952.

Disorders of the Heart

30. Insomnia

Excess patterns
Liver *qi* stagnation
Heart Fire
Stomach disharmony
Phlegm Heat
Stagnant Blood

Deficient patterns
Heart and Spleen deficiency
Heart and Kidney *yin* deficiency
Heart and Gall Bladder deficiency
Liver *yin* and Blood deficiency

30 INSOMNIA
bu mei 不寐

Insomnia describes a variety of different symptoms associated with sleep disturbance, including inability to sleep, difficulty falling asleep, frequent waking, restlessness at night, disordered sleep cycle and dream disturbed sleep.

Approximately one third of all adults experience occasional or persistent sleep disturbances. Sleep deprivation or disruption of circadian rhythm can lead to serious impairment of daytime functioning. Most adults sleep 7 to 8 hours per night, although the timing, duration and internal structure of sleep vary considerably among apparently healthy individuals and as a function of age.

When assessing a patient complaining of insomnia, it is important to distinguish true insomnia from transitory insomnia due to external or temporary changes. Outside noise, sudden weather changes, inappropriate bedroom temperatures, consumption of coffee or other stimulants prior to bedtime, eating late, recent emotional upsets, vigorous exercise and the disordered biorhythms of shiftworkers may all cause a person to sleep poorly. Once these factors are removed, sleep usually returns to normal and the sleep disturbance cannot be considered true insomnia. Similarly, sleep disturbance due to pain, itching, asthma and breathing disorders should not be diagnosed as insomnia.

In TCM, insomnia is associated with instability or agitation of the *shen*. This can occurs because:

- the *shen* is not adequately anchored and secured due to deficiency of Blood or *yin*
- overstimulation and agitation by Heat prevent the *shen* from settling quietly when the time comes for sleep
- the *shen* is 'locked in' and agitated by constraint from *qi* and/or Blood stagnation

Shen

The *shen* is at the most rarefied end of the spectrum of the densities of *qi*. The most condensed is *jing*, in between are the various functional types of *qi* (*zong qi*, *wei qi*, *zang fu qi* etc.) These three aspects of *qi* are termed the 'three treasures' (Fig 30.2) and are the subject of considerable philosophical debate and the focus of daoist meditation techniques. Indeed, it is the transformation of *jing* into *shen* that preoccupies some of the daoist and other esoteric schools of Chinese philosophical thought and practice. Blood and *yin* are more condensed (and therefore material) than *qi*, but less dense than *jing*.

The *shen* plays a key role in higher mental functions, including many of

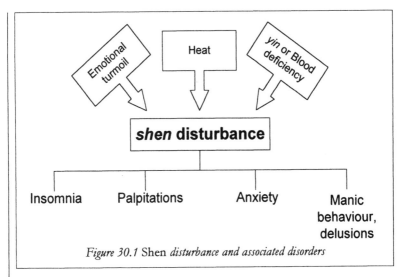

Figure 30.1 Shen *disturbance and associated disorders*

the intellectual and spiritual aspects of consciousness. In practical terms, the *shen* is most closely associated with our conscious awareness, and is essentially our ability to perceive, interact and communicate with our world clearly. In addition, the *shen* and the Heart share an intimate and interdependent relationship (TCM describes the Heart as the residence of the *shen*). *Shen* pathology is therefore associated with disturbances of consciousness and perception, and some aspects of Heart function.

Consciousness is the province of *shen*, however *shen* can be divided into a number of subgroups, each with its own particular facet of consciousness and association with an organ system. That aspect of *shen* especially disturbed by the rising *qi* of anger or repression of emotion is termed the *hun* 魂, and is linked to the Liver. The *hun* is implicated in some types of sleep disturbance, particularly that involving sleepwalking. Other facets of *shen* are the *yi* (意, associated with the Spleen), *po* (魄, Lungs), and *zhi* (志, Kidneys).

Because *shen* is so refined and subtle it must be anchored by the more material *jing* (or Blood and *yin*), otherwise it has a tendency to float away. The interaction of

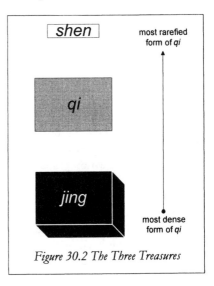

Figure 30.2 *The Three Treasures*

jing and *shen* produces the 'light' of consciousness. It is this interaction that is observed in the twinkle of a clear eye–in Chinese the *jing shen* (精神). Observation of an individuals *jing shen* is the first indication of the state of their consciousness and ultimately their health or capacity to recover from illness. This lightness and subtleness, however, means that *shen* is the least stable form of *qi*, and thus easily unsettled.

There are two broad categories of *shen* disturbance, deficiency and excess. The deficiency patterns are mostly due to the *shen* not being anchored by Heart *yin* or Blood, so it simply 'floats away', or is dissipated instead of resting in the Heart. These patterns usually manifest with symptoms like insomnia, dream disturbed sleep, anxiety with palpitations, phobias and disorientation.

Excess patterns are mostly associated with Heat and Phlegm. The Heat can directly affect the Heart (as in Heart Fire) or be more systemic (as in Heat in the Blood). Either way, the *shen* is continually agitated by the presence of the Heat, and restlessness, agitation, and delusional or manic behaviour result.

Due to the Heart's central position as the 'emperor' of the *zang* organs, it (and the resident *shen*) are affected by all emotional patterns. Some are more damaging than others, particularly prolonged worry and anxiety, or severe shock or terror. Ultimately, however, any emotional imbalance will involve the Heart and *shen*.

Insomnia may accompany many syndromes and disorders, and can be a major obstacle to recovery if it is severe. Insomnia may be a symptom of such conditions as neurological and psychiatric disorders, neurosis, hypertension, cerebral arteriosclerosis, hyperthyroidism, various fevers, hepatitis, menopausal and premenstrual syndrome and anaemia.

AETIOLOGY
Liver *qi* stagnation, stagnant Heat, Liver Fire
Frustration, anger, resentment, prolonged emotional turmoil, repressed emotions and stress disrupt the circulation of Liver *qi*. When Liver *qi* stagnates it can disrupt the generative cycle (*sheng* 生, p.70) of the five phases (*wu xing* 五行) resulting in a poor supply (of *qi* and Blood) to the Heart. Liver *qi* stagnation constrains the *hun* and *shen* causing tension and insomnia. Long term *qi* stagnation can also lead to Blood stagnation with the same, albeit more severe, result.

When *qi* stagnates for any length of time, the resulting pressure can generate Heat, which at a certain intensity may be redefined as Fire. Here the Heat takes over as the primary agitator of the *shen*. Liver Fire is more likely in those with a *yang* or hot constitution, and in those with a diet rich in heating substances.

Heart Fire

Prolonged worry, anxiety and depression, or a sudden shock can retard the movement of Heart *qi*. The resulting accumulation of *qi* creates a focus of pressure in the chest, which then generates Heat, further affecting the Heart. This type of *qi* accumulation is slightly different to Liver *qi* stagnation in that the focus of Liver *qi* stagnation is usually below the diaphragm (although its effects may be systemic). Heart Fire may also develop if Fire is transmitted from the Liver to the Heart. Heart Fire (like Liver Fire) is more likely to occur in those with some pre-existing Heat, whether from diet or congenital factors.

A different type of Heart Fire may occur during severe febrile diseases. This occurs when external Heat penetrates deep into the body, lodging at the *ying* or Blood level (of the Four Levels, pp.38-43). In this situation, high fever is accompanied by delirium and disordered consciousness as the Fire severely disturbs the *shen*.

Heart *yin* deficiency, especially if prolonged, is often associated with Heart Fire. Mixtures of Fire and *yin* deficiency are clinically more common than pure Heart Fire. If the insomnia is very chronic, it may develop into the Heart and Kidney *yin* deficient pattern.

Stomach disharmony

This syndrome is usually due to overindulgence or irregular dietary habits (eating late at night, midnight snacks, eating while upset, eating too quickly etc.) that weaken the Spleen and Stomach so that digestion is impaired. It is essentially a type of food stagnation. If bad dietary habits persist, it can become more severe and overlap with the next pattern, Phlegm Heat.

Phlegm Heat

Phlegm Heat can be generated in several ways. Dampness and Phlegm can be the result of Spleen weakness or overconsumption of Phlegm producing foods (rich, greasy, sweet, spicy foods and alcohol), which then causes stagnation and the generation of Heat. Any pre-existing Heat in the body, whether from Liver *qi* stagnation with stagnant Heat or Fire, *yin* deficiency or external pathogen, can congeal fluids into Phlegm, and subsequently Phlegm Heat. This pattern often occurs in the convalescent stage of a febrile illness, after external Heat has concentrated fluids into Phlegm.

Failure of fluid metabolism as a result of *qi* or *yang* deficiency (affecting Kidney, Spleen or Heart) can lead to accumulation of fluids, which over time congeal into Phlegm. Once Phlegm is present, Heat can be generated by the resulting obstruction.

Heart Blood and Spleen *qi* deficiency

Overwork, physical and mental exhaustion, worry, irregular diet and too much cold, raw or sweet food can damage the Spleen, which then fails to generate sufficient *qi* and Blood. Similarly, any situation that overwhelms the Spleen's ability to replace *qi* and Blood, like a prolonged or severe illness can lead to *qi* and Blood deficiency. The primary weakness in this pattern is in the Spleen, which is unable to generate enough Blood to nourish the Heart and anchor the *shen*.

Heart Blood and Spleen *qi* weakness can be more acute, following a post partum haemorrhage or difficult pregnancy and labour. This pattern is common in women who return to work too soon following pregnancy, without fully recovering their investment of *qi* and Blood. It also occurs in those who breast-feed for lengthy periods of time while expending energy working or looking after demanding children (and husbands). The elderly are another group who frequently suffer from insufficient *qi* and Blood.

Heart and Kidney *yin* deficiency

In Chinese medicine the relationship between the Heart and Kidney is one of the fundamental relationships of the body and mind. This relationship functions on both a physical and a mental level. On the physical level Kidney Water (*yin*) keeps Heart Fire in check, preventing a runaway blaze and overheating, and Heart Fire catalyses Kidney Water, preventing stagnation and accumulation of fluids. On the mental level, the Fire of the *shen* arises from a stable base of Kidney *jing* (summed up in the sparkle of *jing shen* in the eyes), and *jing* and *shen* rely on each other for clear expression of mental consciousness.

If Kidney *yin* is damaged (by overwork, excess sexual activity, insufficient rest and sleep, ageing etc.) there may be a breakdown in the relationship between the Heart and Kidney (via the controlling cycle), whereby Kidney Water no longer keeps Heart Fire in check. The uncontrolled blazing of Heart Fire causes agitation of the *shen* and the resulting insomnia can be severe. If Heart Fire remains unchecked Heart *yin* will be damaged. The *shen* then has no 'anchor' and insomnia can become chronic. Heart *yin* may also be damaged by stimulant and recreational drugs (including coffee) or excessive mental stress. This is a very common cause of insomnia and one characterised by quite severe mental restlessness, anxiety and occasionally total inability to sleep.

At a more superficial level, the communication between the Heart (*shen*) and Kidneys (*zhi*) can be severed by major shock or trauma. This can occur in otherwise robust individuals, in which case the insomnia (and usually anxiety or panic attacks) is accompanied by fewer systemic symptoms since the *yin* of the organs is not damaged. It may also occur in someone with pre-existing *yin* damage, in which case their condition is suddenly greatly exacerbated.

Liver *yin* and Blood deficiency

As well as the various activities and events that can damage Heart and Kidney *yin* (see above), Liver *yin* and Blood can also be weakened by prolonged *qi* stagnation and the generation of stagnant Heat or Fire, overuse of the eyes and chronic Liver disease.

Heart and Gall Bladder deficiency

Heart and Gall Bladder deficiency describes a personality type that may be congenital or acquired. When congenital, it may be due to a significant shock that damaged the developing foetal *shen* during the mother's pregnancy. The pattern may be acquired easily in children (the *shen* is unstable when young) who are brought up in an abusive or fearful environment, or in adults or children who experience a violent or extreme shock or fright. It may also

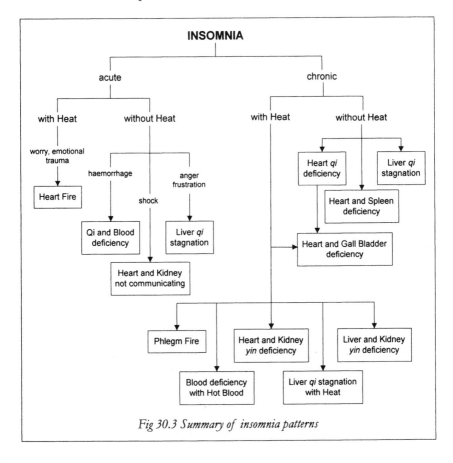

Fig 30.3 Summary of insomnia patterns

> **BOX 30.1 KEY DIAGNOSTIC POINTS**
>
> These are general guides only:
> - difficulty falling asleep, but once asleep stays asleep - Blood deficiency
> - waking frequently during the night, often feeling hot - *yin* deficiency
> - repeated waking around 2-4am, worse when stressed - Liver *qi* stagnation, stagnant Heat or Fire
> - lots of wild dreaming - possible involvement of the *hun*
> - talking during sleep, sleepwalking - possible involvement of the *hun*
> - recurrent frightening dreams that cause waking - Heart and Gall Bladder deficiency
> - waking with palpitations and panic attacks - Heart and Kidney *yin* deficiency
> - chronic insomnia with feverishness at night but no sweating - Blood stagnation

sometimes follow other debilitating illnesses that plunder *qi*.

Because the *shen* is so destabilised it cannot cope easily with change and can be easily disturbed by trivial events, so even a minor change in routine may be enough to trigger episodes of sleeplessness.

The involvement of the Gall Bladder here refers to the timidity and 'lack of gall' (that is, fearfulness) which characterise patients with this pattern. In the Chinese language (as in English) there is an implicit understanding of the relationship between the Gall Bladder and courage, indeed to be bold and courageous is to have a 'big Gall Bladder' (*da dan* 大胆).

Blood stagnation

Blood stagnation insomnia usually follows some external trauma, extreme emotional shock or head injury. It can also be the result of other chronic disorders that eventually cause Blood stagnation, especially extreme or prolonged emotional turmoil and *qi* stagnation. When associated with trauma the insomnia is usually acute, otherwise there is usually a long history of persistent insomnia. Blood stagnation frequently co-exists with other patterns, such as *qi*, *yin* or *yang* deficiency, etc.

TREATMENT

Treatment with acupuncture and herbs usually produces a reliable result in most types of insomnia. Many patients with chronic insomnia will be taking sedative medication of some sort (often benzodiazepines, see anxiety p.868), and they should be slowly weaned off the drugs over a period of weeks or months as the TCM treament takes effect. Adjuvant therapy is useful in most types of insomnia, particularly relaxation or meditation to calm the mind.

The most important distinction is between excess and deficient types of insomnia. The excess varieties tend to be more difficult to treat than the deficient varieties, as in excess patterns there are often complicating lifestyle features—like unhappiness or stress at home or at work and habitual mental emotional responses that have to be dealt with for a satisfactory result. The deficiency patterns generally respond quite well to treatment, although herbal and/or acupuncture treatment may need to be combined with an appropriate nourishing diet. Obvious and easily modifiable aggravating factors, such as coffee, excessive visual stimulation at night (like staying up late watching television), heavy exercise at night and excessive alcohol should be avoided.

30.1 LIVER *QI* STAGNATION, STAGNANT HEAT, FIRE

肝气郁滞

郁热

肝火

Pathophysiology
- Liver *qi* stagnation, *qi* stagnation with stagnant Heat and Liver Fire are a continuum of conditions with similar aetiology and escalating severity. Typically, Liver *qi* stagnation precedes the development of Heat, which at a certain intensity is redefined as Fire. All patterns have emotional turmoil, especially anger, resentment and frustration as common aetiological features, with Liver Fire exacerbated by a Hot constitution and/or a diet rich in alcohol and heating foods. Liver *qi* stagnation without Heat is less likely to cause insomnia than with Heat, and Liver Fire is the more likely cause.
- *Qi* stagnation alone causes insomnia by disrupting the smooth flow of *qi* in the chest, restricting the unhindered movement of the *shen*. When there is Heat, the *shen* is continually being agitated and disturbed.

Clinical features
- difficulty falling asleep, insomnia, dream disturbed sleep, waking in the early hours of the morning (typically between 2 and 4 am), worse when stressed
- depression, irritability, moodiness
- frontal or temporal headaches, shoulder and neck tension, teeth grinding at night
- hypochondriac tension or discomfort
- frequent sighing
- dizziness
- sensation of something lodged in the throat ('plum stone *qi*')
- irregular menstruation, premenstrual syndrome and breast tenderness
- poor appetite
- alternating constipation and diarrhoea

T unremarkable or dark (*qing* 青) with a thin white or yellow coat, or with red edges and a thick yellow coat with Heat or Fire

P wiry

Treatment principle
Soothe Liver *qi*, Calm the *shen*

Prescription

XIAO YAO SAN 逍遥散
(*Bupleurum and Dang Gui Formula*) modified

This prescription is selected when there is *qi* stagnation without Heat.
    chai hu (Radix Bupleuri) 柴胡 9g
    dang gui (Radix Angelicae Sinensis) 当归 9g

cu bai shao (vinegar fried Radix Paeoniae Lactiflora)
醋白芍 9g
bai zhu (Rhizoma Atractylodis Macrocephalae) 白术 9g
fu ling (Sclerotium Poriae Cocos) 茯苓 9g
bo he (Herba Mentha Haplocalycis) 薄荷 6g
suan zao ren (Semen Zizyphi Spinosae) 酸枣仁 15g
he huan pi (Cortex Albizziae Julibrissin) 合欢皮 12g

Method: Decoction or as powder. When the formula is decocted, **bo he** should be added at the end of cooking (*hou xia* 后下).

DAN ZHI XIAO YAO SAN 丹栀逍遥散
(Bupleurum and Paeonia Formula) modified

This formula is selected when *qi* stagnation has generated some Heat. The clinical features are the same as for Liver *qi* stagnation, with the additional features of red, sore eyes, facial flushing, irritability, anger, bitter taste in the mouth, red edges on the tongue and a wiry, rapid pulse.

chai hu (Radix Bupleuri) 柴胡 12g
dang gui (Radix Angelicae Sinensis) 当归 9g
cu bai shao (vinegar fried Radix Paeoniae Lactiflora)
醋白芍 12g
bai zhu (Rhizoma Atractylodis Macrocephalae) 白术 9g
fu ling (Sclerotium Poriae Cocos) 茯苓 9g
shan zhi zi (Fructus Gardeniae Jasminoidis) 山栀子 9g
mu dan pi (Cortex Moutan Radicis) 牡丹皮 9g
bo he (Herba Mentha Haplocalycis) 薄荷 6g
ren dong teng (Ramulus Lonicerae Japonicae) 忍冬藤 9g
ye jiao teng (Caulis Polygoni Multiflori) 夜交藤 12g
zhen zhu mu^ (Concha Margaritaferae) 珍珠母 15g

Method: Decoction or as powder. When the formula is decocted, **zhen zhu mu** should be decocted for 30 minutes prior to the other herbs (*xian jian* 先煎), **bo he** should be added at the end of cooking (*hou xia* 后下). (Source: *Shi Yong Zhong Yi Nei Ke Xue*)

LONG DAN XIE GAN TANG 龙胆泻肝汤
(Gentiana Combination) modified

This formula is selected for Liver Fire. At this stage the Heat is severe. The clinical features include insomnia, extreme restlessness and frequent waking, all worse with emotional stress, irritability, short temper, thirst with desire to drink, bitter taste in the mouth, red, sore eyes, severe temporal headaches, concentrated or painful urination, constipation, a red tongue with a thick yellow coat and a wiry, forceful and rapid pulse.

long dan cao (Radix Gentianae Longdancao) 龙胆草 9g

sheng di (Radix Rehmanniae Glutinosae) 生地 12g
huang qin (Radix Scutellariae Baicalensis) 黄芩 9g
shan zhi zi (Fructus Gardeniae Jasminoides) 山栀子 9g
dang gui (Radix Angelicae Sinensis) 当归 9g
ze xie (Rhizoma Alismatis Orientalis) 泽泻 9g
che qian zi (Semen Plantaginis) 车前子 9g
chai hu (Radix Bupleuri) 柴胡 9g
mu tong (Caulis Mutong) 木通 3g
gan cao (Radix Glycyrrhizae Uralensis) 甘草 3g
zhen zhu mu^ (Concha Margaritaferae) 珍珠母 30g
ye jiao teng (Caulis Polygoni Multiflori) 夜交藤 20g
he huan pi (Cortex Albizziae Julibrissin) 合欢皮 12g

Method: Decoction. **Che qian zi** is decocted in a cloth bag (*bao jian* 包煎).
(Source: *Zhong Yi Nei Ke Lin Chuang Shou Ce*)

Modifications (applicable to all prescriptions)
- In severe cases, add **bai zi ren** (Semen Biotae Orientalis) 柏子仁 12g.
- With fullness and discomfort in the chest and hypochondrium, add **xiang fu** (Rhizoma Cyperi Rotundi) 香附 6g, **yu jin** (Tuber Curcumae) 郁金 9g and **zhi ke** (Fructus Citri Aurantii) 枳壳 6g.
- If easily awoken, startled and frightened, add **long chi**^ (Dens Draconis) 龙齿 10g or **ci shi** (Magnetitum) 磁石 10g.

Patent medicines
Xiao Yao Wan 逍遥丸 (Xiao Yao Wan)
Jia Wei Xiao Yao Wan 加味逍遥丸 (Jia Wei Xiao Yao Wan)
  - with stagnant Heat
Shu Gan Wan 舒肝丸 (Shu Gan Wan)
Long Dan Xie Gan Wan 龙胆泻肝丸 (Long Dan Xie Gan Wan)
  - Liver Fire
Chai Hu Jia Long Gu Mu Li San 柴胡加龙骨牡蛎散
    (Bupleurum and Dragon Bone Combination) - for robust individuals with *qi* stagnation and Heat or Fire causing extreme restlessness, insomnia, agitation and palpitations

Acupuncture
Liv.3 (*tai chong* -), PC.6 (*nei guan*), Bl.18 (*gan shu*), Bl.15 (*xin shu*), GB.20 (*feng chi* -), Ht.7 (*shen men*), an mian (N-HN-54), yin tang (M-HN-3)
- with lateral headaches, add SJ.5 (*wai guan* -) and GB.39 (*xuan zhong* -)
- with teeth grinding or aching jaw, add St.6 (*jia che*)
- with digestive weakness, add Sp.6 (*san yin jiao*)
- with 'plum stone *qi*', add PC.5 (*jian shi*)
- with Heat or Fire, add Liv.2 (*xing jian* -) and GB.44 (*zu qiao yin*)

Clinical notes

- The insomnia of this pattern may be associated with disorders such as stress induced insomnia, hypertension, menopausal syndrome, bipolar mood disorder, depression and premenstrual syndrome.
- Liver *qi* stagnation type insomnia has an excellent prognosis particularly if the source of external stress can be resolved. Acupuncture is often the treatment of choice for moving stagnant *qi* and if the insomnia is relatively recent, one course (or less) of acupuncture should effect a cure. Longer term insomnia or insomnia that is associated with more complex patterns may need several courses of acupuncture combined with herbs.
- Relaxation and stress management techniques are useful in people with ongoing sources of stress.

30.2 HEART FIRE

Pathophysiology
- Any Heat pattern that affects the Heart will quickly unsettle the *shen* and cause relatively severe insomnia, nightmares and restlessness. Clinically, pure excess Heart Fire is not as common as the mixed excess (Fire) and deficiency (of *yin*) pattern, although it may be seen in certain acute states of anxiety or psychosis and some febrile conditions. If Fire persists then Heart *yin* will be damaged, eventually leading to the very common Heart and Kidney *yin* deficiency pattern (p.852).

Clinical features
- insomnia, frequent waking with nightmares
- restlessness, agitiation or anxiety
- palpitations
- thirst with a desire for cold fluids
- bitter taste in the mouth
- mouth and tongue ulcers
- red complexion
- concentrated or painful urination

T red with a redder tip and yellow coat
P full and rapid

Treatment principle
Clear Heart Fire, calm the *shen*

Prescription

HUANG LIAN JIE DU TANG 黄连解毒汤
(*Coptis and Scute Combination*) modified

This formula is suitable for uncomplicated Heart Fire.

huang lian (Rhizoma Coptidis) 黄连	9g
huang qin (Radix Scutellariae Baicalensis) 黄芩	6g
huang bai (Cortex Phellodendri) 黄柏	6g
shan zhi zi (Fructus Gardeniae Jasminoides) 山栀子	9g
dan zhu ye (Herba Lophatheri Gracilis) 淡竹叶	9g
lian zi xin (Plumula Nelumbinis Nuciferae) 莲子心	6g
deng xin cao (Medulla Junci Effusi) 灯心草	3g

Method: Decoction. (Source: *Shi Yong Zhong Yi Nei Ke Xue*)

DAO CHI SAN 导赤散
(*Rehmannia and Akebia Formula*)

This formula is selected if there are minor signs of underlying *yin* deficiency, dysuria, or if the condition has persisted for some time.

sheng di (Radix Rehmanniae Glutinosae) 生地 15-30g
mu tong (Caulis Mutong) 木通 3-6g
dan zhu ye (Herba Lophatheri Gracilis) 淡竹叶 3-6g
gan cao shao (tips of Radix Glycyrrhizae Uralensis)
甘草梢 3-6g

Method: Decoction. (Source: *Formulas and Strategies*)

HUANG LIAN E JIAO TANG 黄连阿胶汤
(Coptis and Ass-Hide Gelatin Decoction)

This formula is selected when Heart *yin* deficiency follows a febrile disease - a type of *shao yin* syndrome. The correct treatment is to clear Fire, nourish *yin*, stop irritability and calm the *shen*.

huang lian (Rhizoma Coptidis) 黄连 12g
huang qin (Radix Scutellariae Baicalensis) 黄芩 6g
e jiao^ (Gelatinum Corii Asini) 阿胶 9g
bai shao (Radix Paeoniae Lactiflora) 白芍 6g
ji zi huang^ (egg yolk) .... 2 yolks

Method: Decoction. E jiao is melted in the hot strained decoction (*yang hua* 烊化). The egg yolks are stirred into the strained decoction. (Source: *Shi Yong Zhong Yi Nei Ke Xue*)

ZHU YE SHI GAO TANG 竹叶石膏汤
(Lophatherus and Gypsum Decoction)

This formula is used to treat lingering fever with restlessness, irritability and insomnia in the aftermath of a Summer Heat or febrile illness. Residual Heat remains lodged in the chest and diaphragm (the *qi* level). The insomnia is characterised by extreme restlessness before sleep and fitful broken sleep thereafter. The patient also experiences dryness of the throat, lips and mouth and a stifling sensation in the chest. This sometimes occurs following incorrect use of antibiotics for a viral illness. The antibiotics are cooling, but do not disperse the Heat pathogen.

dan zhu ye (Herba Lophatheri Gracilis) 淡竹叶 15g
shi gao (Gypsum) 石膏 30g
ban xia* (Rhizoma Pinelliae Ternatae) 半夏 9g
mai dong (Tuber Ophiopogonis Japonici) 麦冬 9g
dang shen (Radix Codonopsis Pilosulae) 党参 15-30g
geng mi (Semen Oryzae) 粳米 15g
gan cao (Radix Glycyrrhizae Uralensis) 甘草 3g

Method: Decoction. (Source: *Shi Yong Zhong Yao Xue*)

ZHU SHA AN SHEN WAN 朱砂安神丸
(Cinnabar Pill to Calm the Spirit)

This formula is powerfully sedative and is selected when the insomnia is accompanied by severe palpitations and anxiety. Because it contains a large dose of **zhu sha** it is not suitable for prolonged use, and once the condition is under control, other formulae should be selected.

huang lian (Rhizoma Coptidis) 黄连	45g
zhu sha* (Cinnabaris) 朱砂	30g
dang gui (Radix Angelicae Sinensis) 当归	30g
sheng di (Radix Rehmanniae Glutinosae) 生地	30g
fu ling (Sclerotium Poriae Cocos) 茯苓	30g
suan zao ren (Semen Zizyphi Spinosae) 酸枣仁	30g
yuan zhi (Radix Polygalae Tenuifoliae) 远志	15g
zhi gan cao (honey fried Radix Glycyrrhizae Uralensis) 炙甘草	15g

Method: Grind the herbs (except **zhu sha**) to a powder and form into 3-gram pills with honey. Coat the outside of the pills with the **zhu sha**. The dose is 1-2 pills daily. May also be decocted with a 60% reduction in dosage. The dose of **huang lian** is reduced by 90%. If the formula is decocted the **zhu sha** (0.5g) is taken with the strained decoction (*chong fu* 冲服). (Source: *Shi Yong Zhong Yao Xue*)

Patent medicines

Huang Lian Jie Du Wan 黄连解毒丸 (Huang Lian Jie Du Wan)
Niu Huang Jie Du Pian 牛黄解毒片 (Peking Niu Huang Chieh Tu Pien)
Dao Chi Pian 导赤片 (Tao Chih Pien)
Xiao Er Qi Xing Cha 小儿七星茶 (Xiao Er Qi Xing Cha)
 - especially good for infants and children

Acupuncture

Ht.8 (*shao fu*), Ht.9 (*shao chong* ↓), (PC.8 (*lao gong* -), Ht.7 (*shen men*), Bl.15 (*xin shu* -), Sp.6 (*san yin jiao* +), Kid.6 (*zhao hai* +), *an mian* (N-HN-54), *yin tang* (M-HN-3)

Clinical notes

- The insomnia of this pattern may be associated with disorders such as anxiety neurosis, depression, panic attacks, glossitis, bipolar mood disorder, schizophrenia, febrile disease and post febrile disease.
- Symptoms of Heart Fire, such as insomnia, generally respond well to treatment with either acupuncture or herbs, however when associated with biomedical conditions like schizophrenia and bipolar mood disorder, the prognosis is poorer.

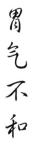

30.3 STOMACH DISHARMONY

Pathophysiology
- Stomach disharmony describes a type of food stagnation that causes insomnia by obstructing the natural descent of Stomach *qi* or by generating Heat, both of which can rise and affect the Heart. It is most common in those who eat late at night, eat too much or who attempt to sleep on a full Stomach. If bad dietary habits persist, it can become more severe and overlap with the next pattern, Phlegm Heat.

Clinical features
- insomnia with fullness, discomfort, gurgling, bloating or a blocked feeling in the epigastric region, relieved by belching or vomiting
- acid reflux
- nausea
- indeterminate gnawing hunger
- bad breath, belching
- loose, foul smelling stools or constipation
- abdominal distension and pain

T thick white or yellow greasy coat
P wiry and slippery or slippery and rapid

Treatment principle
Relieve food stagnation and harmonise the Stomach
Calm the *shen*

Prescription

BAO HE WAN 保和丸
(*Citrus and Crategus Formula*) modified

shan zha (Fructus Crataegi) 山楂	10g
fu ling (Sclerotium Poriae Cocos) 茯苓	15g
shen qu (Massa Fermentata) 神曲	10g
ban xia* (Rhizoma Pinelliae Ternatae) 半夏	10g
chen pi (Pericarpium Citri Reticulatae) 陈皮	10g
mai ya (Fructus Hordei Vulgaris Germinantus) 麦芽	12g
lian qiao (Fructus Forsythia Suspensae) 连翘	30g
lai fu zi (Semen Raphani Sativi) 莱服子	20g
ye jiao teng (Caulis Polygoni Multiflori) 夜交藤	30g
suan zao ren (Semen Zizyphi Spinosae) 酸枣仁	15g

Method: Grind herbs to a powder and form into 9-gram pills with water. The dose is 1 pill twice daily. May also be decocted. (Source: *Zhong Yi Nei Ke Lin Chuang Shou Ce*)

Modifications
- If excessive meat was consumed, double the dose of **shan zha**.
- If starchy foods, like noodles and grains, double the dose of **lai fu zi**.
- If vomiting is severe, double the dose of **ban xia***, and add **sheng jiang** (Rhizoma Zingiberis Officinalis) 生姜 10g.
- With constipation, double the dose of **lai fu zi**, or add **da huang** (Radix et Rhizoma Rhei) 大黄 6-9g.
- With Heat (irritability, red tongue tip and sides), add **shan zhi zi** (Fructus Gardeniae Jasminoides) 山栀子 10g and **huang lian** (Rhizoma Coptidis) 黄连 6g.

Variations and additional prescriptions
- In severe cases, a few doses of a mild purge, like **TIAO WEI CHENG QI TANG** (*Regulate the Stomach and Order the qi Decoction* 调胃承气汤) may be useful first, to clear the Stomach and Intestines and promote the correct downward movement of Stomach *qi*.

    da huang (Radix et Rhizoma Rhei) 大黄 12g
    gan cao (Radix Glycyrrhizae Uralensis) 甘草 6g
    mang xiao (Mirabilitum) 芒硝 9-12g
    Method: Decoction. Cook **da huang** and **gan cao** together for 20 minutes and dissolve **mang xiao** in the strained decoction (*chong fu* 冲服). (Source: *Formulas and Strategies*)

Patent medicines
Bao He Wan 保和丸 (Bao He Wan)
Jian Pi Wan 健脾丸 (Jian Pi Wan)
  - with *qi* deficiency
Mu Xiang Shun Qi Wan 木香顺气丸 (Aplotaxis Carminative Pills)
  - with *qi* stagnation
Liu He Bao He Wan 六合保和丸 (Bo Wo Yuen Medical Pills)

Acupuncture
Ren.12 (*zhong wan* -), St.25 (*tian shu* -), St.40 (*feng long* -), PC.6 (*nei guan* -), St.43 (*xian gu* -), St.44 (*nei ting* -), St.45 (*li dui*), Sp.1 (*yin bai*), St.34 (*liang qiu* -), GB.34 (*yang ling quan* -)

Clinical notes
- This is a disorder of overindulgence and/or inappropriate timing of eating. In isolation it needs no treatment other than adopting a sensible approach to eating, however if bad habits persist it can become a more entrenched problem.

30.4 PHLEGM HEAT

Pathophysiology
- Phlegm Heat has both the cloying nature of Phlegm and the *shen* agitating quality of Heat. The Phlegm in this pattern (usually the insubstantial type), can 'obstruct (or mist) the orifices of the Heart', weighing down the more rarefied *shen* causing clouding of consciousness, vagueness and woolly headedness. This pattern may develop from the previous one, appear as a complication of Heart and Gall Bladder *qi* deficiency (p.856), or follow a febrile illness that has congealed Fluids into Phlegm. Typically, there will be accompanying symptoms of Stomach *qi* disturbance.

Clinical features
- insomnia or fitful sleep with much dreaming, or waking in the early hours of the morning (typically around 4am), unable to fall back to sleep
- palpitations with anxiety and nervousness
- irritability and restlessness
- dizziness and vertigo
- heavy or woolly headedness
- fullness and discomfort in the chest
- poor appetite, belching, acid reflux, bitter taste in the mouth
- nausea, vomiting or indeterminate gnawing hunger

T red body or tip and a greasy yellow coat
P wiry or slippery and rapid

Treatment principle
Clear Heat and transform Phlegm
Harmonise the Stomach and calm the *shen*

Prescription

WEN DAN TANG 温胆汤
(*Bamboo and Hoelen Combination*) modified

ye jiao teng (Caulis Polygoni Multiflori) 夜交藤	30g
suan zao ren (Semen Zizyphi Spinosae) 酸枣仁	15g
fu ling (Sclerotium Poriae Cocos) 茯苓	15g
ban xia* (Rhizoma Pinelliae Ternatae) 半夏	10g
chen pi (Pericarpium Citri Reticulatae) 陈皮	10g
zhu ru (Caulis Bambusae in Taeniis) 竹茹	10g
shan zhi zi (Fructus Gardeniae Jasminoides) 山栀子	10g
huang lian (Rhizoma Coptidis) 黄连	6g
yuan zhi (Radix Polygalae Tenuifoliae) 远志	6g
gan cao (Radix Glycyrrhizae Uralensis) 甘草	3g

Method: Decoction. (Source: *Zhong Yi Nei Ke Lin Chuang Shou Ce*)

Modifications

- With palpitations, panic attacks, or if the patient is easily startled, add **zhen zhu mu**ˆ (Concha Margaritaferae) 珍珠母 30g, **duan long gu**ˆ (calcined Os Draconis) 煅龙骨 15g and **duan mu li**ˆ (calcined Concha Ostreae) 煅牡蛎 15g.
- With severe Phlegm Heat (thick yellow greasy coat, woolly headedness, dizziness), add **tian zhu huang** (Concretio Silicea Bambusae Textillis) 天竺黄 9g, **zhu li** (Succus Bambusae) 竹沥 10g and **dan nan xing*** (Pulvis Arisaemae cum Felle Bovis) 胆南星 6g.
- With food stagnation or obvious digestive disharmony, add two or three of the following herbs: **jiao shen qu** (baked Massa Fermentata) 焦神曲 10g, **jiao shan zha** (baked Fructus Crataegi) 焦山楂 10g, **chao mai ya** (dry fried Fructus Hordei Vulgaris Germinantus) 炒麦芽 10g or **chao lai fu zi** (dry fried Semen Raphani Sativi) 炒莱服子 15g.
- With constipation, add **da huang** (Radix et Rhizoma Rhei) 大黄 6-9g and **gua lou ren** (Semen Trichosanthis) 栝楼仁 15g.

Variations and additional prescriptions

- In resistant cases a stronger prescription that may be useful is **QING HUO DI TAN TANG** (*Clear Fire, Wash Away Phlegm Decoction* 清火涤痰汤).

dan shen (Radix Salviae Miltiorrhizae) 丹参	12g
fu shen (Sclerotium Poriae Cocos Pararadicis) 茯神	12g
ju hua (Flos Chrysanthemi Morifolii) 菊花	9g
chen pi (Pericarpium Citri Reticulatae) 陈皮	9g
mai dong (Tuber Ophiopogonis Japonici) 麦冬	9g
bai zi ren (Semen Biotae Orientalis) 柏子仁	9g
zhe bei mu (Bulbus Fritillariae Thunbergii) 浙贝母	9g
dan nan xing* (Pulvis Arisaemae cum Felle Bovis) 胆南星	6g
jiang canˆ (Bombyx Batryticatus) 僵蚕	6g
xing ren* (Semen Pruni Armeniacae) 杏仁	6g
zhu li (Succus Bambusae) 竹沥	6g
sheng jiang (Rhizoma Zingiberis Officinalis) 生姜	3pce

Method: Decoction. (Source: *Shi Yong Zhong Yi Nei Ke Xue*)

Patent medicines

Er Chen Wan 二陈丸 (Er Chen Wan) plus *Huang Lian Jie Du Wan* 黄连解毒丸 (Huang Lian Jie Du Wan)
Hu Po Bao Long Wan 琥珀抱龙丸 (Po Lung Yuen Medical Pills)
Niu Huang Qing Huo Wan 牛黄清火丸 (Niu Huang Qing Huo Wan)
   - severe cases

Chai Hu Jia Long Gu Mu Li San 柴胡加龙骨牡蛎散
(Bupleurum and Dragon Bone Combination) - for robust individuals with *qi* stagnation and Heat or Fire causing palpitations, extreme restlessness, fullness in the chest, agitation and insomnia

Acupuncture

Du.20 (*bai hui*), Ren.12 (*zhong wan* -), St.25 (*tian shu* -), Sp.1 (*yin bai*), St.40 (*feng long* -), St.36 (*zu san li* -), PC.6 (*nei guan*), St.43 (*xian gu* -), St.45 (*li dui*)
- with Stomach discomfort, add St.34 (*liang qiu* -)
- with dizziness, add GB.43 (*xia xi* -)
- with anxiety, add Du.19 (*hou ding*) and Du.24 (*shen ting*)

Clinical notes

- The insomnia of this pattern may be associated with disorders such as chronic gastritis, peptic ulcer disease, post febrile disease or neurosis.
- Phlegm Heat type insomnia can also appear in the convalescent stage of a febrile illness.
- This type of insomnia responds well to treatment although treatment needs to continue until all signs of Phlegm are cleared. In particular, until the tongue coat becomes normal. Herbs may be more efficient at clearing entrenched Phlegm although acupuncture itself often starts to improve sleep patterns quickly, especially on the day of treatment.
- The use of sleeping pills is not uncommon for this type of insomnia and significantly complicates and exacerbates a Phlegm Heat pattern. Their withdrawal is strongly recommended, although this must be done gradually and with close supervision.

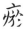

30.5 BLOOD STAGNATION

Pathophysiology
- Blood stagnation type insomnia can be acute or chronic. When acute it often follows some trauma (either physical or emotional) or head injury, or may follow overenthusiastic use of styptic herbs to quell bleeding. When chronic there will usually be a long history of insomnia or some other problem, that over time caused Blood stasis. Blood stagnation frequently co-exists with other patterns such as Liver *qi* stagnation, various deficiencies and Phlegm.
- Stagnant Blood causes insomnia because the *shen* is agitated either by being constrained and prevented from free movement, or from the Heat that may be generated by the stagnation, or both.

Clinical features
- persistent insomnia with much dreaming and restlessness
- irritablity, short temper, depression, mood swings
- low grade fever at night
- fixed sharp pains, particularly in the head and upper body
- dry scaly skin
- broken vessels or spider naevi on the face, trunk, inner knee and ankle
- purplish lips, sclera, conjunctiva and nail beds
- dark rings around the eyes

T in acute cases the tongue body may be unremarkable; in chronic cases dark or red purple with brown or purple stasis spots and a thin white coat; sublingual veins are distended and dark

P deep and choppy or wiry, or intermittent

Treatment principle
Invigorate the circulation of Blood, regulate *qi*
Eliminate stagnant Blood, calm the *shen*

Prescription

XUE FU ZHU YU TANG 血府逐瘀汤
(*Achyranthes and Persica Combination*) modified

sheng di (Radix Rehmanniae Glutinosae) 生地	12g
tao ren (Semen Persicae) 桃仁	12g
dang gui (Radix Angelicae Sinensis) 当归	9g
hong hua (Flos Carthami Tinctorii) 红花	9g
niu xi (Radix Achyranthis Bidentatae) 牛膝	9g
zhi ke (Fructus Citri Aurantii) 枳壳	6g
chi shao (Radix Paeoniae Rubrae) 赤芍	6g

chai hu (Radix Bupleuri) 柴胡 6g
jie geng (Radix Platycodi Grandiflori) 桔梗 6g
chuan xiong (Radix Ligustici Chuanxiong) 川芎 6g
dan shen (Radix Salviae Miltiorrhizae) 丹参 15g
suan zao ren (Semen Zizyphi Spinosae) 酸枣仁 20g

Method: Decoction. (Source: *Zhong Yi Nei Ke Lin Chuang Shou Ce*)

Modifications

- For severe insomnia, add **he huan pi** (Cortex Albizziae Julibrissin) 合欢皮 12g
- With headache, add **man jing zi** (Fructus Viticis) 蔓荆子 9g and **bai ji li** (Fructus Tribuli Terrestris) 白蒺藜 9g.
- With Heat in the Liver, add **yu jin** (Tuber Curcumae) 郁金 9g.
- With pain, add **yan hu suo** (Rhizoma Corydalis Yanhusuo) 延胡索 9g, **mo yao** (Myrrha) 没药 6g, **ru xiang** (Gummi Olibanum) 乳香 6g.
- With Heart *qi* deficiency, delete **chai hu**, **jie geng** and **zhi ke**, and add **dang shen** (Radix Codonopsis Pilosulae) 党参 30g, **huang jing** (Rhizoma Polygonati) 黄精 12g, and **huang qi** (Radix Astragali Membranacei) 黄芪 30g.
- With *yang* deficiency or Cold, delete **chai hu** and **jie geng**, and add **zhi fu zi*** (Radix Aconiti Carmichaeli Praeparata) 制附子 6g, **rou gui** (Cortex Cinnamomi Cassiae) 肉桂 3g, **xian ling pi** (Herba Epimedii) 仙灵脾 12g and **ba ji tian** (Radix Morindae Officinalis) 巴戟天 9g.
- With *yin* deficiency, delete **chai hu**, **jie geng**, **chuan xiong** and **zhi ke**, and add **mai dong** (Tuber Ophiopogonis Japonici) 麦冬 10g, **yu zhu** (Rhizoma Polygonati Odorati) 玉竹 10g, **nu zhen zi** (Fructus Ligustri Lucidi) 女贞子 10g and **han lian cao** (Herba Ecliptae Prostratae) 旱莲草 10g.
- With Blood deficiency, add **shu di** (Radix Rehmanniae Glutinosae Conquitae) 熟地 15g, **gou qi zi** (Fructus Lycii) 枸杞子 15g and **he shou wu** (Radix Polygoni Multiflori) 何首乌 15g.

Patent medicines

Xue Fu Zhu Yu Wan 血府逐瘀丸 (Xue Fu Zhu Yu Wan)
Dan Shen Pian 丹参片 (Dan Shen Pills)
Guan Xin An Kou Fu Ye 冠心安口服液 (Guan Xin An Kou Fu Ye)
Jian Kang Wan 健康丸 (Sunho Multi Ginseng Tablets)
Sheng Tian Qi Pian 生田七片 (Raw Tian Qi Ginseng Tablets)
Fu Ke Wu Jin Wan 妇科乌金丸 (Woo Garm Yuen Medical Pills)

Acupuncture

Bl.17 (*ge shu* -), Sp.6 (*san yin jiao* -), LI.4 (*he gu* -), *an mian* (N-HN-54),

Bl.15 (*xin shu* +), Sp.10 (*xue hai* -), *yin tang* (M-HN-3), Ht.7 (*shen men*)
- with trauma add points of pain on the head (*ah shi*)
- with depression combine LI.4 (*he gu*) and Liv.3 (*tai chong*)

Clinical notes

- The insomnia of this pattern may be associated with disorders such as post-concussion syndrome, post traumatic insomnia and post traumatic stress syndrome.
- Clinically, in some cases there may in fact be few objective signs of Blood stasis and diagnosis is arrived at by a process of elimination, when other treatments to calm and nourish the Blood and *yin*, Heart and *shen* or clear Heat are ineffective.
- Acute cases respond well. Acupuncture, especially applied to sites of obstruction (*ah shi* points), on the head can produce rapid results and few treatments should be required. Chronic cases can respond reasonably well but treatment will need to be prolonged and herbs may be necessary.

30.6 HEART BLOOD AND SPLEEN *QI* DEFICIENCY

心脾两虚

Pathophysiology
- This very common type of insomnia occurs because the *shen* is not anchored by Heart Blood and remains active when it should be settling down into its *yin* phase. In contrast to the *yin* deficiency with Heat pattern, the major difficulty here is falling asleep. However, once asleep the patient may stay asleep as there is no Heat to continue disturbing the *shen*.

Clinical features
- insomnia, with particular difficulty falling asleep (and switching off the mind) and dream disturbed sleep
- palpitations, with or without anxiety
- anxiety, phobias, panic attacks
- forgetfulness, poor memory, poor concentration
- postural dizziness, light-headedness, blurred vision
- fatigue and lethargy
- poor appetite, abdominal distension after eating
- pale, sallow complexion
- easy bruising, or heavy or prolonged menstrual periods

T pale with a thin white coat
P thready and weak

Treatment principle
Strengthen and nourish the Heart and Spleen
Tonify *qi* and Blood, calm the *shen*

Prescription

GUI PI TANG 归脾汤
(Ginseng and Longan Combination)

zhi huang qi (honey fried Radix Astragali Membranacei) 黄芪	15g
suan zao ren (Semen Zizyphi Spinosae) 酸枣仁	12g
fu ling (Sclerotium Poria Cocos) 茯苓	12g
dang shen (Radix Codonopsis Pilosulae) 党参	12g
chao bai zhu (dry fried Rhizoma Atractylodes Macrocephalae) 炒白术	9g
dang gui (Radix Angelicae Sinensis) 当归	9g
long yan rou (Arillus Euphoriae Longanae) 龙眼肉	9g
yuan zhi (Radix Polygalae Tenuifoliae) 远志	6g
mu xiang (Radix Aucklandiae Lappae) 木香	6g

zhi gan cao (honey fried Radix Glycyrrhizae Uralensis)
炙甘草 6g

Method: Decoction. (Source: *Shi Yong Zhong Yi Nei Ke Xue*)

Modifications

- With severe insomnia, add two or three of the following herbs: **wu wei zi** (Fructus Schizandrae Chinensis) 五味子 6g, **bai zi ren** (Semen Biotae Orientalis) 柏子仁 9g, **ye jiao teng** (Caulis Polygoni Multiflori) 夜交藤 30g, **he huan pi** (Cortex Albizziae Julibrissin) 合欢皮 9g, **long chi^** (Dens Draconis) 龙齿 10g, **mu li^** (Concha Ostreae) 牡蛎 30g to settle the *shen*, and **mai ya** (Fructus Hordei Vulgaris Germinantus) 麦芽 15g to protect the Stomach from damage by the mineral drugs.
- With Liver Heat, add **shan zhi zi** (Fructus Gardeniae Jasminoidis) 山栀子 9g and **chai hu** (Radix Bupleuri) 柴胡 6g.
- When Heart Blood deficiency is prominent (palpitations, anxiety, and forgetfulness), add **shu di** (Radix Rehmanniae Glutinosae Conquitae) 熟地 30-50g, **bai shao** (Radix Paeoniae Lactiflora) 白芍 15g and **e jiao^** (Gelatinum Corii Asini) 阿胶 15g to nourish Blood, and **sha ren** (Fructus Amomi) 砂仁 6g to aid the digestion of the **shu di**.
- With abdominal and epigastric fullness, poor appetite and a greasy or glossy tongue coat, add **ban xia*** (Rhizoma Pinelliae Ternatae) 半夏 10g and **chen pi** (Pericarpium Citri Reticulatae) 陈皮 10g.

Patent medicines

Gui Pi Wan 归脾丸 (Gui Pi Wan)
Bai Zi Yang Xin Wan 柏子养心丸 (Bai Zi Yang Xin Wan)
Dang Gui Ji Jing 当归鸡精 (Tang Kuei Essence of Chicken)
Bu Nao Wan 补脑丸 (Cerebral Tonic Pills)
Yang Xin Ning Shen Wan 养心宁神丸
      (Ning San Yuen Medical Pills)

Acupuncture

Sp.6 (*san yin jiao* +), Ht.7 (*shen men* +), St.36 (*zu san li* +), Bl.15 (*xin shu* +), PC.6 (*nei guan* +), Bl.17 (*ge shu* +), Bl.20 (*pi shu* +), Du.19 (*hou ding*), *an mian* (N-HN-54), *yin tang* (M-HN-3)

- with forgetfulness, add Du.20 (*bai hui*) and Bl.52 (*zhi shi*)
- with much dreaming, add Bl.42 (*po hu*)
- with bruising or heavy periods add Sp.10 (*xue hai*) and Sp.1 (*yin bai* ▲)
- with palpitations add Ht.5 (*tong li*)
- with dizziness add Du.20 (*bai hui* ▲)

Clinical notes

- The insomnia of this pattern may be associated with disorders such as neurosis, anaemia, thrombocytopoenia, neuresthenia, chronic fatigue syndrome, post partum insomnia, insomnia with menstrual periods and eating disorders.
- Heart and Spleen deficiency patterns respond well to treatment, which should continue until it is clear the Spleen is strong enough to make sufficient Blood. Careful diet and eating patterns will enhance the result. A strictly regular bedtime routine should be adhered to. Avoidance of all caffeinated drinks and stimulant drugs is strongly recommended.
- Acupuncture can be very effective at tonifying Spleen *qi* but if the patient is already very Blood deficient, herbs will probably be necessary as well. The recommended unmodified prescription includes only two blood tonic herbs so as not to tax the weak Spleen. If the herbs are well tolerated, more Blood tonic herbs can be added cautiously.
- In women who lose blood (and thus Heart Blood) through heavy periods, Blood tonics and Blood replenishing and iron rich foods should be taken after each period. Iron supplements are also useful.

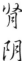

30.7 HEART AND KIDNEY *YIN* DEFICIENCY

Pathophysiology
- At night and during sleep the dynamic *yang* aspect of body function subsides while the quiescent *yin* aspect becomes more prominent. This deep and internal *yin* houses and grounds the *shen* at night so the mind can rest. When the *yin* is damaged, not only is it no longer able to secure the *shen*, but the accompanying *yin* deficient Heat agitates it, causing restlessness and frequent waking.
- In contrast to the Blood deficiency patterns, the Heat here keeps disturbing the *shen*, so frequent waking feeling hot and restless is common. This pattern may follow prolonged or untreated Heart Fire (p.838).

Clinical features
- insomnia, with frequent waking, or waking feeling hot or sweaty
- restlessness, agitation, panic attacks
- palpitations
- sensation of heat in the palms and soles ('five hearts hot')
- night sweats
- dry mouth and throat
- dizziness, tinnitus
- forgetfulness
- lower back ache

T red with little or no coat
P thready and rapid

Treatment principle
Nourish Heart and Kidney *yin*
Clear Heat, calm the *shen*

Prescription

TIAN WANG BU XIN DAN 天王补心丹
(*Ginseng and Zizyphus Formula*)

This is the representative formula for Heart and Kidney *yin* deficiency and is excellent for *yin* deficiency patterns characterised by *shen* disturbance.

    sheng di (Radix Rehmanniae Glutinosae) 生地 .... 120 (24)g
    tian dong (Tuber Asparagi Cochinchinensis) 天冬 .... 30 (12)g
    mai dong (Tuber Ophiopogonis Japonici) 麦冬 .... 30 (12)g
    suan zao ren (Semen Zizyphi Spinosae) 酸枣仁 .... 30 (12)g
    xuan shen (Radix Scrophulariae) 玄参 .... 15 (12)g
    dan shen (Radix Salviae Miltiorrhizae) 丹参 .... 15 (12)g
    fu ling (Sclerotium Poriae Cocos) 茯苓 .... 15 (12)g

    dang gui (Radix Angelicae Sinensis) 当归 .... 30 (9)g
    wu wei zi (Fructus Schizandrae Chinensis) 五味子 .... 30 (9)g
    bai zi ren (Semen Biotae Orientalis) 柏子仁 .... 30 (9)g
    ren shen (Radix Ginseng) 人参 .... 15 (9)g
    jie geng (Radix Platycodi Grandiflori) 桔梗 .... 15 (9)g
    yuan zhi (Radix Polygalae Tenuifoliae) 远志 .... 15 (6)g
    zhu sha* (Cinnabaris) 朱砂 (optional) .... 6 (0.5)g
    Method: Grind herbs (except **zhu sha**) to a powder and form into 9-gram pills with honey. If used, coat the outside of the pills with the **zhu sha**. The dose is one pill 2-3 times daily. May also be decocted with the dosage in brackets. When decocted the **zhu sha** is taken as powder with the strained decoction (*chong fu* 冲服). This is an excellent formula for long term use in treating *yin* deficiency with *shen* disturbance, in which case the **zhu sha** is deleted. (Source: *Shi Yong Zhong Yi Nei Ke Xue*)

GUI ZHI JIA LONG GU MU LI TANG 桂枝加龙骨牡蛎汤
(*Cinnamon and Dragon Bone Combination*) modified

This formula is selected following a major shock or trauma that causes insomnia or dream or nightmare disturbed sleep, palpitations with anxiety, hair loss, loss of appetite, dizziness, depression, lack of motivation and a weak, hollow, slow pulse. This is typical of severed communication between the Heart and Kidneys due to shock. Here the physiological symptoms are mild and the mental emotional symptoms are prominent.

    gui zhi (Ramulus Cinnamomi Cassiae) 桂枝 9g
    bai shao (Radix Paeoniae Lactiflora) 白芍 9g
    long gu^ (Os Draconis) 龙骨 15-30g
    mu li^ (Concha Ostreae) 牡蛎 15-30g
    sheng jiang (Rhizoma Zingiberis Officinalis) 生姜 9g
    da zao (Fructus Zizyphi Jujubae) 大枣 4pce
    gan cao (Radix Glycyrrhizae Uralensis) 甘草 6g
    he huan pi (Cortex Albizziae Julibrissin) 合欢皮 12g
    Method: Decoction. (Source: *Formulas and Strategies*)

Variations and additional prescriptions

Following a febrile illness
- If symptoms of *yin* deficient Fire are severe or the disorder occurs following a febrile disease, the correct treatment is to nourish *yin* and clear Fire with **HUANG LIAN E JIAO TANG** (*Coptis and Ass-Hide Gelatin Decoction* 黄连阿胶汤, p.839).

In severe cases
- Insomnia accompanied by severe palpitations and anxiety may require a

more sedative formula to quickly bring the symptoms under control. **ZHU SHA AN SHEN WAN** (*Cinnabar Pill to Calm the Spirit* 朱砂安神丸, p.840) is suitable. Because it contains **zhu sha** it is not suitable for prolonged use, and once the condition is under control other formulae should be used.

Patent medicines

Tian Wang Bu Xin Dan 天王补心丹 (Tian Wang Bu Xin Dan)
 - excellent for Heart *yin* deficiency with *shen* disturbance
Zuo Gui Wan 左归丸 (Zuo Gui Wan)
Sheng Mai Wan 生脉丸 (Sheng Mai Wan)
Liu Wei Di Huang Wan 六味地黄丸 (Liu Wei Di Huang Wan)
 - a general Kidney *yin* tonic formula
Suan Zao Ren Tang Pian 酸枣仁汤片 (Tabellae Suanzaoren)

Acupuncture

PC.8 (*lao gong*), PC.7 (*da ling*), Kid.3 (*tai xi* +), Ht.7 (*shen men* +), Liv.3 (*tai chong*), Bl.15 (*xin shu* +), Bl.14 (*jue yin shu* +), Bl.23 (*shen shu* +), *an mian* (N-HN-54), *yin tang* (M-HN-3), Sp.6 (*san yin jiao* +)
- with dizziness, add Du.20 (*bai hui*)
- with tinnitus, add SI.19 (*ting gong*) and SJ.3 (*zhong zhu*)
- with arrhythmias, add Ht.5 (*tong li*)

Clinical notes

- The insomnia of this pattern may be associated with disorders such as menopausal syndrome, neuresthenia, hyperthyroidism, anxiety neurosis, fever of unknown origin, convalescence following a febrile disorder and post traumatic shock syndrome.
- This pattern generally responds well to correct treatment, however for it to be long lasting the *yin* will have to be replenished and this takes time. TCM treatment for at least several months will be necessary, although signs of improvement can usually be expected within a few weeks. Long term resolution may depend on the biomedical syndrome the patient presents with. For example, hyperthyroid conditions can be difficult to cure with TCM and may need to be controlled by drugs or surgery if TCM treatment is ineffective, before lasting results can be acheived.
- Acupuncture can be very useful in settling the mind sufficiently to allow sleep and if the insomnia is severe, then daily acupuncture may be desirable.
- Avoidance of all caffeinated drinks and stimulant drugs is strongly recommended. A strictly regular bedtime routine should be adhered to.

Care with other aggravating factors like sex, excessive lifting and standing and dehydration.
- Active pursuit of relaxation should be encouraged. This means that a gentle and positive relaxation routine should be built into the day. Activities such as *tai qi* or yoga nidra are a good way to calm the mind.

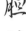

30.8 HEART AND GALL BLADDER *QI* DEFICIENCY

Pathophysiology
- In Heart and Gall Bladder *qi* deficiency the *shen* is congenitally unstable or severely disrupted by shock or fright and consequently unable to settle to sleep at night. During the day this manifests in excessive anxiety and worry, easy fright and fear, suspicion and timidity. In many patients with this pattern there will be a lifelong history of timidity, anxiety and fearfulness.

Clinical features
- insomnia or frequent waking, often early in the morning, unable to fall back to sleep; the patient is easily frightened and startled, and easily unsettled by seemingly trivial events
- anxiety and palpitations
- shortness of breath
- lethargy, fatigue, depression
- spontaneous sweating

T normal or with a pale body and a thin white coat; in congenital or long standing cases there may be a deep narrow crack to the tip
P wiry and thready

Treatment principle
Strengthen *qi* and alleviate fearfulness
Calm the *shen* and mind

Prescription

AN SHEN DING ZHI WAN 安神定志丸
(*Calm the shen, Settle the Emotions Pill*) modified

ren shen (Radix Ginseng) 人参	9g
fu shen (Sclerotium Poriae Cocos Pararadicis) 茯神	15g
fu ling (Sclerotium Poriae Cocos) 茯苓	15g
yuan zhi (Radix Polygalae Tenuifoliae) 远志	15g
long chi^ (Dens Draconis) 龙齿	15g
shi chang pu (Rhizoma Acori Graminei) 石菖蒲	15g
chao suan zao ren (dry fried Semen Zizyphi Spinosae) 炒酸枣仁	15g
ye jiao teng (Caulis Polygoni Multiflori) 夜交藤	15g
mu li^ (Concha Ostreae) 牡蛎	20g
zhu sha* (Cinnabaris) 朱砂 (optional)	5g

Method: Decoction. Grind herbs (except **zhu sha**) to a powder and form into 9-gram pills with honey. If used, coat the outside of the pills with the **zhu sha**. The dose is 1 pill twice daily. May also be decocted. If decocted, the **zhu sha** (0.5g) is taken with the strained decoction (*chong fu* 冲服). (Source: *Shi Yong Zhong Yi Nei Ke Xue*)

Patent medicines
Bu Nao Wan 补脑丸 (Cerebral Tonic Pills)
Ding Xin Wan 定心丸 (Ding Xin Wan)
Yang Xin Ning Shen Wan 养心宁神丸 (Ning San Yuen Medical Pills)

Acupuncture
Du.20 (*bai hui*), PC.7 (*da ling*), Ht.7 (*shen men*), GB.40 (*qiu xu*), Bl.7 (*tong tian*), St.36 (*zu san li*), Bl.23 (*shen shu*), Bl.52 (*zhi shi*), Bl.47 (*hun men*), *an mian* (N-HN-54), *yin tang* (M-HN-3)

Clinical notes
- The insomnia of this pattern may be associated with disorders such as anxiety neurosis, neuresthenia, involutional psychosis, premenstrual syndrome, sinus tachycardia, depression and panic attacks.
- This pattern often overlaps with Phlegm Heat. See also p.843.
- In congenital cases, prolonged acupuncture and herbal treatment, in conjuction with appropriate psychotherapy or other confidence building treatment, may help stabilise the *shen* to some degree.

30.9 LIVER *YIN* (BLOOD) DEFICIENCY

Pathophysiology
- The *hun* 魂 (the aspect of conscious awareness related to the Liver) is contained at night by Liver *yin* and Blood. Weak *yin* and Blood cannot anchor the *hun* to the Liver adequately, and at night it wanders restlessly. At the same time, when the structural components (*yin* and Blood) of the Liver are deficient, the functional aspect (Liver *qi*) will be in relative excess (and therefore prone to stagnation), and can agitate the *hun*. Liver deficiency will also affect the Heart (and *shen*) via the generative (*sheng* 生, p.70) cycle.

Clinical features
- insomnia with difficulty falling asleep or frequent waking, much dreaming and fitful sleep; there may be talking during sleep or, in severe cases, sleep walking
- irritability, quick temper
- forgetfulness
- waking with a dry throat or thirst
- night sweats
- sore, gritty, dry eyes, or visual disturbances
- dizziness
- palpitations

T red and dry
P wiry or thready and rapid

Treatment principle
Soothe the Liver and nourish *yin* Blood
Calm the *hun* (and *shen*) and clear Heat

Prescription

SUAN ZAO REN TANG 酸枣仁汤
(*Zizyphus Combination*)

    suan zao ren (Semen Zizyphi Spinosae) 酸枣仁 15g
    fu ling (Sclerotium Poriae Cocos) 茯苓 15g
    zhi mu (Rhizoma Anemarrhenae Asphodeloidis) 知母 9g
    chuan xiong (Radix Ligustici Chuanxiong) 川芎 6g
    gan cao (Radix Glycyrrhizae Uralensis) 甘草 3g
    Method: Decoction. (Source: *Formulas and Strategies*)

Modifications
- If the insomnia is severe, add one two of the following herbs: **mu lí** (Concha Ostreae) 牡蛎 15g, **ci shi** (Magnetitum) 磁石 15g, **long gǔ**

(Os Draconis) 龙骨 15g, **zhen zhu mu^** (Concha Margaritaferae) 珍珠母 15g or **zi shi ying** (Fluoritum) 紫石英 15g.
- With rising Liver *yang*, add **gou teng** (Ramulus Uncariae) 钩藤 12g.
- With sore gritty eyes, add **gou qi zi** (Fructus Lycii) 枸杞子 12g, **ju hua** (Flos Chrysanthemi Morifolii) 菊花 9g, **mi meng hua** (Flos Buddleiae Officinalis Immaturus) 蜜蒙花 9g and **shi jue ming^** (Concha Haliotidis) 石决明 12g.
- With Liver Heat, add **shan zhi zi** (Fructus Gardeniae Jasminoidis) 山栀子 9g and **chai hu** (Radix Bupleuri) 柴胡 6g.
- With deficient Heat, add **nu zhen zi** (Fructus Ligustri Lucidi) 女贞子 9g and **han lian cao** (Herba Ecliptae Prostratae) 旱莲草 9g.
- With night sweats, add **mu li^** (Concha Ostreae) 牡蛎 15g, **ma huang gen** (Radix Ephedrae) 麻黄根 9g and **fu xiao mai** (Semen Tritici Aestivi Levis) 浮小麦 15g.

Variations and additional prescriptions

With Liver qi stagnation
- If Liver *yin* deficiency is complicated by *qi* stagnation, with the above symptoms plus hypochondriac and chest pain, acid reflux and teeth grinding, the correct treatment is to nourish Liver *yin* and spread Liver *qi* with **YI GUAN JIAN** (*Linking Decoction* 一贯煎, p.790).

Patent medicines

Xiao Yao Wan 逍遥丸 (Xiao Yao Wan)
Suan Zao Ren Tang Pian 酸枣仁汤片 (Tabellae Suanzaoren)

Acupuncture

Liv.3 (*tai chong* +), Bl.18 (*gan shu* +), Bl.15 (*xin shu* +), Bl.17 (*ge shu*), Bl.23 (*shen shu* +), PC.6 (*nei guan*), GB.20 (*feng chi*), Ht.7 (*shen men* +), *an mian* (N-HN-54), *yin tang* (M-HN-3)
  - with Liver Heat add Liv.2 (*xing jian* -)

Clinical notes

- The insomnia of this pattern may be associated with disorders such as stress response, menopausal syndrome, premenstrual syndrome, somnambulism, hyperthyroidism, hypertension and chronic hepatitis.
- Responds reasonably well to correct treatment.
- It is important to avoid stimulants, including alcohol and spicy foods, generally and especially close to bed time. As much as possible stressful situations should be avoided and stress management practices instituted.

SUMMARY OF GUIDING FORMULAE FOR INSOMNIA

Excess patterns

Liver *qi* stagnation - *Xiao Yao Wan* 逍遥丸
- with stagnant Heat - *Dan Zhi Xiao Yao San* 丹栀逍遥散
- Liver Fire - *Long Dan Xie Gan Tang* 龙胆泻肝汤

Heart Fire - *Huang Lian Jie Du Tang* 黄连解毒汤
- with underlying deficiency - *Dao Chi San* 导赤散
- following a febrile disease - *Huang Lian E Jiao Tang* 黄连阿胶汤
- severe insomnia with anxiety and palpitations - *Zhu Sha An Shen Wan* 朱砂安神丸

Stomach disharmony - *Bao He Wan* 保和丸
- with constipation - *Tiao Wei Cheng Qi Tang* 调胃承气汤

Phlegm Heat - *Wen Dan Tang* 温胆汤
- in resistant cases - *Qing Huo Di Tan Tang* 清火涤痰汤

Stagnant Blood - *Xue Fu Zhu Yu Tang* 血府逐瘀汤

Deficient patterns

Heart Blood and Spleen *qi* deficiency - *Gui Pi Tang* 归脾汤

Heart and Kidney *yin* deficiency - *Tian Wang Bu Xin Dan* 天王补心丹
- following a febrile disease - *Huang Lian E Jiao Tang* 黄连阿胶汤
- severe insomnia with anxiety and palpitations - *Zhu Sha An Shen Wan* 朱砂安神丸

Heart and Gall Bladder *qi* deficiency - *An Shen Ding Zhi Wan* 安神定志丸

Liver *yin* (Blood) deficiency - *Suan Zao Ren Tang* 酸枣仁汤
- with *qi* stagnation - *Yi Guan Jian* 一贯煎

Endnote

For more information regarding herbs marked with an asterisk*, an open circle° or a hat ˆ, see the tables on pp.944-952.

Disorders of the Heart

31. Somnolence

Excess patterns
Dampness wrapping the Spleen
Phlegm obstruction
Blood stagnation

Deficient patterns
Spleen *qi* deficiency
Spleen and Kidney *yang* deficiency

31 SOMNOLENCE
duo mei 多寐

The term *duo mei* (literally too much sleep) refers to a particular type of tiredness, specifically mental fatigue and an inability to stay alert during the day. By convention, this chapter is usually addended to insomnia in the Heart section of the text, however there is little or no Heart pathology associated with *duo mei*. As we have seen in the previous chapter, inability to sleep is largely due to disturbance of the *shen*, that aspect of conscious awareness associated with the Heart. The mechanism of its corollary, however, has little to do with the *shen* or the Heart directly (although of course the final outcome does reflect some lack of expression of the *shen*). Rather, somnolence may be said to be a direct repercussion of the failure of clear *yang* to reach the head. The pathological patterns responsible tend to involve the Spleen more than the Heart.

Duo mei may cover some aspects of the fatigue our patients so often complain about when they say they are chronically tired or have low energy. It should be remembered though that *duo mei* refers specifically to mental fatigue and inability to think clearly, not just low physical energy. Low physical energy is often related to *qi* and/or Blood deficiency and does not involve a specific failure of *yang qi* to reach the head.

AETIOLOGY
Phlegm Damp
External Damp may affect people who have prolonged exposure to a damp climate or environmental damp (for example living in damp-affected houses). Alternatively, factors that weaken the Spleen (see below), enable the generation of internal Dampness, which eventually congeals into Phlegm. Such *yin* pathogens can obstruct the flow of *qi* and the ascent of clear *yang*.

Spleen *qi* deficiency
Excessive mental activity, irregular dietary habits (particularly excessive consumption of cold or raw food), or prolonged illness can drain Spleen *qi*. When the Spleen is not functioning properly, there will be inadequate generation of *qi* and Blood with consequent underfunctioning of all organ systems. In this case, inadequate *qi* means inadequate nourishment of the brain and senses.

Spleen and Kidney *yang* deficiency
Prolonged exposure to cold, excessive sexual activity, overwork and excessive consumption of cold raw foods drain Spleen and Kidney *yang*. The elderly,

chronically ill, and those with a constitutional tendency to Kidney weakness often exhibit a lack of *yang*. *Yang* is the dynamic and motivating aspect of normal physiology, and a lack of *yang* energy will manifest in its opposite–a relative excess of *yin*.

Blood stagnation

Head injury is the most common cause of drowsiness due to Blood stagnation. However, Blood stagnation from other causes, for example severe shock, chronic stagnation of *qi*, Phlegm or Damp, long term illness or old age can cause drowsiness and dulled mental activity

---

BOX 31.1 SOME BIOMEDICAL CAUSES OF SOMNOLENCE

- narcolepsy
- sleep apnoea
- hypoglycaemia
- food allergies
- chronic fatigue syndrome
- hypothyroidism
- psychological defense after shock or a physical reaction to trauma or injury (including surgery)
- bereavement
- alcohol excess
- antihistamines
- narcotic analgesics
- β-blockers

DIAGNOSIS

In broad terms, somnolence is due to a failure of *yang qi* invigorating the senses. This lack may be local or systemic. It may be due to systemic deficiency of *yang* or *qi* (a deficient pattern) or an obstruction to the flow of *yang* by Phlegm, Dampness or stagnant Blood (an excess pattern). In most cases there will be a mixture of deficiency and excess, for example, Spleen deficiency underlying Dampness or Phlegm.

BOX 31.2 KEY DIAGNOSTIC POINTS

Fatigue and sleepiness
- better for exercise - excess pattern
- worse for exertion - deficient pattern
- following trauma or shock - Blood stagnation

Tongue
- thick tongue coat - Dampness or Phlegm
- purple tongue or with brown or purple spots - Blood stagnation
- swollen and pale with a thin coat - Spleen *qi* deficiency
- swollen, pale or bluish with a moist coat - Spleen and Kidney *yang* deficiency

31.1 DAMPNESS WRAPPING THE SPLEEN

湿邪因脾多寐

Pathophysiology
- The presence of Dampness impedes the normal circulation of *yang qi*, in this case to the head and extremities. Without adequate *yang* to invigorate the brain and brighten the eyes, the patient experiences mental dullness, difficulty thinking clearly and the eyes wanting to close.

Clinical features
- Sleepiness and drowsiness, particularly after eating and more so after lunch. Depending on the degree of deficiency, however, there may also be difficulty sleeping at night (p.870).
- variable fatigue–may feel better for activity and exertion
- woolly headedness (like having the head wrapped in a damp towel), difficulty concentrating
- dizziness
- heavy tired limbs
- fullness and discomfort, or a feeling of blockage in the chest and epigastrium, abdominal distension
- poor appetite, loss of taste
- nausea, acid reflux
- loose stools

T swollen with a thick, white greasy coat
P soft and soggy or slippery

Treatment principle
Dry Dampness, strengthen the Spleen

Prescription

PING WEI SAN 平胃散
(*Magnolia and Ginger Formula*) modified

cang zhu (Rhizoma Atractylodis) 苍术	15g
hou po (Cortex Magnoliae Officinalis) 厚朴	12g
chen pi (Pericarpium Citri Reticulatae) 陈皮	9g
shi chang pu (Rhizoma Acori Graminei) 石菖蒲	9g
huo xiang (Herba Agastaches seu Pogostemi) 藿香	9g
sheng jiang (Rhizoma Zingiberis Officinalis) 生姜	3pce
da zao (Fructus Zizyphi Jujubae) 大枣	1pce
zhi gan cao (honey fried Radix Glycyrrhizae Uralensis) 炙甘草	6g

Method: Grind the herbs into powder and take 9-grams as a draft on an empty stomach. May also be decocted. (Source: *Shi Yong Zhong Yi Nei Ke Xue*)

Modifications
- With woolly headedness and poor concentration, add **yuan zhi** (Radix Polygalae Tenuifoliae) 远志 6g.
- With nausea, add **ban xia*** (Rhizoma Pinelliae Ternatae) 半夏 9g.
- With Cold, add **gan jiang** (Rhizoma Zingiberis Officinalis) 干姜 6g and **rou gui** (Cortex Cinnamomi Cassiae) 肉桂 3g.
- Prolonged stagnation of Dampness can generate Heat giving rise to a greasy yellow tongue coat, bitter taste in the mouth, yellow urine, irritability and a rapid pulse. Delete **huo xiang** and add **huang qin** (Radix Scutellariae Baicalensis) 黄芩 9g, **shan zhi zi** (Fructus Gardeniae Jasminoides) 山栀子 9g, **tong cao** (Medulla Tetrapanacis Papyriferi) 通草 6g and **yi ren** (Semen Coicis Lachryma-jobi) 苡仁 15g.
- With Spleen deficiency (loss of appetite, pale tongue, weak pulse), add **huang qi** (Radix Astragali Membranacei) 黄芪 12g, **bai zhu** (Rhizoma Atractylodis Macrocephalae) 白术 9g and **shan yao** (Radix Dioscoreae Oppositae) 山药 12g. See also p.870.

Patent medicines
Ping Wei San 平胃散 (Ping Wei San)
Er Chen Wan 二陈丸 (Er Chen Wan)
Xiang Sha Liu Jun Zi Wan 香砂六君子丸 (Xiang Sha Liu Jun Wan)
Xing Jun San 行军散 (Marching Powder, Five Pagodas Brand)
  - a powerful Damp dispersing agent, useful in small doses for difficult or resistent cases

Acupuncture
St.40 *(feng long -)*, Sp.3 *(tai bai)*, Du.20 *(bai hui)*, Bl.62 *(shen mai)*, Kid.6 *(zhao hai)*, Sp.9 *(yin ling quan)*, Sp.6 *(san yin jiao)*, Ren.12 *(zhong wan)*, St.36 *(zu san li +)*, GB.20 *(feng chi)*

Clinical notes
- The somnolence in this pattern may be associated with disorders such as narcolepsy, food allergies, hypoglycaemia, chronic fatigue syndrome and intestinal infection by candida albicans.
- This pattern can respond well to correct and prolonged treatment. Graded exercises are useful in some cases. Care with diet and avoidance of certain foods, if there is intolerance or allergy, is important.

31.2 PHLEGM OBSTRUCTION

痰浊痹阻多寐

Pathophysiology
- This pattern is similar to the previous one, except it occurs in people who exhibit a strong constitutional tendency to Phlegm accumulation. Consequently it tends to become a more chronic and stubborn condition. The Phlegm obstructs the rise of *yang* to the head causing sleepiness and unclear thinking.

Clinical features
- chronic and continuous somnolence, heavy sleep, difficult to rouse
- tendency to obesity
- glossy or greasy skin
- woolly headedness (like having the head wrapped in a damp towel)
- poor concentration
- dizziness
- heavy tired limbs
- fullness and discomfort, or a feeling of blockage in the chest and epigastrium

T flabby, with a thick greasy coat
P slippery

Treatment principle
Transform Phlegm, open channels to the head

Prescription

DI TAN TANG 涤痰汤
(*Scour Phlegm Decoction*) modified

dang shen (Radix Codonopsis Pilosulae) 党参	12g
ban xia* (Rhizoma Pinelliae Ternatae) 半夏	9g
fu ling (Sclerotium Poriae Cocos) 茯苓	9g
zhu ru (Caulis Bambusae in Taeniis) 竹茹	9g
chen pi (Pericarpium Citri Reticulatae) 陈皮	6g
dan nan xing* (Pulvis Arisaemae cum Felle Bovis) 胆南星	6g
shi chang pu (Rhizoma Acori Graminei) 石菖蒲	6g
zhi shi (Fructus Immaturus Citri Aurantii) 枳实	6g
gan cao (Radix Glycyrrhizae Uralensis) 甘草	3g
sheng jiang (Rhizoma Zingiberis Officinalis) 生姜	3pce
da zao (Fructus Zizyphi Jujubae) 大枣	4pce

Method: Decoction. (Source: *Shi Yong Zhong Yao Xue*)

Modifications
- With no Heat, delete **zhu ru**, and substitute **tian nan xing*** (Rhizoma Arisaematis) 天南星 6g for **dan nan xing**.
- With Heat, add **huang lian** (Rhizoma Coptidis) 黄连 6g, **qing dai** (Pulverata Indigo) 青黛 3g and **huang qin** (Radix Scutellariae Baicalensis) 黄芩 9g.

Patent medicines
Er Chen Wan 二陈丸 (Er Chen Wan)
Xiang Sha Liu Jun Zi Wan 香砂六君子丸 (Xiang Sha Liu Jun Wan)

Acupuncture
St.40 (*feng long* -), Sp.3 (*tai bai* -), Du.20 (*bai hui*), Sp.9 (*yin ling quan* -), Sp.6 (*san yin jiao*), St.25 (*tian shu*), Ren.12 (*zhong wan*), Bl.20 (*pi shu*), St.36 (*zu san li* +), Liv.3 (*tai chong*), GB.20 (*feng chi*), Bl.62 (*shen mai*), Kid.6 (*zhao hai*)

Clinical notes
- The somnolence in this pattern may be associated with disorders such as narcolepsy, chronic fatigue syndrome, systemic candidiasis or morbid obesity
- Because of the contitutional tendency to Phlegm in this pattern, treatment generally takes a long time. Appropriate dietary and lifestyle changes (such as weight loss and exercise) are necessary for satisfactory results.

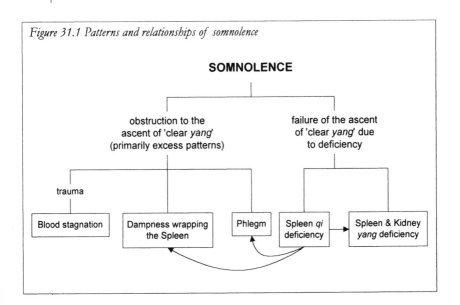

Figure 31.1 Patterns and relationships of somnolence

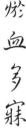

31.3 BLOOD STAGNATION

Pathophysiology
- Blood stagnation type somnolence usually follows a head injury or other trauma. In acute cases the history is the key feature, as classical Blood stagnation signs and symptoms may not be apparent. Blood stagnation may also follow other chronic pathologies, especially prolonged *qi* stagnation, in which case there will usually be objective signs of stagnant Blood.

Clinical features
- persistent daytime drowsiness, mental confusion and unclear thinking
- recurrent fixed headache
- chronic tinnitus
- dizziness
- low grade fever at night
- broken vessels or spider naevi on the face, trunk, inner knee and ankle
- darkish complexion
- dark rings around the eyes, purplish lips, sclera, conjunctiva and nail beds
- depression, mood swings

T in acute cases may be unremarkable; in chronic cases dark or purplish with brown or purple stagnation spots
P choppy or wiry and thready

Treatment principle
Invigorate the circulation of Blood
Open the channels and collaterals

Prescription

TONG QIAO HUO XUE TANG 通窍活血汤
(*Unblock the Orifices and Invigorate the Blood Decoction*) modified

This formula is quite specific for stagnant Blood affecting the head and in particular the senses.

tao ren (Semen Persicae) 桃仁	9g
hong hua (Flos Carthami Tinctorii) 红花	9g
chi shao (Radix Paeoniae Rubrae) 赤芍	6g
chuan xiong (Radix Ligustici Chuanxiong) 川芎	6g
cong bai (Bulbus Allii Fistulosi) 葱白	3g
da zao (Fructus Zizyphi Jujubae) 大枣	7pce
sheng jiang (Rhizoma Zingiberis Officinalis) 生姜	9g
she xiang° (Secretio Moschus) 麝香	0.15g

Method: Decoction. **She xiang** is usually taken separately or added to the strained decoction. (Source: *Shi Yong Zhong Yi Nei Ke Xue*)

XUE FU ZHU YU TANG 血府逐瘀汤, p.821
(Achyranthes and Persica Combination)

This is an excellent general formula for generalised *qi* and Blood stagnation, particularly that affecting the upper body. It is selected when there are systemic signs of Blood stasis.

Modifications (apply to both prescriptions, where not already included)
- With *qi* stagnation, add **qing pi** (Pericarpium Citri Reticulatae Viride) 青皮 9g, **chen pi** (Pericarpium Citri Reticulatae) 陈皮 6g, **xiang fu** (Rhizoma Cyperi Rotundi) 香附 9g and **zhi ke** (Fructus Citri Aurantii) 枳壳 9g.
- With *qi* deficiency, add **huang qi** (Radix Astragali Membranacei) 黄芪 12g and **dang shen** (Radix Codonopsis Pilosulae) 党参 12g.
- With *yin* deficiency, add **sheng di** (Radix Rehmanniae Glutinosae) 生地 12g, **dan shen** (Radix Salviae Miltiorrhizae) 丹参 12g and **mu dan pi** (Cortex Moutan Radicis) 牡丹皮 9g.
- With Cold or *yang* deficiency, add **gui zhi** (Ramulus Cinnamomi Cassiae) 桂枝 9g and **zhi fu zi*** (Radix Aconiti Carmichaeli Praeparata) 制附子 6g.
- With Heat, add **huang qin** (Radix Scutellariae Baicalensis) 黄芩 9g and **shan zhi zi** (Fructus Gardeniae Jasminoides) 山栀子 9g.
- With Phlegm, add **ban xia*** (Rhizoma Pinelliae Ternatae) 半夏 9g, **chen pi** (Pericarpium Citri Reticulatae) 陈皮 6g and **bai jie zi** (Semen Sinapsis Albae) 白芥子 6g.

Patent medicines
Xue Fu Zhu Yu Wan 血府逐瘀丸 (Xue Fu Zhu Yu Wan)

Acupuncture
Local points of pain on the head plus Bl.15 (*xin shu* -), LI.4 (*he gu* -), Bl.17 (*ge shu* -), Sp.6 (*san yin jiao* -), Sp.10 (*xue hai* -), GB.20 (*feng chi* -), Bl.62 (*shen mai*), SI.3 (*hou xi*), Kid.6 (*zhao hai*), Liv.3 (*tai chong*), *si shen cong* (M-HN-1)
- with shock, add Du.26 (*ren zhong*)

Clinical notes
- The somnolence in this pattern may be associated with disorders such as concussion, post concussion syndrome, cerebral tumours, post stroke, post shock or post trauma of any sort including surgery.
- This pattern can be difficult to treat when chronic; acute cases generally respond better to treatment.

31.4 SPLEEN *QI* (AND BLOOD) DEFICIENCY

脾气不足多寐

Pathophysiology
- In Spleen deficiency somnolence, it is deficiency rather than obstruction that prevents the brain and senses from receiving sufficient *qi* so there is sleepiness and a lack of alertness accompanied by physical fatigue.

Clinical features
- daytime drowsiness and desire for sleep which is worse for exertion and eating
- paradoxically, if the Blood has become significantly depleted, Blood deficient insomnia may develop at night (see p.849)
- mental and physical fatigue
- weakness and tiredness in the limbs
- sallow, pale complexion
- poor appetite, nausea
- abdominal distension
- loose stools

T pale and swollen with tooth marks and a thin white coat
P deficient and weak

Treatment principle
Strengthen the Spleen and tonify *qi*
Dry Dampness (if necessary)

Prescription

XIANG SHA LIU JUN ZI TANG 香砂六君子汤
(*Saussurea and Cardamon Combination*) modified

bai zhu (Rhizoma Atractylodis Macrocephalae) 白术	12g
fu ling (Sclerotium Poriae Cocos) 茯苓	12g
ban xia* (Rhizoma Pinelliae Ternatae) 半夏	9g
chen pi (Pericarpium Citri Reticulatae) 陈皮	6g
ren shen (Radix Ginseng) 人参	6g
sha ren (Fructus Amomi) 砂仁	6g
mu xiang (Radix Aucklandiae Lappae) 木香	6g
shi chang pu (Rhizoma Acori Graminei) 石菖蒲	6g
zhi gan cao (honey fried Radix Glycyrrhizae Uralensis) 炙甘草	3g

Method: Decoction. **Sha ren** is added towards the end of cooking time (*hou xia* 后下). (Source: *Shi Yong Zhong Yi Nei Ke Xue*)

Modifications
* With food stagnation, add two or three of the following herbs: **jiao shen qu** (baked Massa Fermentata) 焦神曲 10g, **jiao shan zha** (baked Fructus Crataegi) 焦山楂 10g, **chao mai ya** (dry fried Fructus Hordei Vulgaris Germinantus) 炒麦芽 10g or **chao lai fu zi** (dry fried Semen Raphani Sativi) 炒莱服子 15g.
* With cold extremities, add **gan jiang** (Rhizoma Zingiberis Officinalis) 干姜 6g.
* With thin watery mucus, add **gan jiang** (Rhizoma Zingiberis Officinale) 干姜 6g and **hou po** (Cortex Magnoliae Officinalis) 厚朴 6g.
* With spontaneous sweating, add **mu li^** (Concha Ostreae) 牡蛎 15g, **ma huang gen** (Radix Ephedrae) 麻黄根 9g, **fu xiao mai** (Semen Tritici Aestivi Levis) 浮小麦 12g.

Variations and additional prescriptions
* If Spleen *qi* is sinking, with symptoms such as rectal prolapse or haemorrhoids use **BU ZHONG YI QI TANG** (*Ginseng and Astragalus Combination* 补中益气汤, p.394).
* If *qi* and Blood are both deficient, with shortness of breath, palpitations, and a lustreless complexion use either **REN SHEN YANG YING TANG** (*Ginseng Nutritive Combination* 人参养营汤, p.887) or **SHI QUAN DA BU TANG** (*Ginseng and Dang Gui Ten Combination* 十全大补汤, p.529).

Patent medicines
Xiang Sha Liu Jun Zi Wan 香砂六君子丸 (Xiang Sha Liu Jun Wan)
Ping Wei San 平胃散 (Ping Wei San)
 - combine with the above patent medicine with significant Dampness
Er Chen Wan 二陈丸 (Er Chen Wan)
 - combine with the above patent medicine with significant Phlegm

Acupuncture
Du.20 (*bai hui*), Sp.6 (*san yin jiao* +), Ren.12 (*zhong wan* +), Bl.62 (*shen mai*), Kid.6 (*zhao hai*), St.40 (*feng long* -), Sp.3 (*tai bai* +), St.36 (*zu san li* +), Bl.20 (*pi shu* +), *si shen cong* (M-HN-1)

Clinical notes
* The somnolence in this pattern may be associated with disorders such as narcolepsy, hypoglycaemia, chronic fatigue syndrome, food allergies or systemic candidiasis.
* The mental fatigue of this pattern responds well to correct treatment, although chronic fatigue syndrome itself can take a long time to treat successfully.

- Some foods should be avoided if there are allergies or intolerances. To maintain steady blood sugar, small frequent meals (containing protein and complex carbohydrate) should be taken. Sugar and caffeine, the old standbys for people with fatigue and sleepiness, should be strictly avoided by patients in this category until Spleen function is strengthened and blood sugar regulated.

31.5 SPLEEN AND KIDNEY *YANG* DEFICIENCY

Pathophysiology
- *Yang* is the dynamic and motivating aspect of normal physiology, thus lack of *yang* will manifest in its opposite–an excess of *yin*–in this case dulled sensorium and drowsiness. *Yang* deficiency is especially pronounced in the daytime, the time when the body should be at its most *yang*.

Clinical features
- constant drowsiness and desire to sleep, the patient sleeps curled up
- mental and physical exhaustion
- apathy and depression
- soft voice, reluctance to speak
- forgetfulness
- lower back ache
- low libido, impotence
- digestive weakness
- cold intolerance and extremities

T pale or bluish and swollen with a thin moist coat
P deep, thready and weak

Treatment principle
Benefit *qi*, warm *yang*
Strengthen the Spleen and Kidney

Prescription

FU ZI LI ZHONG WAN 附子理中丸
(*Aconite, Ginseng and Ginger Formula*)

This formula is selected when the primary deficiency affects the Spleen. The main features are somnolence with digestive weakness and loss of appetite and diarrhoea.

zhi fu zi* (Radix Aconiti Carmichaeli Praeparata) 制附子 9g
gan jiang (Rhizoma Zingiberis Officinalis) 干姜 9g
ren shen (Radix Ginseng) 人参 9g
bai zhu (Rhizoma Atractylodis Macrocephalae) 白术 9g
zhi gan cao (honey fried Radix Glycyrrhizae Uralensis)
炙甘草 9g

Method: Grind herbs into powder and form into 3-gram pills with honey. The dose is one pill 2-3 times daily on an empty stomach. May also be prepared as a decoction, in which case **zhi fu zi** is cooked for 30 minutes prior to the other herbs (*xian jian* 先煎).

阳气虚衰多寐

JIN KUI SHEN QI WAN 金匮肾气丸
(Rehmannia Eight Formula)

This formula is selected when Kidney *yang* deficiency is prominent. The main features are somnolence with urinary dysfunction, lower back ache and oedema of the lower extremities.

shu di (Radix Rehmanniae Glutinosae Conquitae) 熟地 240g
shan yao (Radix Dioscoreae Oppositae) 山药 120g
shan zhu yu (Fructus Corni Officinalis) 山茱萸 120g
fu ling (Sclerotium Poria Cocos) 茯苓 90g
ze xie (Rhizoma Alismatis Orientalis) 泽泻 90g
mu dan pi (Cortex Moutan Radicis) 牡丹皮 90g
zhi fu zi* (Radix Aconiti Carmichaeli Praeparata) 制附子 60g
rou gui (Cortex Cinnamomi Cassiae) 肉桂 40g

Method: Grind the herbs into powder and form into 9-gram pills with honey. The dose is 2-3 pills daily. May be decocted with a 90% reduction in dosage. When decocted **zhi fu zi** is cooked for 30 minutes before the other herbs (*xian jian* 先煎). (Source: *Shi Yong Zhong Yi Nei Ke Xue*)

Variations and additional prescriptions
♦ In severe cases with evidence of both *yang* and *yin* deficiency, use prescriptions that have a stronger *jing* nourishing effect, like **YOU GUI WAN** (*Eucommia and Rehmannia Formula* 右归丸, p.559) or **GUI LU ER XIAN JIAO** (*Tortise Shell and Deer Antler Syrup* 龟鹿二仙胶, p.920).

Patent medicines
Fu Zi Li Zhong Wan 附子理中丸 (Li Chung Yuen Medical Pills)
Li Zhong Wan 理中丸 (Li Zhong Wan)
Jin Kui Shen Qi Wan 金匮肾气丸 (Sexoton Pills)

Acupuncture
Bl.23 (*shen shu* +▲), Bl.20 (*pi shu* +▲), Du.4 (*ming men* ▲), Kid.3 (*tai xi* +), Bl.52 (*zhi shi*), Ren.6 (*qi hai* +▲), Du.20 (*bai hui*), Bl.62 (*shen mai*), Kid.6 (*zhao hai*), St.36 (*zu san li* +▲)

Clinical notes
• The somnolence in this pattern may be associated with disorders such as narcolepsy, chronic fatigue syndrome, old age, post illness recovery or hypothyroidism.
• Symptoms of *yang* deficiency generally respond well to correct treatment, although profound or long term deficiency always needs long term therapy.

SUMMARY OF GUIDING FORMULAE FOR SOMNOLENCE

Excess patterns
Dampness wrapping the Spleen - *Ping Wei San* 平胃散

Turbid Phlegm obstruction - *Di Tan Tang* 涤痰汤

Stagnant Blood - *Tong Qiao Huo Xue Tang* 通窍活血汤

Deficient patterns
Spleen *qi* deficiency - *Xiang Sha Liu Jun Zi Tang* 香砂六君子汤

Spleen and Kidney *yang* deficiency
- with primary Spleen deficiency - *Fu Zi Li Zhong Wan* 附子理中丸
- with primary Kidney deficiency - *Jin Kui Shen Qi Wan* 金匮肾气丸
- with *yang* and *yin* deficiency - *You Gui Wan* 右归丸

Endnote

For more information regarding herbs marked with an asterisk*, an open circle° or a hatˆ, see the tables on pp.944-952.

Disorders of the Heart

32. Forgetfulness

Heart and Spleen deficiency
Heart and Kidney not communicating
Kidney *jing* deficiency
Phlegm and Blood stagnation

32 FORGETFULNESS
jian wang 健忘

According to TCM theory, memory depends on the balanced interaction of various aspects of the Heart, Spleen and Kidney. Those aspects of healthy mental functioning which operate to allow clear and enduring memory, are the *yi* 意, *zhi* 志, *shen* 神 and *jing* 精.

Shen (Heart) is responsible for clarity of thought and perception in general. The *yi* (Spleen) controls the ability to focus and concentrate. Understanding or analysis of factual material or ideas is the domain of the *shen* and the *zhi* (Kidneys), while the laying down of memories in the grey matter (Marrow) depends on *jing*.

TCM THEORY OF MEMORY

Processing of perceptions into memory happens every waking moment of life through the effort of *yi* and the awareness of *shen*, thus very many layers of memory are laid down in the body's store of *jing*. As new memories are processed, they are stored (like holographic images) in the substrata of *jing*, the earliest memories at the deepest levels. Long term memory and indeed our collective ancestral memory is related to the quality and quantity of *jing*. It is the transfer of *jing* from one generation to the next that maintains the continuous link to our primordial roots.

Loss of short term memory, such as that following a shock or trauma, is usually related to severe destabilisation of the *shen* or a severing of the communication between the *shen* and *zhi*, while loss of long term memory reflects a more deep seated disorder affecting the *jing* and Marrow. The loss of short term memory typical of advancing age, however, is related to the amount of *jing* remaining. As ageing inexorably consumes *jing*, converting it into *shen* in the process, the most deeply buried memories are uncovered. Thus the very elderly often have very clear memories of their childhood or events of the distant past but very little capacity for short term memory. At this stage of life the amount of *jing* remaining is small, and therefore the amount that can be converted to *shen* is small–clarity of *shen* is reduced and short term memory lost.

This chapter covers memory disorders ranging from the vagueness and poor concentration seen in some neurological diseases and during convalescence, to the amnesia associated with trauma or concussion and full blown dementia with loss of short and long term memory.

AETIOLOGY
Heart Blood and Spleen *qi* deficiency
Excessive mental activity and/or irregular dietary habits can drain Spleen *qi*. This can lead to inadequate generation of *qi* and Blood and consequent underfunction of all organ systems. Spleen weakness leads to instability of the *yi* and therefore to an inability to focus and concentrate, causing short attention span and poor capacity to memorise. Heart weakness, usually as the result of mental stress or shock, or in this case Blood deficiency, causes a *shen* imbalance and a tendency to unclear thinking, poor short term memory and inarticulate speech. Heart and Spleen deficiency often follows inadequate recovery following childbirth or a severe post partum (or other) haemorrhage.

Heart and Kidney not communicating
The relationship between the Heart and Kidney, one of the fundamental relationships of the body and mind, can be disturbed in a number of ways. At a deep level it involves a breakdown of the controlling (*ke* 克, p.70) cycle, where Kidney water prevents a runaway blaze of Heart Fire. Heart and Kidney *yin* are damaged by overworking (especially while under stress), insufficient sleep, febrile diseases, ageing, excessive ejaculation, many pregnancies and abuse of recreational drugs. Prolonged or excessive use of these drugs is quite a common and important cause of forgetfulness and memory loss. The most commonly abused substances in the West are alcohol, cannabis, amphetamine and cocaine. Most likely to consume Heart and Kidney *yin* are cannabis, amphetamines and cocaine. Alcohol tends to clog the brain with Damp Heat. Other drugs that damage *yin* are the anxiolytic benzodiazepines, withdrawal from which can cause memory loss.

At a more superficial level, disconnection of Heart and Kidney may occur as the result of a major shock or trauma, severing the communication between the *zhi* and the *shen*. Clinically, this situation presents primarily with mental symptoms and few, if any, physical symptoms.

Decline of *jing*
The elderly are prone to forgetfulness due to the decline of *jing*. *Jing* is responsible for the maintenance of the Marrow and brain, and for the storage of memory. As the basis of the body's *yin* and *yang*, *jing* is consumed as part of the natural process of ageing. A weakness of *jing* may also be inherited. *Jing* deficiency patterns are not restricted to the elderly or those who inherit poor quality *jing*. Excessive ejaculation, many pregnancies, miscarriages or terminations, severe illness and drug abuse can also consume *jing*.

Blood and Phlegm stagnation

Stagnant Blood and/or Phlegm will obstruct the passage of 'clear *yang*' to the head, affecting the clarity of many mental functions. It may occur as a result of an acute trauma, whether this be injury to the head or a sudden shock, or as a result of chronic or long term *qi* stagnation or accumulation of Phlegm or Damp. Blood and Phlegm stagnation may appear as a complication of any long term illness or simply because of old age.

心脾两虚健忘

32.1 HEART BLOOD AND SPLEEN *QI* DEFICIENCY

Pathophysiology
- When Heart Blood is weak, the *shen* is unanchored and becomes unstable. When Spleen *qi* is deficient, the *yi* will be weak. Depending on whether the Heart or the Spleen is more affected, the patient will exhibit either more forgetfulness or poor attention span and inability to concentrate.

Clinical features
- forgetfulness, poor memory, absent-mindedness, short attention span, inability to concentrate
- insomnia, with particular difficulty falling asleep (and switching off the mind) and dream disturbed sleep
- palpitations with or without anxiety
- anxiety, phobias, panic attacks
- postural dizziness
- blurring vision
- fatigue and weakness
- poor appetite
- abdominal distension after eating
- sallow, pale complexion
- easy bruising
- heavy or prolonged menstrual periods

T pale with a thin white coat
P thready and weak

Treatment principle
Strengthen and nourish the Heart and Spleen
Tonify *qi* and Blood, calm the *shen*

Prescription

GUI PI TANG 归脾汤
(*Ginseng and Longan Combination*) modified

huang qi (Radix Astragali Membranacei) 黄芪	15g
bai zhu (Rhizoma Atractylodis Macrocephalae) 白术	12g
fu shen (Sclerotium Poriae Cocos Pararadicis) 茯神	12g
suan zao ren (Semen Ziziphi Spinosae) 酸枣仁	12g
long yan rou (Arillus Euphoriae Longanae) 龙眼肉	9g
dang gui (Radix Angelicae Sinensis) 当归	9g
ren shen (Radix Ginseng) 人参	6g
mu xiang (Radix Aucklandiae Lappae) 木香	6g
shi chang pu (Rhizoma Acori Graminei) 石菖蒲	6g

yuan zhi (Radix Polygalae Tenuifoliae) 远志 6g
zhi gan cao (honey fried Radix Glycyrrhizae Uralensis)
炙甘草 6g

Method: Decoction. (Source: *Shi Yong Zhong Yi Nei Ke Xue*)

Modifications

- With marked Heart Blood deficiency (severe forgetfulness, palpitations and anxiety), add **shu di** (Radix Rehmanniae Glutinosae Conquitae) 熟地 30-50g, **bai shao** (Radix Paeoniae Lactiflora) 白芍 15g and **e jiao^** (Gelatinum Corii Asini) 阿胶 15g. Add **sha ren** (Fructus Amomi) 砂仁 6g to aid digestion of the rich Blood tonics.
- With marked Spleen *qi* deficiency, it may be necessary to initially reduce the dose of (or delete) the richer Blood tonics (**long yan rou** and **dang gui**) until the Spleen is strong enough to digest them properly.
- With severe insomnia, add two or three of the following herbs: **wu wei zi** (Fructus Schizandrae Chinensis) 五味子 6, **bai zi ren** (Semen Biotae Orientalis) 柏子仁 9g, **ye jiao teng** (Caulis Polygoni Multiflori) 夜交藤 30g, **he huan pi** (Cortex Albizziae Julibrissin) 合欢皮 9g, **long chi^** (Dens Draconis) 龙齿 10g or **mu li^** (Concha Ostreae) 牡蛎 30g, and **mai ya** (Fructus Hordei Vulgaris Germinantus) 麦芽 15g to protect the Stomach from damage by the mineral drugs.
- With Liver Heat, add **shan zhi zi** (Fructus Gardeniae Jasminoidis) 山栀子 9g and **chai hu** (Radix Bupleuri) 柴胡 6g.
- With Dampness causing abdominal and epigastric fullness, poor appetite and a greasy or glossy tongue coat, add **ban xia*** (Rhizoma Pinelliae Ternatae) 半夏 10g and **chen pi** (Pericarpium Citri Reticulatae) 陈皮 10g.

Patent medicines

Gui Pi Wan 归脾丸 (Gui Pi Wan)
Bai Zi Yang Xin Wan 柏子养心丸 (Bai Zi Yang Xin Wan)
Dang Gui Ji Jing 当归鸡精 (Tang Kuei Essence of Chicken)
Bu Nao Wan 补脑丸 (Cerebral Tonic Pills)

Acupuncture

Du.20 (*bai hui* +), Bl.52 (*zhi shi* +), Ht.3 (*shao hai*), Ht.7 (*shen men* +), Bl.15 (*xin shu* +), Bl.17 (*ge shu* +), Bl.20 (*pi shu* +), *yin tang* (M-HN-3), Sp.6 (*san yin jiao* +), St.36 (*zu san li* +), Ren.4 (*guan yuan* +)
- with much dreaming add Bl.42 (*po hu*)

Clinical notes

- The fogetfulness of this pattern may be associated with disorders such as anaemia, neuresthenia, post-concussion syndrome, post-illness

convalescence, depression, drug abuse or multiple sclerosis.
- The forgetfulness and other symptoms of Heart and Spleen deficiency generally respond well to correct treatment; when the deficiency is severe or prolonged, however, long term treatment will be necessary. In the case of a disease like multiple sclerosis of a Heart and Spleen deficiency type, the prognosis is much less certain.
- Spleen *qi* needs to be supported with regular eating habits and easily digested mild foods. Good quality and sufficient sleep is essential, so a strictly regular bedtime routine should be adhered to.
- In women who lose blood (and thus Heart Blood) through heavy periods (or post partum haemorrhage), Blood tonics and Blood replenishing and iron rich foods should be taken after each period. Iron supplements are also useful.
- Activities to calm the *shen* and exercise the *yi* are useful. For example the gentle exercise of *tai qi*, yoga or regular walking are excellent to calm the mind and gradually build *qi*. The *yi* can be exercised by concentration training, like doing crosswords or meditation.
- Treatment with herbs may be important to build the Blood, but acupuncture treatment, especially with points like Du.20 (*bai hui*), will often be requested by the patient once they have expereinced its effect of lifting *qi* to the head and stimulating the mind.

32.2 HEART AND KIDNEY *YIN* DEFICIENCY

Pathophysiology
- Heart and Kidney *yin* deficiency type forgetfulness (also known as Heart and Kidney not communicating) is due to a breakdown in the relationship between the *shen* and *zhi*, such that the mind loses stability and the capacity to remember clearly. The breakdown of this fundamental relationship can occur because Kidney *yin* fails to nourish Heart *yin* and balance Heart Fire, which then blazes out of control. It can also occur following a major trauma or shock.

Clinical features
- forgetfulness
- insomnia, with frequent waking, or waking feeling hot or sweaty
- restlessness
- palpitations
- anxiety, panic attacks
- sensation of heat in the palms and soles ('five hearts hot')
- night sweats
- dry mouth and throat
- dizziness and tinnitus
- lower back ache

T red with little or no coat
P thready and rapid

Treatment principle
Nourish Heart and Kidney *yin*
Clear Heat, calm the *shen*

Prescription

TIAN WANG BU XIN DAN 天王补心丹
(*Ginseng and Zizyphus Formula*)

sheng di (Radix Rehmanniae Glutinosae) 生地	120 (24)g
tian dong (Tuber Asparagi Cochinchinensis) 天冬	30 (12)g
mai dong (Tuber Ophiopogonis Japonici) 麦冬	30 (12)g
suan zao ren (Semen Zizyphi Spinosae) 酸枣仁	30 (12)g
xuan shen (Radix Scrophulariae) 玄参	15 (12)g
dan shen (Radix Salviae Miltiorrhizae) 丹参	15 (12)g
fu ling (Sclerotium Poriae Cocos) 茯苓	15 (12)g
dang gui (Radix Angelicae Sinensis) 当归	30 (9)g
wu wei zi (Fructus Schizandrae Chinensis) 五味子	30 (9)g
bai zi ren (Semen Biotae Orientalis) 柏子仁	30 (9)g

ren shen (Radix Ginseng) 人参	15 (9)g
jie geng (Radix Platycodi Grandiflori) 桔梗	15 (9)g
yuan zhi (Radix Polygalae Tenuifoliae) 远志	15 (6)g
zhu sha* (Cinnabaris) 朱砂 (optional)	6 (0.5)g

Method: Grind herbs (except **zhu sha**) to a powder and form into 9-gram pills with honey. If used, coat the outside of the pills with the **zhu sha**. The dose is one pill 2-3 times daily. May be decocted with the dosage in brackets. When decocted the **zhu sha** is taken as powder with the strained decoction. This is an excellent formula for long term use in treating *yin* deficiency with *shen* disturbance (in which case the **zhu sha** is deleted). (Source: *Shi Yong Zhong Yi Nei Ke Xue*)

Variations and additional prescriptions

Severe Heat, or following a febrile illness
* If symptoms of *yin* deficient Fire are severe, or the disorder occurs following a febrile disease the correct treatment is to nourish *yin* and clear Fire with **HUANG LIAN E JIAO TANG** (*Coptis and Ass-Hide Gelatin Decoction* 黄连阿胶汤, p.839).

Following a major shock or trauma
* If forgetfulness (or in severe cases amnesia) follows a major shock or trauma (other than head injury, see p.890) this indicates that communication between the Heart and Kidneys has been severed. Typically, the characteristic symptoms of *yin* deficiency may be absent and instead the forgetfulness is accompanied by, insomnia and dream- or nightmare–disturbed sleep, flashbacks, panic attacks, palpitations, hair loss, loss of appetite, dizziness, depression, lack of motivation, a slightly pale tongue and a hollow, slow pulse. A useful formula is **GUI ZHI JIA LONG GU MU LI TANG** (*Cinnamon and Dragon Bone Combination* 桂枝加龙骨牡蛎汤, p.814), with the addition of **shi chang pu** (Rhizoma Acori Graminei) 石菖蒲 6g and **yuan zhi** (Radix Polygalae Tenuifoliae) 远志 6g.

With Kidney yin *deficiency*
* If Kidney *yin* is particularly weak, the main principle is to nourish Kidney *yin*, calm the *shen*, and promote memory with **SHENG HUI TANG** (*Promote Wisdom Decoction* 生慧汤).

shu di (Radix Rehmanniae Glutinosae Conquitae) 熟地	18-30g
suan zao ren (Semen Zizyphi Spinosae) 酸枣仁	15g
shan zhu yu (Fructus Corni Officinalis) 山茱萸	12g
bai zi ren (Semen Biotae Orientalis) 柏子仁	12g
fu shen (Sclerotium Poriae Cocos Pararadicis) 茯神	12g
ren shen (Radix Ginseng) 人参	9g
yuan zhi (Radix Polygalae Tenuifoliae) 远志	6g

    shi chang pu (Rhizoma Acori Graminei) 石菖蒲 6g
    bai jie zi (Semen Sinapsis Albae) 白芥子 6g
    Method: Decoction. (Source: *Shi Yong Zhong Yi Nei Ke Xue*)

Patent medicines
Tian Wang Bu Xin Dan 天王补心丹 (Tian Wang Bu Xin Dan)
 - excellent for Heart *yin* deficiency with *shen* disturbance
Zuo Gui Wan 左归丸 (Zuo Gui Wan)
Sheng Mai Wan 生脉丸 (Sheng Mai Wan)
Liu Wei Di Huang Wan 六味地黄丸 (Liu Wei Di Huang Wan)
 - a general Kidney *yin* tonic formula
Suan Zao Ren Tang Pian 酸枣仁汤片 (Tabellae Suanzaoren)

Acupuncture
PC.6 (*nei guan* +), PC.7 (*da ling* +), Kid.3 (*tai xi* +), Ht.7 (*shen men* +), Ht.8 (*shao fu*), Bl.52 (*zhi shi* +), Du.20 (*bai hui*), Bl.15 (*xin shu* +), Bl.23 (*shen shu* +), Bl.14 (*jue yin shu* +), Liv.3 (*tai chong*), *yin tang* (M-HN-3)
 • with arrhythmias add Ht.5 (*tong li*)

Clinical notes
• The fogetfulness of this pattern may be associated with disorders such as menopausal syndrome, neuresthenia, hyperthyroidism, anxiety neurosis, fever of unknown origin, convalescence following a febrile disorder, drug abuse (for example anxiolytic drugs or chronic marijuana use) or post traumatic shock syndrome.
• Heart and Kidney *yin* deficiency patterns generally respond well to correct treatment, however for it to be long lasting the *yin* will have to be replenished and this takes time. Although some improvment may be observed in a few weeks, treatment should continue for several months. Herbs are generally more useful at replenishing *yin* than acupuncture, although acupuncture should be considered to help control any anxiety or restlessness associated with this pattern.
• Proper rest and regular sleep is essential to recovery, and a strict bedtime routine should be adhered to, even in those patients with sleep disturbance. Sleep will gradually improve with treatment.
• Care with other aggravating factors like sex, excessive lifting and standing and dehydration.
• Active pursuit of relaxation should be encouraged. Particularly good for calming the mind are gentle exercises such as *tai qi* and yoga.

32.3 KIDNEY *JING* DEFICIENCY

Pathophysiology
- This pattern is most common in the elderly and is due to gradual consumption of *jing* with ageing. It can also occur in younger people who have inherited insufficient *jing*, or who have lost it through illness, excessive sex or drug use.

Clinical features
- poor memory, in severe cases (usually the elderly) loss of recognition of close relatives, forgetting events instantly, dulled sensorium
- generalised weakness, emaciation
- greying, falling, lifeless hair, or early balding
- soreness and weakness of the lower back and lower extremities
- poor libido, impotence, infertility
- frequent urination, nocturia
- tinnitus, loss of hearing
- loss of visual acuity

T pale with a thin white coat
P thready and weak

Treatment principle
Nourish and tonify the Kidney, *qi* and Blood
Consolidate *jing*

Prescription

REN SHEN YANG YING TANG 人参养营汤
(*Ginseng Nutritive Combination*)

shu di (Radix Rehmanniae Glutinosae Conquitae) 熟地	12g
huang qi (Radix Astragali Membranacei) 黄芪	12g
ren shen (Radix Ginseng) 人参	12g
bai zhu (Rhizoma Atractylodis Macrocephalae) 白术	9g
fu ling (Sclerotium Poriae Cocos) 茯苓	9g
bai shao (Radix Paeoniae Lactiflora) 白芍	9g
dang gui (Radix Angelicae Sinensis) 当归	9g
wu wei zi (Fructus Schizandrae Chinensis) 五味子	6g
chen pi (Pericarpium Citri Reticulatae) 陈皮	6g
yuan zhi (Radix Polygalae Tenuifoliae) 远志	6g
zhi gan cao (honey fried Radix Glycyrrhizae Uralensis) 炙甘草	6g
rou gui (Cortex Cinnamomi Cassiae) 肉桂	3g
sheng jiang (Rhizoma Zingiberis Officinalis) 生姜	3pce
da zao (Fructus Zizyphi Jujubae) 大枣	4pce

Method: Decoction. (Source: *Shi Yong Zhong Yi Nei Ke Xue*)

Modifications

- In most cases the formula is improved by the addition of one or two of the following *jing* tonifying herbs: **lu jiao jiao**^ (Cornu Cervi Gelatinum) 鹿角胶 10g, **gui ban jiao**° (Plastri Testudinis Gelatinum) 龟板胶 10g, **wu jia pi** (Cortex Acanthopanacis Gracilistyli) 五加皮 10g, **ba ji tian** (Radix Morindae Officinalis) 巴戟天 10g or **zi he che fen**^ (powdered Placenta Hominis) 紫河车粉 3g. Combining with a patent formula such as **GUI LU ER XIAN JIAO** (*Tortise Shell and Deer Antler Syrup* 龟鹿二仙胶, p.920) is also useful.
- With signs of Blood stagnation, add **dan shen** (Radix Salviae Miltiorrhizae) 丹参 12g and **mu dan pi** (Cortex Moutan Radicis) 牡丹皮 9g.
- With Cold or *yang* deficiency add **gui zhi** (Ramulus Cinnamomi Cassiae) 桂枝 9g and **zhi fu zi*** (Radix Aconiti Carmichaeli Praeparata) 制附子 6g, boiled for 30 minutes before the other herbs (*xian jian* 先煎).
- With Heat, add **huang qin** (Radix Scutellariae Baicalensis) 黄芩 9g and **shan zhi zi** (Fructus Gardeniae Jasminoides) 山栀子 9g.
- With Phlegm, add **ban xia*** (Rhizoma Pinelliae Ternatae) 半夏 9g, **chen pi** (Pericarpium Citri Reticulatae) 陈皮 6g and **bai jie zi** (Semen Sinapsis Albae) 白芥子 6g.

Patent medicines

You Gui Wan 右归丸 (You Gui Wan)
Jin Kui Shen Qi Wan 金匮肾气丸 (Sexoton Pills)
Ren Shen Lu Rong Wan 人参鹿茸丸 (Jen Shen Lu Yung Wan)
Gui Lu Er Xian Jiao 龟鹿二仙胶 (Tortise Shell and Deer Antler Syrup)

Acupuncture

Kid.3 (*tai xi* +▲), Bl.23 (*shen shu* +▲), Bl.52 (*zhi shi*), Du.20 (*bai hui*), Ren.4 (*guan yuan* +▲), Du.4 (*ming men* +▲), Ht.7 (*shen men* +), Bl.15 (*xin shu* +▲), Kid.6 (*zhao hai*), Bl.62 (*shen mai*), SI.3 (*hou xi*), Kid.1 (*yong quan*)

Clinical notes

- The fogetfulness of this pattern may be associated with disorders such as Alzheimer's disease, senile dementia, sequelae to severe trauma or severe illness or drug abuse.
- This pattern can be very difficult to treat, especially in the elderly. Even in the event they remember to turn up for treatment or take the medication, results are generally poor. In younger people, supplementing *jing* may improve the symptoms to a reasonable degree.

32.4 BLOOD AND PHLEGM STAGNATION

Pathophysiology
- Blood and Phlegm stagnation is a complication of chronic disease, and is common in the elderly. It can also follow a traumatic head injury. Mental functioning will remain impaired unless the stagnation can be removed and the 'clear *yang*' circulation to the brain re-established.

Clinical features
- forgetfulness, poor memory, absent-mindedness, short attention span, inability to concentrate
- slow speech, dulled sensorium, blank expression

T dark or pale purple with brown or purple stasis spots and a greasy white coat; sublingual veins are distended and dark

P generally slippery or thready and choppy

Treatment principle
Transform Phlegm
Invigorate Blood and eliminate stagnant Blood

Prescription

SHOU XING WAN 寿星丸
(*God of Longevity Pills*) modified

This formula is selected for Blood and Phlegm stagnation from causes other than trauma.

huang qi (Radix Astragali Membranacei) 黄芪	15g
bai zhu (Rhizoma Atractylodis Macrocephalae) 白术	12g
fu ling (Sclerotium Poriae Cocos) 茯苓	12g
dang gui (Radix Angelicae Sinensis) 当归	9g
sheng di (Radix Rehmanniae Glutinosae) 生地	9g
bai shao (Radix Paeoniae Lactiflora) 白芍	9g
yuan zhi (Radix Polygalae Tenuifoliae) 远志	6g
ren shen (Radix Ginseng) 人参	6g
chen pi (Pericarpium Citri Reticulatae) 陈皮	6g
tian nan xing* (Rhizoma Arisaematis) 天南星	6g
wu wei zi (Fructus Schizandrae Chinensis) 五味子	6g
rou gui (Cortex Cinnamomi Cassiae) 肉桂	3g
hu po (Succinum) 琥珀	3g
zhi gan cao (honey fried Radix Glycyrrhizae Uralensis) 炙甘草	3g
zhu sha* (Cinnabar) 朱砂 (optional)	3g

Method: Grind herbs (except **zhu sha**) to a powder and form into 9-gram pills with ginger juice. If used, coat the outside of the pills with the **zhu sha**. The dose is one pill 2-3 times daily. May be decocted, in which case the **zhu sha** (0.5g), and **hu po** are taken with the strained decoction (*chong fu* 冲服). (Source: *Shi Yong Zhong Yi Nei Ke Xue*)

Modifications

- Blood stagnation is usually a complication of other pathological conditions and is frequently found with chronic Liver *qi* stagnation, Cold, *yang* and *yin* deficiency etc., and prescription should take these mechanisms into account. Appropriate herbs may be added to the guiding formula, keeping in mind that Blood moving herbs are also dispersing.
- If Cold or *yang* deficiency is responsible for the slowing down and stasis of Blood, warm Blood invigorating herbs like **chuan xiong** (Radix Ligustici Chuanxiong) 川芎 6g, **jiang huang** (Rhizoma Curcumae Longae) 姜黄 9g, **hong hua** (Flos Carthami Tinctorii) 红花 9g, **ru xiang** (Gummi Olibanum) 乳香 9g and **yue ji hua** (Flos et Fructus Rosae Chinensis) 月季花 6g should be included.
- When Heat or *yin* deficiency dry the Blood and increase its viscosity, Blood cooling and regulating herbs are indicated such as **chi shao** (Radix Paeoniae Rubrae) 赤芍 9g, **dan shen** (Radix Salviae Miltiorrhizae) 丹参 15g and **yu jin** (Tuber Curcumae) 郁金 9g.
- *Qi* and Blood deficiency should be addressed with Blood nourishing and regulating herbs like **ji xue teng** (Radix et Caulis Jixueteng) 鸡血藤 15g.
- With prominent Phlegm, add **ban xia*** (Rhizoma Pinelliae Ternatae) 半夏 9g, **zhi shi** (Fructus Immaturus Citri Aurantii) 枳实 9g and **bai jie zi** (Semen Sinapsis Albae) 白芥子 6g.

Variations and additional prescriptions

Following a head injury or trauma

- If the forgetfulness follows a head injury, the correct treatment is to invigorate *qi* and Blood in the Head with **XUE FU ZHU YU TANG** (*Achyranthes and Persica Combination* 血府逐瘀汤) modified.

dan shen (Radix Salviae Miltiorrhizae) 丹参	15g
sheng di (Radix Rehmanniae Glutinosae) 生地	12g
tao ren (Semen Persicae) 桃仁	12g
dang gui (Radix Angelicae Sinensis) 当归	9g
hong hua (Flos Carthami Tinctorii) 红花	9g
chi shao (Radix Paeoniae Rubrae) 赤芍	9g
yan hu suo (Rhizoma Corydalis Yanhusuo) 延胡索	9g
zhi ke (Fructus Citri Aurantii) 枳壳	6g
chai hu (Radix Bupleuri) 柴胡	6g
chen xiang (Lignum Aquilariae) 沉香	6g
niu xi (Radix Achyranthis Bidentatae) 牛膝	6g

shi chang pu (Rhizoma Acori Graminei) 石菖蒲 6g
gan cao (Radix Glycyrrhizae Uralensis) 甘草 3g
Method: Decoction. (Source: *Zhong Yi Nei Ke Lin Chuang Shou Ce*)

Patent medicines
Xue Fu Zhu Yu Wan 血府逐瘀丸 (Xue Fu Zhu Yu Wan)
Sheng Tian Qi Pian 生田七片 (Raw Tian Qi Ginseng Tablets)
Jin Gu Die Shang Wan 筋骨跌伤丸 (Chin Koo Tieh Shang Wan)
Nei Xiao Luo Li Wan 内消瘰疬丸 (Nei Xiao Luo Li Wan)
Fu Ke Wu Jin Wan 妇科乌金丸 (Woo Garm Yuen Medical Pills)

Acupuncture
Bl.15 (*xin shu* -), Bl.23 (*shen shu*), Bl.52 (*zhi shi*), Bl.17 (*ge shu* -),
PC.4 (*jian shi* -), Sp.6 (*san yin jiao* -), LI.4 (*he gu* -), Du.20 (*bai hui*),
si shen cong (M-HN-1), St.40 (*feng long*), Sp.3 (*tai bai*)
  • if from trauma add points of pain on the head (*ah shi*) and GB.20 (*feng chi*)

Clinical notes
  • The fogetfulness of this pattern may be associated with disorders such as Alzheimer's disease, senile dementia and concussion.
  • This pattern can be very difficult to treat when associated with senile dementia or Alzheimer's disease. If associated with concussion, it may respond reasonably well to correct TCM treatment.
  • Acupuncture should always be considered if there is a history of trauma causing stagnation of *qi* and Blood in the channels and points of tenderness (*ah shi*) needled.

SUMMARY OF GUIDING FORMULAE FOR FORGETFULNESS

Heart Blood and Spleen *qi* deficiency - *Gui Pi Tang* 归脾汤

Heart and Kidney *yin* deficiency - *Tian Wang Bu Xin Dan* 天王补心丹
- following a febrile disease - *Huang Lian E Jiao Tang* 黄连阿胶汤
- with prominent Kidney deficiency - *Sheng Hui Tang* 生慧汤

Kidney *jing* deficiency - *Ren Shen Yang Rong Tang* 人参养荣汤

Blood and Phlegm stagnation - *Shou Xing Wan* 寿星丸
- following head injury - *Xue Fu Zhu Yu Tang* 血府逐瘀汤

Endnote

For more information regarding herbs marked with an asterisk*, an open circle° or a hat^, see the tables on pp.944-952.

Disorders of the Heart

33. Anxiety

Heart *qi* deficiency
Heart *qi* and *yin* deficiency
Heart and Kidney *yin* deficiency
Heart Blood and Spleen *qi* deficiency
Heart and Gall Bladder deficiency
Phlegm Heat

33 | ANXIETY
you lü 忧虑

Anxiety is a normal human emotion and most people will experience it to some degree as a normal response to stress. Anxiety becomes pathological when it repeatedly interferes with daily life, is irrational, excessively prolonged or out of proportion with the cause. In TCM, anxiety is the emotion most frequently associated with disorders of the Heart and instability of the *shen*. The *shen* is easily agitated by Heat and easily destabilised if Heart *qi*, *yin* or Blood are weak.

AETIOLOGY
Heart *qi* deficiency
Heart *qi* is most easily damaged by prolonged or excessive sadness, depression or grief. Heart *qi* deficiency may also develop over time if the Spleen fails to produce adequate *qi* for the body's needs. In some individuals excessive coffee consumption will damage Heart *qi*. This is due to the dispersing action of the bitter flavour. Profuse sweating due to fever, high environmental temperature or excessive diaphoresis can damage Heart *qi* (and *yang*, *yin* and Blood), as sweat is the fluid of the Heart.

Heart Blood deficiency
Heart Blood deficiency may develop in much the same way as Heart *qi* deficiency - through prolonged or intense emotions or through inadequate production of Blood by the Spleen. In addition, any deficiency of Liver Blood will eventually lead to Heart Blood deficiency, via the generative (*sheng* 生, p.70) cycle. Significant blood loss can cause Heart Blood deficiency, particularly if the haemorrhage is from the uterus, because the *bao mai* links the Heart and uterus directly. Similarly, significant loss of fluid as sweat can damage Heart Blood.

Heart and Kidney *yin* deficiency
In TCM, the relationship between the Heart and Kidney is one of the fundamental relationships of the body and mind. This relationship functions on both a physical and a mental level. On the physical level, Kidney Water (*yin*) keeps Heart Fire in check, preventing a runaway blaze and overheating, and Heart Fire catalyses Kidney Water, preventing stagnation and accumulation of fluids. On the mental level, the Fire of *shen* arises from a stable base of Kidney *jing* (summed up in the sparkle of *jing shen* in the eyes), and *jing* and *shen* rely on each other for clear expression of mental consciousness.

If Kidney *yin* is damaged (by overwork, excess sexual activity, insufficient rest and sleep, ageing etc.), there may be a breakdown in relationship between the Heart and Kidney (via the controlling cycle), whereby Kidney Water no longer keeps Heart Fire in check. The uncontrolled blazing of Heart Fire causes agitation of the *shen* and the resulting anxiety can be severe. If Heart Fire remains unchecked, Heart *yin* will be damaged. The *shen* then has no 'anchor' and anxiety can become chronic. Heart *yin* may also be damaged by stimulant and recreational drugs (including coffee) or excessive mental stress.

At a more superficial level, the communication between the Heart (*shen*) and Kidneys (*zhi*) can be severed by major shock or trauma. This can occur in otherwise robust individuals, in which case anxiety is accompanied by few systemic symptoms since the *yin* of the organs is not damaged. It may also occur in someone with pre-existing *yin* damage, in which case, their condition is suddenly greatly exacerbated.

> **BOX 33.1 SOME BIOMEDICAL CAUSES OF ANXIETY**
>
> - hyperthyroidism
> - pheochromocytoma
> - temporal lobe epilepsy
> - hypoglycaemia
> - depression
> - neurosis
> - menopausal syndrome
> - premenstrual syndrome
> - stress
> - post-traumatic stress disorder
>
> **Drugs**
> - withdrawal from or dependence on benzodiazepine, alcohol and other drugs of addiction
> - amphetamines
> - bronchodilators
> - caffeine excess
> - ephedrine
> - levodopa
> - thyroxine

Heart and Gall Bladder deficiency

Heart and Gall Bladder *qi* deficiency describes a personality type which may be congenital or acquired. When congenital, it may be due to a significant shock that damaged the developing foetal *shen* during the mother's pregnancy. The pattern may be acquired easily in children (the *shen* is unstable when young) who are brought up in an abusive or fearful environment, or in adults or children who experience a violent or extreme shock or fright. It may also sometimes follow other debilitating illnesses that consume *qi*.

The involvement of the Gall Bladder here refers to the timidity and 'lack of gall' (that is, fearfulness) which characterises people with this pattern. In the Chinese language (as in English) there is an implicit understanding of the relationship between the Gall Bladder and courage, indeed to be bold and courageous is to have a 'big Gall Bladder' (*da dan* 大胆).

Phlegm Heat

Phlegm Heat can be generated in several ways. First, the presence of Phlegm or Dampness due to Spleen weakness or overconsumption of Phlegm producing foods causes stagnation and Heat. Second, overconsumption of Phlegm Heat foods (rich, greasy, sweet, spicy food and alcohol) can directly cause Phlegm Heat buildup. Finally, any pre-existing Heat in the body, due to Liver *qi* stagnation with stagnant Heat or Fire, *yin* deficiency or external invasion can congeal fluids into Phlegm, and subsequently Phlegm Heat. This pattern can also occur in the aftermath of a serious disease or febrile illness that has concentrated Fluids into Phlegm Heat.

ANXIOLYTIC DRUGS

The conventional drugs used to treat anxiety disorders deserve a special mention here because they are so widely used (for this and other conditions) and because they create dependence and are a source of the problem they were designed to treat. Anxiety has in recent times too often been deemed pathological and medicated inappropriately by health professionals who do not have the time or skills to address the feeling or emotions behind the anxiety. Women in particular have often been prescribed sedatives for distress following bereavement or resulting from intolerable domestic or work situations. Such overprescribing and abuse of tranquillisers and anxiolytic agents (most commonly benzodiazepines[1]) has brought with it its own problems. Prolonged use of benzodiazepines in particular has many unpleasant side effects and severe withdrawal symptoms[2]. This class of drug acts in a similar fashion to the heavy mineral substances[3] that are used in TCM to suppress rising *yang* and sedate and anchor the *shen*. The consequences of prolonged use of a single (and unbalanced substance) such as this are several; their bitter cool nature damages Heart and Kidney *yin*, weakens the Spleen, congests the Liver and further destabilises the *shen*.

Depending on the clinical manifestations in such cases, the relevant acupuncture and herbal treatment from this chapter may be applied to ameliorate the heightened anxiety and other withdrawal symptoms experienced when withdrawing from prescription medication.

---

1. Benzodiazapenes include drugs such as diazepam (Valium), nitrazepam (Mogadon) and chlordiazepoxide (Librium)
2. Withdrawal symptoms from benzodiazepines include anxiety, hallucinations, hypersensitivity, seizures, paranoid delusions, tremors, insomnia, palpitations, gastrointestinal upset
3. **long gu** (Os Draconis) 龙骨, **dai zhe shi** (Haematitum) 代赭石 etc.

> **BOX 33.2 KEY DIAGNOSTIC POINTS**
>
> **Tongue**
> • pale - *qi* and/or Blood deficiency
> • red - *yin* deficiency
> • thick yellow coat - Phlegm Heat
>
> **Pulse**
> • irregularly irregular - Heart *qi* and *yin* deficiency
> • thready and rapid - *yin* deficiency
> • rapid and slippery, or wiry - Phlegm Heat
> • thready and weak (especially in the distal position) - Heart *qi* deficiency
>
> **Aggravation**
> • with tiredness - deficiency
> • with loud noises, changes of routine - Heart and Gall Bladder *qi* deficiency

TREATMENT

For obvious reasons, patients with anxiety need to be treated with special care and gentleness. Many will be phobic and may have a major fear of acupuncture, so the technical and communication skills of the therapist are of utmost importance in reassuring the patient and engaging them in a program of treatment. At the same time, many patients will be medicated. Any anxiolytic medication should be withdrawn gradually, while constitutional treatment to support their *yin*, *qi* etc. proceeds. In our experience, acupuncture is especially good for calming the *shen* and the repeated application of needles on a weekly or twice-weekly basis ensures the momentum of the treatment. At the same time, herbs are particularly good at replenishing *yin* and Blood and providing the anchor for the *shen*. Together, acupuncture and herbs are effective at ameliorating the withdrawal effects of conventional medications, and at the same time dealing with the problem that gave rise to the anxiety in the first place.

It is important to remember that other drugs may be responsible for anxiety, and to elicit the full list of medications and other potential aggravating substances the patient is taking. In addition to the benzodiazepines and recreational drug noted above, other drugs like appetite suppressants and caffeine may be implicated. Excessive use of caffeine (in coffee, chocolate and cola drinks) is a reasonably common cause of anxiety and easy to overlook.

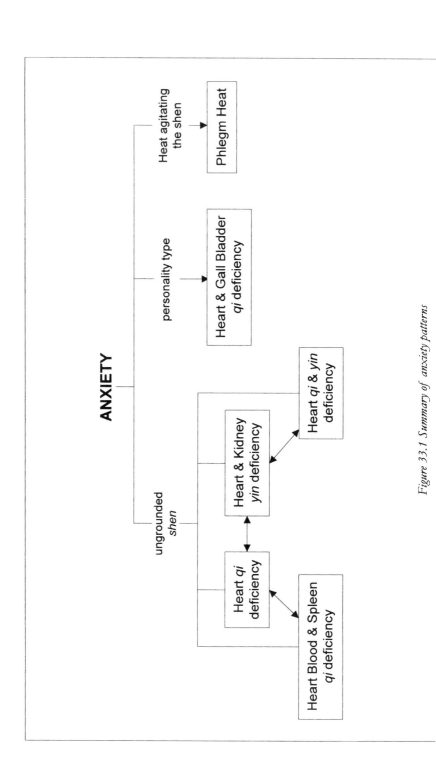

Figure 33.1 Summary of anxiety patterns

33.1 HEART *QI* DEFICIENCY

心气虚忧虑

Pathophysiology
- When there is insufficient Heart *qi* to protect the *shen*, it becomes easily vulnerable, disorientated and unstable, and this results in feelings of anxiety, unease and apprehension.

Clinical features
- anxiety, apprehension, constant worry
- palpitations
- poor concentration
- fitful sleep, insomnia
- shortness of breath
- dizziness
- physical and mental fatigue
- pale complexion
- spontaneous sweating

T pale with a thin white coat
P thready and weak

Treatment principle
Tonify and nourish Heart *qi*
Calm the *shen*

Prescription

MIAO XIANG SAN 妙香散
(*Marvellously Fragrant Powder*)

ren shen (Radix Ginseng) 人参	15g
shan yao (Radix Dioscoreae Oppositae) 山药	30g
huang qi (Radix Astragali Membranacei) 黄芪	30g
fu ling (Sclerotium Poriae Cocos) 茯苓	30g
fu shen (Sclerotium Poriae Cocos Pararadicis) 茯神	30g
yuan zhi (Radix Polygalae Tenuifoliae) 远志	30g
zhu sha* (Cinnabaris) 朱砂	9g
mu xiang (Radix Aucklandiae Lappae) 木香	75g
she xiang° (Secretion Moschus) 麝香	3g
jie geng (Radix Platycodi Grandiflori) 桔梗	15g
zhi gan cao (honey fried Radix Glycyrrhizae Uralensis) 炙甘草	3g

Method: Grind herbs into powder and form into 6-gram pills with honey. The dose is 2-3 pills daily. **Zhu sha** is not suitable for prolonged use. (Source: *Formulas and Strategies*)

Patent medicines
Gui Pi Wan 归脾丸 (Gui Pi Wan)
Sheng Mai Wan 生脉丸 (Sheng Mai Wan)
Bai Zi Yang Xin Wan 柏子养心丸 (Bai Zi Yang Xin Wan)
Ding Xin Wan 定心丸 (Ding Xin Wan)
Yang Xin Ning Shen Wan 养心宁神丸 (Ning San Yuen Medical Pills)
Bu Nao Wan 补脑丸 (Cerebral Tonic Pills)

Acupuncture
Bl.15 (*xin shu* +), PC.5 (*jian shi* +), Ht.7 (*shen men* +), PC.6 (*nei guan*), Ren.14 (*ju que* +), St.36 (*zu san li* +), *yin tang* (M-HN-3), Du.19 (*hou ding*), Du. 24 (*shen ting*)
Ear points: *shen men*, Heart, subcortex, sympathetic. Ear seeds may be left in place between treatments.
- with spontaneous sweating, add Bl.43 (*gao huang shu*)

Clinical notes
- The anxiety in this pattern may be associated with disorders such as anxiety neurosis and anaemia.
- This pattern generally responds well to treatment, however there may be elements of constitutional weakness that predispose people to worry. If so, the tongue may have a deep narrow crack up to the tip and successful treatment is more difficult.
- Avoidance of mental stress is important. This includes violent or otherwise disturbing images from television or movies. In addition coffee and other stimulants should be avoided.
- Active pursuit of relaxation should be encouraged. This means that a gentle and positive relaxation routine should be built into the day (rather than the 'just doing nothing' type or relaxation). Activities such as *tai qi*, yoga nidra, walking or swimming are a good way to calm the mind and gradually build *qi*.

33.2 HEART AND KIDNEY *YIN* DEFICIENCY

心肾不通忧虑

Pathophysiology
- This pattern can cause anxiety in two ways—Heart *yin* depletion failing to anchor and ground the *shen*, and the resulting deficient Heat agitating the *shen*. This pattern often emerges during the withdrawal phase of long term sedative or anxiolytic drug use.

Clinical features
- anxiety or panic attacks with palpitations, easily brought on by a start or fright
- insomnia, often waking to anxiety or panic, or sleep with nightmares
- restlessness, irritability
- sensation of heat in the palms and soles ('five hearts hot')
- night sweats
- dry mouth and throat
- dizziness, light-headedness
- tinnitus
- forgetfulness
- lower back ache

T red and dry with little or no coat
P thready and rapid

Treatment principle
Nourish Heart *yin*, calm the *shen*
Clear Heat

Prescription

TIAN WANG BU XIN DAN 天王补心丹
(*Ginseng and Zizyphus Formula*)

sheng di (Radix Rehmanniae Glutinosae) 生地	120 (24)g
tian dong (Tuber Asparagi Cochinchinensis) 天冬	30 (12)g
mai dong (Tuber Ophiopogonis Japonici) 麦冬	30 (12)g
suan zao ren (Semen Zizyphi Spinosae) 酸枣仁	30 (12)g
xuan shen (Radix Scrophulariae) 玄参	15 (12)g
dan shen (Radix Salviae Miltiorrhizae) 丹参	15 (12)g
fu ling (Sclerotium Poriae Cocos) 茯苓	15 (12)g
dang gui (Radix Angelicae Sinensis) 当归	30 (9)g
wu wei zi (Fructus Schizandrae Chinensis) 五味子	30 (9)g
bai zi ren (Semen Biotae Orientalis) 柏子仁	30 (9)g
ren shen (Radix Ginseng) 人参	15 (9)g
jie geng (Radix Platycodi Grandiflori) 桔梗	15 (9)g

yuan zhi (Radix Polygalae Tenuifoliae) 远志 ...... 15 (6)g
zhu sha* (Cinnabaris) 朱砂 (optional) .... 6 (0.5)g
Method: Grind herbs (except **zhu sha**) to a powder and form into 9-gram pills with honey. If used, coat the outside of the pills with the **zhu sha**. The dose is one pill 2-3 times daily. May also be decocted with the dosage in brackets. When decocted the **zhu sha** is taken as powder with the strained decoction. This is an excellent formula for long term use in treating *yin* deficiency with *shen* disturbance, in which case the **zhu sha** is deleted. (Source: *Shi Yong Zhong Yi Nei Ke Xue*)

Variations and additional prescriptions
Following a febrile illness
- If symptoms of *yin* deficient Fire are severe, or the disorder occurs following a febrile disease with lingering Heat use **HUANG LIAN E JIAO TANG** (*Coptis and Ass-Hide Gelatin Decoction* 黄连阿胶汤, p.839).

In severe cases
- With severe or continuous anxiety or panic attacks, accompanied by palpitations, insomnia and Heat, a more sedative formula is required to control the symptoms quickly. This is intense Heart Fire on a background of *yin* deficiency. The correct treatment is to sedate the Heart, calm the *shen*, drain Fire and nourish *yin with* **ZHU SHA AN SHEN WAN** (*Cinnabar Pill to Calm the Spirit* 朱砂安神丸, p.840). Because it contains **zhu sha** it is not suitable for prolonged use, and once the condition is under control other formulae should be used.

After a major shock or trauma
- Occasionally following a major shock or trauma there is anxiety, insomnia and dream or nightmare disturbed sleep, palpitations, hair loss, loss of appetite, dizziness, depression, lack of motivation, a slightly pale tongue and a hollow, slow pulse. This is typical of severed communication between the Heart and Kidneys due to shock. The correct formula is **GUI ZHI JIA LONG GU MU LI TANG** (*Cinnamon and Dragon Bone Combination* 桂枝加龙骨牡蛎汤, p.814).

Patent medicines
Tian Wang Bu Xin Dan 天王补心丹 (Tian Wang Bu Xin Dan)
  - excellent for Heart *yin* deficiency with *shen* disturbance
Zuo Gui Wan 左归丸 (Zuo Gui Wan)
Sheng Mai Wan 生脉丸 (Sheng Mai Wan)
Liu Wei Di Huang Wan 六味地黄丸 (Liu Wei Di Huang Wan)
  - a general Kidney *yin* tonic formula
Suan Zao Ren Tang Pian 酸枣仁汤片 (Tabellae Suanzaoren)
Ci Zhu Wan 磁朱丸 (Ci Zhu Wan)
  - this pill is usually combined with one of the other formulae above

Acupuncture

Bl.23 (*shen shu* +), Kid.3 (*tai xi* +), Bl.15 (*xin shu* -), Du.19 (*hou ding*), Ht.7 (*shen men* -), PC.7 (*da ling* -), Ren.14 (*ju que*), *yin tang* (M-HN-3), Du. 24 (*shen ting*)

Ear points: shen men, Kidney, Heart, subcortex, sympathetic.

Clinical notes

- The anxiety in this pattern may be associated with disorders such as hyperthyroidism, menopausal syndrome, post traumatic shock syndrome, anxiety neurosis, post febrile disease
- The anxiety in this pattern generally responds well to correct treatment, however for it to be long lasting the *yin* will have to be replenished and this takes time. TCM treatment for at least several months will be necessary, although signs of improvement can usually be expected within a few weeks. Long term resolution may depend on the biomedical syndrome with which the anxiety is associated. For example, hyperthyroid conditions can be difficult to cure with TCM and may need to be controlled by drugs or surgery if TCM treatment is ineffective, before lasting results can be acheived.
- Acupuncture at times of anxiety or acute panic attacks is very useful at alleviating symtoms and calming the mind. In severe cases acupuncture can be given once or twice per day.
- Avoidance of disturbing images from the television or movies, and stimulants like coffee and other drugs, and chillies, is important. A strictly regular bedtime routine should be adhered to, even in patients unable to sleep well. The training of the internal clock to a regular sleep routine may take a while but is worth the effort as it contributes greatly to recovery.
- Care with other aggravating factors like sex, excessive lifting and standing and dehydration.
- Active pursuit of relaxation should be encouraged. This means that a gentle and positive relaxation routine should be built into the day (rather than the 'just doing nothing' type or relaxation). Activities such as *tai qi*, yoga nidra, walking and swimming are a good way to calm the mind and gradually build *qi*.

33.3 HEART BLOOD AND SPLEEN *QI* DEFICIENCY

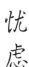

Pathophysiology
- Heart Blood (and *yin*) anchor and ground the *shen*. Spleen *qi* supports and manufactures Heart Blood. When the Heart and Spleen become deficient the *shen* is unanchored and becomes unstable. Clinically, the mixture of deficiency can be equally shared, or tend towards either the Heart or Spleen. In all cases supporting Spleen function in addition to tonifying Blood is essential so the Spleen can continue to manufacture Blood.

Clinical features
- anxiety, phobias, panic attacks
- palpitations
- insomnia, with difficulty falling asleep or dream disturbed sleep
- forgetfulness, poor memory, poor concentration
- postural dizziness
- blurring vision, spots in the visual field
- fatigue and weakness
- poor appetite
- abdominal distension after eating
- sallow complexion
- easy bruising, or heavy or prolonged menstrual periods

T pale with a thin white coat
P thready and weak

Treatment principle
Strengthen and nourish the Heart and Spleen
Tonify *qi* and Blood, calm the *shen*

Prescription

GUI PI TANG 归脾汤
(*Ginseng and Longan Combination*)

huang qi (Radix Astragali Membranacei) 黄芪	30g
bai zhu (Rhizoma Atractylodis Macrocephalae) 白术	30g
fu shen (Sclerotium Poriae Cocos Pararadicis) 茯神	30g
long yan rou (Arillus Euphoriae Longanae) 龙眼肉	30g
suan zao ren (Semen Zizyphi Spinosae) 酸枣仁	30g
dang shen (Radix Codonopsis Pilosulae) 党参	15g
mu xiang (Radix Aucklandiae Lappae) 木香	6g
dang gui (Radix Angelicae Sinensis) 当归	6g
yuan zhi (Radix Polygalae Tenuifoliae) 远志	6g

zhi gan cao (honey fried Radix Glycyrrhizae Uralensis)
炙甘草 6g

Method: Decoction. (Source: *Zhong Yi Nei Ke Lin Chuang Shou Ce*)

Modifications

- If Heart Blood deficiency is more prominent, add **shu di** (Radix Rehmanniae Glutinosae Conquitae) 熟地 30-50g, **bai shao** (Radix Paeoniae Lactiflora) 白芍 15g and **e jiao**^ (Gelatinum Corii Asini) 阿胶 15g (dissolved in the strained decoction), and **sha ren** (Fructus Amomi) 砂仁 6g to aid the digestion of the **shu di**.
- With severe Spleen *qi* deficiency, it may be necessary to initially reduce the dose of (or delete) the richer Blood tonics (**long yan rou** and **dang gui**) until the Spleen is strong enough to digest them properly.
- With Heat, add **shan zhi zi** (Fructus Gardeniae Jasminoidis) 山栀子 9g and **chai hu** (Radix Bupleuri) 柴胡 6g.
- With severe insomnia, add two or three of the following herbs: **wu wei zi** (Fructus Schizandrae Chinensis) 五味子 6g, **bai zi ren** (Semen Biotae Orientalis) 柏子仁 9g, **ye jiao teng** (Caulis Polygoni Multiflori) 夜交藤 30g, **he huan pi** (Cortex Albizziae Julibrissin) 合欢皮 9g, **long chi**^ (Dens Draconis) 龙齿 10g, **mu li**^ (Concha Ostreae) 牡蛎 30g, and **mai ya** (Fructus Hordei Vulgaris Germinantus) 麦芽 15g to protect the Stomach from damage by the mineral drugs.
- If there is abdominal and epigastric fullness, poor appetite, a greasy or glossy tongue coat add **ban xia*** (Rhizoma Pinelliae Ternatae) 半夏 10g and **chen pi** (Pericarpium Citri Reticulatae) 陈皮 10g.

Variations and additional prescriptions

- If *qi* and Blood deficiency is systemic then a more general tonic may be useful. Consider **REN SHEN YANG RONG TANG** (*Ginseng Nutritive Combination* 人参养营汤, p.887) or **SHI QUAN DA BU TANG** (*Ginseng and Dang Gui Ten Combination* 十全大补汤, p.529).

Patent medicines

Gui Pi Wan 归脾丸 (Gui Pi Wan)
Bai Zi Yang Xin Wan 柏子养心丸 (Bai Zi Yang Xin Wan)
Dang Gui Ji Jing 当归鸡精 (Tang Kuei Essence of Chicken)
Bu Nao Wan 补脑丸 (Cerebral Tonic Pills)
Yang Xin Ning Shen Wan 养心宁神丸 (Ning San Yuen Medical Pills)

Acupuncture

Sp.6 (*san yin jiao* +), St.36 (*zu san li* +), Ht.7 (*shen men* +),
Ren.12 (*zhong wan* +), Bl.15 (*xin shu* +), Bl.17 (*ge shu* +),
Bl.20 (*pi shu* +), *yin tang* (M-HN-3), Du.19 (*hou ding*), Du.24 (*shen ting*)

Ear points: *shen men*, Spleen, Heart, subcortex, sympathetic. Ear seeds may be left in place between treatments.

Clinical notes
- The anxiety in this pattern may be associated with disorders such as include anxiety neurosis, thrombocytopoenia and anaemia.
- This pattern responds well to correct treatment; to make it last Spleen *qi* needs to be supported with regular eating habits and easily digested mild foods.
- As in all anxiety patterns, avoidance of disturbing images from the television or movies, as well as stimulants like coffee, is important. A strictly regular bedtime routine should be adhered to.
- In women who lose blood (and thus Heart Blood) through heavy periods, Blood tonics and Blood replenishing and iron rich foods should be taken after each period. Iron supplements are also useful.

33.4 HEART *QI* AND *YIN* DEFICIENCY

Pathophysiology
- The cause of the anxiety in this pattern is a combination of the two previous patterns—*qi* deficiency and *yin* (Blood) deficiency. The *shen* is both vulnerable and ungrounded, and may in addition be agitated by deficient Fire. The most distinctive feature of this pattern is in the pulse—typically irregularly irregular.

Clinical features
- anxiety accompanied by palpitations
- insomnia
- irritability
- shortness of breath
- dry stools or constipation
- dry mouth and throat

T depending on the balance of *qi* or *yin* deficiency, pale pink or red and swollen, with surface cracks and little or no coat

P knotted, intermittent or irregular pulse, particularly if *qi* deficiency is prominent

Treatment principle
Nourish *yin* and Blood
Tonify *qi*, calm the *shen*

Prescription

ZHI GAN CAO TANG 炙甘草汤
(Baked Licorice Combination)

sheng di (Radix Rehmanniae Glutinosae) 生地	24g
zhi gan cao (honey fried Radix Glycyrrhizae Uralensis) 炙甘草	12g
ren shen (Radix Ginseng) 人参	6g
gui zhi (Ramulus Cinnamomi Cassiae) 桂枝	9g
mai dong (Tuber Ophiopogonis Japonici) 麦冬	9g
e jiao^ (Gelatinum Corii Asini) 阿胶	6g
huo ma ren (Semen Cannabis Sativae) 火麻仁	9g
sheng jiang (Rhizoma Zingiberis Officinalis) 生姜	9g
da zao (Fructus Zizyphi Jujubae) 大枣	5pce

Method: Decoction. **E jiao** is melted in the hot strained decoction (*yang hua* 烊化). (Source: *Formulas and Strategies*)

心气阴虚忧虑

Patent medicines
Gui Pi Wan 归脾丸 (Gui Pi Wan)
Sheng Mai Wan 生脉丸 (Sheng Mai Wan)
Bai Zi Yang Xin Wan 柏子养心丸 (Bai Zi Yang Xin Wan)
Yang Xin Ning Shen Wan 养心宁神丸 (Ning San Yuen Medical Pills)
Bu Nao Wan 补脑丸 (Cerebral Tonic Pills)

Acupuncture
Bl.15 (*xin shu* +), Ht.5 (*tong li*), Ht.6 (*yin xi* -), Ht.7 (*shen men* +), PC.5 (*jian shi* +), PC.6 (*nei guan* +), Ren.14 (*ju que* +), St.36 (*zu san li* +), *yin tang* (M-HN-3), Du.19 (*hou ding*), Du. 24 (*shen ting*)
Ear points: *shen men*, Spleen, Heart, subcortex, sympathetic. Ear seeds may be left in place between treatments.
- with spontaneous sweating, add Bl.43 (*gao huang shu*)

Clinical notes
- The anxiety in this pattern may be associated with disorders such as neuresthenia, hyperthyroidism, cardiac arrhythmia and sick sinus syndrome.
- The anxiety in this pattern responds well to correct treatment, although good constitutional results generally take some months.
- As in all anxiety patterns avoidance of disturbing images from the television or movies, as well as stimulants like coffee, is important. A strictly regular bedtime routine should be adhered to.
- Active pursuit of relaxation should be encouraged. This means that a gentle and positive relaxation routine should be built into the day (rather than the 'just doing nothing' type or relaxation). Activities such as *tai qi*, yoga nidra, walking and swimming are a good way to calm the mind and gradually build *qi*.

33.5 HEART AND GALL BLADDER *QI* DEFICIENCY

Pathophysiology
- Acute anxiety and frequent panic attacks are a key feature of Heart and Gall Bladder *qi* deficiency. This pattern represents a deep seated or constitutional *shen* instability combined with Heart *qi* deficiency. This pattern may also be precipitated by a severe shock or trauma.

Clinical features
- frequent severe anxiety, panic attacks, apprehension, fearfulness, inappropriate worry, easily frightened, timidity and phobias
- palpitations
- insomnia, nightmares, waking terrified
- restlessness, forgetfulness

T normal or with a pale body and a thin white coat; in congenital or long standing cases there may be a deep narrow crack to the tip

P weak, thready and rapid or thready and wiry

Treatment principle
Calm the *shen*, nourish and tranquilise the Heart

Prescription

DING ZHI WAN 定志丸
(*Settle the Emotions Pill*) modified

ren shen (Radix Ginseng) 人参 90g
fu ling (Sclerotium Poriae Cocos) 茯苓 90g
shi chang pu (Rhizoma Acori Graminei) 石菖蒲 60g
yuan zhi (Radix Polygalae Tenuifoliae) 远志 60g
long gu^ (Os Draconis) 龙骨 60g
hu po (Succinum) 琥珀 30g

Method: Grind herbs to a powder and form into 9-gram pills with honey. The dose is one pill twice daily. May also be decocted with a 90% reduction in dosage, in which case **hu po** is taken with the strained decoction (*chong fu* 冲服). (Source: *Formulas and Strategies*)

Modifications
- With Blood deficiency, add **dang gui** (Radix Angelicae Sinensis) 当归 60g and **bai shao** (Radix Paeoniae Lactiflora) 白芍 60g.
- With significant insomnia and palpitations, add one or two of the following herbs: **wu wei zi** (Fructus Schizandrae Chinensis) 五味子 60g, **bai zi ren** (Semen Biotae Orientalis) 柏子仁 90g, **ye jiao teng** (Caulis Polygoni Multiflori) 夜交藤 60g, **he huan pi** (Cortex Albizziae Julibrissin) 合欢皮 60g, **mu li^** (Concha Ostreae) 牡蛎 60g to settle the *shen*, and **mai ya**

(Fructus Hordei Vulgaris Germinantus) 麦芽 60g to protect the Stomach from damage by the mineral drugs.
- If the patient is depressed add **he huan pi** (Cortex Albizziae Julibrissin) 合欢皮 60g.
- With severe *qi* deficiency, add one or two of the following herbs: **dang shen** (Radix Codonopsis Pilosulae) 党参 60g, **huang jing** (Rhizoma Polygonati) 黄精 60g, and **huang qi** (Radix Astragali Membranacei) 黄芪 60g.
- With spontaneous sweating, add **mu li^** (Concha Ostreae) 牡蛎 60g, **ma huang gen** (Radix Ephedrae) 麻黄根 40g, **fu xiao mai** (Semen Tritici Aestivi Levis) 浮小麦 40g.

Variations and additional prescriptions
- Sometimes following a major shock or trauma (such as a car accident), anxiety, insomnia and dream–or nightmare–disturbed sleep, palpitations, hair loss, loss of appetite, dizziness, depression, lack of motivation, a slightly pale tongue and a hollow, slow pulse may occur. These symptoms are typical of severed communication between the Heart and Kidneys. This pattern can also be considered an acquired form of Heart and Gall Bladder *qi* deficiency. The correct formula is **GUI ZHI JIA LONG GU MU LI TANG** (*Cinnamon and Dragon Bone Combination* 桂枝加龙骨牡蛎汤, p.814).

Patent medicines
Bu Nao Wan 补脑丸 (Cerebral Tonic Pills)
Ding Xin Wan 定心丸 (Ding Xin Wan)
Yang Xin Ning Shen Wan 养心宁神丸 (Ning San Yuen Medical Pills)

Acupuncture
GB.39 (*xuan zhong*), SJ.5 (*wai guan*), Bl.15 (*xin shu*), PC.6 (*nei guan*), Ht.7 (*shen men*), Ren.14 (*ju que*), Ht.9 (*shao chong*), Du.19 (*hou ding*), Du. 24 (*shen ting*)
Ear points: shen men, Liver, Gall Bladder Heart, subcortex, sympathetic. Ear seeds may be left in place between treatments.

Clinical notes
- The anxiety in this pattern may be associated with disorders such as anxiety neurosis, mental disorders or post natal depression.
- This pattern can be quite difficult to treat and if any result is to be achieved, prolonged therapy is usually necessary. If the pattern is congenital, a combination of TCM treatment with psychotherapy of some sort may be beneficial.

33.6 PHLEGM HEAT

痰热忧虑

Pathophysiology
- Phlegm has a particular affinity with the Heart, indeed the Heart is subject to 'mists' of insubstantial Phlegm that obscure reason and consciousness. The Heat associated with this pattern can agitate the *shen* causing anxiety.
- Phlegm Heat type anxiety can be a chronic response to Phlegm Heat in the body (usually from diet), but can can also be more acute, occurring in the convalescent stage of a febrile disease that has congealed Fluids into Phlegm.

Clinical features
- anxiety and nervousness
- palpitations
- dizziness and vertigo
- insomnia, with waking in the early hours of the morning (typically around 4am) unable to fall back to sleep
- irritability and restlessness
- nausea, vomiting or indeterminate gnawing hunger
- poor appetite
- belching, acid reflux
- bitter taste in the mouth
- abdominal distension

T greasy yellow coat
P rapid and slippery or wiry

Treatment principle
Clear Heat, transform Phlegm
Harmonize the Stomach, calm the *shen*

Prescription

SHI YI WEI WEN DAN TANG 十一味温胆汤
(*Eleven Ingredient Decoction to Warm the Gall Bladder*)

ye jiao teng (Caulis Polygoni Multiflori) 夜交藤	30g
zhu ru (Caulis Bambusae in Taeniis) 竹茹	12g
fu ling (Sclerotium Poriae Cocos) 茯苓	15g
shi chang pu (Rhizoma Acori Graminei) 石菖蒲	9g
ban xia* (Rhizoma Pinelliae Ternatae) 半夏	9g
chen pi (Pericarpium Citri Reticulatae) 陈皮	9g
zhi shi (Fructus Immaturus Citri Aurantii) 枳实	6g
huang lian (Rhizoma Coptidis) 黄连	6g
gan cao (Radix Glycyrrhizae Uralensis) 甘草	6g
yuan zhi (Radix Polygalae Tenuifoliae) 远志	6g

Method: Decoction. (Source: *Formulas and Strategies*)

Modifications
- If the anxiety is severe, add **hu po** (Succinum) 琥珀 1-3g and **suan zao ren** (Semen Zizyphi Spinosae) 酸枣仁 12g.

Patent medicines
Er Chen Wan 二陈丸 (Er Chen Wan) plus *Huang Lian Jie Du Wan* 黄连解毒丸 (Huang Lian Jie Du Wan)
Hu Po Bao Long Wan 琥珀抱龙丸 (Po Lung Yuen Medical Pills)

Acupuncture
Ht.6 (*yin xi*), St.40 (*feng long* -), GB.34 (*yang ling quan* -), St.41 (*jie xi* -), *yin tang* (M-HN-3), Bl.15 (*xin shu*), Liv.3 (*tai chong*), Du.19 (*hou ding*), Du.24 (*shen ting*)
Ear points: *shen men*, Spleen, Heart, subcortex, sympathetic. Ear seeds may be left in place between treatments.

Clinical notes
- The anxiety in this pattern may be associated with disorders such as convalesence following fever, anxiety neurosis or post viral syndrome.
- This pattern generally responds well to correct treatment. Once the Phlegm has cleared the anxiety and associated symptoms will abate. However, the source of the Phlegm will determine how rapidly that can be achieved. Post febrile Phlegm Heat responds quickly.
- Avoidance of Phlegm Heat producing foods (dairy products, alcohol and fatty foods) is essential.

SUMMARY OF GUIDING FORMULAE FOR ANXIETY

Heart *qi* deficiency - *Miao Xiang San* 妙香散

Heart and Kidney *yin* deficiency - *Tian Wang Bu Xin Dan* 天王补心丹

Heart *qi* and *yin* deficiency - *Zhi Gan Cao Tang* 炙甘草汤

Heart Blood and Spleen *qi* deficiency - *Gui Pi Tang* 归脾汤

Heart and Gall Bladder *qi* deficiency - *Ding Zhi Wan* 定志丸
- as a result of shock - *Gui Zhi Jia Long Gu Mu Li Tang* 桂枝加龙骨牡蛎汤

Phlegm Heat - *Shi Yi Wei Wen Dan Tang* 十一味温胆汤

Endnote

For more information regarding herbs marked with an asterisk*, an open circle° or a hat^, see the tables on pp.944-952.

Appendix A: Original Unmodified Formulae

AN GONG NIU HUANG WAN 安宫牛黄丸
(Calm the Palace Pill with Cattle Gallstone)
    niu huang^ (Calculus Bovis) 牛黄
    xi jiao° (Cornu Rhinoceri) 犀角
    she xiang° (Secretio Moschus) 麝香
    huang lian (Rhizoma Coptidis) 黄连
    huang qin (Radix Scutellariae Baicalensis) 黄芩
    shan zhi zi (Fructus Gardeniae Jasminoides) 山栀子
    xiong huang (Realgar) 雄黄
    bing pian (Borneol) 冰片
    yu jin (Tuber Curcumae) 郁金
    zhu sha* (Cinnabaris) 朱砂
    zhen zhu^ (Margarita) 珍珠

BAO HE WAN 保和丸 *(Citrus and Crategus Formula)*
    chao shan zha (dry fried Fructus Crategi) 炒山楂
    shen qu (Massa Fermentata) 神曲
    ban xia* (Rhizoma Pinelliae Ternatae) 半夏
    fu ling (Sclerotium Poriae Cocos) 茯苓
    chen pi (Pericarpium Citri Reticulatae) 陈皮
    lai fu zi (Semen Raphani Sativi) 莱服子
    lian qiao (Fructus Forsythia Suspensae) 连翘

BAO YUAN TANG 保元汤 *(Preserve the Basal Decoction)*
    ren shen (Radix Ginseng) 人参
    huang qi (Radix Astragali Membranacei) 黄芪
    rou gui (Cortex Cinnamomi Cassiae) 肉桂
    zhi gan cao (honey fried Radix Glycyrrhizae Uralensis) 炙甘草

BAO ZHEN TANG 保真汤 *(Preserve the True Decoction)*
    ren shen (Radix Ginseng) 人参
    huang qi (Radix Astragali Membranacei) 黄芪
    bai zhu (Rhizoma Atractylodis Macrocephalae) 白术
    fu ling (Sclerotium Poriae Cocos) 茯苓
    da zao (Fructus Zizyphi Jujubae) 大枣
    tian dong (Tuber Asparagi Cochinchinensis) 天冬
    mai dong (Tuber Ophiopogonis Japonici) 麦冬
    sheng di (Radix Rehmanniae Glutinosae) 生地
    shu di (Radix Rehmanniae Glutinosae Conquitae) 熟地
    wu wei zi (Fructus Schizandrae Chinensis) 五味子
    dang gui (Radix Angelicae Sinensis) 当归
    bai shao (Radix Paeoniae Lactiflora) 白芍
    lian xu (Stamen Nelumbinis Nucifera) 莲须

di gu pi (Cortex Lycii Chinensis) 地骨皮
  yin chai hu (Radix Stellariae Dichotomae) 银柴胡
  chen pi (Pericarpium Citri Reticulatae) 陈皮
  sheng jiang (Rhizoma Zingiberis Officinalis Recens) 生姜
  huang bai (Cortex Phellodendri) 黄柏
  zhi mu (Rhizoma Anemarrhenae Asphodeloides) 知母
  gan cao (Radix Glycyrrhizae Uralensis) 甘草

BEI XIE FEN QING YIN 萆解分清饮 (*Tokoro Combination*)
  bei xie (Rhizoma Dioscoreae Hypoglaucae) 萆解
  yi zhi ren (Fructus Alpiniae Oxyphyllae) 益智仁
  wu yao (Radix Linderae Strychnifoliae) 乌药
  shi chang pu (Rhizoma Acori Graminei) 石菖蒲

BIE JIA JIAN WAN 鳖甲煎丸 (*Tortise Shell Decoction Pills*)
  bie jia° (Carapax Amydae Sinensis) 鳖甲
  huang qin (Radix Scutellariae Baicalensis) 黄芩
  chai hu (Radix Bupleuri) 柴胡
  gan jiang (Rhizoma Zingiberis Officinalis) 干姜
  da huang (Radix et Rhizoma Rhei) 大黄
  shao yao (Radix Paeoniae) 芍药
  gui zhi (Ramulus Cinnamomi Cassiae) 桂枝
  ting li zi (Semen Descurainiae seu Lepidii) 葶苈子
  shi wei (Folium Pyrrosiae) 石苇
  hou po (Cortex Magnoliae Officinalis) 厚朴
  mu dan pi (Cortex Moutan Radicis) 牡丹皮
  qu mai (Herba Dianthi) 瞿麦
  ban xia* (Rhizoma Pinelliae Ternatae) 半夏
  ren shen (Radix Ginseng) 人参
  e jiao^ (Gelatinum Corii Asini) 阿胶
  tao ren (Semen Persicae) 桃仁
  she gan (Rhizoma Belamcandae) 射干
  feng fang^ (Nidus Vespae) 蜂房
  huo xiao (Niter) 火硝
  qiang lang^ (Dung Beetle) 蜣螂
  di bie chong^ (Eupolyphaga seu Opisthoplatia) 地鳖虫

CANG ER ZI SAN 苍耳子散 (*Xanthium Formula*)
  cang er zi* (Fructus Xanthii Sibirici) 苍耳子
  xin yi hua (Flos Magnoliae) 辛夷花
  bai zhi (Radix Angelicae Dahuricae) 白芷
  bo he (Herba Mentha Haplocalycis) 薄荷

CHAI HU QING GAN TANG 柴胡清肝汤
(*Bupleurum Liver Clearing Decoction*)
    chai hu (Radix Bupleuri) 柴胡
    sheng di (Radix Rehmanniae Glutinosae) 生地
    dang gui (Radix Angelicae Sinensis) 当归
    chi shao (Radix Paeoniae Rubrae) 赤芍
    chuan xiong (Radix Ligustici Chuanxiong) 川芎
    lian qiao (Fructus Forsythia Suspensae) 连翘
    niu bang zi (Fructus Arctii Lappae) 牛蒡子
    huang qin (Radix Scutellariae Baicalensis) 黄芩
    shan zhi zi (Fructus Gardeniae Jasminoidis) 山栀子
    tian hua fen (Radix Trichosanthes Kirilowii) 天花粉
    fang feng (Radix Ledebouriellae Divaricatae) 防风
    gan cao (Radix Glycyrrhizae Uralensis) 甘草

CHAI LING TANG 柴苓汤 (*Bupleurum and Hoelen Combination*)
    chai hu (Radix Bupleuri) 柴胡
    ban xia* (Rhizoma Pinelliae Ternatae) 半夏
    huang qin (Radix Scutellariae Baicalensis) 黄芩
    ren shen (Radix Ginseng) 人参
    ze xie (Rhizoma Alismatis Orientalis) 泽泻
    fu ling (Sclerotium Poriae Cocos) 茯苓
    zhu ling (Sclerotium Polypori Umbellati) 猪苓
    bai zhu (Rhizoma Atractylodis Macrocephalae) 白术
    gui zhi (Ramulus Cinnamomi Cassiae) 桂枝
    zhi gan cao (honey fried Radix Glycyrrhizae Uralensis) 炙甘草

CHEN XIANG SAN 沉香散 (*Aquillaria Powder*)
    chen xiang (Lignum Aquilariae) 沉香
    shi wei (Folium Pyrrosiae) 石苇
    hua shi (Talcum) 滑石
    dang gui (Radix Angelicae Sinensis) 当归
    chen pi (Pericarpium Citri Reticulatae) 陈皮
    bai shao (Radix Paeoniae Lactiflorae) 白芍
    dong kui zi (Semen Abutili seu Malvae) 冬葵子
    wang bu liu xing (Semen Vaccariae Segetalis) 王不留行
    gan cao (Radix Glycyrrhizae Uralensis) 甘草

CONG BAI QI WEI YIN 葱白七味饮 (*Shallot and Seven Herb Drink*)
    cong bai (Bulbus Allii Fistulosi) 葱白
    ge gen (Radix Puerariae) 葛根
    sheng di (Radix Rehmanniae Glutinosae) 生地
    mai dong (Tuber Ophiopogonis Japonici) 麦冬
    dan dou chi (Semen Sojae Preparatum) 淡豆豉
    sheng jiang (Rhizoma Zingiberis Officinalis Recens) 生姜

DA BU YUAN JIAN 大补元煎 (*Great Tonify the Basal Decoction*)
ren shen (Radix Ginseng) 人参
shan yao (Radix Dioscoreae Oppositae) 山药
shu di (Radix Rehmanniae Glutinosae Conquitae) 熟地
du zhong (Cortex Eucommiae Ulmoidis) 杜仲
dang gui (Radix Angelicae Sinensis) 当归
shan zhu yu (Fructus Corni Officinalis) 山茱萸
gou qi zi (Fructus Lycii) 枸杞子
zhi gan cao (honey fried Radix Glycyrrhizae Uralensis) 炙甘草

DAI DI DANG WAN 代抵当丸 (*Substituted Resistance Pill*)
da huang (Radix et Rhizoma Rhei) 大黄
mang xiao (Mirabilitum) 芒硝
tao ren (Semen Persicae) 桃仁
dang gui wei (tail of Radix Angelicae Sinensis) 当归尾
sheng di (Radix Rehmanniae Glutinosae) 生地
chuan shan jia° (Squama Manitis Pentadactylae) 穿山甲
rou gui (Cortex Cinnamomi Cassiae) 肉桂

DAI GE SAN 黛蛤散 (*Indigo and Conch Powder*)
qing dai (Pulverata Indigo) 青黛
hai ge ke fen^ (powdered Concha Cylinae Sinensis) 海蛤壳粉

DAN XI BI YUAN FANG 丹溪鼻渊方
(*Dan Xi's Nasal Congestion Formula*)
dan nan xing* (Pulvis Arisaemae cum Felle Bovis) 胆南星
ban xia* (Rhizoma Pinelliae Ternatae) 半夏
cang zhu (Rhizoma Atractylodis) 苍术
bai zhi (Radix Angelicae Dahuricae) 白芷
jiu huang qin (wine fried Radix Scutellariae Baicalensis) 酒黄芩
shen qu (Massa Fermentata) 神曲
xin yi hua (Flos Magnoliae) 辛夷花
jing jie (Herba seu Flos Schizonepetae Tenuifolia) 荆芥

DANG GUI LIU HUANG WAN 当归六黄丸
(*Dang Gui and Six Yellow Pills*)
dang gui (Radix Angelicae Sinensis) 当归
huang qi (Radix Astragali Membranacei) 黄芪
sheng di (Radix Rehmanniae Glutinosae) 生地
shu di (Radix Rehmanniae Glutinosae Conquitae) 熟地
huang lian (Rhizoma Coptidis) 黄连
huang qin (Radix Scutellariae Baicalensis) 黄芩
huang bai (Cortex Phellodendri) 黄柏

DANG GUI SHAO YAO SAN 当归芍药散
(*Dang Gui and Peonia Formula*)
    dang gui (Radix Angelicae Sinensis) 当归
    bai shao (Radix Paeoniae Lactiflora) 白芍
    fu ling (Sclerotium Poriae Cocos) 茯苓
    bai zhu (Rhizoma Atractylodis Macrocephalae) 白术
    ze xie (Rhizoma Alismatis Orientalis) 泽泻
    chuan xiong (Radix Ligustici Chuanxiong) 川芎

DAO QI TANG 导气汤 (*Conduct the Qi Decoction*)
    chuan lian zi* (Fructus Meliae Toosendan) 川楝子
    mu xiang (Radix Aucklandiae Lappae) 木香
    xiao hui xiang (Fructus Foeniculi Vulgaris) 小茴香
    wu zhu yu (Fructus Evodiae Rutaecarpae) 吴茱萸

DAO TAN TANG 导痰汤 (*Guide Out Phlegm Decoction*)
    ju hong (Pericarpium Citri Erythrocarpae) 橘红
    fu ling (Sclerotium Poria Cocos) 茯苓
    ban xia* (Rhizoma Pinelliae Ternatae) 半夏
    gan cao (Radix Glycyrrhizae Uralensis) 甘草
    zhi shi (Fructus Immaturus Citri Aurantii) 枳实
    tian nan xing* (Rhizoma Arisaematis) 天南星

DING ZHI WAN 定志丸 (*Settle the Emotions Pill*)
    ren shen (Radix Ginseng) 人参
    fu ling (Sclerotium Poriae Cocos) 茯苓
    shi chang pu (Rhizoma Acori Graminei) 石菖蒲
    yuan zhi (Radix Polygalae Tenuifoliae) 远志

DU HUO JI SHENG TANG 独活寄生汤
(*Du Huo and Vaecium Combination*)
    du huo (Radix Angelicae Pubescentis) 独活
    sang ji sheng (Ramulus Sangjisheng) 桑寄生
    xi xin* (Herba cum Radice Asari) 细辛
    fang feng (Radix Ledebouriellae Divaricatae) 防风
    qin jiao (Radix Gentianae Qinjiao) 秦艽
    du zhong (Cortex Eucommiae Ulmoidis) 杜仲
    niu xi (Radix Achyranthis Bidentatae) 牛膝
    rou gui (Cortex Cinnamomi Cassiae) 肉桂
    dang gui (Radix Angelicae Sinensis) 当归
    chuan xiong (Radix Ligustici Chuanxiong) 川芎
    sheng di (Radix Rehmanniae Glutinosae) 生地
    bai shao (Radix Paeoniae Lactiflora) 白芍
    ren shen (Radix Ginseng) 人参

fu ling (Sclerotium Poria Cocos) 茯苓
zhi gan cao (honey fried Radix Glycyrrhizae Uralensis) 炙甘草

ER CHEN TANG 二陈汤 (*Citrus and Pinellia Combination*)
ban xia* (Rhizoma Pinelliae Ternatae) 半夏
chen pi (Pericarpium Citri Reticulatae) 陈皮
fu ling (Sclerotium Poriae Cocos) 茯苓
zhi gan cao (honey fried Radix Glycyrrhizae Uralensis) 炙甘草

ER MIAO SAN 二妙散 (*Two Marvel Powder*)
cang zhu (Rhizoma Atractylodis) 苍术
huang bai (Cortex Phellodendri) 黄柏

GAN JIANG LING ZHU TANG 甘姜苓术汤
(*Licorice, Ginger, Hoelen and Atractylodes Decoction*)
gan cao (Radix Glycyrrhizae Uralensis) 甘草
gan jiang (Rhizoma Zingiberis Officinalis) 干姜
fu ling (Sclerotium Poria Cocos) 茯苓
bai zhu (Rhizoma Atractylodis Macrocephalae) 白术

GAN LU XIAO DU DAN 甘露消毒丹
(*Sweet Dew Special Pill to Eliminate Toxin*)
lian qiao (Fructus Forsythiae Suspensae) 连翘
huang qin (Radix Scutellariae Baicalensis) 黄芩
bo he (Herba Mentha Haplocalycis) 薄荷
she gan (Rhizoma Belamacandae) 射干
chuan bei mu (Bulbus Fritillariae Cirrhosae) 川贝母
hua shi (Talcum) 滑石
mu tong (Caulis Mutong) 木通
yin chen (Herba Artemisiae Yinchenhao) 茵陈
huo xiang (Herba Agastaches seu Pogostemi) 藿香
bai dou kou (Fructus Amomi Kravanh) 白豆蔻
shi chang pu (Rhizoma Acori Graminei) 石菖蒲

GUA LUO XIE BAI BAN XIA TANG 瓜楼薤白半夏汤
(*Trichosanthes, Bakeri and Pinellia Combination*)
gua lou (Fructus Trichosanthis) 栝楼
xie bai (Bulbus Allii) 薤白
ban xia* (Rhizoma Pinelliae Ternatae) 半夏
bai jiu (white wine) 白酒

GUAN XIN SU HE XIANG WAN 冠心苏合香丸
(*Liquid Styrax Pills* for *Coronary Heart Disease*)
su he xiang (Styrax Liquidis) 苏合香

    tan xiang (Lignum Santali Albi) 檀香
    qing mu xiang* (Radix Aristolochiae) 青木香
    bing pian (Borneol) 冰片
    ru xiang (Gummi Olibanum) 乳香

GUI LU ER XIAN JIAO 龟鹿二仙胶
(Tortise Shell and Deer Antler Syrup)
    lu jiao^ (Cornu Cervi) 鹿角
    gui ban° (Plastri Testudinis Gelatinum) 龟板
    gou qi zi (Fructus Lycii) 枸杞子
    ren shen (Radix Ginseng) 人参

GUI ZHI GAN CAO LONG GU MU LI TANG 桂枝甘草龙骨牡蛎汤
(Cinnamon, Licorice, Dragon Bone and Oyster Shell Decoction)
    gui zhi (Ramulus Cinnamomi Cassiae) 桂枝
    zhi gan cao (honey fried Radix Glycyrrhizae Uralensis) 炙甘草
    long gu^ (Os Draconis) 龙骨
    mu li^ (Concha Ostreae) 牡蛎

HE CHE DA ZAO WAN 河车大造丸 *(Placenta Great Creation Pills)*
    zi he che^ (Placenta Hominis) 紫河车
    ren shen (Radix Ginseng) 人参
    du zhong (Cortex Eucommiae Ulmoidis) 杜仲
    huang bai (Cortex Phellodendri) 黄柏
    shu di (Radix Rehmanniae Glutinosae Conquitae) 熟地
    gui ban° (Plastri Testudinis Gelatinum) 龟板
    niu xi (Radix Achyranthis Bidentatae) 牛膝
    tian dong (Tuber Asparagi cochinchinensis) 天冬
    mai dong (Tuber Ophiopogonis Japonici) 麦冬

HEI XI DAN 黑锡丹 *(Lead Special Pill)*
    hei xi (Lead) 黑锡
    liu huang (Sulphur) 硫黄
    chen xiang (Lignum Aquilariae) 沉香
    zhi fu zi* (Radix Aconiti Carmichaeli Praeparata) 制附子
    yang qi shi (Actinolitum) 阳起石
    hu lu ba (Semen Trigonellae Foeni-graeci) 胡芦巴
    xiao hui xiang (Fructus Foeniculi Vulgaris) 小茴香
    bu gu zhi (Fructus Psoraleae Corylifoliae) 补骨脂
    rou dou kou (Semen Myristicae Fragrantis) 肉豆蔻
    chuan lian zi* (Fructus Meliae Toosendan) 川楝子
    mu xiang (Radix Aucklandiae Lappae) 木香
    rou gui (Cortex Cinnamomi Cassiae) 肉桂

HUA YU TANG 化瘀汤 (*Transform Blood Stasis Decoction*)
dang gui (Radix Angelicae Sinensis) 当归
chi shao (Radix Paeoniae Rubrae) 赤芍
mu dan pi (Cortex Moutan Radicis) 牡丹皮
hong hua (Flos Carthami Tinctorii) 红花
tao ren (Semen Persicae) 桃仁
dan shen (Radix Salviae Miltiorrhizae) 丹参
chuan shan jia° (Squama Manitis Pentadactylae) 穿山甲
mu li^ (Concha Ostreae) 牡蛎
ze xie (Rhizoma Alismatis Orientalis) 泽泻
bai zhu (Rhizoma Atractylodis Macrocephalae) 白术
qing pi (Pericarpium Citri Reticulatae Viridae) 青皮

HUANG LIAN JIE DU TANG 黄连解毒汤
(*Coptis and Scute Combination*)
huang lian (Rhizoma Coptidis) 黄连
huang qin (Radix Scutellariae Baicalensis) 黄芩
huang bai (Cortex Phellodendri) 黄柏
shan zhi zi (Fructus Gardeniae Jasminoides) 山栀子

HUO LUO XIAO LING DAN 活络校灵丹
(*Fantastically Effective Pill to Invigorate the Collaterals*)
dan shen (Radix Salviae Miltiorrhizae) 丹参
dang gui (Radix Angelicae Sinensis) 当归
ru xiang (Gummi Olibanum) 乳香
mo yao (Myrrha) 没药

JIE GENG TANG 桔梗汤 (*Platycodon Decoction*)
jie geng (Radix Platycodi Grandiflori) 桔梗
sang bai pi (Cortex Mori Albae Radicis) 桑白皮
zhe bei mu (Bulbus Fritillariae Thunbergii) 浙贝母
dang gui (Radix Angelicae Sinensis) 当归
gua lou ren (Semen Trichosanthis) 瓜楼仁
huang qi (Radix Astragali Membranacei) 黄芪
zhi ke (Fructus Citri Aurantii) 枳壳
gan cao (Radix Glycyrrhizae Uralensis) 甘草
fang ji (Radix Aristolochiae Fangchi) 防己
bai he (Bulbus Lilii) 百合
yi ren (Semen Coicis Lachryma-jobi) 苡仁
wu wei zi (Fructus Schizandrae Chinensis) 五味子
di gu pi (Cortex Lycii Radicis) 地骨皮
zhi mu (Rhizoma Anemarrhenae Asphodeloides) 知母
xing ren* (Semen Pruni Armeniacae) 杏仁
ting li zi (Semen Descurainiae seu Lepidii) 葶苈子

JIE YU DAN 解语丹 (*Relax the Tongue Special Pill*)
    bai fu zi* (Rhizoma Typhonii Gigantei) 白附子
    shi chang pu (Rhizoma Acori Graminei) 石菖蒲
    yuan zhi (Radix Polygalae Tenuifoliae) 远志
    tian ma (Rhizoma Gastrodiae Elatae) 天麻
    quan xie* (Buthus Martensi) 全蝎
    qiang huo (Rhizoma et Radix Notopterygii) 羌活
    tian nan xing* (Rhizoma Arisaemae) 天南星
    mu xiang (Radix Aucklandiae Lappae) 木香
    gan cao (Radix Glycyrrhizae Uralensis) 甘草

JIN FEI CAO SAN 金沸草散 (*Inula Powder*)
    jin fei cao (Herba Inulae) 金沸草
    qian hu (Radix Peucedani) 前胡
    jing jie (Herba seu Flos Schizonepetae Tenuifolia) 荆芥
    xi xin* (Herba cum Radice Asari) 细辛
    fu ling (Sclerotium Poria Cocos) 茯苓
    ban xia* (Rhizoma Pinelliae Ternatae) 半夏
    gan cao (Radix Glycyrrhizae Uralensis) 甘草
    sheng jiang (Rhizoma Zingiberis Officinalis Recens) 生姜
    da zao (Fructus Zizyphi Jujubae) 大枣

LI ZHONG WAN 理中丸 (*Ginseng and Ginger Formula*)
    ren shen (Radix Ginseng) 人参
    gan jiang (Rhizoma Zingiberis Officinalis) 干姜
    bai zhu (Rhizoma Atractylodis Macrocephalae) 白术
    zhi gan cao (honey fried Radix Glycyrrhizae Uralensis) 炙甘草

LING YANG JIAO TANG 羚羊角汤 (*Antelope Horn Decoction*)
    ling yang jiao^ (Cornu Antelopis) 羚羊角
    gui ban° (Plastri Testudinis Gelatinum) 龟板
    sheng di (Radix Rehmanniae Glutinosae) 生地
    mu dan pi (Cortex Moutan Radicis) 牡丹皮
    bai shao (Radix Paeoniae Lactiflorae) 白芍
    chai hu (Radix Bupleuri) 柴胡
    chan tui^ (Periostracum Cicadae) 蝉蜕
    ju hua (Flos Morifolii Chrysanthemi) 菊花
    xia ku cao (Spica Prunellae Vulgaris) 夏枯草
    shi jue ming^ (Concha Haliotidis) 石决明

LIU SHEN WAN 六神丸 (*Six Spirit Pills*)
    niu huang^ (Calculus Bovis) 牛黄
    zhen zhu^ (Margarita) 珍珠
    she xiang° (Secretio Moschus) 麝香
    xiong huang (Realgar) 雄黄

chan su* (Secretio Bufonis) 蟾酥
bing pian (Borneol) 冰片

QIAN GEN SAN 茜根散 (*Rubia Decoction*)
qian cao gen (Radix Rubiae Cordifoliae) 茜草根
huang qin (Radix Scutellariae Baicalensis) 黄芩
e jiao^ (Gelatinum Corii Asini) 阿胶
ce bai ye (Cacumen Biotae Orientalis) 侧柏叶
sheng di (Radix Rehmanniae Glutinosae) 生地
gan cao (Radix Glycyrrhizae Uralensis) 甘草
sheng jiang (Rhizoma Zingiberis Officinalis Recens) 生姜

QIAN ZHENG SAN 牵正散 (*Lead to Symmetry Powder*)
jiang can^ (Bombyx Batryticatus) 僵蚕
quan xie* (Buthus Martensi) 全蝎
bai fu zi* (Rhizoma Typhonii Gigantei) 白附子

QIN JIAO BIE JIA SAN 秦艽鳖甲散
(*Gentiana Qinjiao and Soft-shelled Turtle Powder*)
chai hu (Radix Bupleuri) 柴胡
bie jia° (Carapax Amydae Sinensis) 鳖甲
di gu pi (Cortex Lycii Chinensis) 地骨皮
qin jiao (Radix Gentianae Qinjiao) 秦艽
dang gui (Radix Angelicae Sinensis) 当归
zhi mu (Rhizoma Anemarrhenae Asphodeloides) 知母

QING DAN XIE HUO TANG 清胆泻火汤
(*Clear the Gall Bladder and Drain Fire Decoction*)
chai hu (Radix Bupleuri) 柴胡
huang qin (Radix Scutellariae Baicalensis) 黄芩
ban xia* (Rhizoma Pinelliae Ternatae) 半夏
yin chen (Herba Artemisiae Yinchenhao) 茵陈
shan zhi zi (Fructus Gardeniae Jasminoides) 山栀子
long dan cao (Radix Gentianae Longdancao) 龙胆草
yu jin (Tuber Curcumae) 郁金
mu xiang (Radix Aucklandiae Lappae) 木香
da huang (Radix et Rhizoma Rhei) 大黄
mang xiao (Mirabilitum) 芒硝

QING HUN SAN 清魂散 (*Clear the Hun Powder*)
ren shen (Radix Ginseng) 人参
jing jie (Herba seu Flos Schizonepetae Tenuifolia) 荆芥
ze lan (Herba Lycopi Lucidi) 泽兰
chuan xiong (Radix Ligustici Chuanxiong) 川芎
gan cao (Radix Glycyrrhizae Uralensis) 甘草

QING JIN HUA TAN TANG 清金化痰汤
(*Clear Metal, Transform Phlegm Decoction*)
    huang qin (Radix Scutellariae Baicalensis) 黄芩
    shan zhi zi (Fructus Gardeniae Jasminoidis) 山栀子
    jie geng (Radix Platycodi Grandiflori) 桔梗
    mai dong (Tuber Ophiopogonis Japonici) 麦冬
    sang bai pi (Cortex Mori Albae Radicis) 桑白皮
    zhe bei mu (Bulbus Fritillariae Thunbergii) 浙贝母
    zhi mu (Rhizoma Anemarrhenae Asphodeloides) 知母
    gua lou ren (Semen Trichosanthis) 瓜楼仁
    chen pi (Pericarpium Citri Reticulatae) 陈皮
    fu ling (Sclerotium Poriae Cocos) 茯苓
    gan cao (Radix Glycyrrhizae Uralensis) 甘草

QING YAN NING FEI TANG 清咽宁肺汤
(*Clear the Throat and Calm the Lungs Decoction*)
    sang bai pi (Cortex Mori Albae Radicis) 桑白皮
    huang qin (Radix Scutellariae Baicalensis) 黄芪
    shan zhi zi (Fructus Gardeniae Jasminoidis) 山栀子
    zhi mu (Rhizoma Anemarrhenae Asphodeloides) 知母
    zhe bei mu (Bulbus Fritillariae Thunbergii) 浙贝母
    qian hu (Radix Peucedani) 前胡
    jie geng (Radix Platycodi Grandiflori) 桔梗
    gan cao (Radix Glycyrrhizae Uralensis) 甘草

SAN ZI YANG QIN TANG 三子养亲汤
(*Three Seed Decoction to Nourish One's Parents*)
    su zi (Fructus Perillae Frutescentis) 苏子
    bai jie zi (Semen Sinapsis Albae) 白芥子
    lai fu zi (Semen Raphani Sativi) 莱服子

SANG JU YIN 桑菊饮 (*Morus and Chrysanthemum Formula*)
    sang ye (Folium Mori Albae) 桑叶
    ju hua (Flos Chrysanthemi Morifolii) 菊花
    lian qiao (Fructus Forsythia Suspensae) 连翘
    bo he (Herba Mentha Haplocalycis) 薄荷
    jie geng (Radix Platycodi Grandiflori) 桔梗
    xing ren* (Semen Pruni Armeniacae) 杏仁
    lu gen (Rhizoma Phragmitis Communis) 芦根
    gan cao (Radix Glycyrrhizae Uralensis) 甘草

SANG XING TANG 桑杏汤 (*Morus and Apricot Seed Combination*)
    sang ye (Folium Mori Albae) 桑叶
    shan zhi zi (Fructus Gardeniae Jasminoidis) 山栀子
    dan dou chi (Semen Sojae Preparatum) 淡豆豉

    xing ren* (Semen Pruni Armeniacae) 杏仁
    zhe bei mu (Bulbus Fritillariae Thunbergii) 浙贝母
    nan sha shen (Radix Adenophorae seu Glehniae) 南沙参
    li pi (Fructus Pyri) 梨皮

SHA SHEN MAI MEN DONG TANG 沙参麦门冬汤
(Adenophora and Ophiopogon Combination)
    sha shen (Radix Adenophorae seu Glehniae) 沙参
    mai dong (Tuber Ophiopogonis Japonici) 麦冬
    yu zhu (Rhizoma Polygonati Odorati) 玉竹
    sang ye (Folium Mori Albae) 桑叶
    tian hua fen (Radix Trichosanthes Kirilowii) 天花粉
    bai bian dou (Semen Dolichoris Lablab) 白扁豆
    gan cao (Radix Glycyrrhizae Uralensis) 甘草

SHEN FU ZAI ZAO WAN 参附再造丸
(Ginseng and Aconite Pills for a New Lease on Life)
    ren shen (Radix Ginseng) 人参
    zhi fu zi* (Radix Aconiti Carmichaeli Praeparata) 制附子
    gui zhi (Ramulus Cinnamomi Cassiae) 桂枝
    huang qi (Radix Astragali Membranacei) 黄芪
    xi xin* (Herba cum Radice Asari) 细辛
    qiang huo (Rhizoma et Radix Notopterygii) 羌活
    chuan xiong (Radix Ligustici Chuanxiong) 川芎
    fang feng (Radix Ledebouriellae Divaricatae) 防风
    bai shao (Radix Paeoniae Lactiflora) 白芍
    gan cao (Radix Glycyrrhizae Uralensis) 甘草
    sheng jiang (Rhizoma Zingiberis Officinalis Recens) 生姜
    da zao (Fructus Zizyphi Jujubae) 大枣

SHEN LING BAI ZHU SAN 参苓白术散
(Ginseng and Atractylodes Formula)
    ren shen (Radix Ginseng) 人参
    bai zhu (Rhizoma Atractylodis Macrocephalae) 白术
    fu ling (Sclerotium Poriae Cocos) 茯苓
    zhi gan cao (honey fried Radix Glycyrrhizae Uralensis) 炙甘草
    shan yao (Radix Dioscoreae Oppositae) 山药
    bai bian dou (Semen Dolichos Lablab) 白扁豆
    lian zi (Semen Nelumbinis Nuciferae) 莲子
    yi ren (Semen Coicis Lachryma-jobi) 苡仁
    jie geng (Radix Platycodi Grandiflori) 桔梗
    sha ren (Fructus Amomi) 砂仁

SHI WEI SAN 石苇散 *(Pyrrosia Powder)*
    shi wei (Folium Pyrrosiae) 石苇

dong kui zi (Semen Abutili seu Malvae) 冬葵子
che qian zi (Semen Plantaginis) 车前子
qu mai (Herba Dianthi) 瞿麦
hua shi (Talcum) 滑石

SHOU XING WAN 寿星丸 (*God of Longevity Pills*)
yuan zhi (Radix Polygalae Tenuifoliae) 远志
ren shen (Radix Ginseng) 人参
huang qi (Radix Astragali Membranacei) 黄芪
bai zhu (Rhizoma Atractylodis Macrocephalae) 白术
zhi gan cao (honey fried Radix Glycyrrhizae Uralensis) 炙甘草
dang gui (Radix Angelicae Sinensis) 当归
sheng di (Radix Rehmanniae Glutinosae) 生地
bai shao (Radix Paeoniae Lactiflora) 白芍
fu ling (Sclerotium Poriae Cocos) 茯苓
chen pi (Pericarpium Citri Reticulatae) 陈皮
rou gui (Cortex Cinnamomi Cassiae) 肉桂
tian nan xing* (Rhizoma Arisaematis) 天南星
hu po (Succinum) 琥珀
zhu sha* (Cinnabar) 朱砂
wu wei zi (Fructus Schizandrae Chinensis) 五味子
blood from a pigs heart
ginger juice to form into pills

SI JUN ZI TANG 四君子汤 (*Four Major Herbs Combination*)
ren shen (Radix Ginseng) 人参
bai zhu (Rhizoma Atractylodis Macrocephalae) 白术
fu ling (Sclerotium Poria Cocos) 茯苓
gan cao (Radix Glycyrrhizae Uralensis) 甘草

SI NI JIA REN SHEN TANG 四逆加人参汤
(*Frigid Extremities Decoction plus Ginseng*)
zhi fu zi* (Radix Aconiti Carmichaeli Praeparata) 制附子
gan jiang (Rhizoma Zingiberis Officinalis) 干姜
ren shen (Radix Ginseng) 人参
zhi gan cao (honey fried Radix Glycyrrhizae Uralensis) 炙甘草

SI NI SAN 四逆散 (*Frigid Extremities Powder*)
chai hu (Radix Bupleuri) 柴胡
zhi shi (Fructus Immaturus Citri Aurantii) 枳实
bai shao (Radix Paeoniae Lactiflora) 白芍
zhi gan cao (honey fried Radix Glycyrrhizae Uralensis) 炙甘草

SI WU TANG 四物汤 (*Dang Gui Four Combination*)
shu di (Radix Rehmanniae Glutinosae Conquitae) 熟地
bai shao (Radix Paeoniae Lactiflora) 白芍
dang gui (Radix Angelicae Sinensis) 当归
chuan xiong (Radix Ligustici Chuanxiong) 川芎

TAO HE CHENG QI TANG 桃核承气汤 (*Persica and Rhubarb Combination*)
tao ren (Semen Persicae) 桃仁
da huang (Radix et Rhizoma Rhei) 大黄
gui zhi (Ramulus Cinnamomi Cassiae) 桂枝
mang xiao (Mirabilitum) 芒硝
zhi gan cao (honey fried Radix Glycyrrhizae Uralensis) 炙甘草

TIAN TAI WU YAO SAN 天台乌药散 (*Top Quality Lindera Powder*)
wu yao (Radix Linderae Strychnifoliae) 乌药
mu xiang (Radix Aucklandiae Lappae) 木香
xiao hui xiang (Fructus Foeniculi Vulgaris) 小茴香
qing pi (Pericarpium Citri Reticulatae Viride) 青皮
gao liang jiang (Rhizoma Alpiniae Officinari) 高良姜
bing lang (Semen Arecae Catechu) 槟榔
chuan lian zi* (Fructus Meliae Toosendan) 川楝子
ba dou* (Semen Croton Tiglii) 巴豆

WEI JING TANG 苇茎汤 (*Reed Decoction*)
lu gen (Rhizoma Phragmitis Communis) 芦根
yi ren (Semen Coicis Lachryma-jobi) 苡仁
dong gua ren (Semen Benincasae Hispidae) 冬瓜仁
tao ren (Semen Persicae) 桃仁

WEN FEI ZHI LIU DAN 温肺止流丹 (*Warm the Lungs, Stop the Flow Special Pill*)
ren shen (Panax Ginseng) 人参
jing jie (Herba seu Flos Schizonepetae Tenuifolia) 荆芥
xi xin* (Herba cum Radice Asari) 细辛
he zi (Fructus Terminaliae Chebulae) 诃子
gan cao (Radix Glycyrrhizae Uralensis) 甘草
jie geng (Radix Platycodi Grandiflori) 桔梗
yu nao shi^ (Pseudosciaenae Otolithum) 鱼脑石

WU BI SHAN YAO WAN 无比山药丸 (*Incomparable Dioscorea Pill*)
shan yao (Radix Dioscoreae Oppositae) 山药
rou cong rong (Herba Cistanches Deserticolae) 肉苁蓉
shu di (Radix Rehmanniae Glutinosae Conquitae) 熟地

shan zhu yu (Fructus Corni Officinalis) 山茱萸
fu ling (Sclerotium Poria Cocos) 茯苓
tu si zi (Semen Cuscutae Chinensis) 菟丝子
wu wei zi (Fructus Schizandrae Chinensis) 五味子
chi shi zhi (Halloysitum Rubrum) 赤石脂
ba ji tian (Radix Morindae Officinalis) 巴戟天
ze xie (Rhizoma Alismatis Orientalis) 泽泻
du zhong (Cortex Eucommiae Ulmoidis) 杜仲
niu xi (Radix Achyranthis Bidentatae) 牛膝

WU LIN SAN 五淋散 (*Gardenia and Hoelen Formula*)
    chi fu ling (Sclerotium Poriae Cocos Rubrae) 赤茯苓
    shan zhi zi (Fructus Gardeniae Jasminoidis) 山栀子
    dang gui (Radix Angelicae Sinensis) 当归
    gan cao (Radix Glycyrrhizae Uralensis) 甘草
    chi shao (Radix Paeoniae Rubrae) 赤芍

WU WEI ZI TANG 五味子汤 (*Schizandra Decoction*)
    wu wei zi (Fructus Schizandrae Chinensis) 五味子
    mai dong (Tuber Ophiopogonis Japonici) 麦冬
    huang qi (Radix Astragali Membranacei) 黄芪
    ren shen (Radix Ginseng) 人参
    gan cao (Radix Glycyrrhizae Uralensis) 甘草

WU ZI YAN ZONG WAN 五子衍宗丸
(*Five Seed Ancestral [Qi] Amplifying Pill*)
    gou qi zi (Fructus Lycii) 枸杞子
    tu si zi (Semen Cuscutae Chinensis) 菟丝子
    fu pen zi (Fructus Rubi Chingii) 复盆子
    wu wei zi (Fructus Schizandrae Chinensis) 五味子
    che qian zi (Semen Plantaginis) 车前子

XI JIAO SAN 犀角散 (*Rhinoceros Horn Powder*)
    xi jiao° (Cornu Rhinoceri) 犀角
    huang lian (Rhizoma Coptidis) 黄连
    sheng ma (Rhizoma Cimicifugae) 升麻
    yin chen (Herba Artemisiae Yinchenhao) 茵陈
    shan zhi zi (Fructus Gardeniae Jasminoides) 山栀子

XIAN FANG HUO MING YIN 仙方活命饮
(*Sublime Formula for Sustaining Life*)
    jin yin hua (Flos Lonicerae Japonicae) 金银花
    tian hua fen (Radix Trichosanthis Kirilowii) 天花粉
    dang gui (Radix Angelicae Sinensis) 当归
    chi shao (Radix Paeoniae Rubrae) 赤芍

zhe bei mu (Bulbus Fritillariae Thunbergii) 浙贝母
bai zhi (Radix Angelicae Dahuricae) 白芷
zao jiao ci (Spina Gleditsiae Sinensis) 皂角刺
ru xiang (Gummi Olibanum) 乳香
mo yao (Myrrha) 没药
chuan shan jia° (Squama Manitis Pentadactylae) 穿山甲
fang feng (Radix Ledebouriellae Divaricatae) 防风
chen pi (Pericarpium Citri Reticulatae) 陈皮
gan cao (Radix Glycyrrhizae Uralensis) 甘草

XIAO HUO LUO DAN 小活络丹
(Minor Invigorate the Collaterals Special Pill)
zhi cao wu* (Radix Aconiti Kusnezoffii Praeparata) 制草乌
zhi chuan wu* (Radix Aconiti Carmichaeli Praeparata) 制川乌
tian nan xing* (Rhizoma Arisaematis) 天南星
ru xiang (Gummi Olibanum) 乳香
mo yao (Myrrha) 没药
di long^ (Lumbricus) 地龙

XIAO JI YIN ZI 小蓟饮子 *(Cephalanoplos Decoction)*
sheng di (Radix Rehmanniae Glutinosae) 生地
xiao ji (Herba Cephalanoplos) 小蓟
hua shi (Talcum) 滑石
chao pu huang (dry fried Pollen Typhae) 炒蒲黄
ou jie (Nodus Nelumbinis Nuciferae Rhizomatis) 藕节
dan zhu ye (Herba Lophatheri Gracilis) 淡竹叶
shan zhi zi (Fructus Gardeniae Jasminoidis) 山栀子
dang gui (Radix Angelicae Sinensis) 当归
gan cao shao (tips of Radix Glycyrrhizae Uralensis) 甘草稍
mu tong (Caulis Mutong) 木通

XIAO JIANG QI TANG 小降气汤 *(Minor Descending qi Decoction)*
bai shao (Radix Paeoniae Lactiflora) 白芍
zi su ye (Fructus Perillae Frutescentis) 紫苏叶
wu yao (Radix Linderae Strychnifoliae) 乌药
chen pi (Pericarpium Citri Reticulatae) 陈皮
gan cao (Radix Glycyrrhizae Uralensis) 甘草
sheng jiang (Rhizoma Zingiberis Officinalis Recens) 生姜
da zao (Fructus Zizyphi Jujubae) 大枣

XIAO YU TANG 消瘀汤 *(Eliminate Blood Stasis Decoction)*
bie jia° (Carapax Amydae Sinensis) 鳖甲
mu li^ (Concha Ostreae) 牡蛎
ren shen (Radix Ginseng) 人参
chai hu (Radix Bupleuri) 柴胡

    qing pi (Pericarpium Citri Reticulatae Viridae) 青皮
    zhi ke (Fructus Citri Aurantii) 枳壳
    e zhu (Rhizoma Curcumae Ezhu) 莪术
    san leng (Rhizoma Sparganii Stoloniferi) 三棱
    ji nei jin^ (Endothelium Corneum Gigeriae Galli) 鸡内金
    fu ling (Sclerotium Poriae Cocos) 茯苓
    chi shao (Radix Paeoniae Rubrae) 赤芍

XIE BAI SAN 泻白散 (Morus and Lycium Formula)
    chao sang bai pi (dry fried Cortex Mori Albae Radicis) 炒桑白皮
    di gu pi (Cortex Lycii Radicis) 地骨皮
    geng mi (Semen Oryzae) 粳米
    zhi gan cao (honey fried Radix Glycyrrhizae Uralensis) 炙甘草

XIN JIA XIANG RU YIN 新加香薷饮 (Newly Augmented Elsholtzia Combination)
    xiang ru (Herba Elsholtzia seu Moslae) 香薷
    jin yin hua (Flos Lonicerae Japonicae) 金银花
    bai bian dou (Semen Dolichos Lablab) 白扁豆
    lian qiao (Fructus Forsythia Suspensae) 连翘
    hou po (Cortex Magnoliae Officinalis) 厚朴

YIN CHEN HAO TANG 茵陈蒿汤 (Capillaris Combination)
    yin chen (Herba Artemisiae Yinchenhao) 茵陈
    shan zhi zi (Fructus Gardeniae Jasminoides) 山栀子
    da huang (Radix et Rhizoma Rhei) 大黄

YIN CHEN WU LING SAN 茵陈五苓散 (Capillaris and Hoelen Five Formula)
    yin chen (Herba Artemisiae Yinchenhao) 茵陈
    fu ling (Sclerotium Poria Cocos) 茯苓
    zhu ling (Sclerotium Polypori Umbellati) 猪苓
    ze xie (Rhizoma Alismatis Orientalis) 泽泻
    bai zhu (Rhizoma Atractylodis Macrocephalae) 白术
    gui zhi (Ramulus Cinnamomi Cassiae) 桂枝

YIN CHEN ZHU FU TANG 茵陈术附汤 (Capillaris, Atractylodes and Aconite Combination)
    yin chen (Herba Artemisiae Yinchenhao) 茵陈
    bai zhu (Rhizoma Atractylodis Macrocephalae) 白术
    gan jiang (Rhizoma Zingiberis Officinalis) 干姜
    zhi fu zi* (Radix Aconiti Carmichaeli Praeparata) 制附子
    rou gui (Cortex Cinnamomi Cassiae) 肉桂
    gan cao (Radix Glycyrrhizae Uralensis) 甘草

YU NU JIAN 玉女煎 (*Jade Woman Decoction*)
- **shi gao** (Gypsum) 石膏
- **shu di** (Radix Rehmanniae Glutinosae Conquitae) 熟地
- **mai dong** (Tuber Ophiopogonis Japonici) 麦冬
- **zhi mu** (Rhizoma Anemarrhenae Asphodeloides) 知母
- **niu xi** (Radix Achyranthis Bidentatae) 牛膝

YU ZHEN SAN 玉真散 (*True Jade Powder*)
- **bai fu zi*** (Rhizoma Typhonii Gigantei) 白附子
- **tian nan xing*** (Rhizoma Arisaematis) 天南星
- **qiang huo** (Rhizoma et Radix Notopterygii) 羌活
- **bai zhi** (Radix Angelicae Dahuricae) 白芷
- **fang feng** (Radix Ledebouriellae Divaricatae) 防风
- **tian ma** (Rhizoma Gastrodiae Elatae) 天麻

YUE HUA WAN 月华丸 (*Moonlight Pill*)
- **mai dong** (Tuber Ophiopogonis Japonici) 麦冬
- **tian dong** (Tuber Asparagi cochinchinensis) 天冬
- **sheng di** (Radix Rehmanniae Glutinosae) 生地
- **shu di** (Radix Rehmanniae Glutinosae Conquitae) 熟地
- **bai bu** (Radix Stemonae) 百部
- **shan yao** (Radix Dioscoreae Oppositae) 山药
- **sha shen** (Radix Adenophorae seu Glehniae) 沙参
- **e jiao^** (Gelatinum Corii Asini) 阿胶
- **chuan bei mu** (Bulbus Fritillariae Cirrhosae) 川贝母
- **fu ling** (Sclerotium Poriae Cocos) 茯苓
- **ta gan^** (Iecur Lutrae) 獭肝
- **san qi** (Radix Notoginseng) 三七
- **sang ye** (Folium Mori Albae) 桑叶
- **ju hua** (Flos Chrysanthemi Morifolii) 菊花

ZAN YU DAN 赞育丹 (*Special Pill to Aid Fertility*)
- **zhi fu zi*** (Radix Aconiti Carmichaeli Praeparata) 制附子
- **rou gui** (Cortex Cinnamomi Cassiae) 肉桂
- **rou cong rong** (Cistanches Deserticolae) 肉苁蓉
- **ba ji tian** (Radix Morindae Officinalis) 巴戟天
- **xian ling pi** (Herba Epimedii) 仙灵脾
- **she chuang zi** (Fructus Cnidii Monnieri) 蛇床子
- **jiu zi** (Semen Allii Tuberosi) 韭子
- **xian mao** (Rhizoma Curculiginis Orchioidis) 仙茅
- **shan zhu yu** (Fructus Corni Officinalis) 山茱萸
- **du zhong** (Cortex Eucommiae Ulmoidis) 杜仲
- **shu di** (Radix Rehmanniae Glutinosae Conquitae) 熟地
- **dang gui** (Radix Angelicae Sinensis) 当归
- **gou qi zi** (Fructus Lycii) 枸杞子

bai zhu (Rhizoma Atractylodis Macrocephalae) 白术

ZHENG YANG LI LAO TANG 拯阳理劳汤
(*Rescue yang, Manage Exhaustion Decoction*)
    huang qi (Radix Astragali Membranacei) 黄芪
    bai zhu (Rhizoma Atractylodis Macrocephalae) 白术
    ren shen (Panax Ginseng) 人参
    dang gui (Radix Angelicae Sinensis) 当归
    chen pi (Pericarpium Citri Reticulatae) 陈皮
    wu wei zi (Fructus Schizandrae Chinensis) 五味子
    rou gui (Cortex Cinnamomi Cassiae) 肉桂
    gan cao (Radix Glycyrrhizae Uralensis) 甘草
    sheng jiang (Rhizoma Zingiberis Officinalis Recens) 生姜
    da zao (Fructus Zizyphi Jujubae) 大枣

ZHENG YIN LI LAO TANG 拯阴理劳汤
(*Rescue yin, Manage Exhaustion Decoction*)
    sheng di (Radix Rehmanniae Glutinosae) 生地
    mu dan pi (Cortex Moutan Radicis) 牡丹皮
    dang gui (Radix Angelicae Sinensis) 当归
    mai dong (Tuber Ophiopogonis Japonici) 麦冬
    chen pi (Pericarpium Citri Reticulatae) 陈皮
    yi ren (Semen Coicis Lachryma-jobi) 苡仁
    lian zi (Semen Nelumbinis Nuciferae) 莲子
    wu wei zi (Fructus Schizandrae Chinensis) 五味子
    ren shen (Panax Ginseng) 人参
    bai shao (Radix Paeoniae Lactiflora) 白芍
    zhi gan cao (honey fried Radix Glycyrrhizae Uralensis) 炙甘草
    da zao (Fructus Zizyphi Jujubae) 大枣

ZHONG MAN FEN XIAO WAN 中满分消丸
(*Separate and Reduce Fullness in the Middle Pill*)
    hou po (Cortex Magnoliae Officinalis) 厚朴
    zhi shi (Fructus Immaturus Citri Aurantii) 枳实
    jiang huang (Rhizoma Curcumae Longae) 姜黄
    chao huang qin (dry fried Radix Scutellariae Baicalensis) 炒黄芩
    chao huang lian (dry fried Rhizoma Coptidis) 炒黄连
    gan jiang (Rhizoma Zingiberis Officinalis) 干姜
    ban xia* (Rhizoma Pinelliae Ternatae) 半夏
    zhi mu (Rhizoma Anemarrhenae Asphodeloidis) 知母
    ze xie (Rhizoma Alismatis Orientalis) 泽泻
    zhu ling (Sclerotium Polypori Umbellati) 猪苓
    fu ling (Sclerotium Poriae Cocos) 茯苓
    bai zhu (Rhizoma Atractylodis Macrocephalae) 白术
    ren shen (Radix Ginseng) 人参

sha ren (Fructus Amomi) 砂仁
chen pi (Pericarpium Citri Reticulatae) 陈皮
zhi gan cao (honey fried Radix Glycyrrhizae Uralensis) 炙甘草

ZI SHEN TONG GUAN WAN 滋肾通关丸
(*Nourish Kidney, Open the Gate Pill*)
zhi mu (Rhizoma Anemarrhenae Asphodeloidis) 知母
huang bai (Cortex Phellodendri) 黄柏
rou gui (Cortex Cinnamomi Cassiae) 肉桂

Appendix B: Processing methods for herbs and modifications to prescription

PROCESSING METHODS

Many herbs are processed before use in order to modify their nature. These changes may be carried out by the dispensing herbalist or wholesaler or are specified by the prescribing physician when writing the prescription.

1. ZHI (frying with liquids)

Mixing the herb with a liquid and stir frying.

- Frying with honey (*mi zhi* 蜜炙) increases the tonifying, Lung moistening and cough stopping effects. Usually, if no particular medium is specified, writing *zhi* alone will result in honey frying.
- Frying with vinegar (*cu zhi* 醋炙) increases the effects on the Liver, and enhances the analgesic, astringent and Blood invigorating qualities; it also modifies unpleasant odours and tastes.
- Frying with wine (*jiu zhi* 酒炙) increases Blood invigorating, channel clearing action, and leads the herb to the upper body.
- Frying with salt water (*yan zhi* 盐炙) leads the herb to the Kidney, and can improve the Kidney Fire clearing nature.
- Frying with ginger juice (*jiang zhi* 姜炙) reduces the tendency of bitter and cold herbs to injure Stomach *qi*, can enhance the action of stopping nausea and vomiting and can modify the toxic nature of herbs such as **ban xia** (Rhizoma Pinelliae Ternatae) 半夏, and **tian nan xing** (Rhizoma Arisaema) 天南星.

2. CHAO (dry frying)

Browning and drying the herb in a wok. There are several degrees of dry frying:

- Mild dry frying, the most common method, is denoted by the character **chao** before the herb. The herb is dry fried until a light yellow brown. This method increases the warmth and digestibility of a herb, and improves the Stomach strengthening effect. Commonly used with Spleen tonics.
- Frying over high heat until dark brown or black on the outside. This method is usually used with food stagnation herbs, as it strongly improves digestion. Denoted by the character **jiao** (焦) before the herb.
- Frying over high heat until blackened and charred on the outside. This increases the astringent nature, and is used to improve the haemostatic effect of various herbs. Denoted by the character **tan** (炭) after the herb.

3. DUAN (calcining)

- Calcining involves placing the substance, usually a mineral or shell in a fire until it is heated red hot. It becomes brittle and is easily broken up. The substance's active ingredients are then made more available when decocted.

4. WEI (roasting in ashes)

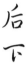

- The herb is wrapped in a coating of wet paper, mud or flour paste and roasted in hot coals until the coating is blackened and cracked; the substance inside has been cooked at a high temperature without burning. Usually used to modify the irritant or toxic natures of certain herbs.

MODIFICATIONS TO PRESCRIPTION

Different terms need to be added to a prescription depending on the specialised treatment some herbs require. The characters denoting these requirements are usually placed in brackets below the herb characters when written from top to bottom in the traditional script format.

1. HOU XIA (added towards the end)

- This instruction is used for herbs and substances that are added at the end of cooking or a few minutes before the end of cooking. These herbs usually contain volatile oils and the short cooking prevents the oils from evaporating off. The herbs are wrapped separately by the dispenser. This group includes light and aromatic herbs and herbs that change in action with different cooking times, like **da huang** (Radix et Rhizoma Rhei) 大黄, which causes a much stronger purge the less it is cooked.

2. XIAN JIAN (cooked first)

- This instruction applies to herbs and substances that require pre-cooking. This group includes toxic herbs like **fu zi** (Radix Aconiti Carmichaeli) 附子 that are rendered safer by long cooking (usually at least one hour), and minerals and shells like **mu li** (Concha Ostrea) 牡蛎, **long gu** (Os Draconis) 龙骨 and **ci shi** (Magnetitum) 磁石. The herbs are wrapped separately by the dispenser and usually cooked for about 30 minutes before the rest of the prescription is added.

3. CHONG FU (added to {or followed by} the strained decoction)

- This instruction applies to herbs and substances that are not cooked at all. They are wrapped separately by the dispensing herbalist, and dissolved in the hot liquid after straining or taken powdered and chased by the decoction. It is used for substances like **mang xiao** (Mirabilitum) 芒硝, **san qi** (Radix Notoginseng) 三七 and **zhu sha** (Cinnabaris) 朱砂.

4. BAO JIAN 包煎 (cooked in a cloth bag)

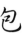

- Due to the presence of hairs or other irritants and the small size of certain seeds, some herbs should be cooked in a cloth or muslin bag. Often the whole formula will be placed in the bag by the dispenser.

5. YANG HUA (melted before adding to the strained decoction)
- Very sticky or viscous substances that may stick to the pot or the other herbs in the decoction are melted separately and added to the strained decoction. These substances can be gently boiled to aid their melting. Herbs that require this treatment include **e jiao** (Gelatinum Corii Asini) 阿胶 and **yi tang** (Saccharum Granorum) 饴糖.

Alteration to standard cooking method	Herbs
added at the end of cooking hou xia 后下 *cooked no more than 5 minutes °cooked no more than 10 minutes	bai dou kou* (Fructus Amomi Kravanh) bo he* (Herba Mentha Haplocalycis) chuan xiong° (Radix Ligustici Chuanxiong) da huang (Radix et Rhizoma Rhei) gou teng° (Ramulus Uncariae cum Uncis) huo xiang° (Herba Agastaches seu Pogostei) qing hao° (Herba Artemisiae Annuae) sha ren* (Fructus seu Semen Amomi)
cooked for 30 minutes before the other herbs xian jian 先煎	bie jia (Carapax Amydae Sinensis) ci shi (Magnetitum) dai zhe shi (Haematitum) fu zi (Radix Aconiti Carmichaeli) gui ban (Plastrum Testudinis) long gu (Os Draconis) mu li (Concha Ostreae) shi gao (Gypsum) shi jue ming (concha Haliotidis) zhen zhu mu (Concha Margaritaferae)
cooked in a muslin bag bao jian 包煎	che qian zi (Semen Plantaginis) hua shi (Talc) pi pa ye (Folium Eryobotryae Japonicae) xuan fu hua (Flos Inulae)
best taken seperately in pill or powder form	bing pian (Borneol) di long (Lumbricus) ge jie (Gecko) hu po (Succinum) ji nei jin (Endothelium Corneum Gigeraiae Galli) ling yang jiao (Cornu Antelopis) lu rong (Cornu Cervi Parvum) niu huang (Calculus Bovis) quan xie (Buthus Martensi) san qi (Radix Pseudoginseng su he xiang (Styrax Liquidis) wu bei zi (Galla Rhois Chinensis) wu gong (Scolopendra Subspinipes) zhu li (Succus Bambusae) zhu sha (Cinnabaris) zi he che (Placenta Hominis)
dissolved in the strained decoction chong fu 冲服	e jiao (Gelatinum Corii Asini) mang xiao (Mirabilitum) yi tang (Maltose)

Appendix C: Delivery methods for herbal medicine

There are numerous methods of getting herbs into a patient, each with its own advantages and disadvantages. Matching the delivery method to the patient and the type of disorder is an important aspect of correct practice and must be carefully considered when prescribing.

DECOCTION

Decoction involves boiling various ingredients in water or a mixture of water and wine for a specific period of time. Decoctions can be taken by mouth or delivered as an enema.

Uses
Most appropriate in acute or severe cases.

Advantages
Swift alteration of prescription, rapid absorption, strong and direct effect, best for acute or severe cases.

Disadvantages
Complexity, different cooking times for different ingredients, time consuming, bad smell and taste, poor patient compliance, cost.

Traditional method
The pot used should be preferably ceramic, although stainless steel is also acceptable. Aluminium, iron and copper pots should not be used. A tight fitting lid is necessary to prevent the escape of volatile oils. Plant materials should be soaked in cold water for at least 20–30 minutes before cooking. This allows the plant cells to expand and to release their contents when boiled. If the herbs are boiled before they are soaked, the boiling water can seal in the active components by toughening the cell walls.

One packet of herbs is usually decocted twice, although tonic herbs may be decocted three times. The amount of water required will vary depending on the type of herbs used and the purpose of the formula, but in general, enough water to cover the herbs by about one centimetre is correct (usually about 3-4 cups) with the aim of providing two cups of decoction per day. Keep in mind that some dry ingredients are very absorbent and will soak up a considerable amount of the water, while others, like minerals and shells, will absorb none. For the first boil the decoction is reduced to about two cups. The decoction is strained and taken one hour either side of a meal. For the second boil, 2½ - 3 cups of water are added to the same herbs and reduced to two cups. The results of the two boilings can be combined to maintain consistency of strength. The dose is two cups daily. In severe or emergency situations, the dose can be doubled and a cup can be taken every two hours. For patients unable to ingest the medicine, the herbs may be give via a nasogastric tube or retention enema. Diaphoretic and purgative formulae are generally discontinued once sweating or purgation occurs.

Practical considerations

For busy people, the traditional decoction method can be time consuming and inconvenient. To increase patient compliance, variations to the traditional decoction regime can be made. Several packets of herbs can be decocted at one time and the second boiling avoided by beginning with more water and boiling for longer (other than for those exceptions listed below). For example, two packets of herbs can be cooked with 9-10 cups of water and reduced to around 8 cups, yielding four days doses (at two cups daily). The strained decoction can be stored in a covered plastic container in the refrigerator and warmed by the addition of boiling water before ingestion. Stored in this way, the herbs will keep for up to a week.

Cooking time

Most general formulae can be cooked for 20-30 minutes. Formulae for dispersing external Wind, clearing Heat or those containing ingredients with volatile oils should be simmered in a lidded pot for a relatively short time, 10-15 minutes. Tonics, minerals and shells can stand long slow simmering (one hour +) to extract all their goodness. Certain groups of herbs (very hard or very delicate herbs) will require different treatment than the bulk of the ingredients and can be packaged separately for convenience (see Appendix B).

PILLS

Pills are finely ground up herbs that are bound with honey, water or some other sticky medium. Depending on the binding medium and the size of the pill, their ingredients are released and absorbed slowly and at a constant rate.

Uses

Pills are best for chronic problems that require lengthy therapy and are particularly good at long term tonification of *yin* and Blood. Pills are also useful for emergency or first aid situations, for example *Su He Xiang Wan* for chest pain, *An Gong Niu Huang Wan* for fever and delirium and *Zi Xue Dan* for febrile convulsions. They are also the preferred method when a formula requires herbs that should not be decocted.

Advantages

Pills are easier to store and take than decoctions. They are generally cheaper and more convenient for travelling or when decocting is impractical. A wide variety of pills are available as prepared patents.

Disadvantages
The ingredients of pills are fixed, so modifications to the prescription are not possible. The amount of pills required in order to achieve a therapeutic result is often large (8-16 pills three times per day for some varieties).

POWDERS

Powders are finely ground herbs sifted through a uniform mesh. They can be taken directly chased with a liquid or boiled and the resulting liquid taken.

Uses
Powders are useful for long term administration in the treatment of chronic disorders. They can be applied externally for skin diseases. They can be blown into the nose or throat for local disorders, or to resuscitate patients from unconsciousness.

Advantages
Powders are easier to store and take than decoctions, can be stored for long periods and can be formulated specifically for individual patients. They can provide a cheaper alternative to traditional decoction, as much less herb is required (due to the greatly increased surface area) to provide a dose. For patients unable to take the powder directly, it can be packed in to gelatin capsules.

Disadvantages
Once powdered, ingredients can not be deleted. If taken directly the possible enhancements to the formula gained by boiling are absent. Raw powders can irritate the gut in some patients.

CONCENTRATED GRANULES/POWDERS

Concentrated granules (*chong ji* 冲剂) are a relatively recent and very popular method of herb preparation that was developed in Japan in the 1950s. It has since become a major method of providing herbs in Japan, Taiwan and the West. Concentrated granules are produced by making large batches of herb formulae as decoctions and then draining the liquid from the dregs. The liquid is then evaporated and concentrated by gentle heating and exposure to a vacuum. The concentrate is added to a corn starch filler or the dregs of the decoction to form a paste. The paste is then spray dried and the remaining water evaporated, leaving a dry powder.

The concentration factor varies from one herb to another and from one formula to another, but on average is around a 6:1 concentration of the ingredients of the crude herbs. What this means is that about 600 grams of raw herbs go into 100 grams of concentrated powder. The typical dose for these granules is from 6-12 grams per day, which is equivalent to about 40-80 grams of raw herb.

Advantages

Because the herbs are concentrated, the daily dose is relatively small and easily tolerated. The production process for the major manufacturers (located in China, Japan, Taiwan and the United States) is regulated by Good Manufacturing Practice (GMP), which ensures quality control, consistency and the presence of active ingredients across batches. Concentrated powders can be packed into gelatin capsules.

Patient compliance is high, and as the powders are often quite bland they are excellent for children. The extraction technology is improving all the time and the quality of these products is usually very high. In Chinese hospitals, concentrated granules are gradually replacing decoctions

Disadvantages

The formulas are fixed and ingredients cannot be deleted. Generally not as good as decoctions for acute or severe disorders (but improving all the time). Products originating from Japan, while of the highest quality may vary significantly from the original prescription. Dosage regimes specified in Japan are often at odds with those preferred in China. The Japanese are fond of smaller doses and frequently change the dose of individual herbs, possibly altering the hierarchy of the formula.

SYRUPS

Syrups are composed of herbs that have been decocted, then concentrated by further cooking or thickened with the addition of honey or malt sugar. Syrups are good for children and most commonly used for coughs and moistening the Lungs.

Appendix D: Herbs that are contraindicated or to be used cautiously during pregnancy

Herbs contraindicated during pregnancy

ba dou* (Semen Croton Tiglii) 巴豆
ban mao^ (Mylabris) 斑蝥
chan su* (Secretio Bufonis) 蟾酥
che qian zi (Semen Plantaginis) 车前子
chuan niu xi (Radix Cyanthulae) 川牛膝
da ji* (Radix Euphorbiae seu Knoxie) 大戟
di bie chong^ (Eupolyphagea seu Opisthoplatiae) 地鳖虫
e wei (Asafoetida) 阿魏
e zhu (Rhizoma Curcumae Zedoariae) 莪术
fan xie ye (Folium Sennae) 番泻叶
fu zi* (Radix Aconiti) 附子
gan sui* (Radix Euphorbiae Kansui) 甘遂
guan zhong (Rhizoma Guanzhong) 贯众
hai long^ (Hailong) 海龙
hai ma^ (Hippocampus) 海马
hong hua (Flos Carmanthi Tinctorii) 红花
liu huang (Sulphur) 硫黄
ma chi xian (Herba Portulacae Oleracae) 马齿苋
ma qian zi (Semen Strychnotis) 马钱子
mang xiao (Mirabilitum) 芒硝
meng chong^ (Tabanus Bivittatus) 虻虫
niu huang^ (Calculus Bovis) 牛黄
qian niu zi (Semen Pharbitidis) 牵牛子
qing fen (Calomelas) 轻粉
qu mai (Herba Dianthi) 瞿麦
san leng (Rhizoma Sparganii) 三棱
shang lu* (Radix Phytolaccae) 商陆
she gan (Rhizoma Belamacandae) 射干
she xiang° (Secretio Moschus Moschiferi) 麝香
shui zhi^ (Hirudo seu Whitmanae) 水蛭
tao ren (Semen Persicae) 桃仁
tian hua fen (Radix Trichosanthis) 天花粉
wu gong* (Scolopendra Subspinipes) 蜈蚣
wu tou* (Radix Aconiti) 乌头
xiong huang (Realgar) 雄黄
xuan ming fen (Natrii Sulphas Exsiccatus) 玄明粉
yan hu suo (Rhizoma Corydalis Yanhusuo) 延胡索

yi mu cao (Herba Leonuri Heterophylli) 益母草
yu li hua (Flos et Fructus Rosae) 月李花
yuan hua (Flos Daphnes Genkwa) 芫花
zao jiao (Fructus Gleditsae Sinensis) 皂角
zhang nao (Camphora) 樟脑

Herbs to be used with caution during pregnancy

bai fu zi* (Rhizoma Typhonii Gigantei) 白附子
ban xia* (Rhizoma Pinelliae Ternatae) 半夏
bing pian (Borneol) 冰片
chang shan (Radix Dichorae Febrifugae) 常山
chuan jiao (Fructus Zanthoxyli Bungeani) 川椒
chuan shan jia° (Squama Manitis Pentadactylae) 穿山甲
da huang (Rhizoma Rhei) 大黄
dai zhe shi (Haematitum) 代赭石
dong kui zi (Semen Abutiloni seu Malvae) 冬葵子
gan jiang (Rhizoma Zingiberis Officinalis) 干姜
hou po (Cortex Magnoliae Officinalis) 厚朴
huai niu xi (Radix Achyranthis Bidentatae) 怀牛膝
hua shi (Talcum) 滑石
lou lu (Radix Rhapontici seu Echinops) 漏芦
lu hui* (Herba Aloes) 芦荟
lu lu tong (Fructus Liquidambaris Taiwanianae) 路路通
mo yao (Myrrha) 没药
mu tong (Caulis Mutong) 木通
pu huang (Pollen Typhae) 蒲黄
quan xie* (Buthus Martensi) 全蝎
rou gui (Cortex Cinnamomi Cassiae) 肉桂
ru xiang (Gummi Olibanum) 乳香
san qi (Radix Pseudoginseng) 三七
su he xiang (Styrax Liquidis) 苏合香
su mu (Lignum Sappan) 苏木
tian nan xing* (Rhizoma Arisaematis) 天南星
tong cao (Medulla Tetrapanacis Papyriferi) 通草
wang bu liu xing (Semen Vaccariae Segetalis) 王不留行
xue jie (Sanguis Draconis) 血竭
yi yi ren (Semen Coicis Lachryma-jobi) 薏苡仁
yu jin (Radix Curcumae) 郁金
yu li ren (Semen Pruni) 郁李仁
ze lan (Herba Lycopi Lucidi) 泽兰
zhi ke (Fructus Citri seu Ponciri) 枳壳
zhi shi (Fructus Citri seu Ponciri Immaturis) 枳实

Appendix E: Incompatible and antagonistic herbs

Eighteen incompatible herbs

These are herbs which, if used together, may cause toxic or strong unwanted effects.

gan cao (Radix Glycyrrhizae Uralensis) 甘草 is incompatible with
    gan sui (Radix Euphorbiae Kansui) 甘遂
    da ji (Radix Euphorbiae seu Knoxiae) 大戟
    yuan hua (Flos Daphnes Genkwa) 芫花
    hai zao (Herba Sargassii) 海藻
wu tou (Radix Aconiti) 乌头 is incompatible with
    ban xia (Rhizoma Pinelliae Ternatae) 半夏
    gua lou (Fructus Trichosanthis) 栝楼
    bei mu (Bulbus Fritillariae) 贝母
    bai lian (Radix Ampelopsis) 白蔹
    bai ji (Rhizoma Bletillae Striatae) 白芨
li lu (Radix Veratrum Nigrum) 藜芦 is incompatible with
    ren shen (Radix Ginseng) 人参
    sha shen (Radix Glehniae Littoralis) 沙参
    dan shen (Radix Salviae Miltorrhizae) 丹参
    ku shen (Radix Sophorae Flavescentis) 苦参
    xi xin (Herba Asari cum Radice) 细辛
    bai shao (Radix Paeoniae Lactiflora) 白芍

Nineteen antagonistic herbs

These are herbs which, if used together, may counteract or neutralize each other's positive effects. The symbol ~ means antagonises.

- **liu huang** (Sulphur) 硫黄 ~ **po xiao** (Mirabilitum Depuratium) 朴硝
- **shui yin** (Hydragyrum) 水银 ~ **pi shuang** (Arsenicum Sublimatum) 砒霜
- **lang du** (Radix Euphorbiae Fischerianae) 狼毒 ~ **mi tuo seng** (Lithargyrum) 密佗僧
- **ba dou** (Semen Croton Tiglii) 巴豆 ~ **qian niu zi** (Semen Pharbitidis) 牵牛子
- **ding xiang** (Flos Caryophilli) 丁香 ~ **yu jin** (Radix Curcumae) 郁金
- **ya xiao** (Nitrum) 牙硝 ~ **san leng** (Rhizoma Sparganii) 三棱
- **chuan wu** (Radix aconiti) 川乌 and **cao wu** (Radix Aconiti Kusnezoffii) 草乌 ~ **xi jiao** (Cornu Rhinoceri) 犀角
- **ren shen** (Radix Ginseng) 人参 ~ **wu ling zhi** (Excrementum Trogopterum) 五灵脂
- **rou gui** (Cortex Cinnamon Cassiae) 肉桂 ~ **chi shi zhi** (Halloysitum Rubrum) 赤石脂

Appendix F. Herbs with potential toxic effects[1,2], noted in the text with an asterisk *

Herb	Safe Dosage Range (g)	Toxic effects of overdose	Comments	Antidote, Treatment[3]
Fu Zi (Wu Tou, Cao Wu, Chuan Wu) (Rhizoma Aconiti Carmichaeli)	3-12	hypersalivation, numbness of the mouth and extremities, dizziness, headache, blurred vision, difficulty speaking, tremors, abdominal pain, vomiting, diarrhoea, cardiac arrhythmia, hypotension, incontinence and in severe cases respiratory depression, cardiogenic shock and death	Very toxic in the raw state. Generally cooked for at least one hour to reduce toxicity. Always supplied in the prepared form, but to be on the safe side *zhi fu zi*, *hei fu zi* · a processing method that renders the root black, or *fu zi pian* · prepared and thinly sliced, should be specified in the prescription. Contraindicated during pregnancy.	~ activated charcoal ~ atropine ~ decoction of ku shen 30g, or decoction of gan cao 15g, huang lian 3g, sheng jiang 15g and jin yin hua 15g
Ban Xia (Rhizoma Pinelliae Ternatae)	3-12	burning, swelling, numbness and stiffness in the tongue, throat and lips, hypersalivation, difficulty speaking, nausea, pressure in the chest	Very toxic in the raw state. The herb dispensed by pharmacies is processed with vinegar, alum or ginger and generally safe. Caution during pregnancy	~ ginger juice or strong ginger decoction ~ vinegar ~ choline
Tian Nan Xing (Rhizoma Arisaematis)	3-10	initially gastrointestinal irritation, burning numbness and stiffness of the tongue, hypersalivation, oral erosion, then neurological symptoms including dizziness, arrythmia, numbness in the limbs, delirium, respiratory distress	Very toxic in the raw state. The herb that is dispensed by pharmacies has been processed to alleviate its toxicity. Caution during pregnancy.	~ strong black tea ~ egg white ~ ginger juice or strong ginger decoction ~ vinegar ~ tannic acid
Ma Huang (Radix Ephedrae)	2-9 grams	hypertension, tachycardia, vasoconstriction, sweating, headache, dizziness, tremors, restlessness, nausea, abdominal pain, urinary retention; in severe cases and susceptible patients ventricular fibrillation and death	The raw herb is most likely to cause side effects; cooking with honey alleviates the diaphoretic effect somewhat.	~ atropine ~ chlorpromazine

1. From *Shi Yong Zhong Yi Nei Ke Xue* and *Zhong Yi Nei Ke Lin Chuang Shou Ce*.
2. Most of these herbs are quite safe *when used correctly*.
3. In severe cases of poisoning, treatment requires hospitalisation, and depending on the herb, gastric lavage, mechanical ventilation, electrolyte and fluid replacement etc. Suggestions given in the antidote/treatment section are not complete measures and may be useful only in non critical cases.

Appendix F: Herbs with potential toxic effects   945

Herb	Safe Dosage Range (g)	Toxic effects of overdose	Comments	Antidotes, Treatment[3]
Xi Xin (Herba cum Radice Asari)	1-3	headache, vomiting, sweating, restlessness, hypertension, panting, stiffness and spasm of the neck and jaw, confusion; in severe cases respiratory paralysis	Toxic effects occur at doses of 15 grams.	~ decoction of ren shen, mai dong and wu wei zi
Ku Xing Ren (Semen Pruni Armeniacae)	5-10	dizziness, hypersalivation, upper abdominal pain, nausea, vomiting, diarrhoea, headache, numbness, dyspnoea, coma	The lethal dose is around 50-60 seeds in adults and 10 in children.	~ activated charcoal ~ ipecac ~ fresh radish juice ~ decoction of gan cao 120g and black beans 120g
Chan Su (Secretio Bufonis)	0.015-0.03	digitalis like effects, nausea, vomiting, hypersalivation, abdominal pain, diarrhoea, palpitations, bradycardia, dropped beats, dizziness, headache, lethargy, slow reflexes, numbness in the limbs, cyanosis, hypotensive shock	Only ever used in pills at tiny doses. Contraindicated during pregnancy.	~ atropine ~ Sheng Mai San decoction (or injection) ~ Shen Fu Tang decoction (or injection) ~ eyewash of zi cao for eye irritation
Quan Xie (Buthus Martensi)	1.5-5	headache, dizziness, palpitations, dyspnoea, cyanosis, confusion, respiratory paralysis	If only the tail is used the dose is 1-1.5 grams. Care during pregnancy.	~ atropine ~ calcium lactate ~ decoction of jin yin hua 30g, ban bian lian 10g, tu fu ling 10g, lu dou 15g and gan cao 10g
Wu Gong (Scolopendra Subspinipes)	2-5	nausea, vomiting, abdominal pain, dyspnoea, confusion, palpitations, bradycardia, collapse	Contraindicated during pregnancy.	
Lu Hui (Herba Aloes)	1-2	nausea, vomiting, haematemesis, abdominal pain, diarrhoea, tenesmus, low back pain, anuria, haematuria, proteinuria, miscarriage	Contraindicated during pregnancy.	~ activated charcoal ~ egg white
Ya Dan Zi (Fructus Brucae Javanicae)	10-30 fruit	nausea, vomiting, abdominal pain, diarrhoea, headache, lethargy, numbness in the limbs; in severe cases paralysis and dyspnoea	Not used in decoction, taken only in capsules or inside longan fruit to mask its exceptional bitterness	~ egg white ~ milk ~ decoction of gan cao and brown sugar ~ cold rice porridge
Bai Guo (Semen Ginkgo Bilobae)	5-10	headache, dizziness, fever, spasms, restlessness, vomiting, dyspnoea, abdominal pain, diarrhoea		~ decoction of gan cao 60g and mung beans 60g

946 CLINICAL HANDBOOK OF INTERNAL MEDICINE

Herb	Safe Dosage Range (g)	Toxic effects of overdose	Comments	Antidote Treatment[3]
Ma Dou Ling (Qing Mu Xiang) (Fructus Aristolochiae)	3-9	abdominal pain, diarrhoea, rectal bleeding, tenesmus, weakness, somnolence, anuria, haematuria, dyspnoea	Qing Mu Xiang is the root of the same plant. Ma Dou Ling frequently causes nausea when taken hot although this can be alleviated by frying in honey.	~ frequent strong tea ~ neostigmine
Chuan Lian Zi (Fructus Meliae Toosendan)	5-10	nausea, vomiting, diarrhoea, dyspnoea, palpitations, dizziness, tremors, spasms, numbness	Also known as Jin Ling Zi	~ activated charcoal ~ egg white
Cang Er Zi (Fructus Xanthii Sibirici)	3-10	headache, nausea, vomiting, abdominal pain, in severe cases weakness and liver damage with hepatomegaly, jaundice and elevated SGPT, oliguria, extensive bleeding, tonic spasms, respiratory distress, coma		~ activated charcoal ~ Vitamin C (with bleeding) ~ decoction of ban lan gen 120g ~ Gan Cao Lu Dou Tang ~ Zhi Bao Dan
Ai Ye (Folium Artemisiae Argyi)	3-10	acute overdose: dry mouth and throat, epigastric pain, vomiting, abdominal distension, epileptiform seizures, cold clammy skin chronic poisoning: tonic spasms, weakened vision, neuritis	These toxic effects only occur with internal use of ai ye.	~ for spasms Zi Xue Dan ~ Wind extinguishing herbs
Wei Ling Xian (Radix Clematis)	3-10	redness and pain of the skin, abdominal pain, diarrhoea, oral erosion, black stools, ; in severe cases dyspnoea, dilated pupils, stiff tongue, slow pulse		~ egg white, gastric lavage ~ atropine ~ decoction of gan cao and brown sugar
Bai Fu Zi (Rhizoma Typhonii Gigantei)	3-5	numbness of the mouth and tongue, dizziness, generalised numbness, spasms, hyersalivation, vomiting	Contraindicated during pregnancy.	~ decoction of gan cao 30 g and ginger 30g
Bai Bu (Radix Stemonae)	5-10	nausea, epigastric opain, diarrhoea; can depress the respiratory centre, in extreme cases causing respiratory paralysis		~ fresh ginger juice or a strong ginger decoction ~ rice vinegar

Appendix F: Herbs with potential toxic effects 947

Herb	Safe Dosage Range (g)	Toxic effects of overdose	Comments	Antidote, Treatment[3]
Ba Dou (Semen Croton Tiglii)	0.1-0.3 in pills or powder	gastrointestinal irritation, inflammation and erosion, hypersalivation, abdominal pain, nausea, vomiting, incessant diarrhoea, dehydration, jaundice, dyspnoea, hypotension, dizziness, cyanosis; in severe cases respiratory and circulatory failure and death	Contraindicated during pregnancy. Extremely toxic in the raw form. When used at all, it is in the defatted form, *ba dou shuang*	~ egg white, milk, activated charcoal ~ peanut oil 100g ~ with severe pain morphine or atropine ~ for incessant diarrhoea huang lian, huang qin and cold rice porridge, fluid replacement ~ for skin irritation soak in huang lian decoction
Shang Lu (Radix Phytolaccae)	2-5	nausea, vomiting, diarrhoea, haemafecia, abdominal pain, spasms in the limbs, inhibition of respiratory and cardiac function, hypotension, dilated pupils, miscarriage; in severe cases delirium, cardiac paralysis and death	This herb is extremely toxic. Contraindicated during pregnancy.	~ vitamin C ~ decoction of fang ji, fang feng, gan cao and gui zhi ~ mechanical ventilation as necessary
Da Ji (Radix Euphorbiae)	0.6-1.5	nausea, vomiting, abdominal pain violent diarrhoea, dizziness, delirium, spasms, dilated pupils, respiratory paralysis	Contraindicated during pregnancy. Frying with vinegar reduces the toxicity of da ji. Mostly used in pill or powder form.	~ decoction of lu gen 120g
Yuan Hua (Flos Daphnes Genkwa)	0.6-1.5	vomiting, violent or bloody diarrhoea, dehydration, muscle spasms, delirium	Contraindicated during pregnancy. Frying with vinegar reduces its toxicity. Generally only used in pill or powder form	~ vitamin C ~ fluid replacement
Gan Sui (Radix Euphorbiae Kansui)	0.6-1.5	nausea, vomiting, palpitations, abdominal pain, dizziness, palpitations, hypotension, low back ache, haematuria	Contraindicated during pregnancy. Generally only used in pill or powder form. When processed (zhi gan sui) its tendency to cause vomiting is reduced.	

Appendix G. Medicinal substances derived from animal species considered potentially or definitely endangered, noted in the text with an open circle °

The issue of endangered species is somewhat confused in regards to some of the animals and plants used in Chinese medicine. Some that are listed by CITES (the Convention on International Trade in Endangered Species), are certainly endangered and should be avoided–these include rhinocerous, tiger and musk deer products. The status of other species is less certain and some species considered endangered in the wild are abundantly cultivated (and may have been for centuries; examples include **du zhong** [Cortex Eucommia] and **huang lian** [Rhizoma Coptidis]), so genetically they are not endangered. In some cases certain genera have multiple listings (for example *Trionyx* spp.), but the specific species noted as the source of the particular medicinal substance by authorities such as Bensky and Gamble (1993) is not listed. This absence from the CITES list does not imply that the animal is not endangered, however, it may simply reflect the difficulty in compiling complete lists. In addition, the CITES lists are being updated continually and new species added as the data on their abundance comes to light.

The CITES lists have three main levels of classification, Appendices 1, 2 and 3. **Appendix I** includes all species threatened with extinction which are or may be affected by trade.

Appendix 2 includes:
  i. all species that although not necessarily now threatened with extinction may become so unless trade in specimens of such species is subject to strict regulation in order to avoid utilisation incompatible with their survival; and
  ii. other species that must be subject to regulation in order that trade in specimens of certain species referred to in sub-paragraph (i) of this paragraph may be brought under effective control.

Appendix 3 includes all species that any country identifies as being subject to regulation within its jurisdiction for the purpose of preventing or restricting exploitation, and as needing the co-operation of other countries in the control of trade.

Appendix G: Medicinal substances derived from endangered species

Table Appendix G. Animal species potentially or definitely endangered that are used in TCM

Animal	Comments	Possible Alternative
Gui Ban (Plastrum Testudinis)	There are several species or turtle that are marketed as this substance and they are definitely endangered in the wild. Turtles which provide the material for this substance are extensively farmed for food in China, but also collected throughout South East Asia. The species noted by Bensky and Gamble (1993) as the source of this substance (*Geoclemys reevesii*) is not listed by CITES, however the fresh water turtle family, Testudinidae, is listed in Appendix 2.	No good substitute for gui ban when deeply enriching the *yin*. Possible alternatives for restraining *yang* include Mu Li (Conchae Ostrea) and Shi Jue Ming (Concha Haliotidis).
Bie Jia (Carapax Amydae Sinensis)	Status uncertain, although may be similar to gui ban and possibly farmed as a food item. The species noted by Bensky and Gamble (1993) as the source of this substance (*Trionyx sinensis*) is not listed by CITES, although other *Trionyx* species are listed in Appendix 1.	Qing Hao (Herba Artemisiae Annuae) and Di Gu Pi (Cortex Lycii Radicis) for night sweats and bone steaming; Xuan Shen (Radix Scrophulariae Ningpoensis) for swellings and masses.
Xi Jiao (Cornu Rhinoceri)	Seriously endangered, in fact very few rhino remain. All products claiming to contain rhino horn should be avoided. All species of *Rhinocerotidae* listed by CITES (Appendix 1).	Shui Niu Jiao (Cornu Bubali).
Ling Yang Jiao (Cornu Antelopis)	The antelope noted by Bensky and Gamble (1993) (*Saiga tatarica*) that provides this substance is listed by CITES (Appendix 2).	Shan Yang Jiao (Cornu Naemorhedis) goat horn.
Chuan Shan Jia (Squama Manitidis)	Pangolins are endangered in the wild, but are farmed for their scales. *Manis* species are listed by CITES (Appendix 2)	Zao Jiao Ci (Spina Gleditsiae Sinensis).
She Xiang (Secretio Moschus)	Definitely endangered in the wild, but the musk deer is farmed and musk allegedly extracted humanely. Film evidence suggests this is not the case. Synthetic substitutes exist. All species (Moschus spp.) listed by CITES (Appendix 1).	Synthetic muscones.
Hu Gu (Os Tigris)	Seriously endangered in the wild, possibly extinct in China. All subspecies (*Panthera tigris*) listed by CITES (Appendix 1).	Pig or dog bone.

950 CLINICAL HANDBOOK OF INTERNAL MEDICINE

Appendix H. Non toxic medicinal substances that are derived from animals, noted in the text with a hat ^.

Any substitutes suggested in these tables should be viewed with caution. In many cases, animal products are unique in action and no adequate vegetable substitute exists.

Substance	Characteristics
E Jiao (Gelatinum Asini) *Equus asinus*	a hard gelatin derived from boiling down donkey skins; a strong Blood tonic, moistening agent and haemostatic
Di Long (Lumbricus) *Pheretima aspergillum* *Allobophora caliginosa*	earthworm; clears Heat and extinguishes Wind to stop convulsions, also for wheezing from Lung Heat, opens the channels for *bi* syndrome and hemiplegia, for painful urination and hypertension from Liver *yang* rising
Yu Nao Shi (Pseudosciaenae Otolithum) *Pseudosciaena crocea*	otolith (ear bones) from the yellow croaker fish; for sinus congestion, otitis and urinary tract stones; alternatives include Bai Zhi (Radix Angelica Dahuricae) and Cang Er Zi (Fructus Xanthii Sibirici) for nasal congestion
Ji Nei Jin (Endothelium Corneum Gigeriae Galli) *Gallus gallus domesticus*	endothelium of chickens gizzard; for food stagnation and dissolving urinary tract and gall bladder stones
Wu Ling Zhi (Excrementum Trogopteri seu Pteromi) *Trogopterus xanthipes*	flying squirrel excrement (one source suggests that Wu Ling Zhi was originally the resinous excretion retrieved from the squirrels nest, apparently some sort of glandular secretion); for dispersing Blood stagnation and stopping pain; possible alternatives include Yan Hu Suo (Rhizoma Corydalis Yanhusuo), Yi Mu Cao (Herba Leonuri Heterophylli) and Pu Huang (Pollen Typhae) for menstrual pain from stagnant Blood
Hou Zao (Calculus Macacae Mulattae) *Macaca mulatta*	macaque gallstone; clears hot Phlegm for childhood febrile convulsions; products containing this substance can usually be substituted with one of the following common patent medicines · BAO YING DAN or HUI CHUN DAN (although depending on the manufacturer, both contain insect drugs).
Jiang Can (Bombyx Batryticatus) *Bombyx mori*	dried silkworm larva that died due to infection with the fungus *Beauveria bassiana* Bals.; extinguishes internal Wind to treat convulsions, spasms and facial paralysis; also Phlegm nodules and itching
Chan Tui (Periostracum Cicadae) *Cryptotympana pastulata*	cicada shell; disperses external Wind for itchy skin lesions and throat disorders, extinguishes internal Wind for febrile convulsions and spasms; possible substitutes for itchy skin disorders include Niu Bang Zi (Fructus Arctii Lappae) and Bai Ji Li (Fructus Tribuli Terrestris)

Appendix H: Medicinal substances derived from animals 951

Substance	Characteristics
Wa Leng Zi (Concha Arcae) *Arca subcrenata, A. granosa, A. inflata*	ark shell; for eliminating Blood stasis and Phlegm in the treatment of nodules and tumours; possible substitutes include Fu Hai Shi (Pumice) for Phlegm nodules; San Leng (Rhizoma Sparganii Stoloniferi) and E Zhu (Rhizoma Curcumae Ezhu) for abdominal and gynaecological masses
Shi Jue Ming (Concha Haliotidis) *Haliotis spp.*	abalone shell; for extinguishing internal Wind and reducing excesssive Liver *yang* and improving vision; possible substitutes include Xia Ku Cao (Spica Prunellae Vulgaris), Jue Ming Zi (Semen Cassiae) and Bai Ji Li (Fructus Tribuli Terrestris)
Zhen Zhu Mu (Concha Margaritaferae) *Pteria martensii, P. margaritifera, Hydiopsis cumingii, Cristaria plicata*	mother of pearl shell; for calming the *shen*, sedating *yang* and improving vision; possible substitutes for calming *yang* and benefiting the eyes include Xia Ku Cao (Spica Prunellae Vulgaris), Jue Ming Zi (Semen Cassiae) and Bai Ji Li (Fructus Tribuli Terrestris)
Mu Li (Concha Ostreae) *Ostrea rivularis, O. gigas, O. talianwhanensis*	oyster shell; an astringent and sedative for *shen* disturbance and rising Liver *yang*, also softens hardness for various types of masses
Hai Ge Ke (Concha Cyclinae Sinensis) *Cyclinae sinensis*	clam shell; clears stubborn Phlegm Heat; can be substituted with Fu Hai Shi (Pumice)
Hai Piao Xiao (Os Sepiae seu Sepiellae) *Sepiella maindroni, S. esculenta*	cuttlefish bone; an astringent for various types of bleeding as well as vaginal discharge, chronic diarrhoea and premature ejaculation; possible substitutes include Bai Ji (Rhizoma Bletillae Striatae) for bleeding from the lungs or stomach, and Bai Zhi (Radix Angelicae Dahuricae) for vaginal discharge
Sang Piao Xiao (Ootheca Mantidis) *Paratenodera sinensis, Statillia maculata, Hierodula saussurei*	praying mantis egg case; an astringent for excessive or frequent urination patterns; possible substitutes for frequent urination, enuresis or nocturia include Sha Yuan Ji Li (Semen Astragali Complanati), Fu Pen Zi (Fructus Rubi Chingii), Tu Si Zi (Semen Cuscutae Chinensis), Yi Zhi Ren (Fructus Alpiniae Oxyphyllae) and Bu Gu Zhi (Fructus Psoraleae Corylifoliae)
Long Gu (Os Draconis)	fossilised bone; astringent, sedative and tranquiliser; a possible substitute for *shen* disturbance or *yang* rising is Zi Shi Ying (Fluoritum)
Long Chi (Dens Draconis)	fossilised teeth; sedative and tranquilliser; possible substitute is Zi Shi Ying (Fluoritum)
Ge Jie (Gecko) *Gecko gecko*	gecko; for Lung and Kidney *yang* deficiency wheezing; a possible substitute is walnut - Hu Tao Ren (Semen Juglandis Regiae)

Substance	Characteristics
Lu Rong (Cornu Cervi Parvum) *Cervus nippon, C. elaphus*	deer velvet and horn; essential for powerfully tonifying *jing*, especially for congenital *jing* deficiency patterns.
Shui Niu Jiao (Cornu Bubali) *Bubalus bubalis*	water buffalo horn; to reduce severe fever, used as a substitute for rhino horn
Dong Chong Xia Cao (Cordyceps Sinensis) *Cordyceps sinensis*	fungus growing in dead silkworm; a popular general tonic for the Lungs and Kidneys
Zi He Che (Placenta Hominis) *Homo sapien*	human placenta; general tonic for the treatment of consumptive diseases, especially of the Lungs
Xue Yu Tan (Crinus Carbonisatus) *Homo sapien*	charred human hair; haemostatic
Niu Huang (Calculus Bovis) *Bos taurus domesticus*	cow gallstone; clears Heat, opens the orifices and extinguishes Wind– an important substance for patterns associated with high fever and disturbances of consciousness; usually already prepared in pills
Wu Shao She (Zaocys Dhumnades) *Zaocys dhumnades*	black tailed snake; for Wind Damp patterns with pain and numbness, stubborn skin diseases and spasms; possible substitutes include Bai Ji Li (Fructus Tribuli Terrestris), Chi Shao (Radix Paeoniae Rubrae) and He Shou Wu (Radix Polygoni Multiflori) for chronic Wind rash; for spasms and *bi* syndrome Tian Ma (Rhizoma Gastrodiae Elatae)
Bai Hua She (Agkistrodon seu Bungarus) *Agkistrodon acutus Bungarus multicinctus*	multibanded krait; same indications as for Wu Shao She
She Tui (Exuviae Serpentis) *Elaphe taeniurus, E. carinata, Zaocys dhumnades*	snake skin; dispels external Wind for itchy skin lesions and extinguishes internal Wind for spasms and convulsions; possible substitutes as for Wu Shao She
Di Bie Chong (Eupolyphaga seu Opisthoplatia) *Eupolyphaga sinensis Opisthoplatia orientalis Steleophaga plancyi*	field cockroach; powerful Blood stagnation remover for severe Blood stasis; closest vegetable substitutes probably San Leng (Rhizoma Sparganii Stoloniferi) and E Zhu (Rhizoma Curcumae Ezhu)
Shui Zhi (Hirudo seu Whitmania) *Hirido nipponica Whitmania pigra*	leech; powerful Blood stagnation remover for severe Blood stasis; closest vegetable substitutes probably San Leng (Rhizoma Sparganii Stoloniferi) and E Zhu (Rhizoma Curcumae Ezhu)

Index

Numbers in bold refer to the original and unmodified version of a formula or main chapter heading.

Conditions described in Volume 2 and 3 may have limited entries in this index and then only subsidiary to the primary diseases of this volume

A

abdomen *see* Vol.2 for full discussion
   distension
      food stagnation and insomnia 841
      in Liver *qi* stagnation 567-568
      in Spleen *qi* def. 870
      in Spleen *yang* def. 56
      in tai *yin* syndrome 56
   fullness and pain 376
   lower, coldness and pain 619
   masses 428
   pain 34, 42, 716, 737, 740, 841
      better with warmth and pressure 56
abscess
   cerebral 723, 725
   peritonsillar 291
   retropharyngeal 291
absences (epileptic) 680, 681, 688, 716
absent-mindedness *see* Forgetfulness
Achyranthes and Persica Combination 105, **522**, **552**, **576**, 698, 781, **821**, 846, 890 *see also Xue Fu Zhu Yu Tang*
Achyranthes and Rehmannia Formula **277**, 347, 557 *see also Zuo Gui Wan*
acid reflux 573, 815, 841, 843, 864
Aconite and Halloysium Pills 775 *see also Wu Tao Chi Shi Zhi Wan*
Aconite, Ginseng and Ginger Formula **56**, 434, 476, 527, 555, 742, 819, **873** *see also Fu Zi Li Zhong Wan*

Acute Exterior Disorders 2
   Damp Heat 14
   Summer Heat and Dampness 12
   Wind Cold 6
   Wind Damp 7
   Wind Dryness 16
   Wind Heat 10
   with Blood deficiency 25
   with *qi* deficiency 20
   with stiff neck 6, 7
   with viral hepatitis 599
   with wheezing 7
   with sore throat 10, 18
   with myalgia 6, 18, 23
   with headache 6, 7, 8, 10, 25
   with blocked nose 6, 10, 18, 20
   with *yang* deficiency 23
   with *yin* deficiency 27
Adenophora and Ophiopogon Combination 114, **925** *see also Sha Shen Mai Men Dong Tang*
Agastache and Pig Bile Pills 243, 245 *see also Huo Dan Wan*
Agastache Formula **13** *see also Huo Xiang Zheng Qi Tang*
AIDS related illness 205
albuminuria 389, 401, 405
alcohol toxicity 517
alcoholism 173, 176
Alzheimer's disease 888, 891
amenorrhoea 316
amnesia 885
amyloidosis 387, 403, 405, 407, 410
An Gong Niu Huang Wan 39, 171, 198, 303, 605, 739, **914**
An Shen Ding Zhi Wan
   epilepsy **691**
   insomnia 856
anaemia 494, 541, 556, 727, 802, 805, 809, 812, 814, 817, 820, 823, 828, 851, 882, 886, 888, 891, 900
   haemolytic 608, **610**
Anemarrhena and Gypsum Combination **32**, 173, 709 *see also Bai Hu Tang*
Anemarrhena, Phellodendron and Rehmannia Formula **177**, 375, 384, 406, **452**, 473, 501, 546 *see also Zhi*

Bai Ba Wei Wan
aneurism
  burst 646
angina pectoris 768, 769, 773, 776, 779, 820, 823
Antelope Horn and Uncaria Decoction 661, 709 *see also Ling Jiao Gou Teng Tang*
Antelope Horn Decoction 543, **922** *see also Ling Yang Jiao Tang*
antibiotics
  nature of 131
Anxiety 894
  chronic, lifetime 909
  following febrile illness 902, 911
  Heart and Kidney *yin* def. 901
  Heart Blood and Spleen *qi* def. 904
  Heart *qi* and *yin* def. 907
  Heart *qi* def. 899
  Phlegm Heat 911
  post traumatic 902
  with digestive symptoms 904, 911
  with irregular pulse 907
anxiety neurosis 60, 141, 809, 814, 817, 840, 854, 886, 900, 903, 912
aortic incompetence 797
appendicitis
  acute 35
appetite, poor *see* Vol.2 for full discussion
  Damp Heat in Liver/Gall Bladder 571
  in *shao yang* syndrome 54
  in *tai yin* syndrome 56
  Liver *qi* stagnation 566
  Spleen and Kidney *yang* def. 818
Apricot Kernel and Perilla Leaf Powder 82 *see also Xing Su San*
apthous ulcers *see* ulcers
Aquillaria Powder 376, 426, **916** *see also Chen Xiang San*
Arouse *yang*, Please the Heart Special Pill 495 *see also Qi Yang Yu Xin Dan*
Arrest Seizures Pill **685**, 688 *see also Ding Xian Wan*
arteriosclerosis
  cerebral 828
arthritis 324, 334, 652 *see also Bi* Syndrome (Vol.3)

ascariasis 603
Ascites 730
  Blood stagnation 740
  Cold Damp 735
  Damp Heat 737
  Liver and Kidney *yin* def. 744
  qi and Damp stagnation 733
  Spleen and Kidney *yang* def. 742
Ass-Hide Gelatin and Mugwort Decoction **178**, 181, 205 *see also Jiao Ai Tang*
Aster Decoction 320 *see also Zi Wan Tang*
asthma 118, 155 *see also* wheezing/cough
  acute 7, 48, 74, 122, 123, 124, 126, 128
  cardiac 153
  chronic, in kids and the elderly 106, 143
  Kidney and Spleen def. 103
  Kidney *yang* def. 103, 150
  Liver *qi* stagnation 138
  Lung and Kidney *yin* def. 147
  Lung and Spleen def. 144
  Lung *qi* and *yin* def. 142
  paediatric **157**
  Phlegm Damp 131, 132, 133
  qi stagnation with Heat 139, 140
  Wind Cold 7, 48, 51, 122, 124
    with internal Heat 126
Astragalus Combination **609** *see also Huang Qi Jian Zhong Tang*
ataxia 655
atherosclerosis 646
Atractylodes and Hoelen Combination 125, 551, **818** *see also Ling Gui Zhu Gan Tang*
Atractylodes Combination **422** *see also Yue Bi Jia Zhu Tang*
Augmented Two Marvel Powder **333** *see also Jia Wei Er Miao San*
aura
  in epilepsy 685

B

Ba Zhen Tang 555, 639, 726
  dizziness 555
  spasms and convulsions 726
  tremors 639

Ba Zheng San **359**, 418, **444**
  painful urination **359**
  urinary difficulty or retention 418
  urinary frequency or incontinence **444**
bad breath 289, 841
Bai He Gu Jin Tang **96**, **147**, 201, 226, 312
  cough **96**
  haemoptysis 201
  loss of voice, hoarseness 226
  wheezing **147**
  tuberculosis 312
Bai Hu Tang **32**, 173, **709**
  convulsions **709**
  epistaxis 173
  Heat in *yang ming* channels **32**
Bai Tou Weng Tang
  spasms, from Hot dysenteric disorder **711**
Baked Licorice Combination **789**, **811**, **907** *see also Zhi Gan Cao Tang*
Bamboo and Hoelen Combination 518, 549, 766, 815, 843 *see also Wen Dan Tang*
Ban Xia Bai Zhu Tian Ma Tang
  dizziness **549**
  tinnitus 520
Ban Xia Hou Po Tang
  wheezing **132**
Bao He Wan 137, 841, **914**
  insomnia 841
  wheezing 137
Bao Ying Dan
  as preventitive for glue ear 520
  paediatric asthma 161
Bao Yuan Tang 785, **914**
  chest pain 785
Bao Zhen Tang 314, **914**
  tuberculosis 314
Behçet's syndrome 364, 467, 469
Becloforte, effect of according to TCM 155
Becotide, effect of according to TCM 155
Bei Xie Fen Qing Yin 386, **915**
  cloudy painful urination syndrome 386
belching 566, 586, 770, 815, 841, 843
Bell's palsy 652, 654, 657, 659

acupuncture treatment 654
benign prostatic hypertrophy (BPH) 435
bi nü **164**
bi qiu **262**
Bi Yun San
  rhinitis **270**
Bie Jia Jian Wan 612, **915**
  jaundice 612
Bie Jia Wan
  hypochondriac pain **577**
Bing Lian San **241**, 245, 248
Bing Peng San **287**
bipolar mood disorder 837, 840
bladder *see also urinary disorders*
  prolapse 395, 430, 455
    acupuncture treatment of 455
  cancer 383, 385, 472, 474
  bleeding *see also epistaxis, haemoptysis, haematuria*
    with ascites 738
    with febrile rashes (Hot Blood) 41
blindness
  monocular, in Wind Stroke 655
blood
  increased viscosity of 646, 755
Blood and Phlegm stagnation
  forgetfulness 889
Blood Deficiency
  with external Wind 25
Blood and *qi* def. *see also qi* and Blood def.
Blood and *yin* def. *see also yin* and Blood def.
Blood stagnation
  ascites 740
  Blood painful urination syndrome 382
  chest pain 781
  cough 105
  difficult urination 428
  dizziness 552
  epilepsy 698
  haematuria 470
  hypochondriac pain 576
  insomnia 846
  jaundice 611
  lower back pain 339
  palpitations 821
  sinusitis, nasal congestion 258
  spasms and convulsions 724

stone painful urination syndrome 367
Blue Cloud Powder 270 *see also Bi Yun San*
blurring vision *see* vision, blurring of
Borneol and Borax Powder 287 *see also Bing Peng San*
Borneol and Coptis Powder 241 *see also Bing Lian San*
botulism 704, 719
Brain Tonic Pills 256 *see also Bu Nao Wan*
Break Into a Smile Powder 771, **782** *see also Shi Xiao San*
breast tenderness 138, 223, 376, 425, 446, 513, 540, 566, 834
Broken Liver Pills 643 *see also Cui Gan Wan*
bronchial asthma *see asthma*
bronchiectasis 89, 92, 99, 110, 113, 134, 137, 196, 203, 227
bronchitis
  acute 11, 19, 51, 53, 79, 86, 92, 95, 110, 113, 125, 127, 137, 169, 188, 190, 196
  asthmatic 110, 116, 125
  chronic 63, 89, 92, 95, 99, 102, 104, 134, 137, 146, 190, 196, 203, 227, 820
  convalescent stage of 116
bruising, easy 180, 475, 554, 611, 740, 810, 849, 881, 904
Bu Fei E Jiao Tang
  cough **98**
Bu Fei Tang
  cough **100**
Bu Gu Zhi Wan
  hearing loss **524**
  tinnitus **524**
bu mei **826**
Bu Nao Wan
  sinusitis, nasal congestion **256**
Bu Tian Da Zao Wan
  tuberculosis **316**
Bu Yang Huan Wu Tang
  Wind stroke **667**
Bu Zhong Yi Qi Tang
  cloudy urine **404**
  dizziness **555**
  exhaustion painful urination syndrome **394**

haematuria 475
hearing loss 526
loss of voice, hoarseness 228
lower back pain 343
shan *qi* 625
sinusitis, nasal congestion 252
somnolence 871
tinnitus 526
urinary difficulty or retention 431
urinary frequency or incontinence 451, 454
wheezing 144
Bupleurum and Cyperus Formula 95, 425, 426, **566**, 587, 733, **770** *see also Chai Hu Shu Gan San*
Bupleurum and Dang Gui Formula 95, **139**, 446, 483, 513, 540, 568, 574, 587, 640, 771, 783, 834 *see also Xiao Yao San*
Bupleurum and Dragon Bone Combination 447, 484, 694, **816** *see also Chai Hu Jia Long Gu Mu Li Tang*
Bupleurum and Hoelen Combination 359, **916** *see also Chai Ling Tang*
Bupleurum and Paeonia Formula **140**, 242, 771, 835 *see also Dan Zhi Xiao Yao San*
Bupleurum and Zhi Shi Formula 95 *see also Si Ni San*
Bupleurum Liver Clearing Decoction 224, **916** *see also Chai Hu Qing Gan Tang*

C

Calm the Palace Pill with Cattle Gallstone 39, 41, 171, 198, 303, 605, 661, 707, 739, **914** *see also An Gong Niu Huang Wan*
Calm the *shen*, Settle the Emotions Pill **691**, 856 *see also An Shen Ding Zhi Wan*
cancer
  abdominal 730
  auditory 522
  bladder 381, 383, 385, 472, 474
  cerebral 522, 723, 725, 869
  liver 578, 613, 730, 741, 745
  lung 106, 199, 203, 205, 227

INDEX 957

prostate 383, 385, 472, 474
testicular 616, 619, 630
candida albicans 865, 867, 871
Cang Er Zi San 240, 268, **915**
  rhinitis 268
  sinusitis, nasal congestion 240
Canopy Powder **74** *see also Hua Gai San*
Capillaris and Hoelen Five Formula 597,
  930 *see also Yin Chen Wu Ling San*
Capillaris, Atractylodes and Aconite
  Combination 607, **930** *see also Yin
  Chen Zhu Fu Tang*
Capillaris Combination 572, 594, 604,
  930 *see also Yin Chen Hao Tang*
caput medusae 740, 744
cardiac arrhythmia 792, 908
Cephalanoplos Decoction 380, 462, 466,
  929 *see also Xiao Ji Yin Zi*
cerebral
  arteriosclerosis 828
  embolism 646
  haemorrhage 659
  thrombosis 659
  tumours 522, 723, 725, 869
cerebral artery
  atherosclerotic occlusion of 646
cerebro-vascular accident 646, 657, 659,
  666
Chai Hu Jia Long Gu Mu Li Tang 447, 484,
  694, **816**
  eneuresis in children 447
  epilepsy 694
  impotence 484
  palpitations **816**
Chai Hu Qing Gan Tang 224, **916**
  loss of voice, hoarseness 224
Chai Hu Shu Gan San 95, 425, 426, **566**,
  587, 733, **770**
  ascites 733
  chest pain **770**
  gallstones 587
  hypochondriac pain **566**
  urinary difficulty or retention 425, 426
Chai Ling Tang 359, **916**
  painful urination 359
channel stroke 647, 652

chan zheng 634
Chen Xiang San 376, 426, **916**
  qi painful urination syndrome 376
  urinary difficulty or retention 426
Cheng Shi Bei Xie Fen Qing Yin
  cloudy urination **402**
  involuntary seminal emission 498
Cheng Ying-mao 590
Chest Pain 748
  Blood stagnation 781
    from trauma 783
  Cold congealing Heart Blood 774
  differential diagnosis of 749, 753
  emergency management of 757
  Heart and Kidney *yin* def. 787
    following febrile disease 788
    with *qi* def. 789
    with irregular pulse 789
    with Liver *yin* def. 790
    prominent Kidney def. 790
    and Blood def. 790
  Heart *qi* def. 785
  Heart *yang* def. 777
    with Kidney *yang* def. 778
  Heat knotting the chest 761
  Phlegm Fluids 764
  Phlegm Heat 765
  psychogenic 763, 773
  qi stagnation 770
    with digestive symptoms 771
    with Heat 771
    with Heat and constipation 771
  Turbid Phlegm 764
  Wind Phlegm 765
Children's Return of Spring Special Pill
  708 *see also Xiao Er Hui Chun Dan*
cholecystitis
  acute 35, 572, 586, 596
  chronic 55, 570, 575, 588
cholelithiasis 572, 581, 596, 603 *see also*
  gallstones
chronic fatigue syndrome 22, 294, 295,
  298, 494, 812, 851, 863, 865, 867,
  871, 874
chronic obstructive airways disease 106,
  143, 149

Chuan Xiong Cha Tiao San 7
chyluria 387, 401, 403, 405, 415
cigarette smoke
   aversion to 594, 597, 599
Cinnabar Pill to Calm the Spirit 767, **807**, **840**, 854, 902 *see also Zhu Sha An Shen Wan*
Cinnamon and Dragon Bone Combination **814**, 853, 885, 902, 910 *see also Gui Zhi Jia Long Gu Mu Li Tang*
Cinnamon Combination 49 *see also Gui Zhi Tang*
Cinnamon, Licorice, Dragon Bone and Oyster Shell Decoction 803, **920** *see also Gui Zhi Gan Cao Long Gu Mu Li Tang*
Cinnamon, Magnolia and Apricot Seed Combination **123** *see also Gui Zhi Jia Hou Po Xing Ren Tang*
cirrhosis 575, 578, 579, 598, 613, 734, 739, 741, 743
   biliary 608, 610
Citrus and Crategus Formula 137, 841, **914** *see also Bao He Wan*
Citrus and Pinellia Combination 87, 132, 136, 519, **919** *see also Er Chen Wan*
Clear Epidemics and Overcome Toxin Decoction **710** *see also Qing Wen Bai Du Yin*
Clear Fire, Wash Away Phlegm Decoction **844** *see also Qing Huo Di Tan Tang*
Clear Metal, Transform Phlegm Decoction 90, 93, **924** *see also Qing Jin Hua Tan Tang*
Clear the Gall Bladder and Drain Fire Decoction 585, 601, **923** *see also Qing Dan Xie Huo Tang*
Clear the *Hun* Powder 553, **923** *see also Qing Hun San*
Clear the Lungs Decoction 423 *see also Qing Fei Yin*
Clear the Throat and Calm the Lungs Decoction 221, 230, **924** *see also Qing Yan Ning Fei Tang*
Clear the Throat, Benefit the Diaphragm Decoction see also 215, 302

Clear the *Ying* Decoction 38, 39, 171, 198, 303, **711** *see also Qing Ying Tang*
closed syndrome
   yang closed syndrome 660
   yin closed syndrome 662
Cloudy Urine 400
   Damp Heat 402
   Kidney *yang* def. 408
      with Heart involvement and less cold 409
   Kidney *yin* def. 406
      with severe Heat 407
   Spleen *qi* def. 404
Cnidium and Thea Formula 8 *see also Chuan Xiong Cha Tiao San*
coffee
   effect of 797
cold
   aversion to 238, 316, 433, 742, 774, 803
   extremities 430, 433, 558, 619, 716, 774, 777, 803, 873
   extremities and abdomen 56
   intolerance 558, 607
Cold congealing Heart blood circulation 774
Cold Damp
   ascites 735
   external Wind Cold Damp
      spasms in 720
   jaundice 607
   lower back pain 330
   shan qi 620
colitis
   chronic 57, 63
coma 660, 662, 663, 665
common cold 8, 11, 19, 51, 76, 83, 125, 169, 188, 192, 194, 213, 512
   during pregnancy 26
   in frail or elderly patients 24, 28
concentration, poor
   Blood stagnation 868
   Blood and Phlegm stagnation 889
   Heart and Spleen def. 810, 849, 881, 899, 904
   Heart *yin* def. 806
   Phlegm Damp 548, 864, 866

INDEX 959

consciousness, disturbances of
    delirium 38, 39, 41, 42, 43, 170, 171, 303, 605, 710, 711, 739
    loss of 39, 303, 660, 662, 665, 685, 688
    concussion 725, 869, 891 *see also* post concussion syndrome
Conduct the *Qi* Decoction 627, **918** *see also Dao Qi Tang*
Cong Bai Qi Wei Yin 25, **916**
    acute exterior disorder 25
congestive cardiac failure 61, 104, 125, 153, 730, 776, 779, 805, 820
conjunctivitis 290
constipation *see* Vol.2 for full discussion
    food stagnation 137
    Heat and Phlegm in *yang ming* 33, 34
    Heat in *yang ming* with Blood stasis 42
    in Damp Heat 737
    internal Heat with external Wind Cold 18, 52, 126
    Lung Fire 85
    Liver Heat 771-772
    Phlegm Heat 658
    qi stagnation with Heat 771
    qi and *yin* deficiency 907
    Stomach Heat 172, 289
convalescence following a febrile disorder 114, 792, 809, 817, 854, 886
Convulsions/Spasms 704
    acute febrile 707
    in children 708
    from *yang ming* syndrome 709
    from epidemic Toxic Heat 710
    from focal Toxic Heat 710
    from dysenteric disorder 711
    from Heat in the Blood 711
    from Liver Heat stirring Wind 709
    Blood stagnation 724
    post acute
        chronic childhood 716
        yin and Blood deficient 713
    Phlegm obstruction 722
    puerperal 712
    Wind Toxin tetany 718
Cool Dryness
    cough 80

Cool the Diaphram Powder **85** *see also Liang Ge San*
Coptis and Ass-Hide Gelatin Decoction **788**, 808, **839**, 853, 885, 902 *see also Huang Lian E Jiao Tang*
Coptis and Magnolia Bark Decoction **14**, 286 *see also Lian Po Yin*
Coptis and Scute Combination 170, 361, 463, 604, 838, **921** *see also Huang Lian Jie Du Tang*
Coptis Decoction to Warm the Gall Bladder 420, 767 *see also Huang Lian Wen Dan Tang*
cor pulmonale 119, 153, 768, 784
coronary artery disease 769, 776, 779, 784, 786, 792, 805, 820, 823
corticosteroids
    effects of, in TCM 155
costochondritis 579, 763
Cough 68
    Blood stagnation 105
    Heat in the Lungs 30, 84
    Kidney and Spleen *yang* def. 103
    Liver Fire invading the Lungs 93
    Lung and Heart *yin* def. 97
    Lung and Kidney *yin* def. 97
    Lung Fire 85
    Lung Heat 84
    Lung *qi* def. 100
    Lung *yin* def. 96
        following febrile illness 98
        persistant post viral 78
    Phlegm and Toxic Heat 91
    Phlegm Damp 87
        with Kidney def. 88-89
        with Spleen deficiency 88
    Phlegm Heat 90
    Whooping *see Whooping cough*
    Wind Cold 74
    Wind Dryness 80
    Wind Heat 77
    with thin watery mucus 6, 48, 50, 74, 87, 88, 100, 103
    with thick yellow or green mucus 10, 30, 52, 77, 90, 109, 111, 126, 135
    with blood streaked mucus 80, 84, 90, 93, 96, 105, 111 *see also haemoptysis*

and Tuberculosis
Coughing of Blood Formula **198** *see also Ke Xur Fang*
cracked lips 16
cramps 713, 722, 724, 726 *see also spasms*
Cui Gan Wan
  tremors **643**
cyanosis 774
cyst
  cerebral 723, 725
cysticercosis 723, 725
cystitis 362, 364, 366, 387, 403, 420, 445, 464
  interstitial 381, 437, 453

D

Da Bu Yin Wan 348, **407**, 636
  lower back pain 348
  cloudy urine **407**
  tremors 636
Da Bu Yuan Jian 696, **917**
  epilepsy 696
Da Chai Hu Tang **585**
Da Cheng Qi Tang **34**
Da Ding Feng Zhu
  convulsions **714**
  tremors **637**
Da Fen Qing Yin
  shan qi **621**
Da Huang Zhe Chong Wan 577, **612**
  jaundice **612**
  palpable hypochondriac masses 577
Da Qin Jiao Tang
  Wind stroke **652**
Da Qing Long Tang 19, **52**, 213
  acute exterior disorder 19, **52**
  loss of voice 213
Dai Di Dang Wan 428, **917**
  urinary difficulty or retention 428
Dai Ge San 93, 197, **917**
  cough 93
  haemoptysis 197
Damp Heat
  ascites 737
  Blood painful urination syndrome 379
  cloudy painful urination syndrome 386
  cloudy urination 402
  difficult urination 418
  frequent urination 444
  gallstones 584
  haematuria 462
  hypochondriac pain 571
  impotence 485
  jaundice
    Damp greater than Heat 597
    Heat greater than Damp 594
    with exterior symptoms 599
  lower back pain 333
  painful urination syndrome 358
  shan qi 621
  stone painful urination syndrome 367
Damp Heat in the Liver and Gall Bladder
  hypochondriac pain 571
Damp Heat in *yang ming* 35
Dampness wrapping the Spleen
  somnolence 864
Dan Dao Qu Hui Tang
  jaundice **602**
  roundworms in the bile duct 572
Dan Shen Yin
  chest pain 771, **783**, 790
Dan Xi Bi Yuan Fang 246, **917**
  sinusitis, nasal congestion 246
Dan Xi's Nasal Congestion Formula see also *Dan Xi Bi Yuan Fang* 246, **917**
Dan Zhi Xiao Yao San **140**, 242, 771, 835
  chest pain 771
  insomnia 835
  sinusitis, nasal congestion 242
  wheezing **140**
Dang Gui and Peonia Formula 258, **918** *see also Dang Gui Shao Yao San*
Dang Gui and Six Yellow Pills 318, **917** *see also Dang Gui Liu Huang Wan*
Dang Gui Blood Tonic Decoction 136, 289, **537** *see also Dang Gui Bu Xue Tang*
Dang Gui Bu Xue Tang 145, 303, **555**
  dizziness, vertigo **555**
  throat abscess 303
  wheezing 145
Dang Gui Decoction for Frigid Extremities **774** *see also Dang Gui Si Ni Tang*

Dang Gui Four Combination 175, 294, **927** *see also Si Wu Tang*
Dang Gui, Gentiana Longdancao and Aloe Pill 543, **771** *see also Dang Gui Long Hui Wan*
Dang Gui Liu Huang Wan
  tuberculosis 318, **917**
Dang Gui Long Hui Wan
  chest pain **771**
  dizziness/vertigo 543
Dang Gui Shao Yao San
  sinusitis, nasal congestion 258, **918**
Dang Gui Si Ni Tang
  chest pain **774**
Dao Chi San 363, 396, 466, **838**
  haematuria 466
  insomnia **838**
  painful urination syndrome 363, 396
Dao Qi Tang 627, **918**
  shan qi 627
Dao Tan Tang 642, **918**
  tremors 642
deafness **506** *see also Tinnitus/Deafness*
Decoction for Expelling Roundworms from the Bile Duct 572, **602** *see also Dan Dao Qu Hui Tang*
Deer Horn Pills to Tonify and Astringe 408 *see also Lu Rong Bu Se Wan*
delirium *see also* consciousness, disturbances of
dengue fever 721
depression
  following shock or trauma 814
  in Blood stagnation 552, 781, 821, 846, 868
  in Heart and Gall Bladder *qi* def. 856
  in Heart Blood and Spleen *qi* def. 883
  in Liver and Kidney *yin* def. 636
  in Liver *qi* stagnation 540, 566, 567, 623, 834
  in *qi* and Blood deficiency 554
  post natal 910
Descurainia and Jujube Decoction to Drain the Lung 125 *see also Ting Li Da Zao Xie Fei Tang*
Di Huang Yin Zi
  dysphasia **673**

Di Tan Tang 663, 693, **767**, 866
  chest pain **767**
  epilepsy 693
  somnolence 866
  Wind stroke 663
dian xian 680
Dian Xian San
  epilepsy **686**
Dianthus Formula 359, 418, **444** *see also Ba Zheng San*
diarrhoea *see* Vol.2 for full discussion, *see also* loose stools
  alternating with constipation 370, 376, 386, 425, 444, 446, 462, 483, 485, 513, 540, 566, 834
  cockcrow 316, 317
  Cold Damp 735
  collapse of *yang* 61
  Damp Heat 14, 35, 711
  in *jue yin* syndrome 62
  Spleen Damp 344
  Spleen *qi* def. 253
  Spleen *yang* def. 56
  Summer Heat 12
  with faecal impaction 34
  with gallstones 585
difficult urination *see* urinary difficulty
Ding Chuan Tang
  wheezing **126**, 160
Ding Xian Wan
  epilepsy **685**, 688
Ding Zhi Wan 813, 909, **918**
  anxiety 909
  palpitations 813
Discharge Pus Powder **303** *see also Tou Nong San*
Dispel Wind, Clear Heat Decoction 214, 285 *see also Shu Feng Qing Re Tang*
Dizziness/Vertigo 534
  Blood stagnation 552
    postpartum 553
  Kidney *yang* def. 558
  Kidney *yin* def. 557
  Liver and Kidney *yin* def. 545
  Liver Fire 542
  Liver *qi* stagnation 540
  Liver *yang* rising 542

Phlegm Damp 548
  with Spleen deficiency 550
  with Spleen *yang* deficiency and thin Fluids 551
  with Heat 549
  postural 529
  qi and Blood def. 554
  post haemorrhage 555
double vision 724
Drain the Yellow Powder 364 *see also Xie Huang San*
Drive Out Blood Stasis Below the Diaphragm Decoction 577, 611 *see also Ge Xia Zhu Yu Tang*
Drive Out Blood Stasis in the Lower Abdomen Decoction 382, 470 *see also Shao Fu Zhu Yu Tang*
drug abuse 883, 886
drug withdrawal 635, 895
drum like abdominal distension, *see* ascites
Du Huo and Vaecium Combination 330, 918 *see also Du Huo Ji Sheng Tang*
Du Huo Ji Sheng Tang 330, **918**
  lower back pain 330
duo mei **862**
dysentery
  amoebic 36, 711
  bacillary 36, 711
  chronic 63
dysmenorrhoea 428
dysphasia 652, 655, 658, 672

E

ears
  discharge from 510, 515, 518, 521
  glue 520, 528
  grommets in 526
  withered 696
ecchymosis 604
echinococcosis 723, 725
eclampsia 544, 711
ectopic pregnancy 43
eczema
  atopic 268
Eleven Ingredient Decoction to Warm the Gall Bladder **911** *see also Shi Yi Wei Wen Dan Tang*

Eliminate Blood Stasis Decoction 744, **929** *see also Xiao Yu Tang*
emphysema 89, 102, 106, 134, 143, 146
encephalitis 11, 33, 39, 40, 42, 171, 173, 188, 338, 710, 711, 715, 721
endometriosis 429
endometritis 43
enteritis 63
enuresis, nocturnal 447, 448, 450, 451
Ephedra, Apricot Seed, Gypsum and Licorice Combination *see* Ma Huang, Apricot Seed, Gypsum and Licorice Combination
Ephedra, Asarum and Prepared Aconite Decoction *see* Ma Huang and Asarum Combination
epididymal cyst 621
epididymo-orchitis 630
epiglottitis 31, 288, 291
Epilepsy 680
  Blood stagnation 698
  chronic 691, 694, 695, 697
  grand mal 681, 685
  Liver and Kidney *yin* deficiency 696
  Liver Fire with Phlegm Heat 693
  petit mal 681, 688
  Spleen deficiency with Phlegm 690
  yang seizure 685
  yin seizures 688
Epilepsy Powder **686** *see also Dian Xian San*
Epistaxis 164
  first aid 166
  Liver and Kidney *yin* def. 177
    with *yang* rising 178
    with Blood deficiency 178
  Liver Fire 174
    premenstrual or menstrual 175
  Lung Heat 168
  Spleen *qi* def. 180
    Spleen and Kidney *yang* def. 181
  Stomach Heat 172
  Toxic Heat 170
  Wind Heat 168
Er Chen Tang 87, 132, 136, 519, **919**
  cough 87
  tinnitus/deafness 519
  wheezing 132, 136

INDEX 963

Er Long Zuo Ci Wan
  deafness 523
  tinnitus 523
Er Miao San 485, **919**
  impotence 485
er long **506**
er ming **506**
erection dysfunction *see* impotence
Eriobotrya and Ophiopogon Combination 81, **129**, 189, 219 *see Qing Zao Jiu Fei Tang*
erysipelas 710
erythema
  faint 38
Escape Restraint Pill 95, **567** *see also Yue Ju Wan*
Eucommia and Rehmannia Formula 181, 256, **347**, 449, 503, **559**, 804, 819, 874 *see also You Gui Wan*
eustachian tube
  congestion of 526
Evodia Combination **63**, 434 *see also Wu Zhu Yu Tang*
Expel Urinary Stones #1 Decoction 372 *see also Niao Lu Pai Shi Tang #1*
Expel Urinary Stones #2 Decoction 370 *see also Niao Lu Pai Shi Tang #2*
Expel Urinary Stones #3 Decoction 373 *see also Niao Lu Pai Shi Tang #3*
Expel Wind and Guide Out the Phlegm Decoction 722 *see also Qu Feng Dao Tan Tang*
exernal pathogenic disorders *see* acute exterior disorders
eyes *see also* vision
  dark rings under 150, 470, 521, 576, 803, 846, 868
  deviation of 667, 718
  dry and sore 573, 696, 858
  itchy, irritated 265
  pressure behind 545, 655
  red and sore 93, 174, 197, 242, 468, 515, 542
  spots before 529

F

facet joint syndrome 340
facial
  muscle spasm 675, 718
  oedema 150, 316, 422, 818
  paralysis 652, 654, 655, 656, 658, 675
  rictus 718
Fading Star Order the Qi Decoction **658** *see also Xing Wu Cheng Qi Tang*
faecal impaction
  with watery diarrhoea 34
Fang Feng Tong Sheng Tang
  tinnitus/deafness **511**
Fang Ji Huang Qi Tang
  difficult urination/retention 423
  lower back pain **344**
Fantastically Effective Pill to Invigorate the Collaterals 339, **921** *see also Huo Luo Xiao Ling Dan*
fats and oils, aversion to 584, 586, 601
febrile convulsions
  acute 707
  post acute 716
febrile disease
  analysis of 2, 30, 46
fei lao **306**
fei yong (Lung abscess) 108
fever *see* Vol.3 for full discussion
  afternoon 13, 35, 310, 314, 358, 402, 418, 444, 462, 473, 501, 557
  bone steaming 201, 312, 407, 473
  in acute external disease 6, 10, 12, 14, 16, 18, 20, 25, 27
  lingering, with drenching nightsweats 114
  mild, lingering or relapsing 37
  post partum 55
  puerperal 26, 43
  tidal 34, 310, 312, 314
  unrelieved with sweating 35
  with acute ear infection 510
  with acute lower abdominal pain and constipation 42
  with acute lower back pain 333, 335, 336, 337

fever and chills, alternating 54, 358, 379, 444, 462, 571, 585, 594, 601
fever of unknown origin 721, 809, 854, 886
filariasis 616, 622
finger clubbing 147
Five Ingredient Decoction to Eliminate Toxin 301, 361, 604, **710** *see also Wu Wei Xiao Du Yin*
Five Milled Herb Decoction 138 *see also Wu Mo Yin Zi*
Five Seed Ancestral *Qi* Amplifying Pill 488, **928** *see also Wu Zi Yan Zong Wan*
flaccid collapse syndrome 665
fluid retention *see* oedema
food allergies 229, 863, 865, 871
food poisoning 14
Forgetfulness 878
    Blood and Phlegm stagnation 889
    following head injury 890
    Heart and Kidney *yin* def. 884
    following febrile disease or with severe Heat 885
    predominant Kidney def. 885
    Heart Blood and Spleen *qi* def. 881
    Kidney *jing* def. 887
Four Major Herbs Combination 294, 570, **926** *see also Si Jun Zi Tang*
Frigid Extremities Decoction **61** *see also Si Ni Tang*
Frigid Extremities Decoction plus Ginseng 152, **926** *see also Si Ni Jia Ren Shen Tang*
Frigid Extremities Powder 95, **926** *see also Si Ni San*
Fu Yuan Huo Xue Tang
    hypochondriac pain **578**
    chest pain 783
Fu Zi Li Zhong Wan **56**, 434, 476, 527, 555, 742, 819, **873**
    ascites 742
    somnolence **873**
    tai yin syndrome **56**
    urinary retention with vomiting 434
    haematuria 476
    tinnitus/deafness 527
    dizziness 555

palpitations 819

G

gallstones 572, 581, 584, 603
    Damp Heat 584
    Liver *qi* stagnation 586
Gan Jiang Ling Zhu Tang
    lower back pain 330, **919**
Gan Lu Xiao Du Dan 599, **919**
    jaundice 599
Gan Lu Yin
    sore throat **293**
Gan Mai Da Zao Tang
    wheezing **139**
gan mao 2
Gardenia and Hoelen Formula 360, **928** *see also Wu Lin San*
Gardenia and Soybean Combination **37** *see also Zhi Zi Dou Chi Tang*
gastric flu 8, 14
gastric ulcer disease 575
gastritis 34, 173, 570
    chronic 57, 229, 845
Gastrodia and Gambir Formula 516, 542, 639, 642, **670** *see also Tian Ma Gou Teng Yin*
gastroenteritis
    acute 14, 36, 50, 64
    chronic 63
Ge Gen Huang Qin Huang Lian Tang
    wen bing **36**
Ge Gen Tang
    acute exterior disorders **7**
    sapasm/convulsions 720
Ge Jie San
    wheezing 148
Ge Xia Zhu Yu Tang
    hypochondriac pain **577**
    jaundice 611
Gecko Powder 148 *see also Ge Jie san*
Generate the Pulse Powder **101**, 133, 255, 789, 790, 807 *see also Sheng Mai San*
genitals
    eczema 365, 468, 622
    herpes 366, 468
    ulceration 365, 468
    swelling and pain *see* testicle

Gentiana Combination 139, 174, 244, **365**, 447, 468, 486, **500**, 515, 543, 569, 571, 595, **621**, 693, 762, 835 *see also Long Dan Xie Gan Tang*
Gentiana Qinjiao and Soft-shelled Turtle Powder 319, **923** *see also Qin Jiao Bie Jia San*
Ginseng and Aconite Pills for a New Lease on Life 23, **925** *see also Shen Fu Zai Zao Wan*
Ginseng and Astragalus Combination 144, 228, 252, 343, **394**, 404, 431, 451, 454, 471, 475, 526, 555, 625, 627 *see also Bu Zhong Yi Qi Tang*
Ginseng and Atractylodes Formula 253, 273, 296, **925** *see also Shen Ling Bai Zhu San*
Ginseng and Dang Gui Eight Combination 555, 639, 726 *see also Ba Zhen San*
Ginseng and Dang Gui Ten Combination 145, 304, **529**, 555, 871, 905 *see also Shi Quan Da Bu Tang*
Ginseng and Gecko Powder **151** *see also Ren Shen Ge Jie San*
Ginseng and Ginger Formula 716, 777, **922** *see also Li Zhong Wan*
Ginseng and Longan Combination 180, 205, 395, 493, **554**, **810**, 849, 881, **904** *see also Gui Pi Tang*
Ginseng and Perilla Combination **21**, 76, 123, 250, 455 *see also Shen Su Yin*
Ginseng and Prepared Aconite Decoction 152, **665**, 775, 779, 805 *see also Shen Fu Tang*
Ginseng and Zizyphus Formula 58, 467, 638, **787**, **806, 852, 884, 901** *see also Tian Wang Bu Xin Dan*
Ginseng Nutritive Combination 789, **887**, 905 *see also Ren Shen Yang Ying Tang*
glandular fever 283, 288, 295, 298
globus hystericus 225, 773
glomerulonephritis 362, 381, 407, 424
  acute 424
  chronic 407
  post streptococcal 424
glossitis 840
glue ear *see* ear
God of Longevity Pills 889, **926** *see also Shou Xing Wan*
gonorrhoeal urethritis 362, 445, 464, 467, 469
Goodpasture's syndrome 381
gout 334
grand mal seizures *see* epilepsy
Great Tonify the Basal Decoction 696, **917** *see also Da Bu Yuan Jian*
Great Tonify the Yin Pill 348, **407**, 636 *see also Da Bu Yin Wan*
Greatest Treasure Special Pill 39, 171, 198, 605, **660**, 707, 739, 762 *see also Zhi Bao Dan*
grommets *see* ear
gu zhang 730
Gua Luo Xie Bai Ban Xia Tang 766, **919**
  chest pain 766
guan ge syndrome 416
Guan Xin Su He Xiang Wan 775, 779, 804, **919**
  chest pain 775, 779
  palpitations 804
Gui Lu Er Xian Jiao 874, 880, **920**
Gui Pi Tang 180, 205, 395, 493, **554**, **810, 849, 881, 904**
  anxiety **904**
  dizziness **554**
  epistaxis 180
  forgetfulness 881
  impotence 493
  insomnia 849
  palpitations **810**
Gui Zhi Gan Cao Long Gu Mu Li Tang 803, **920**
  palpitations 803
Gui Zhi Jia Hou Po Xing Ren Tang
  wheezing **123**
Gui Zhi Jia Long Gu Mu Li Tang 814, 853, 885, 902, 910
  anxiety 902, 910
  insomnia 853
  palpitations **814**
Gui Zhi Tang
  acute exterior disorders **49**

966   INDEX

Guide Out Phlegm Decoction 642, **918**
   see also *Dao Tan Tang*
gums
  atrophy of 177
  bleeding 32, 170, 180, 604
  swollen, ulcerated or bleeding 172
Gun Tan Wan 519, **694**, 767, **816**
  chest pain 767
  epilepsy **694**
  palpitations **816**
  tinnitus **519**

H

haematocoele 621
Haematuria 458
  Blood stagnation 470
    with *qi* def. 471
  Damp Heat 462
    with Toxin Heat 463
  Heart Fire 466
    with *yin* def. 467
  Kidney *yin* def. with Fire 473
  Liver Fire 468
  Spleen and Kidney *yang* (*qi*) def. 475
haemophilia 181, 205, 477
Haemoptysis 184
  diagnosis of 186
  Liver Fire 197
  Lung and Kidney *yin* def. 201
  Lung Dryness 189
  Lung Heat 193
  Phlegm Heat 195
  Spleen *qi* def. 204
  symptomatic treatment of 319
  Wind Cold 191
    persistence following dispersal of Wind Cold 192
  Wind Heat 187
haemorrhoids 475, 871
hair
  dry 529, 554
  greying and lifeless 255, 275
hallucinations 685
hayfever 51, 102, 125, 262, 267
He Che Da Zao Wan 148, **920**
  wheezing 148
head injury *see* trauma

headache (migraine) *see* Vol.3 for full discussion
  Blood stagnation 552, 868
  external Damp 7, 335
  frontal 10, 32, 74, 77, 122, 128, 172, 238, 240, 242, 246, 834
  in *yang ming* syndrome 32
  jue yin 63
  Liver *qi* stagnation 242, 566
  Liver Fire 244
  Liver *yang* rising 542, 545, 655
  maxillary 240, 244
  occipital 6, 18, 48, 50, 52, 74, 122, 126, 191, 212, 238, 336
  Phlegm Damp 548
  Stomach Heat 172
  temporal 174, 197, 242, 244, 365, 468, 834
  vertex 63, 655
  Wind Cold 8
  Wind Dryness 16
  Wind Heat 10
    severe 285
  with hypertension and visual disturbance 655
  with vomiting and cold extremities 63
Hearing Loss 506
  Blood stagnation 521
  Kidney def. 523
  Liver Fire 515
    with *yin* def./*yang* rising 516
  Phlegm Heat 518
    residual Phlegm 501
  qi and Blood def. 519
  Spleen *qi* def. (with Phlegm) 526
  Wind Heat 510
Heart (and Kidney) *yin* deficiency
  chest pain 787
Heart (Lung and Spleen) *qi* deficiency
  chest pain 785
Heart and Gall Bladder *qi* deficiency
  anxiety 909
  impotence 495
  insomnia 856
  palpitations 813

INDEX 967

Heart and Kidney *qi* and *yin* deficiency
  exhaustion painful urination syndrome 396
Heart and Kidney *yang* deficiency
  shang han 59
Heart and Kidney *yin* deficiency
  anxiety 901
  forgetfulness 884
  insomnia 852
  shao yin syndrome 58
Heart Blood and Spleen *qi* deficiency
  anxiety 904
  forgetfulness 881
  impotence 493
  insomnia 849
  palpitations 810
Heart Fire
  haematuria 466
  insomnia 838
  painful urination syndrome 363
Heart *qi* and *yin* deficiency
  anxiety 907
Heart *qi* deficiency
  anxiety 899
  palpitations 801
Heart *yang* deficiency
  chest pain 777
  palpitations 803
Heart *yin* deficiency
  palpitations 806
Heat, external (*wen bing*)
  accumulating in the Stomach and Intestines 32
  causing reckless movement of Blood 41
  entering the Pericardium 38
  in the Blood 41
  in the Blood with Blood stasis 42
  in the Lungs 30
  in the *yang ming* channels 32
  in *yang ming* with constipation 34
  lingering in the chest and diaphragm 37
  with Phlegm in the chest and *yang ming* 33
Heat scorching and knotting the chest
  chest pain 761
heat stroke 33

Hei Xi Dan 152, **920**
  wheezing 152
hemiplegia 667, 765
Henoch Schönlein purpura 381
hepatic encephalopathy 606
hepatic failure 606
hepatitis 541, 570, 731, 828
  acute infectious 572, 596, 598
  acute infectious, early stage of 600
  alcoholic 572, 596, 598
  chronic 575, 578, 608, 610, 613, 734, 736, 739, 743, 859
  fulminant 606
hepatitis C 569
  asymptomatic 569
hepatosplenomegaly 611
hernia *see shan qi*
herpes
  simplex 283
  genitalia 366, 468
hoarse voice *see* Loss of Voice
Hoelen Five Formula **50**, 549, 620, 742
  see also Wu Ling San
***hou bi* 282**
Hua Gai San
  cough **74**
Hua Yu Tang 740, **921**
  ascites 740
***huang dan* 590**
Huang Lian E Jiao Tang **788**, **808**, **839**, 853, 885, 902
  anxiety 902
  chest pain **788**
  forgetfulness 885
  insomnia **839**, 853
  palpitations **808**
Huang Lian Jie Du Tang 170, 361, 463, 604, 838, **921**
  epistaxis 170
  haematuria 463
  insomnia 838
  jaundice 604
  painful urination 361
Huang Lian Wen Dan Tang
  chest pain 767
  urinary difficulty or retention 420

Huang Qi Jian Zhong Tang
   jaundice **609**
Hui Chun Dan **708** *see also Xiao Er Hui Chun Dan*
hun 827
hunger *see also* appetite
   indeterminate gnawing 172, 594, 815, 841, 843, 911
Huo Dan Wan
   sinusitis/nasal congestion 243, 245
Huo Luo Xiao Ling Dan 339, **921**
   lower back pain 323
Huo Xiang Zheng Qi San
   acute exterior disorder **13**
hydrocoele 616, 621, 622, 626
hyperaldosteronism 560
   primary 63
hypercarotenaemia 590
hyperprolactinaemia 481
hypertension 64, 165, 176, 179, 199, 245, 407, 514, 525, 544, 547, 551, 560, 643, 646, 655, 657, 669, 828, 837, 859
   acupuncture treatment for 657
hyperthyroidism 560, 634, 638, 641, 797, 809, 828, 854, 859, 886, 908
hypocalcaemia 715
Hypochondriac Pain 564
   Blood stagnation 576
   Damp Heat in the Liver and Gall Bladder 571
      with roundworms 572
   Liver *qi* stagnation 566
      with Fire 569
      with unresolved Wind Cold 569
      with gallstones 569
      with Blood stagnation 569
      with Spleen def. 570
   Liver *yin* (Blood) deficiency 573
      with *qi* stagnation 574
   traumatic 578
hypoglycaemia 863, 865, 871
hypotension 566, 560
hypothyroidism 63, 435, 451, 489, 560, 874
hysteria 141, 225
hysterical anuria 427

hysterical aphonia 225

I

immune dysfunction
   chronic fatigue 22, 294, 295, 298, 494, 812, 851, 863, 865, 867, 871, 874
   poor 20, 21, 22, 24, 146, 295, 298
impotence **480**
   Damp Heat 485
   Heart and Gall Bladder *qi* def. 495
   Heart and Spleen def. 493
   Kidney *yang* def. 488
   Kidney *yin* def. 490
   Liver *qi* stagnation 483
Incomparable Dioscorea Pill 391, 395, 475, **927** *see also Wu Bi Shan Yao Wan*
Increase the Fluids and Order the *Qi* Decoction **35** *see also Zeng Ye Cheng Qi Tang*
Indigo and Conch Powder 93, 197, **917** *see Dai Ge San*
infertility, male 480, 485, 488, 489, 490, 492
influenza 8, 19, 51, 53, 55, 76, 125, 190, 192, 213, 239, 338, 512, 721
Insomnia 826
   Blood stagnation 846
   Heart and Gall Bladder *qi* def. 856
   Heart and Kidney *yin* def. 852
      after shock or trauma 853
      following febrile disease or with severe Heat 853
      with severe palpitaions and anxiety 853-854
   Heart Blood and Spleen *qi* def. 849
   Heart Fire 838
   Liver *qi* stagnation 834
      with Heat 835
      Liver Fire 835
   Liver *yin* (Blood) def. 858
      with *qi* stagnation 859
   Phlegm Heat 843
      resistant cases 844
   post partum 851
   Stomach disharmony 841
      to purge in severe cases 842

INDEX

intercostal neuralgia 34, 575, 579
internal Wind
   mechanisms of 536, 648
intervertebral disc
   prolapse of 324
intestinal obstruction 35
intestinal tuberculosis 736, 743
Inula Flower Decoction **772** *see also Xuan Fu Hua Tang*
Inula Powder 191, **922** *see also Jin Fei Cao San*
involutional psychosis 814, 857
Iron Whistle Pill **287** *see also Tie Di Wan*

J

Jade Screen Powder 21, 268, 318 *see also Yu Ping Feng San*
Jade Woman Decoction 172, **931** *see also Yu Nu Jian*
Jaundice 590
   Blood stagnation 611
   Cold Damp 607
   Damp Heat
      Damp greater than Heat 597
      Heat greater than Damp 594
      with exterior symptoms 599
      Liver and Gall Bladder stagnant Heat 601
      with roundworms 602
   Spleen *qi* and Blood def. 609
   Toxic Heat 604
      with delerium 605
      with consipation, spasms or convulsions 606
Ji Sheng Shen Qi Wan
   ascites **743**
   urinary difficulty or retention **433**
Jia Jian Wei Rui Tang
   acute exterior disorders **27**
Jia Wei Er Miao San
   lower back pain **333**
***jian wang* 878**
Jiao Ai Tang
   epistaxis **178**, 181
   haemoptysis 205
Jiao Gui Tang
   Cold *shan qi* **618**

Jie Geng Tang 111, **921**
   Lung abscess 111
Jie Yu Dan 672, **922**
   dysphasia 672
Jin Fei Cao San 191, **922**
   haemoptysis 191
Jin Kui Shen Qi Wan **60**, **104**, 125, **150**, 181, 276, 295, **392**, **409**, 476, 778, 804, 819, **874**
   chest pain 778
   cloudy urine **409**
   cough **104**
   epistaxis 181
   exhaustion painful urination syndrome **392**
   haematuria 476
   palpitatations 804, 819
   rhinitis 276
   shang han **56**
   somnolence **874**
   sore throat 295
   wheezing 125, **150**
Jin Suo Gu Jing Wan
   tuberculosis **320**
   cloudy painful urination syndrome 388
***jing bing* 704**
***jing ji* 796**
Jing Fang Bai Du San **6**, 286, **336**
   acute exterior disorders **6**
   lower back pain **336**
   sore throat 286
jing shen 828
Ju He Wan
   shan qi **629**
jue yin channel syndrome 63
jue yin syndrome 62

K

***ke sou* 68**
***ke xue* 184**
Ke Xue Fang
   haemoptysis **198**
Kidney *jing* def.
   forgetfulness 887
   sinusitis, nasal congestion 255
Kidney *qi* def.
   cloudy painful urination syndrome 388

exhaustion painful urination syndrome 391
frequent urination 449
lower back pain 346
Kidney def.
  dizziness 557
  lower back pain 346
  rhinitis 275
  stone painful urination syndrome 367
  tinnitus/deafness 523
Kidney *Qi* Pill [from Formulas to Aid the Living] **433, 743** see *Ji Shen Sheng Qi Wan*
kidney stones 334, 367-375
  acupuncture treatment of 369
Kidney *yang* def.
  cloudy urination 408
  difficult urination 433
  exhaustion painful urination syndrome 392
  frequent urination/incontinence 449
  impotence 488
  lower back pain 346
  rhinitis 275
  wheezing 150
Kidney *yin* def.
  Blood painful urination syndrome 384
  cloudy urination 406
  difficult urination 436
  exhaustion painful urination syndrome 391
  frequent urination 452
  haematuria 473
  impotence 490
  lower back pain 347
  rhinitis 277
  stone painful urination syndrome 374
kidneys
  polycystic 324, 459
  tuberculosis of 459
Kudzu, Coptis and Scute Combination **36** see also *Ge Gen Huang Qin Huang Lian Tang*

L

lacrimation
  excessive 124

laryngitis
  acute 209, 213, 216, 222
  chronic 209, 222, 227, 295
  tuberculous 209
Leach out Dampness Decoction **331** see also *Shen Shi Tang*
Lead Special Pill 152, **920** see also *Hei Xi Dan*
Lead to Symmetry Powder 653, 675, **923** see also *Qian Zheng San*
leptospirosis 596, 600
leukaemia 40, 179
  acute 40, 42
Li Zhong Wan 716, 777, **922**
  chest pain 777
  convulsions 716
Lian Po Yin
  acute exterior disorder **14**
Liang Ge San
  cough **85**
libido
  loss of 480, 483, 488, 523, 558
Licorice and Jujube Combination **139** see also *Gan Mao Da Zao Tang*
Licorice, Ginger, Hoelen and Atractylodes Decoction 330, **919** see also *Gan Jiang Ling Zhu Tang*
Lily Combination **96, 147**, 201, 226, 312 see also *Bai He Gu Jin Tang*
lin zheng 352
Ling Gui Zhu Gan Tang 125, 551, **818**
  dizziness 551
  palpitations **818**
  wheezing 125
Ling Jiao Gou Teng Tang
  convulsions 709
  Wind stroke **661**
Ling Yang Jiao Tang 543, **922**
  dizziness 543
Linking Decoction 573, 744, **790**, 808, 859 see also *Yi Guan Jian*
Liquid Styrax Pill **662** see also *Su He Xiang Wan*
Liquid Styrax Pills for Coronary Heart Disease 775, 779, 805, **919** see also *Guan Xin Su He Xiang Wan*
Liu Jun Zi Tang **88**, 101, 125, 132, 145,

253, 272, 520, 527, 550, 690
cough **88**, 101
dizziness 550
epilepsy 690
hearing loss 520, 527
rhinitis 272
sinusitis/nasal congestion 253
tinnitus/deafness 520, 527
wheezing 125, 132, 145
Liu Shen Wan **922**
Liu Wei Di Huang Wan 255, 293, 388, 342, **391**, 436, 490, 636
  cloudy painful urination syndrome 388
  exhaustion painful urination syndrome **391**
  impotence 490
  lower back pain 342
  sinusitis, nasal congestion 255
  sore throat 293
  tremors 636
  urinary difficulty or retention 436
Liu Wei Tang
  loss of voice, hoarseness **212**
Liver and Gall Bladder Fire
  sinusitis, nasal congestion 244
Liver and Gall Bladder stagnant Heat
  jaundice 601
Liver and Kidney *yin* and *yang* def.
  sequelae of Wind stroke 673
Liver and Kidney *yin* def.
  ascites 744
  epilepsy 696
  epistaxis 177
  tremors 636
Liver and Kidney *yin* def. with *yang* rising
  dizziness 545
  Wind Stroke 655
Liver Fire
  cough 93
  dizziness 542
  epistaxis 174
  haemoptysis 197
  haematuria 468
  insomnia 834
  painful urination syndrome 365
  tinnitus 515
Liver Fire with Phlegm Heat
  epilepsy 693
Liver *qi* stagnation
  chest pain 770
  difficult urination 425
  dizziness 540
  frequent urination 446
  gallstones 586
  hypochondriac pain 566
  impotence 483
  insomnia 834
  loss of voice, hoarseness 223
  lower back pain 341
  painful urination syndrome 376
  shan qi 623
  tinnitus 513
  wheezing 138
Liver *qi* stagnation with Heat
  insomnia 834
  sinusitis, nasal congestion 242
Liver *yang* rising
  dizziness 542
Liver *yang* rising with Blood stagnation
  sequelae of Wind stroke 669
Liver *yin* (Blood) def.
  hypochondriac pain 573
  insomnia 858
lobar pneumonia 31
long bi 398
Long Dan Xie Gan Tang 139, 174, 244, **365**, 447, 468, 486, **500**, 515, 543, 569, 571, 595, **621**, 693, 762, 835
  chest pain 762
  dizziness 543
  epilepsy 693
  epistaxis 174
  haematuria 468
  hearing loss 515
  hypochondriac pain 569, 571
  impotence 486
  insomnia 835
  involuntary seminal emission 500
  jaundice 595
  paediatric eneuresis 447
  painful urination syndrome **365**
  shan qi 621
  sinusitis, nasal congestion 244
  tinnitus 515

wheezing 139
Lonicera and Forsythia Formula
    10, 109, 187, 510 *see also Yin Qiao San*
Lophatherus and Gypsum Decoction **839**
    see also Zhu Ye Shi Gao Tang
Loss of Voice/Hoarse Voice 208
    Liver *qi* stagnation 223
    Lung and Kidney *yin* def. 226
    Lung and Spleen *qi* def. 228
    Lung Dryness 218
        in severe cases 219
    Phlegm Heat 221
    qi, Phlegm and Blood stagnation 230
    Stomach (*yang* ming) Heat 215
    Wind Cold 212
        with pre-existing internal Heat 213
    Wind Heat 214
Lotus Seed Combination **396** *see also Qing Xin Lian Zi Yin*
low sperm count 485, **488**, 489, 490, 491
Lower Back Pain 324
    Blood stagnation 339
    Cold Damp 330
        with residual Damp following expulsion of Cold 331
    Damp Heat 333
    Kidney def. 346
    Liver *qi* stagnation 341
    Spleen def. with Damp 343
    Wind (Damp, Cold or Heat) 335
        Wind Cold 336
        Wind Damp 335
        Wind Heat 337
Lu Rong Bu Se Wan
    cloudy urine **408**
Lung Abscess 108
    convalescent stage 114
    early stage (Wind Heat) 109
    suppuration stage (Toxic Heat) 111
Lung and Kidney *yin* def.
    loss of voice, hoarseness 226
    sore throat 292
    tuberculosis 312
    wheezing 147
Lung and Kidney *yin* def. with Heat

haemoptysis 201
Lung and Spleen *qi* def.
    loss of voice, hoarseness 228
    rhinitis 272
    wheezing 144
Lung and Stomach Heat
    sore throat 289
Lung Dryness
    haemoptysis 189
    loss of voice, hoarseness 218
Lung Heat
    cough 84
    epistaxis 168
    haemoptysis 193
Lung *qi* and *yin* def.
    cough 101
    tuberculosis 314
    wheezing 142
Lung *qi* def.
    cough 100
    rhinitis 268
    sinusitis, nasal congestion 249
Lung *qi* obstruction
    difficult urination 422
Lung *yin* def.
    cough 96
Lung *yin* def. with Heat
    tuberculosis 310
Lungs and Kidney defensive *qi* system 142, 147
Lycium, Chrysanthemum and Rehmannia Formula 546, **574** *see also Qi Ju Di Huang Wan*
lymphangitis 710

M

Ma Huang, Apricot Seed, Gypsum and Licorice Combination 18, **31**, 75, 84, 110, 129, 135, 193 *see also Ma Xing Shi Gan Tang*
Ma Huang, Asarum and Prepared Aconite Decoction **24**, 434 *see also Ma Huang Fu Zi Xi Xin Tang*
Ma Huang Combination *see also Ma Huang Tang* **7**, **48**, **122**, 160
Ma Huang, Forsythia and Aduki Bean Decoction 599 *see also Ma Huang Lian*

INDEX 973

Qiao Chi Xiao Dou Tang
Ma Huang Fu Zi Xi Xin Tang
  acute exterior disorders 24
  urinary difficulty or retention 434
Ma Huang Lian Qiao Chi Xiao Dou Tang
  jaundice 599
Ma Huang Tang 7, **48**, **122**, 160
  acute exterior disorders 7
  shang han **48**
  wheezing **122**, 160
Ma Xing Shi Gan Tang 18, **31**, 75, 84,
    110, 129, 135, 193
  acute exterior disorders 18
  cough 75, 84
  haemoptysis 193
  Lung abscess 110
  wen bing **31**
  wheezing 129, 135
Magnolia and Atractylodes Combination
    344, **431**, 735 *see also Shi Pi Yin*
Magnolia and Ginger Formula 344, 733,
    864 *see also Ping Wei San*
Magnolia and Hoelen Combination 425 *see
    also Wei Ling Tang*
Magnolia Flower Lung Clearing Decoction
    269 *see also Xin Yi Qing Fei Yin*
Magnolia Flower Powder 238 *see Xin Yi
    San*
Mai Wei Di Huang Wan 98, **148**, 227
  cough 98
  loss of voice, hoarseness 227
  wheezing **148**
Major Arrest Wind Pearl 637, **714** *see also
    Da Ding Feng Zhu*
Major Blue Dragon Combination 19,
    52, 213 *see also Da Qing Long Tang*
Major Distinguishing Decoction 621 *see also
    Da Fen Qing Yin*
Major Gentiana Qinjiao Decoction 652 *see
    also Da Qin Jiao Tang*
Major Rhubarb Combination 34 *see also Da
    Cheng Qi Tang*
malaria 55 *see Vol.3 for more detail*
  chronic 579, 730, 739, 741
Man Jing Zi San
  tinnitus **511**
Mantis Egg Case Powder 409, 450 *see also*

Sang Piao Xiao San
Marvellously Fragrant Powder **899** *see also
    Miao Xiang San*
mastitis 55, 710
measles 11, 711
  early stage of 11, 79, 169, 188, 338
melaena 475
memory, poor 58, 177, 255, 275, 523,
    554, 557, 558, 636, 806, 810, 849,
    881, 904 *see also* Forgetfulness
  severe loss of short term 887
Meniere's disease 520, 541, 544, 551, 643
meningeal irritation 723
meningitis 11, 33, 39, 40, 171, 173,
    338, 710
  early stage of 11, 188, 721
  epidemic cerebrospinal 704
  late stage of 715
menopausal syndrome 59, 179, 437,
    828, 837, 859, 903
menstruation, irregular 138, 223, 341,
    376, 425, 446, 513, 540, 566, 834
Metal Lock Pill to Stabilize the Essence
    320, 388 *see also Jin Suo Gu Jin Wan*
Miao Xiang San
  anxiety **899**
migraine *see* headache
miliaria crystallina 14
Minor Blue Dragon Combination **51**, 75,
    124, 265 *see also Xiao Qing Long Tang*
Minor Bupleurum Combination **54**, 78,
    337, 541, 569 *see also Xiao Chai Hu
    Tang*
Minor Descending Qi Decoction 223, **929**
    see also Xiao Jiang Qi Tang
Minor Invigorate the Collaterals Special Pill
    668, **929** *see also Xiao Huo Luo Dan*
Minor Prolong Life Decoction 653 *see also
    Xiao Xu Ming Tang*
Minor Sinking Into the Chest Decoction
    34, 761 *see also Xiao Xian Xiong Tang*
mitral stenosis 205, 797, 809, 823
Modified Yu Zhu Tang 27 *see also Jia Jian
    Wei Rui Tang*
Moisten the Throat Pill 288 *see also Run
    Hou Tang*
Moonlight Pill 97, 202, 310, **931** *see also*

Yue Hua Wan
Morus and Apricot Seed Combination 16, 80, 218, **924** *see also Sang Xing Tang*
Morus and Chrysanthemum Formula 77, 128, 168, 266, **924** *see also Sang Ju Yin*
Morus and Lycium Formula 197, **930** *see also Xie Bai San*
Mother of Pearl and Cow Gallstone Powder 287 *see also Zhu Huang San*
motor dysfunction 655
motor dysfunction of the extremities 652
mouth ulcers *see* ulcers, mouth
Mu Li San
   tuberculosis **318**
Mulberry Leaf and Moutan Decoction to Drain the White **94**, 762 *see also Sang Dan Xie Bai Tang*
multiple sclerosis 415, 441, 883
Mume Pill **62** *see also Wu Mei Wan*
myalgia 6, 23, 48, 50, 52, 74, 122, 126, 212, 599
Mycobacterium tuberculosis 306
myocardial infarction 666, 779, 784, 797
myocarditis 797

N

narcolepsy 863, 865, 867, 869, 871, 874
nasal polyps 272, 274
Nasal Congestion 234, 262 *see also* sinusitis and rhinitis
   acute 6, 10, 18, 48, 238, 240, 244, 246, 265, 268
   Blood stagnation 258
   chronic 249, 252, 255, 258, 268, 272, 275
      white, inoffensive, worse at night 249, 252
      worse with stress 242, 244
   Liver *qi* stagnation with Heat 242
   Lung and Spleen *qi* def. 272
   Lung *qi* def. 249, 268
   Phlegm Heat 246
   Spleen *qi* def. 252
   Wind Cold 6, 238, 265
   Wind Heat 10, 240

nasal discharge 234, 262 *see also* sinusitis and rhinitis
   acute 6, 10, 18, 48, 238, 240, 244, 246, 265, 268
   copious yellow or green mucus 240, 244, 246
   Kidney def. 255, 275
   Liver and Gall Bladder Fire 244
   Lung and Spleen def. 272
   Lung *qi* def. 249, 268
   Phlegm Heat 246
   Spleen *qi* def. 252
   Wind Cold 6, 238, 265
   Wind Heat 10, 240
nausea *see* Vol.2 for full discussion
   in *jue yin* syndrome 63
   in *shao yang* syndrome 54
   in *tai yang* organ syndrome 50
   in *wen bing* 33
   Phlegm Damp 548, 864
   Phlegm Heat 518
   Spleen *qi* def. 88, 132, 870
   Spleen *yang* def. 818
   Summer Heat 12
   with cough 87, 90
   with dizziness 548
   with food stagnation and insomnia 841
neck
   stiffness of 6, 48, 50, 74, 122, 191, 514, 566, 707, 720, 722, 724, 726
nephritis
   acute 50, 424
   chronic 62, 389, 395, 405, 407, 410, 432, 435, 451, 453, 560, 736, 743, 820
nephrotic syndrome 383, 387, 405, 407, 410, 432, 435, 451
neuresthenia 383, 387, 405, 407, 410, 432, 435, 451
neurosis 530, 812, 845, 851
Newly Augmented Elsholtzia Combination 12, **930** *see also Xin Jia Xiang Ru Yin*
Niao Lu Pai Shi Tang #1
   stone painful urination syndrome **372**
Niao Lu Pai Shi Tang #2
   stone painful urination syndrome **370**

Niao Lu Pai Shi Tang #3
   stone painful urination syndrome **373**
***niao xue* 458**
***niao zhuo* 400**
nocturia 59, 60, 103, 150, 346, 408, 449, 488, 502, 523, 558, 818
Nocturnal Seminal Emission 497
   Heat, Damp Heat 498
   Kidney *yang* and *yin* def. 502
   Kidney *yin* def. 501
   Liver Fire 499
   symptomatic treatment of 320
nocturnal enuresis 440, 447, 448, 450, 451
nosebleed *see* epistaxis
Notopterygium Decoction to Overcome Dampness 7, **335**, 720 *see also Qiang Huo Sheng Shi Tang*
Nourish Kidney, Open the Gate Pill 419, **933** *see also Zi Shen Tong Guan Wan*
Nourish the Heart Decoction **786** *see also Yang Xin Tang*
Nuan Gan Jian
   shan qi **619**
numbness
   of one side of the body 667, 669
   of the extremities 636, 639, 653, 655, 672, 673, 765
   of the lower limbs 673

O

obesity 642, 866
oedema *see* Vol.3 for full discussion
   Cold Damp 735
   Heart and Kidney *yang* def. 59, 778, 804
   Kidney *yang* def. 150, 433
   Kidney and Spleen *yang* def. 103, 742, 818
   Kidney *yin* def. 436
   Lung *qi* obstruction 422
   Spleen *qi* def. 296, 343, 344
   Spleen *yang* def. 344, 430
   orbital/facial 150, 394, 404, 422, 454, 818
   pitting 103, 150, 152, 433, 777, 803, 818

pulmonary 104, 152, 205, 778, 804
tai yang organ syndrome 49
Wind Damp 335
Wind oedema 422
Ophiopogon, Schizandra and Rehmannia Formula 98, **148**, 227 *see also Mai Wei Di Huang Wan*
opisthotonos 707, 718
orchitis 366, 403, 616, 622, 630 *see also Shan Qi*
organ stroke 646
orthopnoea 50, 124, 133, 152, 777, 803
otitis 286, 507, 512, 517, 520
Oyster Shell Formula **318** *see also Mu Li San*

P

pain
   abdominal 34, 42, 56, 60, 376, 382, 623
   chest 748 *see also* Chest Pain
      with cough 30, 80, 81, 84, 85, 93, 105, 109, 111, 114, 193, 195, 197, 310, 320
      with injury/trauma 105, 576, 578
      with Lung abscess 109, 111, 114
      with *wen bing*/Heat and Phlegm 33
      with wheezing 138
   ear 510, 515, 518, 521
   epigastric 584
      with Heat and Phlegm 33
   heel 384, 452, 473, 557
   hypochondriac 564 *see also* Hypochondriac pain
      with chronic liver disease 576
      with cough 93, 197
      with gallstones 584, 586
      with *shao yang* syndrome 54
   lower back 324 *see also* Lower Back Pain
      with cloudy urination 402, 406, 408
      with difficult urination 418, 433, 436
      with frequent urination 444, 449, 452
      with haematuria 379, 384, 462, 473, 475
      with loin pain and kidney stones 370, 372, 373, 374

testicles/scrotum 618, 619, 620, 623, 625 *see also Shan Qi*
Painful Urination Syndrome 352
  Blood
    Blood stagnation 382
    Damp Heat, Heat 379
    Kidney *yin* def. 384
  cloudy
    Damp Heat 386
    Kidney *qi* def. 388
  exhaustion
    Heart and Kidney *qi* and *yin* def. 396
    Kidney def. 390
    Spleen *qi* def. 394
  Heat painful urination
    Damp Heat 358
      during pregnancy 360
    Heart Fire 363
    Liver Fire 365
  qi painful urination
    Liver *qi* stagnation 376
  stone painful urination 367
    acupuncture treatment of 368
    asymptomatic 367
    Blood stagnation 372
    Damp Heat 370
    Kidney *qi* def. 373
    Kidney *yin* def. 374
palmar erythema 740
Palpitations 796
  Blood stagnation 821
  Heart and Gall Bladder *qi* def. 813
    following severe shock or trauma 814
  Heart Blood and Spleen *qi* def. 810
    with irregular pulse 811
  Heart *qi* def. 801
  Heart *yang* def. 803
    severe 804
    with Kidney *yang* def. 804
  Heart *yin* def. 806
    with *qi* def. 807
    with severe or continuous palpitations 807
    following febrile disease 808
    with Liver and Kidney *yin* def. 808
  Phlegm Heat 815
    severe cases with constipation 816

  with *qi* stagnation and Fire 816
  Spleen and Kidney *yang* deficiency 818
  with wheezing and oedema 819
pancreatitis 35, 572, 586, 596
panic attacks 58, 493, 806, 810, 814, 840, 849, 852, 857, 881, 904
paralysis 655, 667, 669, 673
parasitic liver disease 565
Parkinson's disease 638, 641
paroxysmal supraventricular tachycardia 797
Patent medicines
  African Sea Coconut Cough Syrup 17, 79
  An Gong Niu Huang Wan 38, 39, 42, 171, 606, 661, 739
  An Shen Bu Nao Wan 812
  Ba Ji Yin Yang Wan 257, 277, 410, 451, 476, 489, 503, 559, 626
  Ba Xian Chang Shou Wan 98, 143, 149, 203, 227, 295
  Ba Zhen Wan 530, 555, 628, 640, 727
  Bai Feng Wan 640
  Bai He Gu Jin Wan 98, 115, 143, 149, 203, 227, 295, 311
  Bai Zi Yang Xin Wan 494, 496, 786, 802, 812, 850, 882, 900, 905, 908
  Ban Lan Gen Chong Ji 11, 79, 286
  Bao He Wan 842
  Bao Ji Wan 14
  Bao Ying Dan 161
  Bi Min Gan Wan 238, 266, 270, 274
  Bi Xie Fen Qing Wan 387, 395, 405
  Bi Yan Ning 241, 243, 245, 247
  Bi Yan Pian 266
  Bu Nao Wan 59, 257, 277, 494, 496, 555, 812, 814, 850, 857, 882, 900, 905, 908, 910
  Bu Yang Huan Wu Wan 654, 668, 676
  Bu Zhong Yi Qi Wan 101, 146, 229, 251, 254, 270, 274, 297, 345, 395, 405, 432, 455, 476, 527, 555, 610, 626, 628
  Chai Hu Jia Long Gu Mu Li San 817, 836, 844
  Chai Hu Shu Gan Wan 140, 224, 243, 342, 377, 427, 447, 484, 541, 570,

588, 624, 772
Chong Cao Ji Jing 229, 257, 277, 313, 315, 317
Chuan Bei Pi Pa Gao 79, 81, 82, 98, 149, 190, 219
Chuan Ke Ling 91, 127
Chuan Xin Lian Kang Yan Pian 36, 85, 95, 110, 112, 130, 194, 247, 286, 290, 311, 313, 315, 317, 361, 364, 366, 380, 387, 403, 420, 445, 463, 467, 469, 486, 499, 500, 516, 520 602, 606, 622, 762
Chuan Xiong Cha Tiao Wan 8, 49, 76, 192, 213, 238, 266, 337, 721
Ci Zhu Wan 809, 902
Cong Rong Bu Shen Wan 489
Da Bai Du Jiao Nang 290, 364, 366
Da Bu Yin Wan 491
Da Chai Hu Wan 602
Dan Shen Pian 106, 429, 700, 772, 822, 847
Dang Gui Ji Jing 555, 610, 640, 812, 850, 882, 905
Dao Chi Pian 33, 361, 364, 366, 387, 403, 420, 445, 463, 467, 840
Die Da Tian Qi Yao Jiu 340
Die Da Zhi Tong Gao 331, 340
Ding Chuan Wan 127, 130, 137
Ding Xin Wan 494, 802, 814, 900, 910
Du Huo Ji Sheng Wan 331, 336
Er Chen Wan 89, 133, 551, 768, 817, 844, 865, 867, 871, 912
Er Long Zuo Ci Wan 524, 546, 558, 574, 715
Fang Feng Tong Sheng Wan 19, 424, 512
Fu Ke Wu Jin Wan 106, 383, 783, 822, 847, 891
Fu Ku Wu Jin Wan 429
Fu Zi Li Zhong Wan 57, 152, 297, 345, 432, 476, 551, 608, 691, 717, 736, 743, 768, 776, 779, 805, 819, 874
Gan Mao Ling 8, 11, 17, 26, 28, 49, 76, 79, 81, 82, 192, 213, 238, 337, 338, 721

Gan Mao Qing Re Chong Ji 8, 76, 123, 125, 192, 213, 336, 337, 721
Gan Mao Zhi Ke Chong Ji 76, 123, 125, 192, 338
Ge Jie Bu Shen Wan 152
Ge Jie Da Bu Wan 205
Guan Xin An Kou Fu Ye 783, 822, 847
Guan Xin Su He Xiang Wan 776, 779
Gui Lu Er Xian Jiao 888
Gui Pi Wan 181, 205, 494, 496, 555, 786, 802, 850, 882, 900, 905, 908
Gui Zhi Fu Ling Wan 578, 612, 630
Hai Zao Wan 621, 630, 723
Hu Po Bao Long Wan 520, 544, 643, 686, 689, 694, 719, 817, 844, 912
Hua Qi Shen Ji Jing 315, 317
Hua Tuo Zai Zao Wan 654, 668, 676
Huang Lian Jie Du Wan 36, 171, 173, 247, 334, 520, 606, 762, 840, 912
Huang Lian Su Pian 36, 112
Hui Chun Dan 708
Huo Dan Wan 245, 247
Huo Xiang Zheng Qi Pian 14, 600, 721
Ji Gu Cao Chong Ji 572, 595, 598, 600
Ji Gu Cao Wan 516, 572, 586, 595, 598, 600, 602
Jia Wei Xiang Lian Pian 36
Jia Wei Xiao Yao Wan 140, 243, 377, 447, 514, 541, 772, 836
Jian Bu Qiang Shen Wan 348
Jian Kang Wan 106, 783, 822, 847
Jian Nao Wan 59, 857
Jian Pi Wan 297, 842
Jin Gu Die Shang Wan 106, 340, 472, 783, 822, 891
Jin Kui Shen Qi Wan 61, 152, 181, 257, 277, 295, 348, 374, 389, 392, 410, 432, 451, 476, 489, 503, 559, 743, 779, 805, 819, 874, 888
Jin Suo Gu Jing Wan 389, 410, 451, 455, 503
Kang Wei Ling 484, 486, 654, 676
Li Dan Pian 572, 586, 595, 598, 600, 602
Li Gan Pian 588
Li Zhong Wan 57, 297, 345, 432, 619,

691, 717, 819, 874
Liu He Bao He Wan 842
Liu Shen Shui 14
Liu Wei Di Huang Wan 257, 277, 295, 313, 348, 391, 407, 437, 453, 474, 491, 502, 524, 558, 715, 791, 809, 854, 886, 902
Long Dan Xie Gan Wan 95, 175, 199, 245, 361, 364, 366, 380, 387, 403, 420, 445, 447, 463, 467, 469, 486, 499, 500, 516, 544, 570, 572, 586, 595, 598, 600, 602, 622, 694, 762, 836
Luo Han Guo Chong Ji 98, 115, 149, 190, 219
Ma Xing Zhi Ke Pian 19, 31, 52, 85, 110, 112, 127, 130, 169, 424
Ming Mu Di Huang Wan 546, 558, 574, 638, 697, 715
Ming Mu Shang Qing Pian 361, 364, 366, 380, 387, 403, 420, 445, 463, 467, 469, 499, 500
Mu Xiang Shun Qi Wan 342, 427, 484, 624, 734, 772, 842
Nan Bao 489
Nei Xiao Luo Li Wan 106, 259, 429, 578, 612, 630, 700, 723, 725, 783, 891
Ning Xin Bu Shen Wan 257, 277, 451
Niu Huang Jie Du Pian 31, 33, 110, 112, 173, 241, 286, 290, 512, 516, 840
Niu Huang Qing Huo Wan 35, 85, 112, 173, 194, 196, 245, 290, 602, 606, 694, 762, 768, 817, 844
Ping Wei San 133, 768, 865, 871
Qi Guan Yan Ke Sou Tan Chuan Wan 89, 133
Qi Ju Di Huang Wan 178, 546, 558, 574, 638, 697, 715
Qian Bai Bi Yan Pian 241, 243, 245, 247
Qian Jin Zhi Dai Wan 334, 387
Qian Lie Xian Wan 377, 420, 427, 429, 432, 437, 447, 451, 453, 486, 499, 500, 622
Qing Fei Yi Huo Pian 31, 34, 35, 85, 91, 95, 110, 112, 130, 137, 169, 171,

173, 188, 194, 196, 199, 245, 762
Qing Qi Hua Tan Wan 34, 91, 95, 112, 115, 130, 137, 196, 222, 520
Qing Yin Wan 215, 219, 222, 295
Ren Shen Lu Rong Wan 152, 888
Ren Shen Yang Ying Wan 101, 205, 527, 628
Sang Ju Yin Pian 17, 81
She Dan Chuan Bei Ye 115, 133, 137
Shen Fu Zai Zao Wan 24
Shen Ling Bai Zhu Wan 229, 251, 254, 270, 274, 297, 405
Shen Qi Da Bu Wan 101, 146, 229, 251, 254, 270, 274
Shen Qu Cha 14
Shen Su Yin 21
Sheng Mai Wan 101, 115, 143, 315, 791, 802, 809, 854, 886, 900, 902, 908
Sheng Tian Qi Pian 106, 383, 429, 472, 522, 783, 822, 847, 891
Shi Lin Tong Pian 368, 371, 372, 374, 375
Shi Quan Da Bu Wan 146, 530, 555, 610, 628, 640
Shi San Tai Bao Wan 26, 28
Shi Xiang Zhi Tong Wan 619
Shu Gan Wan 140, 224, 342, 377, 427, 447, 484, 514, 570, 588, 619, 624, 772, 836
Shu Jin Huo Xue Wan 340
Shuang Liao Hou Feng San 215, 286, 290
Su He Xiang Wan 663
Su Zi Jiang Qi Wan 89, 133
Suan Zao Ren Tang Pian 809, 854, 859, 886, 902
Tao He Cheng Qi San 43, 429, 472
Te Xiao Pai Shi Wan 368, 371, 372, 374, 375
Tian Ma Gou Teng Wan 178, 516, 544, 546, 640, 643, 656, 670, 768
Tian Wang Bu Xin Dan 59, 397, 491, 638, 697, 791, 809, 854, 886, 902
Tong Jing Wan 259, 472
Tong Xuan Li Fei Pian 89
Wan Shi Niu Huang Qing Xin Wan 606,

739
Wu Ji Bai Feng Wan 317, 610
Wu Ling San 734
Wu Pi Wan 734
Wu Zi Yan Zong Wan 489
Xi Gua Shuang 215, 286, 290
Xi Huang Cao 572, 595, 598, 600, 608
Xiang Sha Liu Jun Zi Wan 101, 146, 251, 254, 270, 274, 345, 527, 551, 768, 865, 867, 871
Xiang Sha Yang Wei Wan 570
Xiao Chai Hu Wan 26, 55, 79, 338, 512, 527, 570
Xiao Er Qi Xing Cha 840
Xiao Huo Luo Dan 331, 348, 668, 676, 776, 779, 805
Xiao Qing Long Wan 49, 51, 123, 125
Xiao Shuan Zai Zao Wan 656, 670
Xiao Yao Wan 140, 224, 243, 377, 427, 447, 484, 514, 541, 570, 727, 772, 836, 859
Xin Yi San 238, 243, 266, 270, 274
Xing Jun San 14, 598, 721, 865
Xue Fu Zhu Yu Wan 106, 259, 383, 472, 522, 553, 578, 612, 630, 700, 725, 783, 822, 847, 869, 891
Yang Xin Ning Shen Wan 494, 496, 814, 850, 857, 900, 905, 908, 910
Yang Yin Jiang Ya Wan 178, 544, 516, 546, 656, 670, 768
Yang Yin Qing Fei Wan 98, 115, 149, 190, 203, 219, 227, 311
Yin Qiao Jie Du Pian 11, 17, 79, 81, 130, 188, 215, 286, 338, 512
You Gui Wan 257, 277, 410, 503, 559, 888
Yu Dai Wan 36, 334
Yu Feng Ning Xin Wan 721
Yu Ping Feng Wan 21, 101, 251, 270, 455
Yun Nan Bai Yao 169, 171, 173, 175, 178, 181, 188, 190, 192, 194, 196, 199, 203, 205, 372, 380, 383, 385, 463, 467, 469, 472, 474, 476
Zheng Gu Shui 340
Zhi Bai Ba Wei Wan 178, 257, 277, 295,
313, 348, 375, 385, 391, 397, 407, 437, 453, 474, 491, 502, 546, 558, 638, 697, 715
Zhi Bao Dan 39, 661
Zhi Sou Ding Chuan Wan 19, 52, 85, 424
Zhi Sou Wan 81, 82, 192
Zhu Sha An Shen Wan 791
Zhuang Yao Jian Shen Pian 257, 277, 317, 331, 348, 559, 626
Zi Xue Dan 38, 39, 42, 606, 661, 707, 739
Zuo Gui Wan 397, 407, 502, 638, 697, 791, 809, 854, 886, 902
pelvic inflammatory disease 43, 334
peptic ulcer disease 763, 845
pericarditis 763, 797
Perilla Fruit Combination **88**, 133 *see also Su Zi Jiang Qi Tang*
peritonsillar abscess 291, 304
Persica and Rhubarb Combination 42, **927** *see also Tao He Cheng Qi Tang*
pharyngitis 19, 99, 216, 220, 222, 288, 291, 295
Phlegm and Blood stagnation
  shan qi 629
Phlegm Damp
  cough 87
  dizziness 548
  wheezing 131
Phlegm Fire
  chest pain 767
Phlegm Fluids
  chest pain 766
Phlegm Heat
  anxiety 911
  cough 90
  haemoptysis 195
  insomnia 843
  loss of voice, hoarseness 221
  palpitations 815
  tinnitus 518
  wheezing 135
Phlegm Heat generating Wind
  tremors 642
Phlegm Heat with Wind Phlegm
  Wind stroke 658

Phlegm obstructing Heart *yang*
  chest pain 764
Phlegm obstruction
  somnolence 866
phobias 810, 881, 904
Pill for Deafness that is Kind to the Left 523 *see also Er Long Zuo Ci Wan*
Pinellia and Gastrodia Combination 520, **549** *see also Ban Xia Bai Zhu Tian Ma Tang*
Pinellia and Magnolia Combination **140** *see also Ban Xia Hou Po Tang*
Ping Wei San **344**, 733, 864
  ascites 733
  lower back pain **344**
  somnolence 864
pituitary hypofunction 560
Placenta Great Creation Pills 148, **920** *see also He Che Da Zao Wan*
Plasmodia 731
Platycodon Decoction 111, **921** *see also Jie Geng Tang*
pleurisy 199, 570, 763
plum stone throat 138, 223, 834
pneumonia 19, 31, 53, 86, 92, 95, 110, 113, 127, 130, 137, 169, 171, 188, 190, 196, 199, 711, 763
  convalescent stage of 116
po 801
polycystic kidneys 324, 459
Polyporus Combination **360**, 436 *see also Zhu Ling Tang*
polyps
  nasal 259, 272
  vocal cord 209
post cerebro-vascular accident 663
post concussion syndrome 522, 553, 848, 869, 882
post febrile disease 437, 840
post herpetic neuralgia 579
post illness convalescence 874, 882
post partum
  cold 26
  convalescence 556
  haemorrhage 812
post traumatic shock syndrome 496, 553, 560, 854, 895, 902, 903

post viral syndrome 55, 227, 229, 294, 912
postnasal drip 283
pregnancy
  Wind Cold during 26
  dysuria during 360
premenstrual syndrome 138, 223, 341, 376, 425, 446, 513, 540, 566, 770, 814, 837, 837, 856
premature ectopic beats 802, 812
premature ejaculation 490, 497
Preserve the Basal Decoction 785, **914** *see also Bao Yuan Tang*
Preserve the True Decoction 314, **914** *see also Bao Zhen Tang*
prolapse
  acupuncture treatment of 432, 626
  bladder 395, 430, 432, 455
  uterine 395, 432, 455
  vaginal 395
Promote Wisdom Decoction **885** *see also Sheng Hui Tang*
prostate cancer *see* cancer
prostatic hypertrophy 415, 429, 451
prostatitis 362, 364, 366, 381, 387, 403, 420, 464, 467, 469, 487
Protect the Child Special Pill 161, 520 *see also Bao Ying Dan*
pruritis, generalised 609
Psoraleae Pills **524** *see also Bu Gu Zhi Wan*
Pu Ji Xiao Du Yin
  sore throat 289
Pueraria Combination **7**, 720 *see also Ge Gen Tang*
puerperal fever 43, 544
  early stage of 26
Pulsatilla Decoction **711** *see also Bai Tou Weng Tang*
Purple Snow Special Pill 39, 171, 198, 303, 606, **707** *see also Zi Xue Dan*
purpura 38, 611, 710, 711, 740
pyelonephritis 324, 362, 364, 366, 387, 420, 445, 464, 467
Pyrrosia Powder 368, **925** *see also Shi Wei San*

Q

qi and Blood deficiency
  dizziness 554
  spasms and convulsions 726
  tinnitus 529
  tremors 639
qi and Damp stagnation
  ascites 733
qi and *yin* deficiency
  tuberculosis 314
qi, Blood and Phlegm Stagnation
  loss of voice, hoarseness 230
qi deficiency
  shan qi 625
  with external Wind 20
qi deficiency with Blood stagnation
  sequelae of Wind stroke 667
Qi Ju Di Huang Wan
  dizziness/vertigo 546
  hypochondriac pain **574**
Qi Yang Yu Xin Dan
  impotence **495**
Qian Gen San
  haematuria 471, **923**
Qian Jin Wei Jing Tang
  Lung abscess 111
Qian Zheng San 653, 675, **923**
  facial paralysis 653, 675
Qiang Huo Sheng Shi Tang
  acute exterior disorder 7
  lower back pain **335**
  spasms **720**
Qin Jiao Bie Jia San
  tuberculosis 319, **923**
Qing Dan Xie Huo Tang 585, 601, **923**
  gallstones 585
  jaundice 601
Qing Fei Yin
  difficult urination/retention **423**
Qing Hun San 553, **923**
  dizziness/vertigo 553
Qing Huo Di Tan Tang
  insomnia **844**
Qing Jin Hua Tan Tang 90, 93, **924**
  cough 90, 93

Qing Wen Bai Du Yin
  convulsions **710**
Qing Xin Lian Zi Yin
  exhaustion painful urination **396**
Qing Yan Li Ge Tang
  loss of voice, hoarseness 215
  throat abscess 302
Qing Yan Ning Fei Tang 221, 230, **896**
  loss of voice, hoarseness 212, 230
Qing Ying Tang **38**, 39, 171, 198, 303, **711**
  convulsions **711**
  epistaxis 171
  haemoptysis 198
  throat abscess 303
  wen bing **38**, 39
Qing Zao Jiu Fei Tang **81**, **129**, 189, 219
  cough **81**
  loss of voice/hoarseness 219
  haemoptysis 189
  wheezing **129**
Qu Feng Dao Tan Tang
  convulsions **722**
quinsy 304

R

Red Cross Hospital 583
Reed Decoction 91, 111, 195, **927** *see also Wei Jing Tang*
Regulate the Stomach and Order the *Qi* Decoction **842** *see also Tiao Wei Cheng Qi Tang*
Rehmannia and Akebia Formula 363, 396, 466, **838** *see also Dao Chi San*
Rehmannia Decoction **673** *see also Di Huang Yin Zi*
Rehmannia Eight Formula **60**, **104**, 125, **150**, 181, 276, 295, **392**, **409**, 476, 778, 804, 819, **874** *see also Jin Kui Shen Qi Wan*
Rehmannia Six Formula 255, 293, 342, 388, **391**, 436, 490, 636 *see also Liu Wei Di Huang Wan*
Reiter's syndrome 362, 366, 467, 469
Relax the Tongue Special Pill 672, **922** *see also Jie Yu Dan*
Ren Shen Ge Jie San
  wheezing **151**

Ren Shen Yang Ying Tang
  chest pain 789
  forgetfulness **887**
  somnolence 871
renal tuberculosis 407
Rescue *Yin*, Manage Exhaustion Decoction 202, **932** *see also Zheng Yin Li Lao Tang*
Restore the Left Decoction **790** *see also Zuo Gui Yin*
retained placenta 43
retropharyngeal abscess 283, 291, 301, 304
Return of Spring Special Pill **708** *see also Xiao Er Hui Chun Dan*
Revive Health by Invigorating the Blood Decoction **578**, 783 *see also Fu Yuan Huo Xue Tang*
rheumatic fever 334, 797
Rhinitis 262
  Kidney def. 275
  Lung and Spleen *qi* def. 272
    perennial in children 273
  Lung *qi* deficiency 268
    with stagnant Heat (aggravation with certain foods and wine) 269
  Wind Cold 265
    with signs of Heat 266
Rhinoceros Horn and Rehmannia Decoction **41**, 171, 198, 303 *see also Xi Jiao Di Huang Tang*
Rhinoceros Horn Powder 605, 738, **928** *see also Xi Jiao San*
Rhubarb and Eupolyphaga Pill 577, **612** *see also Da Huang Zhe Chong Wan*
round worms in the bile duct 572
Rubia Decoction 471, **923** *see also Qian Gen San*
Run Hou Wan
  sore throat **288**

S

Salbutamol
  effects of, in TCM 155
Salvia Decoction 771, **783**, 790 *see also Dan Shen Yin*
San Jia Fu Mai Tang
  convulsions, spasms **713**

San Jin Tang 371, 569, **583**, 595, 598
  gallstones 568, **583**, 595, 598
  urinary calculi 371
San Ren Tang
  acute external disorder **13**
  spasms 721
San Zi Yang Qin Tang 132, **924**
  wheezing 132
Sang Dan Xie Bai Tang
  chest pain 762
  cough **94**
Sang Ju Yin 77, 128, 168, 266, **924**
  cough 77
  epistaxis 168
  rhinitis 266
  wheezing 128
Sang Piao Xiao San
  cloudy urine **409**
  urinary frequency or incontinence **450**
Sang Xing Tang 16, 80, 218, **924**
  acute exterior disorder **16**
  cough 80
  loss of voice, hoarseness 218
sarcoidosis 405, 410, 723, 725
scarlet fever 288, 710, 711
schistosomiasis 730, 731, 734, 739
Schizandra Decoction 801, **928** *see also Wu Wei Zi Tang*
Schizonepeta and Ledebouriella Powder to Overcome Pathogenic Influences 6, 286, **336** *see also Jing Fang Bai Du San*
schizophrenia 817, 840
Scour Phlegm Decoction 663, 693, **767**, 866 *see also Di Tan Tang*
scrotum *see also shan qi* and testicles
  eczema of 620, 621
  swollen and hard with loss of sensation 629
  swollen and oedematous 620
Sedate the Liver and Extinguish Wind Decoction 178, 516, **545**, **655**, 669 *see also Zhen Gan Xi Feng Tang*
seizures 680, 689, 694 *see also* Epilepsy and Convulsions
  complex partial 689
  febrile convulsions 707

following head trauma 698
grand mal 685
induced by stress and emotion 693
partial 689
petit mal 689
senile dementia 888, 891
Separate and Reduce Fullness in the Middle Pill 737, **932** *see also Zhong Man Fen Xiao Wan*
septicaemia 39, 42, 171, 606, 710, 711
Settle the Emotions Pill 813, 909, **918** *see also Ding Zhi Wan*
Sha Shen Mai Men Dong Tang 114, **925**
   Lung abscess 114
Shallot and Seven Herb Drink 25, **916** *see also Cong Bai Qi Wei Yin*
Shan Qi 616
   Cold Damp 620
   Damp Heat 621
      Damp Heat affecting the Liver 621
   deficient Cold 619
   excess Cold 618
   foxy 627
   Phlegm and Blood stagnation 629
   qi def. 625
   qi stagnation 623
   watery 620
Shang Han Lun 46
   jue yin syndromes 62
   shao yang syndrome 54
   shao yin syndromes 58
   tai yang syndromes 48
   tai yin syndrome 56
   yang ming syndrome 55
Shao Fu Zhu Yu Tang
   Blood painful urination syndrome **382**
   haematuria 470
shao yin syndrome 58
shao yang syndrome 54
shen
   description of 826
Shen Fu Tang 152, **665**, 775, 779, 805
   chest pain 775, 779
   devastated *yang*/Wind stroke **665**
   palpitations 805
   wheezing 152

Shen Fu Zai Zao Wan 23, **925**
   acute exterior disorder 23
Shen Ling Bai Zhu San 253, 273, 296, **925**
   rhinitis 273
   sinusitis, nasal congestion 253
   sore throat 296
Shen Shi Tang
   lower back pain **331**
Shen Su Yin **21**, 76, 123, 250, 455
   acute exterior disorder **21**
   cough 76
   frequent urination/incontinence 455
   sinusitis/nasal congestion 250
   wheezing 123
Sheng Hui Tang
   forgetfulness **885**
Sheng Mai San **101**, 142, 255, 789, 790, 807
   cough **101**
   chest pain 789, 790
   palpitations 807
   sinusitis, nasal congestion 255
   wheezing 142
Shi Pi Yin
   ascites 735
   lower back pain 344
   urinary difficulty or retention **431**
Shi Quan Da Bu Tang 145, 304, **529**, 555, 871, 905
   anxiety 905
   dizziness/vertigo 555
   somnolence 871
   throat abscess (non-healing) 304
   tinnitus/deafness **529**
   wheezing 145
Shi Wei San 368, **925**
   stone painful urination syndrome 351
Shi Xiao San
   chest pain **782**
Shi Yi Wei Wen Dan Tang
   anxiety **911**
***shi yin* 208**
Shi Zao Tang
   ascites **741**
shingles 565
shock 663, 666
Shou Xing Wan 889, **926**

forgetfulness 889
Shu Feng Qing Re Tang
   loss of voice, hoarseness 214
   sore throat **285**
Shu Gan Li Pi Tang
   hypochondriac pain **569**
Si Jun Zi Tang 294, 570, **926**
   hypochondriac pain 570
   sore throat 294
Si Ni Jia Ren Shen Tang 152, **926**
   severe wheezing 152
Si Ni San 95, **926**
   cough 95
Si Ni Tang
   shang han lun 62
Si Wu Tang 175, 294, **927**
   epistaxis 167
   sore throat 281
Sichuan Pepper and Cinnamon Decoction **618** *see also Jiao Gui Tang*
sick sinus syndrome 812, 908
sickle cell anemia 459
Siler and Platycodon Combination **511** *see also Fang Feng Tong Sheng San*
silicosis 99, 203, 227
sinus tachycardia 802, 814, 857
Sinusitis/Nasal Congestion 234
   Blood stagnation 258
   Kidney def. 255
   Liver and Gall Bladder Fire 244
   Liver *qi* stagnation with Heat 242
   Lung *qi* def. 249
      with Wind Cold 250
   Phlegm Heat 246
   Spleen *qi* def. 252
   Wind Cold 238
   Wind Heat 240
Six Flavour Decoction **212** *see also Liu Wei Tang*
Six Major Herbs Combination **88**, 101, 125, 132, 145, 253, 272, 520, 527, 550, 690 *see also Liu Jun Zi Tang*
Six Spirit Pills **922** *see also Liu Shen Wan*
sleep apnoea 863
smokers throat 295
somnambulism 859

Somnolence 862
   Blood stagnation 868
   Dampness wrapping the Spleen 864
   Phlegm obstruction 866
   Spleen and Kidney *yang* def. 873
      with *yin* and *yang* def. 874
   Spleen *qi* and Blood def. 870
      more severe *qi* and Blood def. 871
      with sinking *qi* 871
Sore Throat 282
   chronic
      worse in the evening 292
      worse in the morning 296
   Kidney *yang* def. 294
   Lung and Kidney *yin* def. 292
      with Blood def. (eg. postpartum) 293
      with *qi* and fluid damage 294
   Spleen *qi* def. 296
   Wind Cold 286
   Wind Heat 285
Spasms 704
   Blood stagnation 724
   Cold Damp 720
      with invasion of Damp Heat 721
      with severe Cold 720
   Phlegm obstruction 722
   qi and Blood deficiency 726
   yin and Blood deficiency 713
Special Pill to Aid Fertility 488, **931** *see also Zan Yu Dan*
spermatocoele 621
Spleen (and Lung) *qi* deficiency
   frequent urination 454
Spleen and Kidney *yang* deficiency
   ascites 742
   cough 103
   epilepsy 688
   haematuria 475
   palpitations 818
   somnolence 873
   wheezing 125
Spleen Damp
   lower back pain 343
Spleen deficiency with Phlegm
   epilepsy 690
Spleen *qi* and Blood deficiency
   jaundice 609

somnolence 870
Spleen *qi* deficiency
  cloudy urination 404
  epistaxis 180
  exhaustion painful urination syndrome 394
  haemoptysis 204
  sinusitis, nasal congestion 252
  sore throat 296
  tinnitus 526
Spleen *yang* deficiency
  chronic childhood convulsions 716
  difficult urination 430
  dizziness/vertigo 551
Spread the Liver and Regulate the Spleen Decoction 569 *see also Shu Gan Li Pi Tang*
stage fright 225
Stephania and Astragalus Combination 344, 423 *see also Fang Ji Huang Qi Tang*
Stomach disharmony
  insomnia 841
Stomach Heat
  epistaxis 172
stools
  black and tarry 42, 740
  dry 18, 126, 244, 406, 436, 452, 473, 490, 501, 658, 713, 907 *see also* constipation
  incontinence of, in Wind stroke 665
  loose *see* Vol.2 for full discussion
    Cold Damp 735
    Damp Heat 485, 571
    Spleen and Kidney *yang* def. 818
    Spleen *qi* def. 253
Stop Coughing Powder 78, 192 *see also Zhi Sou San*
Stop Wheezing Decoction 126, 160 *see also Ding Chuan Tang*
stress incontinence 440
Su He Xiang Wan
  Wind stroke, *yin* closed syndrome 662
Su Zi Jiang Qi Tang
  cough/asthma 88, 133
Suan Zao Ren Tang
  insomnia 858
  palpitations 808

subdural haematoma 725
Sublime Formula for Sustaining Life 302, 928 *see also Xian Fang Huo Ming Yin*
Substituted Resistance Pill 428, 917 *see also Dai Di Dang Wan*
Summer Heat 12
Sun Si-miao 306, 414
sweating *see* Vol.3 for full discussion
  night sweats 318
    Heart and Kidney *yin* def. 58, 787, 806, 852, 884, 901
    in convalescent stage of Phlegm Heat in the Lungs 91, 114
    Kidney *yin* def. 314, 407, 452, 501
    Liver and Kidney *yin* def. 177
    Liver *yin* (Blood) def. 858
    Lung and Kidney *yin* def. 147, 148
    Lung *yin* def. 96
    post febrile disease 91, 114
    symptomatic treatment of 318
    with *shao yin* syndrome 58
  spontaneous
    Heart and Gall Bladder *qi* def. 814
    Heart *qi* def. 801
    Heart *yang* def. 803
    Kidney *yang* and *wei qi* def. 150
    Lung and Spleen *qi* def. 144
    Lung *qi* and *yin* def. 101
    Lung *qi* def. 21, 100
    post febrile disease 114
    Spleen and Kidney *yang* def. 103
    symptomatic treatment of 318
    with acute exterior disorder 20, 23
Sweet Dew Decoction 293 *see also Gan Lu Yin*
Sweet Dew Special Pill to Eliminate Toxin 599, 919 *see also Gan Lu Xiao Du Dan*
systemic lupus erythematosus 366

T

tachycardia 796
tai yang channel syndrome 48
tai yang organ (Urinary Bladder) syndrome 49
tai yin syndrome 56
Tangerine Seed Pill 629 *see also Ju He Wan*
Tao He Cheng Qi Tang 42, 927

wen bing 42
Ten Jujube Decoction **741** *see also Shi Zao Tang*
tetanus 704
Three Golden Herbs Decoction 371, 569, **583**, 595, 598 *see also San Jin Tang*
Three Nut Decoction **13**, 721 *see also San Ren Tang*
Three Seed Decoction to Nourish One's Parents 132, **924** *see also San Zi Yang Qin Tang*
Three Shells Decoction to Restore the Pulse **713** *see also San Jia Fu Mai Tang*
Throat abscess 301
  Toxic Heat 301
    non-healing residual ulceration 303
    with unruptured abscess 303
    with *shen* disturbance 303
thrombocytopoenia 165, 181, 205, 556, 812, 851, 906, 908, 912
thrombosis 646
thrush, oral 283 *see also* candida
Tian Ma Gou Teng Yin 516, 542, 639, 642, **670**
  dizziness/vertigo 542
  Wind stroke **670**
  tinnitus 516
  tremors 639, 642
Tian Tai Wu Yao San 341, 623, **927**
  lower back pain 341
  shan qi 623
Tian Wang Bu Xin Dan **58**, 467, 638, 787, 806, 852, 884, **901**
  anxiety **901**
  chest pain 787
  forgetfulness **884**
  haematuria 467
  insomnia **852**
  palpitations 806
  shao yin syndrome **58**
Tiao Wei Cheng Qi Tang
  insomnia **842**
Tie Di Wan
  sore throat 287
Ting Li Da Zao Xie Fei Tang
  wheezing **125**

Tinnitus/Deafness 506
  Blood stagnation 521
  Kidney def. 523
  Liver Fire 515
    with *yin* def. and *yang* rising 516
  Liver *qi* stagnation 513
  Phlegm Heat 518
    with residual Phlegm Damp following resolution of Heat 519
    with *shen* disturbance and constipation 519
  qi and Blood def. 529
  Spleen *qi* def. (with Phlegm) 526
  Wind Heat 510
TMJ syndrome 514, 522
Tokoro Formula 386, **915** *see also Bei Xie Fen Qing Yin*
Tokoro Formula [from the Cheng Clan] **402**, 498 *see also Cheng Shi Bei Xie Fen Qing Yin*
Tong Qiao Huo Xue Tang **521**, 699, 724, 868
  epilepsy 699
  hearing loss 521
  somnolence 868
  spasms and convulsions 724
  tinnitus 521
tongue
  deviation of 673
  stiffness of 672, 673, 765
  ulcers 806, 838
tonic clonic seizures 681, 685
Tonify Heaven Great Creation Pill **316** *see also Bu Tian Da Zao Wan*
Tonify the Lungs Decoction **100** *see also Bu Fei Tang*
Tonify the Lungs Decoction with Ass-Hide Gelatin **98** *see also Bu Fei E Jiao Tang*
Tonify the *Yang* to Restore Five [Tenths] Decoction **667** *see also Bu Yang Huan Wu Tang*
tonsillitis 11, 19, 79, 83, 169, 188, 194, 199, 216, 220, 222, 282, 285, 288, 289, 291, 295, 298 *see also* Sore Throat
tooth grinding 514, 834
toothache 32

Top Quality Lindera Powder 341, 623,
  927 see also *Tian Tai Wu Yao San*
torticollis 7, 724
Tortise Shell and Deer Antler Syrup 874,
  880, **920** see also *Gui Lu Er Xian Jiao*
Tortise Shell Decoction Pills 612, **915** see
  also *Bie Jia Jian Wan*
Tou Nong San
  throat abscess **303**
Tourette's syndrome 635
Toxic Heat
  epistaxis 170
  jaundice 604
  throat abscess 301
tracheitis 79, 86, 95, 199
Transform Blood Stasis Decoction 740,
  921 see also *Hua Yu Tang*
transient ischaemic attack 517, 544, 547,
  646, 657
transverse myelitis 415
trauma/injury
  chest 105, 576, 578, 781, 783
  groin 382, 470
  head 521, 552, 698, 6724, 846, 868,
    889, 890
  insomnia/palpitations following 814,
    853
  lower back 339, 382, 470
Tremors 634
  benign familial 641
  Liver and Kidney *yin* def. 636
  Phlegm Heat generating Wind 642
  qi and Blood def. 639
    with *qi* stagnation 640
  senile 638
Trichosanthes, Bakeri and Pinellia
  Combination 766, **919** see also *Gua
  Lou Xie Bai Ban Xia Tang*
trigeminal neuralgia 64
trismus 720
True Jade Powder 718, **931** see also *Yu Zhen
  San*
True Warrior Decoction **60**, **103**, 152,
  778, 804, 819 see also *Zhen Wu Tang*
Tuberculosis 306
  anti *Mycobacterium tuberculosis* herbs 309
  Lung and Kidney *yin* def. 312

Lung *yin* def. with Heat 310
qi and *yin* def. 314
symptomatic treatment 318
  night sweats/spontaneous sweats 318
  tidal/bone steaming fever 319
  haemoptysis 319
  cough 320
  chest pain 320
  nocturnal seminal emission 320
yin and *yang* def. 316
Tuberculosis and Haemoptysis Formula
  319 see also *Zhi Fei Jie He Ke Tan Xue
  Fang*
tuberculous laryngitis 209
tuberculous peritonitis 730
tumours see also cancer
Turbid Phlegm
  chest pain 766
  spasms and convulsions 722
Turtle Shell Pills 577 see also *Bie Jia Wan*
Two Marvel Powder 485, **919** see also *Er
  Miao San*

U

ulcers
  apthous 283
  gastric 565, 570, 575, 579
  mouth and tongue 58, 85, 98, 283,
    286, 287, 290, 316, 363, 364, 466,
    806, 838
Unblock the Orifices and Invigorate Blood
  Decoction **521**, 699, 724, 868 see
  also *Tong Qiao Huo Xue Tang*
Universal Benefit Decoction to Eliminate
  the Toxins **289** see also *Pu Ji Xiao Du
  Yin*
upper respiratory tract infection 8, 11,
  17, 19, 53, 76, 79, 83, 127, 130,
  169, 188, 190, 192, 194, 199, 213,
  216, 220, 222 see also Acute Exterior
  Disorder/Cough/Sore Throat
urethral stricture 383, 429
urethritis 362, 364, 366, 387, 403, 420,
  445, 464 see also Painful Urination
  Syndrome
urge incontinence 440

urinary stones 367
Urinary Difficulty or Retention 414
  Blood stagnation 428
  Damp Heat 418
    with Toxic Damp 419
    Damp Heat and *yin* def. 419
  Kidney *yang* def. 433
    with exterior pathogens 434
    with 'Water Toxin' 434
  Liver *qi* stagnation 425
  obstruction of Lung *qi* 422
    persistent, with oedema and sweating 423
  Spleen *yang* def. 430
    with no Cold (i.e. *qi* def.) 431
Urinary Frequency/Incontinence 440
  Damp Heat 444
  Kidney *qi* (*yang*) def. 449
  Kidney *yin* def. 452
  Liver *qi* stagnation 446
    enuresis in hyperactive children 447
  Spleen and Lung *qi* def. 454
    with Wind Cold 455
urinary tract infection 334, 381, 383, 385, 387, 389, 393, 395, 420, 421, 453, 467, 469 *see also* Painful Urination Syndrome/Haematuria/ Cloudy Urination

V

vaginitis
  atrophic 453
Vaporize Phlegm Pill **519**, **694**, 767, **816** *see also Gun Tan Wan*
varicocoele 616, 621, 626
Ventolin 155
vertebral artery
  atherosclerotic occlusion of 646
vertebral disc herniation 340
Vertigo 534 *see* Dizziness
  benign positional 551
Vessel and Vehicle Pill **738**, 741 *see also Zhou Che Wan*
vision *see also* eyes
  blurring of 542, 545, 573, 639, 810, 881, 904
  sudden loss of 655

Vitex Powder **511** *see also Man Jing Zi San*
vocal cord polyps 230
voice, lose of or hoarse *see* Loss of Voice
vomiting *see* Vol.2 for full discussion
  in *jue yin* syndrome 62, 63
  of thin fluids 56
  of worms 62, 572
  with anxiety 911
  with childhood convulsions 716

W

Warm Diseases 30
  wei level 30
  qi level 30
    Heat in the Lungs 30
    Heat in *yang ming* channels 32
    Heat and Phlegm in the chest and *yang ming* 33
    strong Heat in *yang ming* 34
    Damp Heat in *yang ming* 35
    Heat lingering in the chest and diaphragm 37
  ying level 38
    Heat entering the Pericardium 38
    Heat obstructing the Pericardium 39
  Blood level 41
    Heat causing reckless movement of Blood 41
    Hot Blood and Blood stasis 42
Warm Dryness
  cough 80
Warm the Liver Decoction **619** *see also Nuan Gan Jian*
Warm the Lungs Decoction **250** *see also Wen Fei Tang*
Warm the Lungs, Stop the Flow Special Pill 249, 276, **927** *see also Wen Fei Zhi Liu Dan*
Wei Jing Tang 91, 111, 195, **927**
  cough 91
  haemoptysis 195
  Lung abscess 111
Wei Ling Tang
  urinary difficulty or retention 425
wen bing 30 *see* Warm Diseases
  classification of 30
Wen Dan Tang 518, 549, 766, 815, 843

chest pain 766
dizziness 549
insomnia 843
palpitations 815
tinnitus 518
Wen Fei Tang
   sinusitis/nasal congestion **250**
Wen Fei Zhi Liu Dan 249, 276, **927**
   rhinitis 276
   sinusitis, nasal congestion 249
Wheezing 118
   Kidney *yang* def. 150
      with pulmonary oedema 152
   Lung and Kidney *yin* def. 147
   Lung and Spleen *qi* def. 144
      with prominent Spleen def. 145
      following haemorrhage or menstruation 145
   Lung Heat 129
   Lung *qi* and *yin* def. 142
   Phlegm Damp 131
      recurrent, with Kidney def. and Cold invasion 133
      with prominent Spleen def. 132
   Phlegm Heat 135
      wheezing worse with certain foods 137
   qi stagnation 138
      with Heat or Fire 139
   Wind Cold 122
      persistent, after sweating 123
   Wind Cold with internal Heat 126
   Wind Cold with Phlegm Fluids 124
      with Spleen and Kidney *yang* def. 125
      with Heat and Kidney *yang* def. 125
   Wind Heat 128
whooping cough 19, 31, 53, 79, 92, 95, 110, 113, 127, 130, 137, 196, 199
   in adults 199
Wind Cold
   cough 74
   exterior syndrome 6
   haemoptysis 191
   in children 76
   in weak patients 75
   loss of voice, hoarseness 212
   lower back pain 336

rhinitis 265
sinusitis, nasal congestion 238
wheezing 122
with Blood def. 25
with internal Heat 18, 51, 126
with Phlegm Damp 50
with Phlegm Fluids 124
with *qi* def. 20
with *yang* def. 23
Wind Damp
   lower back pain 335
Wind Dryness
   exterior syndrome 16
Wind Heat
   cough 77
   epistaxis 168
   exterior syndrome 10
   haemoptysis 189
   loss of voice, hoarseness 214
   lower back pain 337
   Lung abscess 109
   sinusitis, nasal congestion 240
   sore throat 285
   tinnitus 508
   tinnitus, deafness 510
   wheezing 128
Wind Phlegm 672, 767
   chest pain 767
Wind Stroke 646
   ancient theories 647
   closed syndrome 660
      yang closed syndrome 660
      yin closed syndrome 662
   emptiness of the channels with Wind invasion 652
   flaccid collapse syndrome 665
   Liver and Kidney *yin* def. with rising Liver 655
   Phlegm Heat with Wind Phlegm 658
   sequelae of 667
      dysphasia 672
      facial paralysis 675
      hemiplegia 667
Wonderful Scrophularia Powder **98** *see also Xuan Miao San*
Wu Bi Shan Yao Wan 391, 395, 475, **927**
   painful urination syndrome 391, 395

haematuria 475
Wu Lin San 360, **928**
  painful urination 344
Wu Ling San **50**, 549, 620, 742
  ascites 742
  dizziness/vertigo 549
  shan qi 620
  tai yang organ syndrome **50**
Wu Mei Wan
  jue yin syndrome **62**
Wu Mo Yin Zi
  wheezing **138**
Wu Tou Chi Shi Zhi Wan
  chest pain 775
Wu Wei Xiao Du Yin 301, 361, 604, **710**
  convulsions **710**
  jaundice 604
  painful urination 361
  throat abscess 301
Wu Wei Zi Tang 801, **928**
  palpitations 801
Wu Zhu Yu Tang
  difficult urination 434
  jue yin syndrome **63**
Wu Zi Yan Zong Wan 470, **928**
  impotence 488

X

Xanthium Formula 240, 268, **915** *see also* Cang Er Zi Tang
Xi Jiao Di Huang Tang **41**, 171, 198, 303
  epistaxis 171
  haemoptysis 198
  throat abscess 303
  wen bing **41**
Xi Jiao San 605, 738, **928**
  ascites 738
  jaundice 605
Xian Fang Huo Ming Yin 302, **928**
  throat abscess 302
Xiang Sha Liu Jun Zi Tang
  somnolence 870
Xiao Chai Hu Tang **54**, 78, 338, 541, 569
  cough 78
  dizziness 541
  hypochondriac pain 569
  lower back pain 338

shao yang syndrome **54**
xiao chuan 118
Xiao Er Hui Chun Dan
  infantile convulsions **708**
Xiao Huo Luo Dan 668, **929**
  severe, chronic hemiplegia 668
Xiao Ji Yin Zi 380, 462, 466, **929**
  Blood painful urination syndrome 380
  haematuria 462, 466
Xiao Jiang Qi Tang 223, **929**
  loss of voice, hoarseness 223
Xiao Qing Long Tang 51, **75**, **124**, 265
  cough **75**
  rhinitis **265**
  shang han **51**
  wheezing **124**
Xiao Xian Xiong Tang
  chest pain **761**
  wen bing **34**
Xiao Xu Ming Tang 647, **653**
  channel stroke **653**
Xiao Yao San 95, **139**, 446, 483, 513, 540, 568, 574, 587, 640, 771, 783, 834
  chest pain 771, 783
  dizziness 540
  gallstones (post) 587
  hypochondriac pain 568, 574
  impotence 483
  insomnia 834
  tinnitus 513
  tremors 640
  urinary frequency or incontinence 446
  wheezing **139**
Xiao Yu Tang 744, **929**
  ascites 744
Xie Bai San 197, **930**
  haemoptysis 197
Xie Huang San
  painful urination **364**
xie tong 564
Xin Jia Xiang Ru Yin 12, **930**
  Summer Heat 12
Xin Yi Qing Fei Yin
  rhinitis **269**
Xin Yi San
  sinusitis, nasal congestion **238**

Xing Su San
  dry cough **82**
Xing Wei Cheng Qi Tang
  Wind stroke **658**
xiong bi 748
Xuan Fu Hua Tang
  chest pain **772**
Xuan Miao San
  cough **98**
xuan yun 516
Xue Fu Zhu Yu Tang 105, **522**, **552**, **576**, 698, 781, **821**, 846, 890
  chest pain **781**
  cough **105**
  dizziness **552**
  epilepsy **698**
  forgetfulness after trauma **890**
  hypochondriac pain **576**
  insomnia **846**
  palpitations **821**
  somnolence **869**
  tinnitus, hearing loss **522**

Y

yang deficiency
  with external Wind Cold **23**
yang ming syndrome **55**
yang wei 480
yao tong 324
Yang Xin Tang
  chest pain **786**
yi 878
yi niao 440
Yi Guan Jian 573, 744, **790**, 808, 859
  ascites **744**
  chest pain **790**
  hypochondriac pain **573**
  insomnia **859**
  palpitations **808**
yin and Blood deficiency
  spasms and convulsions **713**
Yin Chen Hao Tang 572, 594, 604, **930**
  hypochondriac pain **572**
  jaundice **594**, **604**
Yin Chen Wu Ling San 597, **930**
  jaundice **597**
Yin Chen Zhu Fu Tang 607, **930**
  jaundice **607**
yin deficiency
  with external Wind **27**
Yin Qiao San **10**, 109, 187, 510
  acute exterior disorder **10**
  fei yong (Lung abscess) **109**
  haemoptysis **187**
  tinnitus **510**
You Gui Wan 181, **256**, 347, 449, 503, 559, 804, 819, 874
  dizziness **559**
  epistaxis **181**
  lower back pain **347**
  nocturnal seminal emission **503**
  palpitations **804**, **819**
  sinusitis, nasal congestion **256**
  somnolence **874**
  urinary frequency or incontinence **449**
you lu 894
Yu Nu Jian 172, **931**
  epistaxis **172**
Yu Ping Feng San **21**, 268, **318**
  acute exterior disorder **21**
  rhinitis **268**
  tuberculosis **318**
Yu Zhen San 718, **931**
  muscular tetany **718**
Yue Bi Jia Zhu Tang
  difficult urination/retention **422**
Yue Hua Wan 97, 202, 310, **931**
  cough **97**
  haemoptysis **202**
  tuberculosis **310**
Yue Ju Wan 95, **567**
  hypochondriac pain **567**
Yun Nan Bai Yao 112, 115, 188, 190, 191, 194, 196, 198, 203, 205, 319

Z

Zan Yu Dan 488, **931**
  impotence **488**
Zeng Ye Cheng Qi Tang
  wen bing **35**
Zhang Zhong-jing 2, 46
Zhen Gan Xi Feng Tang 178, 516, **545**, **655**, 669
  dizziness **545**

epistaxis 178
hemiplegia 669
tinnitus, deafness 516
Wind stroke **655**
Zhen Wu Tang **60**, **103**, 152, 778, 804, 819
  chest pain 778
  cough **103**
  palpitations 804, 819
  shang han **60**
  wheezing 152
zheng chong 796
Zheng Yang Li Lao Tang 204, **932**
  haemoptysis 204
Zheng Yin Li Lao Tang 202, **932**
  haemoptysis 202
zhi 827
Zhi Bai Ba Wei Wan **177**, 375, 384, 406, **452**, 473, 501, 546
  dizziness/vertigo 546
  Blood painful urination syndrome 384
  cloudy urine 406
  epistaxis **177**
  haematuria 473
  nocturnal seminal emission 501
  stone painful urination syndrome 375
  urinary frequency or incontinence **452**
Zhi Bao Dan 39, 171, 198, 605, **660**, 707, 739, 762
  ascites 739
  chest pain 762
  epistaxis 171
  haemoptysis 198
  jaundice 605
  spasms, convulsions 707
  wen bing 39
  Wind stroke, resuscitation **660**
Zhi Fei Jie He Ke Tan Xue Fang
  tuberculosis 319
Zhi Gan Cao Tang 789, **811**, 907
  anxiety **907**
  chest pain **789**
  palpitations **811**
Zhi Sou San
  cough **78**
  haemoptysis 192
zhong feng 646

Zhi Zi Dou Chi Tang
  wen bing **37**
Zhong Man Fen Xiao Wan 737, **932**
  ascites 737
Zhou Che Wan
  ascites **738**, 741
Zhu Huang San
  sore throat **287**
Zhu Ling Tang
  painful urination **360**
  urinary difficulty or retention **436**
Zhu Sha An Shen Wan 767, **807**, 840, 854, 902
  anxiety 902
  chest pain 767
  insomnia **840**, 854
  palpitations **807**
Zhu Ye Shi Gao Tang
  insomnia **839**
Zi Shen Tong Guan Wan 419, **933**
  urinary difficulty or retention 419
Zi Wan Tang
  tuberculosis **320**
Zi Xue Dan 39, 171, 198, 303, 606, **707**
  epistaxis 171
  febrile convulsions **707**
  haemoptysis 198
  jaundice 606
  throat abscess 303
  wen bing 39
Zizyphus Combination 808, **858** *see also Suan Zao Ren Tang*
Zuo Gui Wan **277**, 347, 557
  dizziness 557
  lower back pain 347
  rhinitis 277
Zuo Gui Yin
  chest pain **790**

BIBLIOGRAPHY

Chinese language sources

Ji Zheng Zhen Jiu 急症针灸
(Emergency Acupuncture) 1988
Zhang Ren, Peoples Medical Publishing Company, Beijing

Shi Yong Zhong Yi Nei Ke Xue 实用中医内科学
(Practical Traditional Chinese Internal Medicine) 1984
Huang Wen-Chen (Supervising editor), Shanghai Science and Technology Press

Shi Yong Zhong Yi Fu Ke Xue 实用中医妇科学
(Practical Traditional Chinese Gynaecology) 1985
Zhou Feng-Wu (ed.), Shandong Science and Technology Press, Shandong

Shi Yong Zhong Yi Wai Ke Xue 实用中医外科学
(Practical Traditional Chinese External Medicine) 1985
Gu Bo-Hua (Supervising editor), Shanghai Science and Technology Press

Shi Yong Zhong Yi Xue Ye Bing Xue 实用中医血液病学
(Practical Traditional Chinese Treatment of Blood Diseases) 1992
Wu Han-Xiang (Supervising editor), Shanghai Science and Technology Press

Shi Yong Zhong Yao Xue 实用中药学
(Practical Chinese Herbs) 1985
Zhou Feng-Wu (ed.), Shandong Science and Technology Press, Shandong

Shi Yong Fang Ji Xue 实用方剂学
(Practical Chinese Herbal Formulas) 1989
Zhou Feng-Wu (ed.), Shandong Science and Technology Press, Shandong

Shi Yong Zhong Yi Wai Ke Xue 实用中医外科学
(Practical Traditional Chinese External Medicine) 1985
Shang De-Jun (ed.), Shandong Science and Technology Press, Shandong

Shi Yong Zhong Yi Er Ke Xue 实用中医儿科学
(Practical Traditional Chinese Paediatrics) 1987
Jin Zu-Peng (ed.), Shandong Science and Technology Press, Shandong

Zhong Yi Nei Ke Ji Zheng Zheng Zhi 中医内科急症证治
(Proven TCM Treatments for Acute Internal Disorders) 1985
Huang Xing-Yuan (ed.), Peoples Medical Publishing Company, Beijing

Zhong Yi Nei Ke Lin Chuang Shou Ce 中医内科临床手册
(Clinical Handbook of Tradtional Chinese Internal Medicine) 1984
Dang You-Lian (ed.), Henan Science and Technology Press

Zhong Yi Er Bi Hou Ke Xue 中医耳鼻喉科学
(Traditional Chinese Otonasopharyngology) 1985
Wang De-Jian (ed.), Peoples Medical Publishing Company, Beijing

Zhong Yi Tan Bing Xue 中医痰病学
(Study od TCM Phlegm Diseases) 1984
Zhu Ceng-Bo, Hubei Science and Technology Press

Zhen Jiu Zhi Liao Xue 针灸治疗学
(Acupuncture Therapeutics) 1985
Yang Zhang-Sen (ed.), Shanghai Science and Technology Press

Zhong Guo Zhong Yi Mi Fang Da Quan 中国中医秘方大全
(A Compendium of Secret Chinese Medicine Formulas) 1991
Hu Xi-Ming (ed.), Wenhui Publishing

Zhong Yi Nei Ke Shou Ce 中医内科手册
(Handbook of TCM Internal Medicine) 1997
Chao En-Xiang (ed.), Fujian Science and Technology Press, Fujian

English sources and references

Baldry PE (1993) *Acupuncture, Trigger Points and Musculoskeletal Pain*, Churchill Livingstone, Edinburgh

Bensky D and Gamble A (1993) *Chinese Herbal Medicine: Materia Medica*, Eastland Press, Seattle, Washington

Bensky D and Barolet R (1990) *Chinese Herbal Medicine: Formulas and Strategies*, Eastland Press, Seattle, Washington

Brown V (1984) The Differentiation and Treatment of Epigastric Pain by Acupuncture. The Journal of Chinese Medicine, 16:2-17

Clavey S (1995) *Fluid Physiology and Pathology in Traditional Chinese Medicine*, Churchill Livingstone, Melbourne

Edwards CRW et al. (1995) *Davidson's Principles and Practice of Medicine* (17th Ed), Churchill Livingstone, Edinburgh

Fruehauf H (1998) *Gu* syndrome. The Journal of Chinese Medicine, 57:10-17

Gascoigne S (1995) *The Manual of Conventional Medicine for Alternative Practitioners*, Jigme Press, Dorking, Surrey

Hsu HY (1980) *Commonly Used Chinese Herbal Formulas with Illustrations*, Oriental Healing Arts Institute, Los Angeles, California

Legge D (1997) *Close to the Bone*, Sydney College Press, Sydney

Lorenz P (1997) *Differential Diagnosis* (4th ed.) Social Science Press, Katoomba, NSW, Australia

Naeser M (1992) *Outline to Chinese Herbal Patent Medicines in Pill Form* (2nd ed.), Boston Chinese Medicine

Maciocia G (1994) *The Practice of Chinese Medicine*, Churchill Livingstone, Edinburgh

Maclean W (2000) *The Clinical Manual of Chinese Patent Medicines*, Pangolin Press, Sydney

Murtagh J (1996) *General Practice*, McGraw Hill Book Company, Sydney

Pitchford P (1993) *Healing with Whole Foods: Oriental Traditions and Modern Nutrition*. North Atlantic Books, Berkeley, California

Scott JP (1985) The Treatment of Diarrhoea and Constipation by Acupuncture. The Journal of Chinese Medicine, 19:2-11

Scott JP (1991) *Acupuncture in the Treatment of Children*, Eastland Press, Seatlle

Travell JG and Simons DG (1983) *Myofacial Pain and Dysfunction. The Trigger Point Manual*, Williams and Wilkins, Baltimore

Zhang Zhong-Jing (c. 210AD) Treatise on Febrile Diseases Caused By Cold with 500 Cases (Shang Han Lun). Translated by Luo Xi-Wen (1993) New World Press, Beijing, China